AMBULATORY PEDIATRICS

III

MORRIS GREEN, M.D.

Perry W. Lesh Professor and Chairman, Department of Pediatrics,
Indiana University School of Medicine;
Physician-in-Chief, James Whitcomb Riley Hospital for Children,
Indianapolis, Indiana

ROBERT J. HAGGERTY, M.D.

President, William T. Grant Foundation;
Clinical Professor of Pediatrics,
The New York Hospital–Cornell Medical Center,
New York, New York

W. B. SAUNDERS COMPANY

PHILADELPHIA / LONDON / TORONTO / MEXICO CITY / RIO DE JANEIRO / SYDNEY / TOKYO

W. B. Saunders Company: West Washington Square
Philadelphia, PA 19105

1 St. Anne's Road
Eastbourne, East Sussex BN21 3UN, England

1 Goldthorne Avenue
Toronto, Ontario M8Z 5T9, Canada

Apartado 26370—Cedro 512
Mexico 4, D.F., Mexico

Rua Coronel Cabrita, 8
Sao Cristovao Caixa Postal 21176
Rio de Janeiro, Brazil

9 Waltham Street
Artarmon, N.S.W. 2064, Australia

Ichibancho, Central Bldg., 22-1 Ichibancho
Chiyoda-Ku, Tokyo 102, Japan

Library of Congress Cataloging in Publication Data

Main entry under title:

Ambulatory pediatrics III.

1. Pediatrics. 2. Ambulatory medical care for children. I. Green, Morris. II. Haggerty, Robert J. [DNLM: 1. Ambulatory—Care—In infancy and childhood. 2. Pediatrics. WS 200 A497]

RJ47.A43 1984 618.92 83–14393

ISBN 0–7216–4237–3

Ambulatory Pediatrics—III ISBN 0-7216-4237-3

Last digit is the print number: 9 8 7 6 5 4 3 2

Dedication

This book is affectionately dedicated to
our wives, Janice and Muriel,
and to our children

CONTRIBUTORS

JOEL J. ALPERT, M.D.

Professor and Chairman of Pediatrics, Boston University School of Medicine. Director of Pediatric Services, Boston City Hospital, Boston, Massachusetts.

School Absence

ROBERT L. BAEHNER, M.D.

Hugh McK. Landon Professor of Pediatrics and Professor of Clinical Pathology, and Director, Pediatric Hematology/Oncology, Indiana University School of Medicine. Attending Physician, James Whitcomb Riley Hospital for Children, Indianapolis, Indiana.

Blood Disorders: Anemia and Hemorrhage

ABRAHAM B. BERGMAN, M.D.

Professor of Pediatrics, University of Washington. Pediatrician-in-Chief, Harborview Medical Center, Seattle, Washington.

Sudden Infant Death Syndrome and Infantile Apnea

JERRY M. BERGSTEIN, M.D.

Professor of Pediatrics, Indiana University School of Medicine. Director, Section of Nephrology, James Whitcomb Riley Hospital for Children, Indianapolis, Indiana.

Urinary Tract Infection

DOUGLAS A. BOENNING, M.D.

Assistant Professor of Pediatrics, University of Pennsylvania School of Medicine. Assistant Physician, Children's Hospital of Philadelphia, Philadelphia, Pennsylvania.

Animal Bites

MARTIN D. BROFF, M.D.

Clinical Instructor of Pediatrics, Harvard Medical School. Assistant in Allergy, Children's Hospital Medical Center, Boston, Massachusetts.

Insect Stings and Bites

PATRICK H. CASEY, M.D.

Assistant Professor, Department of Pediatrics, University of Arkansas College of Medicine. Medical Director, Arkansas Children's Developmental Center and Growth and Development Clinic, Arkansas Children's Hospital, Little Rock, Arkansas.

Health Promotion in Preschool Aged Children

CLAIRE CHAFEE-BAHAMON, M.S.

Coordinator, Planning and Evaluation, Massachusetts Poison Control System, Boston, Massachusetts.

Poisoning in Children and Adolescents

JOSEPH H. CLARK, M.D.

Lecturer in Pediatrics, Indiana University School of Medicine. Pediatric Gastroenterologist, James Whitcomb Riley Hospital for Children, Indianapolis, Indiana.

Vomiting; Diarrhea; Inflammatory Bowel Disease

DONALD J. COHEN, M.D.

Professor of Pediatrics and Psychiatry, Yale University School of Medicine. Director, Yale Child Study Center, New Haven, Connecticut.

Tics

ELLA COPOULOS, M.D.

Visiting Fellow in Adolescent Medicine, Department of Pediatrics, Columbia University College of Physicians and Surgeons. Visiting Fellow (A), Presbyterian Hospital (Babies Hospital), New York, New York.

Depression in Childhood and Adolescence

CATHERINE DE ANGELIS, M.D.

Associate Professor of Pediatrics, The Johns Hopkins University School of Medicine. Director, Pediatric Primary Care and Adolescent Medicine, Johns Hopkins Hospital, Baltimore, Maryland.

Health Care for the Elementary School Age Child

G. PAUL DEROSA, M.D.

Professor of Pediatric Orthopaedic Surgery, Indiana University School of Medicine. Attending Pediatric Orthopaedic Surgeon, James Whitcomb Riley Hospital for Children, Indiana University Hospitals and Affiliates, Indianapolis, Indiana.

Musculoskeletal Disorders

HOWARD EIGEN, M.D.

Associate Professor of Pediatrtics, Indiana University School of Medicine. Director, Section of Pulmonology, and Director, Pediatric Intensive Care Unit, James Whitcomb Riley Hospital for Children, Indianapolis, Indiana.

Asthma and Allergic Rhinitis

PEGGY C. FERRY, M.D.

Professor of Pediatrics and Neurology, University of Arizona College of Medicine. Chief, Section of Child Neurology, University Hospital, Arizona Health Sciences Center, Tucson, Arizona.

Learning Problems

JOSEPH F. FITZGERALD, M.D.

Professor of Pediatrics, Indiana University School of Medicine. Pediatric Gastroenterologist, James Whitcomb Riley Hospital for Children, Indianapolis, Indiana.

Vomiting; Diarrhea; Hepatitis; Constipation; Inflammatory Bowel Disease

GILBERT B. FORBES, M.D.

Professor of Pediatrics, University of Rochester School of Medicine and Dentistry. Pediatrician, Strong Memorial Hospital, Rochester, New York.

Obesity

STANFORD B. FRIEDMAN, M.D.

Professor of Psychiatry and Human Development, and Professor of Pediatrics, University of Maryland School of Medicine. Director, Division of Child and Adolescent Psychiatry; Head, Division of Behavioral Pediatrics, University of Maryland, Medical School Teaching Facility, Baltimore, Maryland.

Adolescent Out-of-Control Behavior

CARL W. FULLER, Ph.D.

Professor Emeritus of Audiology, Indiana University School of Medicine, Indianapolis, Indiana.

Speech and Hearing Problems

RAIF S. GEHA, M.D.

Associate Professor of Pediatrics, Harvard Medical School. Chief, Division of Allergy, Children's Hospital Medical Center, Boston, Massachusetts.

Insect Stings and Bites

MORRIS GREEN, M.D.

Perry W. Lesh Professor and Chairman, Department of Pediatrics, Indiana University School of Medicine. Physician-in-Chief, James Whitcomb Riley Hospital for Children, Indianapolis, Indiana.

The Pediatric Clinician; Fainting; Delirium; Biopsychosocial-Developmental Disorders; The Pediatric Interview; Mothering Disabilities; Breath-Holding Spells; Pica; Psychogenic Pain Disorders; Sleep Disorders; Enuresis; School Refusal (Avoidance); Conversion Symptoms; Hyperventilation Syndrome; Toddler Out-of-Control Behavior; Pediatric Psychotherapeutic Skills; Children and Divorce; Failure to Gain, Failure to Thrive, Weight Loss; Hyperactivity, Attentional Deficit; The Management of Children with Chronic Disease; Encopresis; Headaches; Chronic Fatigue

JOHN F. GRIFFITH, M.D.

Professor and Chairman, Department of Pediatrics, University of Tennessee College of Medicine. Medical Director, Le Bonheur Children's Hospital, Memphis, Tennessee.

Seizures

JAY L. GROSFELD, M.D.

Layfayette F. Page Professor and Director, Section of Pediatric Surgery, Indiana University School of Medicine. Surgeon-in-Chief, James Whitcomb Riley Hospital for Children, Indianapolis, Indiana.

The Skin: Lacerations, Abrasions, and Burns

HERBERT J. GROSSMAN, M.D.

Professor in the Departments of Pediatrics, Neurology, and Psychiatry, University of Michigan Medical School. Attending Physician, the University of Michigan Hospitals, Ann Arbor, Michigan.

Mental Retardation

ROBERT J. HAGGERTY, M.D.

Clinical Professor of Pediatrics, The New York Hospital–Cornell Medical Center. President, William T. Grant Foundation, New York, New York.

The Pediatric Clinician; Health Promotion; Episodic Disorders; Family Crisis and Intervention

KATHERINE A. HALMI, M.D.

Associate Professor of Psychiatry, Cornell University Medical College, New York, New York. Associate Attending Psychiatrist, New York Hospital, Westchester Division, White Plains, New York.

Anorexia Nervosa

MARGARET C. HEAGARTY, M.D.

Associate Professor of Pediatrics, Columbia University College of Physicians and Surgeons. Director of Pediatrics, Harlem Hospital Center, New York, New York.

Providing Health Services for the Underserved

KAREN HEIN, M.D.

Assistant Professor of Pediatrics and Director, Division of Adolescent Medicine, Columbia University College of Physicians and Surgeons. Assistant Attending Pediatrician, Presbyterian Hospital (Babies Hospital), New York, New York.

Depression in Childhood and Adolescence

EUGENE M. HELVESTON, M.D.

Coleman Professor and Chairman, Department of Ophthalmology, Indiana University School of Medicine. Staff Physician, indiana University Hospitals, Indianapolis, Indiana.

Screening Eye Examination

MARGARET W. HILGARTNER, M.D.

Professor of Pediatrics, Cornell University Medical College. Director, Division of Pediatric Hematology/Oncology, and Attending Physician, New York Hospital, New York, New York.

Current Care for Hemophilia

E. LAWRENCE HODER, M.D.

Assistant Professor of Pediatrics, Yale University School of Medicine. Staff, Yale Child Study Center, New Haven, Connecticut.

Tics

SIDNEY HURWITZ, M.D.

Clinical Professor of Pediatrics and Dermatology, Yale University School of Medicine. Attending Physician in Pediatrics and Dermatology, Yale–New Haven Medical Center and St. Raphael's Hospital, New Haven, Connecticut.

Pediatric Dermatology

CHARLES E. IRWIN, Jr., M.D.

Assistant Professor of Pediatrics, University of California, San Francisco, School of Medicine. Director, Adolescent Medicine Unit, University of California Hospital, San Francisco, California.

Sexually Transmitted Diseases in Adolescents

MARTIN B. KLEIMAN, M.D.

Associate Professor of Pediatrics, Section of Pediatric Infectious Diseases, Indiana University School of Medicine. Attending Physician, Indiana University Hospitals and Wishard Memorial Hospital. Consulting Physician, St. Vincent Hospital and Health Care Center, Indianapolis, Indiana.

Immunization; Fever; Recurrent Infections

BARBARA M. KORSCH, M.D.

Professor of Pediatrics, University of Southern California School of Medicine. Attending Physician, Children's Hospital of Los Angeles, Los Angeles, California.

Compliance

HERMAN W. LIPOW, M.D.

Pediatric Pulmonologist, Children's Hospital Medical Center and Bruce Lyon Memorial Research Laboratory, Oakland, California.

Respiratory Tract Infections

IRIS F. LITT, M.D.

Associate Professor of Pediatrics, Stanford University School of Medicine. Director, Division of Adolescent Medicine, Children's Hospital at Stanford, Stanford, California.

Adolescent Health Care

FREDERICK H. LOVEJOY, Jr., M.D.

Associate Professor of Pediatrics, Harvard Medical School. Associate Physician-in-Chief, The Children's Hospital Medical Center; director, Massachusetts Poison Control System, Boston, Massachusetts.

Poisoning in Children and Adolescents

LYLE J. MICHELI, M.D.

Instructor in Orthopedic Surgery, Harvard Medical School. Director, Division of Orthopedic Surgery, Children's Hospital Medical Center, Boston, Massachusetts.

Musculoskeletal Trauma in Children

MICHAEL E. MITCHELL, M.D.

Associate Professor of Urology, and Head of Section of Pediatric Urology, Indiana University School of Medicine. Head, Department of Pediatric Urology, James Whitcomb Riley Hospital for Children, Indianapolis, Indiana.

The Acute Scrotum; Undescended Testis

LAWRENCE F. NAZARIAN, M.D.

Clinical Associate Professor of Pediatrics, The University of Rochester School of Medicine and Dentistry. Senior Associate Pediatrician, Strong Memorial Hospital, Rochester, New York.

The Well-Equipped Office

MICHAEL L. NETZLOFF, M.S., M.D.

Associate Professor of Pediatrics and Human Development, Michigan State University College of Human Medicine. Attending Physician, Michigan State University Clinical Center, Ingham Medical Center, Edward W. Sparrow Hospital, and St. Lawrence Hospital, and Consultant Staff, Lansing Osteopathic Hospital, Lansing, Michigan.

Diabetes Mellitus

MURRAY H. PASSO, M.D.

Assistant Professor of Pediatrics and Director of Pediatric Rheumatology, Indiana University School of Medicine. Attending Physician, Wishard Memorial Hospital and Indiana University Hospitals, Indianapolis, Indiana.

Juvenile Rheumatoid Arthritis and Dermatomyositis; Musculoskeletal Aches and Limb Pain

PATRICIA J. SALISBURY, R.N., M.S.N.

Assistant Professor, Department of Pediatrics and Human Development, Michigan State University College of Human Medicine. Active Staff, Michigan State University Clinical Center, East Lansing, Michigan.

Diabetes Mellitus

BARTON D. SCHMITT, M.D.

Associate Professor of Pediatrics, University of Colorado Health Sciences Center. Attending Physician, University Hospital, The Denver Children's Hospital, and Denver General Hospital, Denver, Colorado.

Physical Abuse; Sexual Abuse (Incest); Ambulatory Pediatric Drugs

S. KENNETH SCHONBERG, M.D.

Associate Professor of Pediatrics, Albert Einstein College of Medicine of Yeshiva University. Director, Division of Adolescent Medicine, Montefiore Hospital and Medical Center, Bronx, New York.

Alcohol and Drug Abuse

RICHARD L. SCHREINER, M.D.

Professor of Pediatrics, Indiana University School of Medicine. Director, Section of Neonatal-Perinatal Medicine, Indiana University School of Medicine and the James Whitcomb Riley Hospital for Children, Indianapolis, Indiana.

The Death of a Newborn

PETER H. SCOTT, M.D.

Assistant Professor of Pediatrics, Indiana University School of Medicine, Indianapolis, Indiana.

Asthma

MARY-ANN B. SHAFER, M.D.

Assistant Professor of Pediatrics, University of California, San Francisco, School of Medicine. Associate Director, Adolescent Medicine Unit, University of California Hospital, San Francisco, California.

Sexually Transmitted Diseases in Adolescents

ROBERT J. SHAFFER, M.A.

Adjunct Instructor, Department of Pediatrics and Human Development, Michigan State University College of Human Medicine, East Lansing, Michigan.

Diabetes Mellitus

JOHN SHILLITO, Jr., M.D.

Professor of Surgery, Harvard Medical School. Associate Chief of Neurosurgery, Children's Hospital Medical Center, Boston, Massachusetts.

Head Injuries

JAMES E. SIMMONS, M.D.

Arthur B. Richter Professor and Director of Child Psychiatry, Indiana University School of Medicine. Attending Staff, Indiana University Hospitals (including James Whitcomb Riley Hospital for Children), and Consulting Staff, Wishard Memorial Hospital, LaRue D. Carter Memorial Hospital, Indianapolis, Indiana.

Childhood Psychosis; Lying, Stealing, and Firesetting; Parents who Suffer Psychosis; Pediatric Psychotherapeutic Skills

ERNEST E. SMITH, M.D.

Assistant Professor of Pediatrics, Indiana University School of Medicine. Director, Riley Child Development Program, James Whitcomb Riley Hospital for Children, Indianapolis, Indiana.

Prenatal/Infancy—The First 24 Months; Developmental Assessment: Office Developmental Screening

NATHAN J. SMITH, M.D.

Professor of Pediatrics and Orthopedics, University of Washington, Seattle, Washington.

Sports Medicine

BARBARA STARFIELD, M.D., M.P.H.

Professor, The Johns Hopkins University Schools of Hygiene and Public Health and Medicine. Medical Staff, The John Hopkins Hospital Department of Pediatrics, Baltimore, Maryland.

Social Factors in Child Health

LARRY TAFT, M.D.

Professor and Chairman, Department of Pediatrics, College of Medicine and Dentistry of New Jersey—Rutgers Medical School. Attending Staff, Middlesex General–University Hospital, New Brunswick, New Jersey.

Cerebral Palsy

DEBORAH KLEIN WALKER, Ed.D.

Assistant Professor of Human Development, Harvard School of Public Health, and Assistant Professor of Education, Harvard Graduate School of Education, Boston, Massachusetts.

Runaways

THOMAS R. WEBER, M.D.

Assistant Professor of Pediatric Surgery, Indiana University School of Medicine. Attending Surgeon, James Whitcomb Riley Hospital for Children, Indianapolis, Indiana.

The Skin: Lacerations, Abrasions, and Burns

WILLIAM B. WEIL, Jr., M.D.

Professor of Pediatrics and Human Development, Michigan State University College of Human Medicine. Active Staff, Michigan State University Clinical Center, Ingham Medical Center, Edward W. Sparrow Hospital, and St. Lawrence Hospital, Lansing, Michigan.

Diabetes Mellitus

MICHAEL WEITZMAN, M.D.

Assistant Professor of Pediatrics, Boston University School of Medicine. Assistant Visiting Physician for Pediatrics, Boston City Hospital, Boston, Massachusetts.

School Absence

MORRIS A. WESSEL, M.D.

Clinical Professor of Pediatrics, Yale University School of Medicine. Attending Pediatrician, Yale–New Haven Hospital, New Haven, Connecticut.

Helping a Child Cope with the Death of a Loved One; The Pediatrician and Adoption

BRUCE E. WILSON, M.D.

Clinical and Research Fellow in Pediatric Endocrinology, Department of Pediatrics/Human Development, Michigan State University College of Human Medicine. Active Staff, St. Lawrence Hospital, and Fellowship Appointments, Michigan State University Clinical Center and Ingham Medical Center, Lansing, Michigan.

Diabetes Mellitus

PAUL H. WISE, M.D., M.P.H.

Instructor, Department of Pediatrics, Harvard Medical School. Director, Emergency and Primary Care Services, Children's Hospital Medical Center, Boston, Massachusetts.

Principles of Emergency Medical Care

JAMES WRIGHT, M.D.

Associate Professor, Department of Pediatrics, Indiana University School of Medicine. Director, Endocrine Service, James Whitcomb Riley Hospital for Children, Indianapolis, Indiana.

Short Stature

PREFACE

Six years have elapsed since the publication of the second edition of *Ambulatory Pediatrics*. Because of the rapid progress in the field, we believe that it is time for a new edition to reflect the advancing medical knowledge.

The Report of the Task Force on Pediatric Education, the Residency Review Committee for Pediatrics revised Special Requirements for residency training in pediatrics, The Robert Wood Johnson Foundation Programs to prepare academic general pediatricians and to consolidate health services for young people, the Federal Manpower Grants for Primary Care Residency Training, and the W. T. Grant Foundation Grants for Residency Training in Behavioral and Developmental Pediatrics have contributed importantly to the steady evolution of ambulatory pediatrics. Few aspects of pediatric education have received as great an emphasis in recent years. Continuity care clinics, augmented attention to the psychosocial aspects of pediatrics, adolescent medicine, school health, community pediatrics, and child development are now integral parts of accredited three-year general pediatrics residency programs.

Along with these changes in education in pediatrics, the practice of ambulatory pediatrics has also changed. Although initially identified with the outpatient departments of teaching hospitals, and of marginal academic vitality, ambulatory pediatrics, now viewed as an integral part of general pediatrics, is in the mainstream of pediatric education. Having reached the stage of generativity, it is actively subdividing into academic areas of special interest: primary care; psychosocial or behavioral pediatrics; child development; the care of children with handicaps; adolescent medicine; consultation; child welfare, including child abuse and foster care; community pediatrics; health services research; school health; and emergency care. Ambulatory and general pediatrics have come of age!

Pediatric practice in the community is also changing, as reflected in the trend to practice in groups and in smaller communities, the development by practitioners of special pediatric interest areas, and the occurrence of more prenatal and adolescent pediatric visits. Hospital emergency rooms have increasingly become deliverers of primary services, even for families with a regular source of pediatric care. Cooperative arrangements between pediatricians are also developing in the form of independent practice associations and after-hours clinics staffed by pediatric practitioners. Health supervision visits are being examined in efforts to (1) broaden their scope; (2) adapt them to the changing needs of families; (3) prove that prevention works; and (4) improve the remuneration for this service.

The consumer of pediatric care is also different. Divorce, one-parent families, working mothers, alternative lifestyles, substance abuse, teenage pregnancies, child abuse and neglect, and the mounting stresses of everyday life have become part of the rapidly changing pediatric scene. That the profile of problems encountered also now includes more behavioral complaints is recognized in a special section on Psychosocial-Developmental Disorders. In addition to this new section, other chapter groupings include the Clinician's Job; Health Promotion; Episodic Biomedical Disorders; and Persistent, Recurrent, and Long-Term Disorders. New chapters deal with childhood depression, vandalism, the out-of-control adolescent, hyperactivity, contraception, food fads, girls' sports, alcohol and drug abuse, sports injuries, sexually transmitted diseases, runaways, sexual abuse, and learning problems.

This organization parallels, we reason, what happens in practice. Children are brought to see the physician because of problems or symptoms, usually acute and often not yet labeled; for the management of an already diagnosed chronic or long-term disorder; or by age groups for health promotion needs. While this arrangement of content does not avoid all duplication, we hope that it will facilitate finding what the reader wants. As in the previous editions, no pretense of complete coverage is made. Each section is introduced by a theme chapter written by the editors. These discussions provide a general orientation to the chapters that follow by including a presentation of concepts, background, assumptions, review of the pertinent literature, and a perspective on how such material fits into the clinician's job.

Child health care is the responsibility of many persons, including pediatricians, family physicians, nurses, physician associates, social workers, allied health workers, teachers, and especially parents and children. Because we hold that a group alliance, including the most important contributions of parents and children, is necessary for the best child health, we hope that this book will be useful to them all.

As a means to introduce different points of view, some of the chapters are written by authors new to this book. To them and to those with whom we have been privileged to work before, the editors express their heartfelt appreciation. In addition to expressing our thanks to our colleagues, to our secretaries (Mrs. Glenna Clark at Indiana, and Mrs. Nancy Bennett and Ms. Pat Owen in New York), and to Mr. Albert Meier of the W. B. Saunders Company, we wish also to express publicly our indebtedness to our colleagues, house staff, and students for the constant stimulation and gratification they provide.

MORRIS GREEN
ROBERT J. HAGGERTY

CONTENTS

SECTION I

THE PEDIATRIC CLINICIAN

In this book on the role of the pediatric practitioner in the personal health care of children, the editors have sought to include those facts, attitudes, and behaviors thought useful in an ambulatory setting. This introductory chapter deals with the scope of comprehensive child health services and the pediatric clinician's job. It is a topic rarely addressed during residency training. The principles apply equally to office-based and to hospital-based practice.

THE SCOPE OF CHILD HEALTH SERVICES

In his daily work, whether that be prevention, treatment, or health promotion, the pediatrician is concerned with biological and psychosocial homeostasis in the child. Figure 1 presents a model, which we have termed a *homeogram,* that we have found useful in the assessment of homeostasis broadly defined. The intent of this model is to demonstrate the interrelatedness of the child, his family, and the environment and to convey the multiple causality of health and disease. These factors are so interrelated that, as Alan Gregg once wrote:

> . . . no part can be changed without changing in some way and in some measure all the others. . . . It is intellectual weakness that prompts us to ascribe a given result to only one sufficient cause. We ignore the value of suspecting that a result may be due to a convergence of several "causes" which separately or in some other sequence will not produce the result we seek to explain. This tendency to overlook convergent or multiple causation seduces us as an unrecognized temptation in our enthusiasm as teachers to make things "clear."

On one axis of the homeogram are listed the clinician's major assessment areas: illness, vulnerabilities, potentialities, and strengths. Problems and vulnerabilities are actively or potentially disruptive of homeostasis, whereas strengths and potentialities promote that balance necessary for health. In addition to the assessment of these factors within the host—the individual child—the clinician must similarly assess the family and the environment. Although the number of variables in this model is almost without limit, the pertinent ones can be readily identified by history and observation in the course of one or more pediatric interviews. There are no simple questionnaires available for this assessment.

THE COMPONENTS OF CHILD HEALTH CARE

PROBLEMS

As used in the homeogram, problems are those illnesses, symptoms, deficits, and impairments of functioning that arise in the physical, social, emotional, or cognitive aspects of a child's development when something has gone wrong. Problems in the family and the environ-

HOMEOGRAM

		Child	Family	Environment
+	Strengths			
(+)	Potentialities			
(−)	Vulnerabilities			
−	Problems			

Figure 1. A model for the assessment of biological and psychosocial homeostasis.

ment obviously may have an adverse effect on the health of a child.

VULNERABILITIES

Vulnerabilities represent potential precursors of problems. Preventive pediatrics, perhaps better called health promotion, seeks to avoid the overt expression of these precursors as illnesses and now occupies about 50 per cent of the practicing pediatrician's time in the United States. The number and nature of these vulnerabilities depend on multiple factors such as genetic inheritance, psychological background, chronological and developmental age, environment, socioeconomic status, family constellation, past experiences, life style, and long-term illness. Once the specific biomedical and psychosocial vulnerabilities of a child, his family, and his environment are identified, the clinician's role is to help the child and his family utilize their potential resources and strengths to contain these health risks.

STRENGTHS

Strengths in the child and the family are synonymous with health, well-being, competence, achievement, and ability to cope and to adapt. Table 1 contains a list of strengths in the

Table 1. STRENGTHS: THE CHILD

- Able to communicate well
- Able to express feelings
- Able to relate positively to others
- Regards the visit to the doctor as a good idea
- Has physical fitness, endurance, vigor
- Has personal achievements, successes, special interests, hobbies, or talents in relation to music, art, athletics, writing, school work, cheerleading, or working with animals
- Has the ability to form realistic and constructive assessments of his own capacities
- Has a wide social support network
- Is able to form trusting relationships
- Has one or more close friends
- Attends to personal grooming
- Demonstrates readiness to accept help
- Has a history of compliance with medical advice
- Spontaneously raises the possibility that life stresses may have contributed to the problem and seeks mastery over these stresses
- Has an understanding of health
- Feels responsible for his own health
- Has had experiences of joy
- Able to enjoy life
- Has the capacity to cope with stress and life change
- Interested in self-improvement

Table 2. STRENGTHS: THE FAMILY

- Close family ties
- Communicates well
- Good health
- Economically secure
- Parents are knowledgeable about child health and are psychologically and developmentally minded
- Good social support systems
- Interacts with community; group associations
- Parent(s) accompany child for visit
- Have reared other children successfully
- Parents reared in supportive families

child and Table 2 those in the family. Environments also have their strengths—those persons, institutions, and services that support the child and his family, elements that need to be mobilized to help children and families cope with problems and contain vulnerabilities. Where environmental strengths are lacking, the clinician will want to work to improve these social environments of children; however, in most situations, he must be content to help coordinate those that are available.

POTENTIALITIES

The term *potentialities* is used here to represent those potential, latent, unrealized, or previously unidentified strengths and those human aspirations that can become activated as *new capabilities* and *improved function.* Potentialities are analogous to what Caplan has termed *mastery,* i.e.,

> . . . behavior by the individual that (1) results in reducing to tolerable limits physiological and psychological manifestations of emotional arousal during and shortly after a stressful event and (2) mobilizes the individual's internal and external resources and develops new capabilities in him that lead to his changing his environment or his relation to it, so that he reduces the threat or finds alternate sources of satisfaction for what is lost.

Senn phrased the concept this way:

> In formulating a treatment program or one of prevention, the physician and nurse need to know the potentialities for growth and change which are inherent within the human being, and which need to be mobilized for overcoming ill health of any kind and in maintaining good health.

The sources of such vulnerability to stress are a combination of innate biological factors, experience, and maturation. Among the resources contributing to what she has termed "resiliency," Werner has identified "*adaptability* on the biological, psychological, social, and cultural levels; *profound* ties to *concrete* immediate others; and formal or informal *ties* between the *individual* and his or her *community.*" Other synonyms for potentiality include *plasticity, reserve,* and *invulnerability.* A major task for pediatricians in the future will be to help children develop such mastery through education, behavioral approaches, crisis intervention, and other supports. This frontier for pediatric research, care, and education is relatively unexplored.

THE CONSTITUENCIES OF CHILD HEALTH SERVICES

CHILDREN

The child is the primary focus of pediatric care. Systematic, periodic collection of data about a child's problems, vulnerabilities, and strengths, beginning prenatally and continuing through adolescence, contributes to the delivery of child health care at an optimal level. While there are few research data to support the thesis that such care improves health, there is evidence that it reduces the use of curative health services, including use of medicines and diagnostic tests. On the basis of current knowledge, we have no hesitation in endorsing the comprehensive health care outlined in this book while at the same time recommending research on its efficacy. Such periodic assessments constitute a pediatric diary or biography of an individual child. Before birth, information about a child's family and environment permits anticipation, if not prediction, of what will appear in the first chapters of that biography, just as the accumulation of data in the early months and years may permit some notion of what will be evident at adolescence.

FAMILIES

The family, the one social unit to which most children relate, must be understood in order to provide personal and comprehensive child health care. The pediatrician has an unique opportunity to contribute to the strengths of families by promoting parental self-reliance, participation of the father in child rearing, parent education, and the use of those community resources that contribute to family intactness and health. Asking about the health of the parents and about life events in the family are ways to do this. Such a focus in care obviously has benefit in the management of chronic disease, psychosocial and developmental problems, and family crises and health promotion.

THE ENVIRONMENT

The environment, including the community, has long been a consideration in pediatric practice. Indeed, pediatrics may be defined as family and community medicine applied to a child. Since the family is often more influenced by the community—its resources, strengths, and weaknesses—than it is independent, the body of knowledge termed "community pediatrics" has a real contribution to make to pediatric practice. This approach focuses on *all* children in a defined area, not only those with the resources and initiative to seek help. In order to provide optimal care for his patient, the doctor needs to know the special vulnerabilities associated with specific groups of children and how to deploy strengths and resources in the community as well as to be aware of its problems and weaknesses. Environmental manipulation is an important therapeutic option.

There is need today for the practitioner to be conversant with the risks of exposure of children to noxious agents in chemical dumps, sanitation landfills, and industrial pollution as well as to the physical and psychological hazards of nuclear plant disasters.

We would differentiate here the community orientation of the practitioner in the care of an individual child from what might be termed the practice of community pediatrics. The personal pediatrician in an office setting is not in a position to practice community pediatrics unless he also serves part-time with a community organization, as by providing services or consultations to an organization that serves a population of children (schools, health centers, adoption agencies) or through joining with other citizens in advocacy for the improvement of services in the community.

THE PEDIATRICIAN'S IDENTITY

With the exception of those whose careers are in research, in a subspecialty, or in community pediatrics, the editors believe that the professional ontogeny of most pediatricians recapitulates the growth and development of pediatrics as a specialty. Initially, there is usually a major investment in illness, hospital pediatrics, subspecialty care, the biomedical aspects of child health, and the individual patient. Somewhat later, the clinician becomes more involved with ambulatory and general pediatric care and with the behavioral and psychosocial aspects of child health and the family. A little later, a health team–family relationship evolves, and the physician becomes involved more in teaching of other health professionals. With further maturation, an interest in community pediatrics and administration may develop. Although there are many exceptions, the pediatrician's patients tend to increase in age as he does, from an early predominance of infants to an increase in the number of adolescents later and, finally, a decrease in newborn and young infants.

This process of professional development reflects that of pediatrics itself. Historically, the primary emphasis on illness was followed by interest in prevention and then in optimal health. The initial focus on the individual patient was followed by a concern with families and the environment, and the early concentration on in-hospital training was followed by the evolution of a more balanced educational experience.

The pediatrician's interest in children as children, his personal advocacy for their welfare, and his feelings of empathy and warmth probably derive more from his personal than from his professional identity, and, we believe, largely antedate the latter. The educational experiences of the pediatric house officer generally do not prepare him to become an advocate for children unless he becomes personally and emotionally involved in appropriate clinical situations or has a continuing and close exposure to admired role models who have such commitments.

We believe that everyone who works in child health should have a background in human developmental biology, including human behavior, and in the behavioral and social sciences. Every clinician should also have solid experience with hospital pediatrics not only to learn how to manage patients with a variety of illnesses but also to help the physician master such upsetting experiences as the death of a patient, the birth of a child with a serious congenital anomaly, the lack of gratitude associated with the care of some patients, the hostile parent, the minimal effect that one's therapy has upon a good many conditions, the family with overwhelming problems, the lack of crucial community resources, needless drugs and procedures, unnecessary hospitalizations, and the lack of compliance by some families. All these should be experienced by the physician-in-training at a time when he can, with help, learn how to cope with them effectively and with some equanimity.

The editors believe "training for uncertainty" is a necessary part of learning in ambulatory pediatrics so that the clinician can proceed in the management of the patient with reasonable confidence. Much of what is presented in this book does not have a firm empirical basis but rather is based on what experienced clinicians believe is the best approach today. This does not mean that the recommendations might not change nor that there is no need for research in this area. Indeed, the lack of a firm empirical base is a good reason for more emphasis upon research in ambulatory pediatrics.

It is also important for the resident to recognize that medicine does not have the answer to most of the pressing problems of children—poor housing, discrimination, inadequate schools, delinquency, school dropouts, drugs, divorce, and poverty. Changes in training that center on and allow discussion of these problems with seasoned faculty may lessen some of the practitioner's later psychological discomforts and distress and help avoid simplistic proposals to solve these problems.

DETERMINANTS OF THE CLINICIAN'S JOB

Approximately 33 per cent of the visits now made to pediatricians' offices are for acute, especially respiratory, illnesses. Although these do not often lead to death or disability, the physician must alleviate discomfort while being alert to diagnose and treat rare, life-threatening complications such as meningitis. Undoubtedly this kind of role will continue. The care of children with chronic illness consumes only 3 to 10 per cent of the average pediatrician's time today, but long-term disorders, which require different sets of skills, therapeutic goals, and time, will attract more attention and effort of the pediatrician in the future. The extent of the general clinician's involvement with secondary or tertiary hospital care will vary, depending upon his training and the practice setting, but in most cases he will be responsible for some hospital as well as ambulatory care, including attention to a wide scope of biomedical, psychosocial, developmental, and educational problems.

It has been helpful in the past to define three levels of medical care—primary, secondary, and tertiary. It appears timely to categorize general ambulatory care in three levels based on the following determinants:

1. Length of time required for the specific service.
2. Level of competence required to provide the service.
3. Complexity of the problem.
4. The professional cast, i.e., the pediatrician acting alone or sharing roles with other health and nonhealth disciplines.
5. The setting of the service.
6. The specific needs of the target population.

These three levels of general ambulatory pediatric care may be characterized as follows:

Level I Care

A. Requires up to 30 minutes of professional time for delivery.

B. Provided by the pediatrician solely, by the pediatrician and the nurse jointly, or by the nurse solely.

C. Includes health supervision visits, acute illness or trauma care, continuity visits for patients with chronic handicaps/diseases, and home visits.

D. Professional activities include the pediatric interview, the physical examination, screening procedures, prescription of medications, brief procedures (injections), explanation, anticipatory guidance, education, clarification, and suggestions for environmental changes. Audio- and videotapes, brochures, and group sessions with parents may be additional modalities for the delivery of Level I care.

All general pediatricians provide Level I care.

Level II Care

A. Requires up to 40 minutes of professional time per session.

B. Provided solely by pediatrician, shared with nurse or other professional (psychologist, social worker) in the office, or provided in collaboration with other health and nonhealth professionals in the community.

C. Includes more thorough health supervision visits; some continuity visits for chronic disease/handicap; consultations from other physicians, professionals, and community agencies;

procedures such as suturing; family crisis visits; and Level II special interest or subspecialty care.

The amount of Level II care given by an individual general pediatrician will depend upon his or her special interests, the comprehensiveness of the health supervision packages offered, and the patients' needs. In addition to Level I care, most general pediatricians will provide some Level II care. Although the percentage of time spent in Level I and Level II care will vary widely among practitioners, the trend will be toward increased delivery of Level II care, especially in the special interest areas of child development, the psychosocial aspects of pediatrics, developmental disabilities, adolescence, and school problems.

Level III Care

A. Requires up to 60 minutes of professional time per session.

B. Provided solely by the pediatrician, shared with the nurse or other professional (psychologist, social worker) in the office, provided in collaboration with other health or nonhealth professionals in the community, or provided by an interdisciplinary or multidisciplinary group at a regional center.

C. Includes consultations, family crisis visits, Level III special interest or subspecialty problems, and diagnostic/evaluation sessions in regional centers and child guidance clinics. Community advocacy for children, consultation with courts, schools, agencies and government are other Level III activities.

General pediatricians may provide some Level III care for general or special interest problems, participate in a regional center for the care of children who are chronically ill or handicapped, and continue with Level I or II care when Level III care for a specific child is given by a regional team under the direction of another physician. Some pediatric subspecialists, who provide chiefly Level II and III care, may also deliver some Level I care.

A different perspective from which to view growth and differentiation in pediatrics is presented in Figure 2. The symbolic triangle on the left portrays, without quantification, hospital-based care with its greatest involvement in tertiary and secondary care and least participation in the delivery of primary health services. While further differentiation may be anticipated within this setting, significant growth or expansion is unlikely to occur. This prediction is much in contrast to the situation on the right, which depicts the concept of three levels of office-based or ambulatory care. Here there is considerable potential for growth and differentiation beyond the present frontier at all three levels. At Level I, the growth will come from prenatal visits, adolescent health care, sports medicine, and more sophisticated health supervision, which includes attention to psychosocial and developmental factors. Growth at Levels II and III will result from differentiation of general pediatrics into areas of special interest. Figure 3 projects how all this may eventually fit together.

General pediatrics is dividing into areas of special interest, and it is likely that the pediatric practitioner of the future will be prepared to practice both general and special-interest pediatrics. The general pediatric care matrix shown in Figure 4 acknowledges the docu-

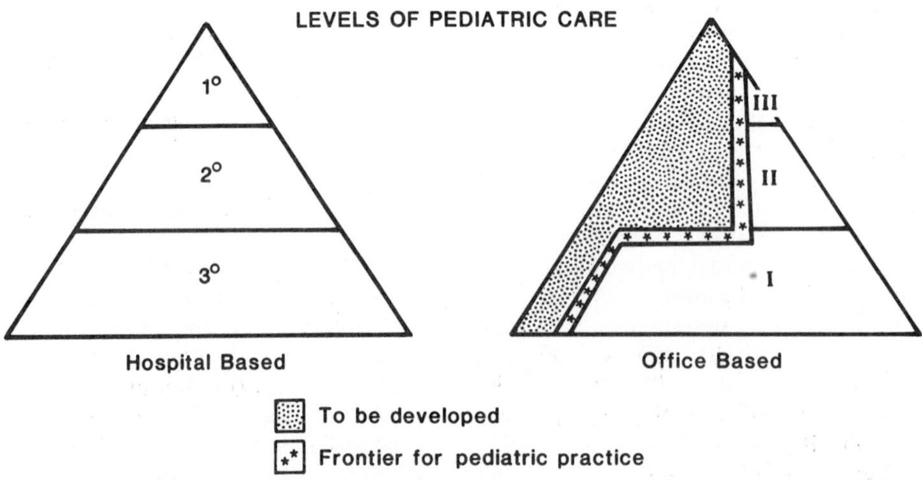

Figure 2. Categorization of pediatric general ambulatory care.

LEVELS OF PEDIATRIC CARE

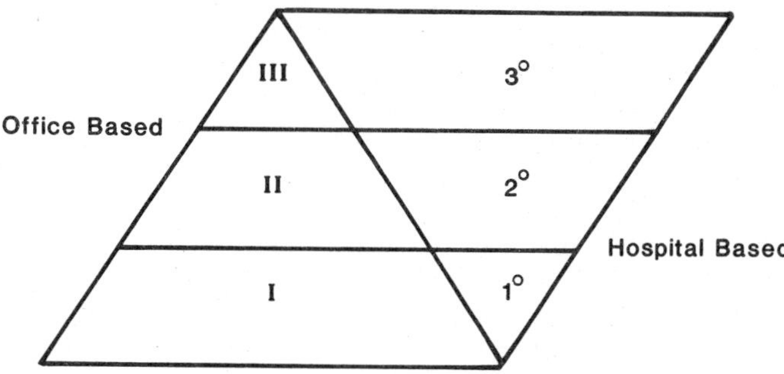

The Complete Spectrum

Figure 3. The organization of pediatric care.

mented readiness of pediatric practitioners to develop both a general and a special competence—or expressed differently, their interest in seeing patients with more complex problems while continuing health supervision, a role for which they profess great professional satisfaction. The vertical slices represent special interest areas, while the horizontal divisions depict the three levels of ambulatory general care. The first vertical slice on the left is intended to represent the activities of a general pediatrician. Using sleep patterns of infants as an example, at Level I the anticipatory guidance given as part of the periodic pediatric assessment visit would be concerned with what the parents might expect in the way of a baby's reluctance to go to sleep and prospective advice as to how appropriate sleep practices might be best fostered. Advice concerning the management of a moderate sleep problem would be a Level II activity, whereas attention to a more persistent sleep problem linked to maternal depression and marital discord would be a Level III problem.

The next vertical segment (G-CD) would represent the general pediatrician with a special interest in child development. As an example, Level I care would be the developmental evaluation provided as part of a periodic pediatric assessment; Level II care would be given to an infant with a developmental delay in language; and Level III care would be given to an infant with general developmental delay and evidence of spasticity. The other vertical slices apply to other areas of special interest such as allergy, behavior, neurology, and developmental dis-

THE MATRIX OF GENERAL PEDIATRIC AMBULATORY CARE

LEVELS OF CARE									
	III								
	II								
	I								
Special Interests		Gen.	Gen. + C. Dev.	G. + P. Soc.	Gen. + Neur.	Gen. + Allergy	Gen. + D.D.		Gen. + Adol.

Figure 4. Integration of general and special interest pediatrics.

abilities. Table 3 provides examples of Level I, II, and III psychosocial problems, some of which may be managed by the general pediatrician, by the pediatrician with a special interest in child development and the psychosocial aspects of child and family health, or by the child psychiatrist or other mental health professional.

In the delivery of personal health services, the clinician's practice fits along the several spectra depicted in Figure 5. It is useful to think of a practice profile for each clinician which depends on the time spent in illness care and health promotion; primary care and secondary or tertiary care; acute and chronic illness; ambulatory and hospital care; Level I, II or III ambulatory care; hospital care of newborns or sick infants and children; biomedical and psychosocial problems; independent and complementary activity; office and community collaborative activity; individual patients and community activities; purely medical activities or management and administrative demands; services or research; and direct services or educational activities. The pediatrician may be satisfied with or wish to change his current profile.

Except for the small town where there are not enough patients for more than one pediatrician or for the very individualistic physician, there are compelling reasons to practice together. A group seems essential to share knowledge, have easy access to consultation, have someone with whom to share concerns, avoid fatigue, have opportunities for continuing education, engage in a subspecialty, or participate in a community child health program. These other activities serve to reduce the pressure of practice for brief periods and to create new and refreshing intellectual challenges. Because of the low prevalence of chronic pediatric disorders, only in a very unusual setting, such as a group practice or in a teaching hospital, can the general clinician expect to deliver subspecialty care for problems other than those of a behavioral, allergic, neurological, educational, developmental, or dermatological character. In a group, the style and content of one's work will be influenced by whether the practice consists solely of pediatricians or includes other physicians—internists, family physicians, obstetricians, and other medical and surgical subspecialists. Some pediatricians find it more comfortable to practice in the same building but maintain separate practices, arranging for collaboration only through night and weekend coverage.

Whether practicing independently or in a

Table 3. LEVELS OF PSYCHOSOCIAL PROBLEMS

Level I	Level II	Level III
Feeding problems →		
Breath-holding spells →		
Temper tantrums →		
Sleep disorders →		
Discipline problems →		
Separation difficulties →		
Enuresis →		
	Failure to thrive	
	Rumination	
	Development delay	
	School avoidance →	
	School underachievement →	
	Family crisis →	
	Psychogenic pain →	
	Conversion disorders →	
	Suicide gesture →	
	Anorexia nervosa →	
	Adolescent sexual problems, including teenage pregnancy →	
	←	Conduct disorder
	←	Suicide attempt
	←	Chronic depression
		Infantile autism
		Failure, maternal attachment
		Gender identity disorder
		Delinquency

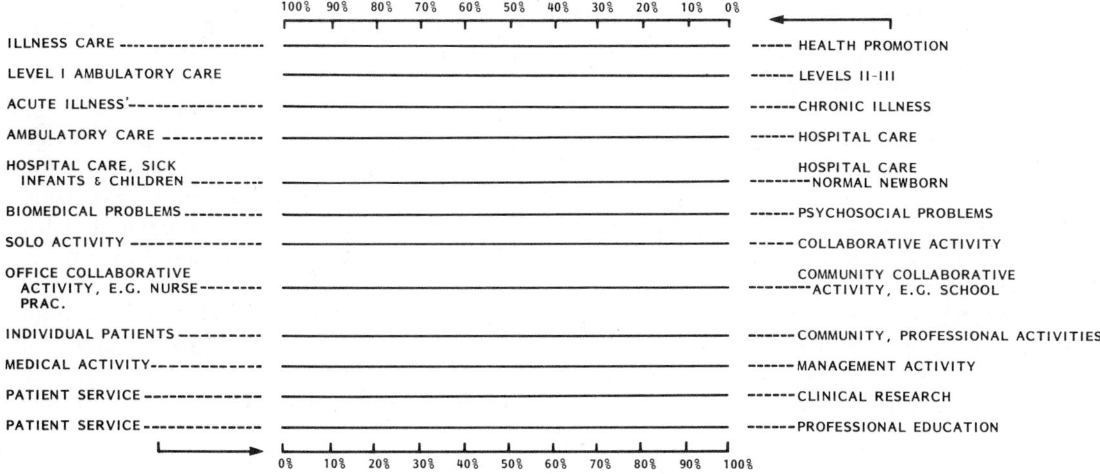

Figure 5. A clinical pediatric practice profile.

group, the pediatrician will need to work closely with others, both to augment the scope of care available and to integrate the diverse services received by his patients. Just as he needs to have subspecialists available for biomedical disorders, either within the group setting, by phone consultation, or through ready referral, he also needs community facilities and services in order to care for children with psychosocial, developmental, and educational problems.

In the traditional model of pediatric practice, the pediatrician is personally responsible for the diagnosis and management of the child's problem, with most of the required services provided in the office by himself or his associates. When hospitalization is indicated, e.g., for pneumonia or croup, the pediatrician usually gives total care. When he cannot, e.g., for patients who need open heart surgery or care of end-stage renal disease, he maintains communication and coordination between the family and the subspecialists but continues primary responsibility for the care of the child. In progressive ambulatory care with Level I, II, and III activities, some services are given in the physician's office through the use of nurse practitioners, social workers, or psychologists, while others are arranged collaboratively with other community services such as schools, family service agencies, marriage counselors, family therapists, community mental health centers, developmental day care centers, psychological assessments, and special education programs in the school, recreational programs for retarded children, respite centers, parent education programs, parent groups, clergymen, and juvenile courts.

As the psychosocial and developmental aspects of child health care become more prominent in the next decade, the "developmental therapist"—a new professional prepared in child development and in parent education—may evolve to complement the pediatric nurse in the pediatric office of tomorrow. Forward-looking community hospitals will move to assist the pediatric practitioners on their staffs to practice Level II and III general pediatric care by sharing with them other health professionals such as the psychologist, social worker, nutritionist, occupational therapist, physical therapist, and speech therapist and by offering, on a scheduled basis, itinerent office suites in the hospital in which the pediatrician can see by appointment those Level II and Level III patients whose management requires collaboration with other health disciplines available in that hospital setting.

In relation to school health the physician might have several different functions. Most commonly, he is involved in the assessment and management of disease or of learning and developmental problems. In addition, he has a role in health education, in environmental programs in school, and in the continuing professional education of the teacher. Finally, some clinicians provide primary health care in the school setting.

In addition to children in his practice, the practitioner may provide care in health centers, adoption agencies, day care, and Head Start programs. The pediatrician may also be asked to serve as a consultant for an individual child or to help community agencies evaluate overall programs and plan new services.

The average pediatrician cares for about 2000 patients (ranging from 1000 to over 4000) each year, including about 100 newborns. With the decline in the birth rate in recent years (now stabilized), the pediatrician now has more time available for management of older children and adolescents, those with chronic disease, and those with psychosocial and developmental problems.

The setting of a practice is a major determinant of the way in which a pediatrician practices. How things are done in a community may have a greater influence on the pediatrician's role than his training. Changes in pediatric practice come either when there is a sufficient number of individual clinicians who practice in new ways, when there is a change in the expectations of the consumers, when there is a change in the practice mix, or when there is a change in method of remuneration.

In a rural area or medium-sized city, the pediatrician functions as a generalist-consultant (Level II ambulatory care) as well as a provider of Level I primary care, whereas in larger cities and suburbs he will be more of a personal primary care physician (Level I ambulatory care) for children while providing Level II care in an area of special interest.

Parents, already a major factor in determining the character of practice, will play a larger role in the future. Their social class, desires, insurance or government health benefits, attitudes,

Table 4. THE CLINICIAN'S STRENGTHS

- An understanding of his personal and professional identities
- Biomedical, psychological, managerial, and technical competence
- Personal warmth and openness
- Knowledge of the developmental needs of children and parents
- Ability to deal comfortably with both biomedical and biosocial illness
- Skill as an interviewer
- Skill as a perceptive observer
- Degree of empathy and awareness of feelings in himself, the child, and the family
- Excellence of clinical judgment
- Ability to develop working alliances with a child, parents, and others
- Availability
- Recognition that many burdens have to be accepted as part of the privilege of being a physician
- Ability to call for help with comfort
- Ability to avoid situations in which the physician has no constructive role, i.e., recognition of the boundaries of one's competence
- No discomfort about fee arrangements
- Ability to set limits on demands made on him
- Respect for the dignity of children and their parents
- Ability to inspire trust and confidence
- Sense of responsibility for the patient
- Ability to define and persist in achieving objectives
- Ability to deal with strengths and resources of parents rather than just their weaknesses
- Interest in children and parents as individuals
- Scientific curiosity about human behavior
- Access to and use of continuing education
- Opportunities for change of pace, e.g., work in a university, community health project, research in practice or professional organization at the community, state, or national level
- Special interest in an age group, organ subspecialty, chronic disease, or community project
- Ability to use time effectively and efficiently
- Recognition of areas of gratification in practice
- Satisfaction gained from watching children and families grow from infancy to adulthood
- Ability to work well with nurses, social workers, psychologists, and allied health professionals
- Avoidance of professional isolation
- Recognition that physicians as well as patients have emotional needs
- Ability to identify personal and professional stresses
- Opportunity to discuss problems encountered in practice in study groups of pediatricians who meet regularly to discuss their problems with patients, and to learn new and to sharpen old diagnostic and treatment skills
- Development of a sense of accomplishment and pride in daily work
- Interest in improving existing clinical skills and acquiring new ones
- Ability to be enthusiastic, encouraging, and optimistic
- Recognition and acceptance that much of what clinicians do is routine and repetitive service
- Ability to tend to personal and family needs

Table 5. THE CLINICIAN'S VULNERABILITIES AND PROBLEMS

- Some problems in physical and emotional health
- Excessive use of alcohol or drugs, problems in marriage, problems with authority, anxieties, feelings of anger and guilt
- Insensitivity to patient's feelings
- Tendency to create undue dependency
- Difficulty in keeping up with advances
- Lack of understanding of human behavior
- Feeling of being trapped in a process that cannot be changed
- Feeling that he has to do everything
- Insufficient training in some areas such as adolescent medicine or behavioral pediatrics
- Inability to function well with other disciplines in a team
- Not seeing, denying, or avoiding problems rather than realistically resolving them
- Conflicts between career commitments and role as husband or wife, father or mother
- Expecting too much from oneself
- Lack of time due to pressure of number of patients
- Lack of variety
- Professional isolation
- Ceaseless demands
- Lack of gratitude of some patients
- Failure of patient compliance
- Incongruity between needs of a child as seen by the pediatrician and the concerns and desires of the parents

expectations of care, and decisions as to the timing of medical attention and whom to call for it are obvious examples of this. In urban areas, families have increasingly taken their children to emergency rooms at night and on weekends even when they have a family pediatrician. In response to this, pediatric practitioners may offer evening office hours or evening clinics staffed on a rotating schedule.

The physician who has a special interest, either in a specific age group (e.g., adolescence), chronic illness, school health, or the like, will have a significantly different practice from one who does not. The kinds, extent, and frequency of services to be offered by the clinician will depend upon the benefit packages that the physician is able to offer and what the consumer either desires or can afford. The method of reimbursement, whether prepaid or fee-for-service, will have great impact on the character of the practice.

For those who live near a medical center, one day or so per week spent caring for children in a specialty clinic or teaching can be professionally satisfying and stimulating. Even those who do not live near such resources find that joining together for continuing education programs can be rewarding. Many community hospital departments of pediatrics have found it useful to coordinate their continuing education with that of the American Academy of Pediatrics PREP (Pediatric Review and Education Program) and its special review journal, "Pediatrics In Review."

The physician, in his role as health counselor, constantly evaluates his patients in order to help ensure their health. The editors believe that the physician would benefit from the opportunity to look at himself, and to assess his own strengths, vulnerabilities, and problems (Tables 4 and 5). Defining his professional and personal objectives and characteristics, he can take steps to achieve the kind of practice and life style that he and his family value. Such practice would not be devoid of stress—practice is demanding—but it would bring significant gratification. There is no established tradition for such self-evaluation. Growth in personal and professional capacities and the discovery of unrealized potenial may be facilitated by discussions with a senior colleague, an admired teacher, or small group of colleagues or by sessions with a new kind of counselor interested in the health, practice, and life style of physicians.

REFERENCES

Burnett, R. D., and Bell, L. S.: Projecting pediatric practice patterns. Pediatrics, *62*:627, 1978.

Caplan, G.: Mastery of stress: Psychosocial aspects. Am. J. Psychiatry, *138*:4, 1981.

Green, M.: Coming of Age in Pediatrics. Submitted for publication. Pediatrics, in press.

Gregg, A.: Multiple causation and organismic and integrative approaches to medical education. Presented at Conference on Psychiatric Education, American Psychiatric Association, Washington, D.C., 1951.

Senn, M. J. E.: The contribution of psychiatry to child health services. Am. J. Orthopsychiatry, *21*:138, 1951.

Werner, E. E., and Smith, R. S.: Vulnerable, but Invincible: A Longitudinal Study of Resilient Children and Youth. New York, McGraw-Hill, 1981.

Morris Green, M.D.,
and Robert J. Haggerty, M.D.

1

SOCIAL FACTORS IN CHILD HEALTH

Barbara Starfield, M.D.

In the final analysis, disease is a social phenomenon. Social factors have always played a large role in the genesis and course of illness. Biomedical knowledge that makes it possible to prevent disease, to diagnose it earlier, or to prevent or reverse its progression is useless unless translated into health services, and the organization and delivery of health services are social as well as technical phenomena.

Most of the extensive literature on this subject deals with either theoretical formulations or epidemiological studies in adult populations (see references listed at the end of this chapter). This chapter will focus almost exclusively on children, referring to the larger body of knowledge only when necessary for adequate interpretation.

Social context is the relationship between classes of people and the environment in which they live and work. This environment has both physical and social aspects, which include the relationship people have with those around them.

HISTORICAL VIEWS OF THE CAUSE OF ILLNESS

Until the Renaissance, disease was an individual phenomenon, generally attributed to poor living habits or the sinfulness of the individual unfortunate enough to develop an illness. The invention of the compound microscope in the sixteenth century, revelations about the anatomy of the human body, and the discovery of microbes and their role in disease causation resulted in increasingly narrow concepts of disease. Illness came to be viewed as a derangement in parts of the body, a concept reflected in a system of taxonomy that fragments illness into specific diseases related to organ systems or pathophysiological processes involving specific organ systems. For those who subscribe to this approach, disease is conquerable primarily by attacking the pathologic process associated with it.

Some, however, saw illness largely as a social phenomenon, a viewpoint that had its origins in the Industrial Revolution, when epidemics were traceable to industrialization and urbanization.

The opposing forces crystallized when increasing knowledge and the harnessing of social resources made it possible, for the first time, to attack systematically the roots and manifestations of illness. Biologically oriented scientists, relying on the germ theory, focused on the individual; socially oriented scientists (the "hygienists") maintained that more would be gained by controlling the environment.

The effect of social conditions on child health was well recognized by the 1840s. Frederick Engels documented high rates of mortality in infants and children of the working class as compared with children of the higher classes, and he commented on the cumulative effects of class and urbanism on childhood mortality. His publications documented the higher death rates from smallpox, measles, scarlet fever, and pertussis among working class compared to upper class children. He linked the greater likelihood of childhood falls, drownings, and burns to lack of suitable child care in families where both mother and father had to work. He also decried the lack of medical care and the promotion of inappropriate medications among this group.

Virchow also noted that morbidity and mortality and especially infant mortality rates were much higher in working class districts of cities than in wealthier areas. The particular relationship between infant mortality and social conditions has always been noticeable, at least in part because the risk of death is relatively high in the first year of life.

Figure 1–1 demonstrates the per cent changes in infant mortality rates in the United States between 1915 and 1980. From 1915 to 1930 there was not much improvement in either the neonatal (first month of life) or postneonatal (mortality in the second through eleventh months of life). In the 1930s, increased access to medical care as a result of legislation was associated with an accelerated decline in both components of infant mortality. This phenomenon continued into the 1940s, with generally rising living standards at that time. However, there were substantial decreases in the rate of declines of mortality in both components during the 1950s; by 1960 the rate of decline in neonatal mortality was extremely small, and postneonatal mortality did not decline at all. Recovery occurred only after the mid 1960s, when the "War on Poverty" legislation provided financing for care of the poor. In the late 1960s the rate of decline in postneonatal mortality was greater than at any time since 1915. Since 1970, the rate of decline in neonatal mortality has increased, probably as a result of better neonatal intensive care, but the rate of decline in postneonatal mortality has slowed markedly. From 1977 to 1979, there was no decrease in postneonatal mortality, and in some areas of the country it increased.

THE SOCIAL ENVIRONMENT AND HEALTH

Four types of factors are involved in the cause and progression of disease: the social and physical environment, genetic structure, individual behavior, and medical and public health interventions. Although the process by which they influence disease involves interactions among them, this chapter will address only the first (Fig. 1–2).

Of the various social influences on health, the most salient is social class. Although the measurement and specification of social class is a subject of great interest and debate, most researchers designate social class by family income, education, or occupation. Sometimes proxies for these (such as characteristics of housing) are used, and often these factors are combined into an index.

Poverty constitutes one of the major social factors related to ill health. Using poverty as an example, this chapter demonstrates how social factors influence the cause, manifestations, and sequelae of illness in childhood and why it is necessary for health care practitioners to be aware of and deal with them.

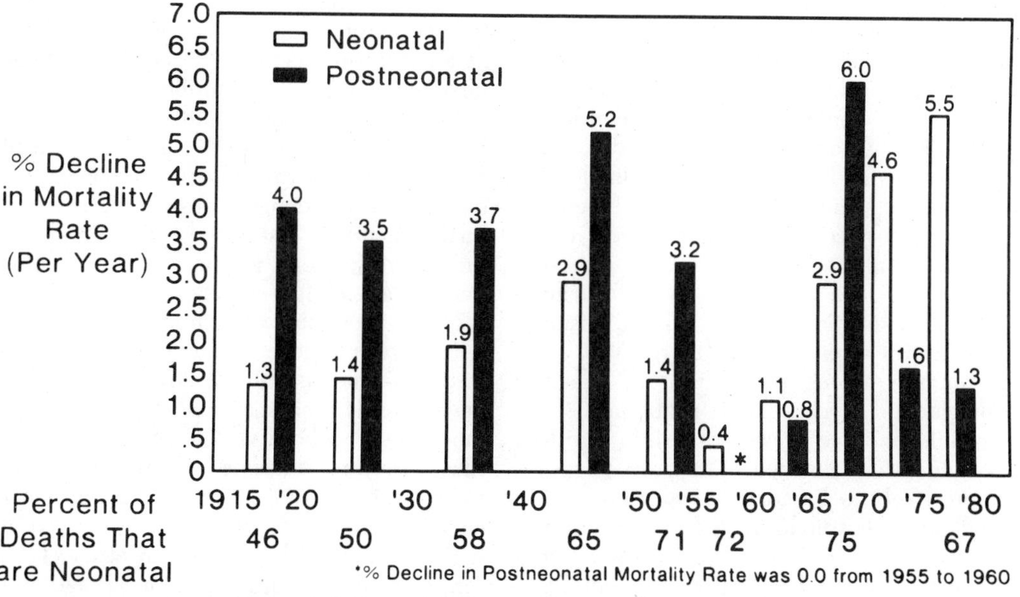

Figure 1–1. Per cent decline in infant mortality, 1915–1980.

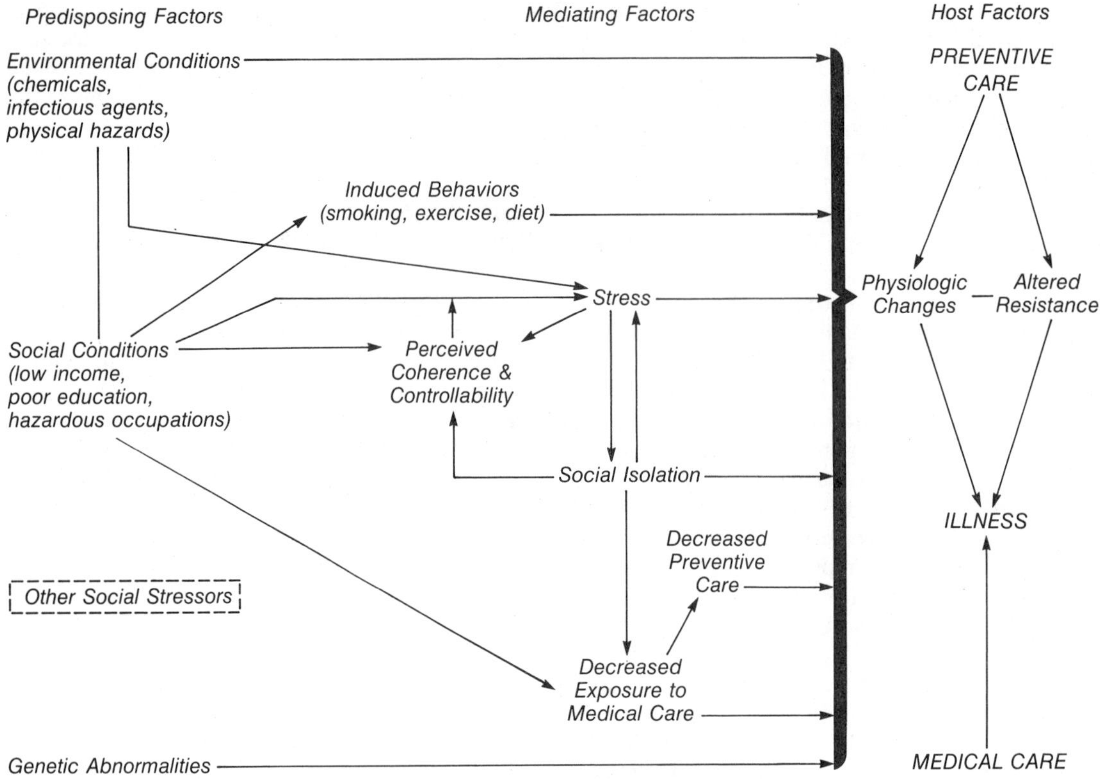

Figure 1–2. Pathogenesis of illness.

Poverty and the Health of Children

Most of the common illnesses of childhood are more frequent among poor children. Children in poor families are much more likely to be small at birth, primarily because of intrauterine growth retardation. They are more likely than other children to have congenital anomalies, and the most common congenital infection (cytomegalic inclusion disease) is more common among poor children. Poor children are more likely to contract infectious diseases such as measles and rubella and less likely to be immunized against them. Iron-deficiency anemia (the most common hematological disorder in children) is more common among these children, as is lead poisoning. Both hearing disorders and functionally poor vision (vision tested with the child's usual correction) are more common among poor children, as are psychosocial and psychosomatic problems.

Poor children have greater disability due to illness than other children. They are 75 per cent more likely to be admitted to a hospital. Even when not hospitalized, they have 30 per cent more days when their activity is restricted and 40 per cent more days lost from school due to acute illness. They are more likely to be reported by their parents as having one or more chronic health problems and much more likely to be reported by their teachers to have a chronic problem interfering with their school work. In a national examination of children of all types, the proportion of poor children found to have significant abnormalities on examination by a physician was higher in families with lower incomes than in other families.

Not only are poor children more likely to become ill, but when they do, they are likely to be sicker and to suffer more adverse consequences. For example, perinatal stress or low birth weight is associated with markedly reduced subsequent intellectual functioning of lower class children, whereas there are few sequelae in upper class children. When hospitalized, poor children spend twice as much time in the hospital as affluent children. When they have chronic illnesses such as asthma, they are more likely to be disabled by the condition so that they cannot attend school, and are likely to be more seriously ill from the condition. Poor children are much more likely to have very high levels of body toxins than other children. Their death rates are higher in all age groups.

They have poorer survival from some life-threatening conditions. Even when the occurrence of the condition is not greater among the poor, death rates from the condition may be greater. This is the case, for example, for childhood leukemia.

Mechanisms by which Poverty Exerts an Effect on Health Levels

The effect of poverty on ill health is real and not due either to an artifact resulting from the process of measurement or to adverse selection of ill individuals into low income groups by virtue of their decreased ability to earn an income. The literature on social medicine provides important clues to mechanisms by which phenomena such as poverty exert their effect.

Disease states are always the outcome of a constellation of factors. Although disease can occur directly as a response to a single stimulus, in most circumstances a single cause is insufficient. This phenomenon explains why some people become ill and others do not, even when exposed to the same pathogenic agent. It also provides a basis for the assertion that the occurrence of disease might be reduced by altering any of several relatively unrelated phenomena, instead of putting all emphasis on the discovery of "magic bullets" for specific diseases.

In the search for explanations of the effect of poverty on ill health, it is therefore important to take into consideration the interactions among the variety of circumstances that are associated with economic deprivation. Figure 1–2 shows the pathways for which there is evidence derived from scientific studies.

For some types of disease, the conditions of living and working are of prime importance in the genesis of illness. This is the case for problems arising from environmental exposure to toxins, infectious agents, excessive noise, radiation, and unsafe or overcrowded housing, neighborhoods, and living conditions that do not provide adequate heat, light, refrigeration, or ventilation. Occupational hazards may also exert adverse effects with a high probability of producing illness, as demonstrated by lead poisoning in children of individuals who work in industries involving contact with lead.

Even in these cases, illness does not develop in all individuals similarly exposed. Other factors make it possible for individuals to either resist or capitulate to external threats. These inciting, predisposing, and ameliorating factors include genetic heritage, environmental conditions, stress, social isolation, individual behavior, and medical care. The next section will show how illness can either result from or be resisted through their mediation.

Environmental Conditions Predisposing to Childhood Illness

Lead poisoning is the most well-known of the environmental causes of illness in children. Major sources of lead include lead-based paint, which was in common use until banned for in-home use. As houses painted with lead-based paint age, paint chips become loosened and subject to ingestion, particularly by toddlers. Automobile exhaust, especially in the absence of regulations requiring automobiles to use low-lead gasoline, contains lead, which accumulates in the soil and dust of heavily trafficked neighborhoods. Children of parents who work with old storage batteries are also subject to poisoning from exposure to lead in these batteries. Although lead may be associated with an acute and sometimes fulminant toxic encephalopathy, the damage from chronic low-level exposure is more insidious and more widespread, with adverse effects on cognitive and neurological performance. It is largely a lower social class problem.

Infant mortality, neonatal mortality, and fetal mortality are higher in areas with high pollution, measured either by particulate matter or by sulfates, even when analyses are controlled for other important contributors to mortality.

Other studies have shown significant relationships between air pollution and respiratory disease in school children. Data collected from examinations of a representative national sample of children in the United States show that blood carbon monoxide levels are higher in individuals living in congested urban areas; the effect is most marked for children, particularly poor children.

Exposure to constant noise produces a variety of effects predisposing to health problems. It leads to a narrowed focus of attention, to a reduction in perception of control over the environment, and to physiological alterations that are characteristic of generalized stress reactions. Several studies in Europe have shown that children living in noisy environments show blood pressure abnormalities, higher-than-average pulse rates, and other cardiovascular effects. A study among school children in the United States (Los Angeles) showed similar effects on blood pressure as well as cognitive and motivational effects, even after controlling for a variety of other social factors. Not all of the effects were reversed when the noise was abated.

The effects of environmental agents can exert themselves in utero. Although evidence is just beginning to accumulate, it is apparent that these effects are not limited to teratogenic drugs such as diethylstilbestrol and substances such as alcohol and inhalation anesthetics. The harm done by chemicals such as PCBs (polychlorinated biphenyls) is being documented with increasing frequency. Now restricted by governmental regulation, PCBs were formerly used in everything from pesticide extenders to carbon paper and are still present in the environment.

That children suffering from some types of malignant brain tumors are more likely to have parents who are occupationally exposed to chemicals than children of similar characteristics who have parents in other occupations suggests that at least some brain tumors are more common in children of certain types of workers.

Stress, Social Isolation, and Perceived Unpredictability as Mediators of Illness

Life for everyone is generally stressful. In fact, without a certain amount of challenge to stability it is unlikely that civilization would advance. Stressors produce tension, and if the individual fails to manage this tension well enough to deal with the stressors, the dysfunctional state known as stress results (see Chapter 47, pg. 305). Stress heightens susceptibility to a wide variety of illnesses. The means by which individuals deal with tension produced by stressors is known as coping. Genetic predispositions to endocrine responsiveness, to immunological competence, and to neural mechanisms influencing circulatory, metabolic, and psychological processes have all been demonstrated, suggesting that biological factors play a role in reaction to stressors. However, it is equally clear that psychosocial forces also elicit the same types of secretory, motor, and other bodily changes. Among the most important of these psychosocial forces is social support. A wide variety of studies demonstrate conclusively that individuals with social supports are much less likely to become ill than individuals who are socially isolated. The classic pediatric study of this phenomenon concerned pregnancy and birth complications. Neither the presence of stressful events nor the absence of social supports alone was related to these complications. However, the combination of stressors and lack of social supports was very highly predictive of the occurrence of complications.

The other (and related) psychosocial factor of great importance is the individual's perceptions of things as coherent and predictable. Individuals who tend to view their surroundings as unpredictable and life events as largely uncontrollable are more likely to have difficulty with their tensions and avoiding the physiological and psychological response that is known as stress. Absence of social support, lack of a sense of predictability and coherence, and failure to cope with tensions are important in enhancing susceptibility to disease and are more likely among families of lower social class. In contrast, presence of strong social support networks and a sense that events are predictable and controllable are important mechanisms by which disease is resisted.

Individual Behavior as a Mediator of Illness

Although studies have shown that health practices are capable of explaining only a part of the environment-disease association and that other mechanisms must also be involved, there is little question that certain behaviors do predispose to ill health, at least in adults. The relationship between smoking and increased risk of a wide variety of conditions is well accepted, and evidence is accumulating that physical activity can reduce risks of certain illnesses. There is little evidence either for or against the hypothesis that the behavior per se of children is an important factor in the genesis of illness in childhood, or that it is an important factor in predisposing or protecting against illness later in life. However, behaviors that are conditioned by the environment in which children live may greatly increase the vulnerability of poor children. For example, poor children whose families do not have the means to move from urban ghettos to safe neighborhoods and who therefore must ride their bicycles in much more dangerous places are at much greater risk of accidents.

Poverty and Increased Susceptibility to Disease

As the above discussion has demonstrated, disease is generally multifactorial in origin. Although it can be initiated directly by single causes, there is almost always a spectrum of susceptibility to insult and a spectrum of ability to resist the insult. There is much evidence that individuals from lower socioeconomic classes are less able to resist threats to health and more likely to succumb to illnesses with exposure to an insult.

The effect of poverty in increasing the likelihood of illness is only partly a result of more adverse biological characteristics such as very young maternal age or high parity. Risks of illness among the poor are greater even when these characteristics are controlled.

Although rates of accidents to children of working mothers are not higher than those among children whose mothers are at home in the population as a whole, poor children whose mothers work are more likely to have an accident, presumably because their mothers cannot afford another caretaker or because their social networks are too limited for them to find adequate help.

Poor children are more likely to be exposed to environmental toxins because of the neighborhoods in which they live. For example, a nationwide survey of carbon monoxide levels in children showed that blood levels of carbon monoxide are higher in crowded urban environments and in poor children. Moreover, air pollution increases the risk of respiratory problems in lower class children to a much greater extent than it does in upper class children, even when the exposure is equal. Both British and American researchers have concluded that genetic factors provide the basis for a variety of congenital defects but that environmental factors act as the triggering mechanisms for their manifestation. These conclusions derive from work on major central nervous system malformations and spina bifida.

Although major life events causing stress predispose to physical as well as emotional disease in all children (as well as adults), chronic stress associated with urban poverty predicts maladjustment of children more strongly than other types of stresses. Among poor children, those who are on welfare are more likely to be maladjusted in school than other poor children, but the effects of life stress in predisposing to maladjustment are greatest for poor children whose families are not on welfare. It is likely that the enormous struggle of some working poor families and perhaps their lesser access to social and medical supports has a particularly adverse effect on their children's health.

How Can Health Professionals Deal with the Social Aspects of Illness?

The range of opportunities for influencing the occurrence and progression of illness, particularly among those most predisposed to it by virtue of social disadvantage, is great. Recall of the pathways in Figure 1–2 suggests the various ways. The traditional medical care approach through biomedical mechanisms enables the recognition of biological risk states that predispose to disease, facilitates the detection of disease before it becomes symptomatic, permits early management of symptomatic disease, and provides for rehabilitation when disease is already advanced. But even traditional biomedical approaches must confront social phenomena, because medical care services occur in a social context. How do we ensure that efficacious medical regimens, whether they are screening, diagnostic, or therapeutic, are made available to all who need and want them? How should society organize its resources to make sure that this occurs? Medical care can make a difference. In the decade after access to medical care for the poor was facilitated by the availability of federal funding, the gap in infant mortality between the poor and the nonpoor narrowed, particularly for that component which is most susceptible to sustained social and medical management.

Practitioners can make a major contribution to the early recognition and management of illness and in doing so reduce the disparities in health status between poor and nonpoor children. Children with recurrent absences from school or with frequent illnesses (even if each one by itself is relatively trivial) are prime targets for concern, because if the factors that are responsible for recurrences are not identified and managed, these children are very likely to persist in their vulnerability to a wide variety of health problems (see Chapter 55, page 324). All practitioners periodically should review the records of each patient in their practice; those children who are visiting more frequently than the average for the practice should be evaluated carefully for evidence of environmental or social stressors.

In working with poor children, it is especially important to monitor such things as immunization status rather than to assume that the children have received the indicated preventive procedures in medical care administered elsewhere. Awareness that poor children are particularly prone to conditions such as anemia, symptomatic and asymptomatic lead poisoning, dental caries, and hearing and vision disorders should lead practitioners to look carefully for evidence of such problems and to make special efforts to tailor their therapy to the special needs and constraints of families with limited financial resources. Special efforts at follow-up and reassessment are also needed to make sure that the problem has responded to management. When problems seem to be resistant to medical interventions, it may be appropriate to reach out to other resources such as schools, religious organizations or community groups for guidance and collaboration.

Health professionals can also help influence the mediators of disease and wellness. The opportunities are perhaps greater in childhood than at any other time in life, as patterns of responding to stressors may not yet be so firmly set. Children need to gain an understanding of events that surround them and to be given an opportunity to develop some control over them. Experience in sensing mastery of anxiety and frustration is essential in building immunity against learned helplessness. Children who for whatever reason constantly experience inability to control things in their environment quickly learn that nothing they do matters. Unless this pattern of response is altered, their vulnerability to illness will stay with them from childhood through life. Because most illness stems directly from social conditions, simply giving children knowledge and encouraging them to take more responsibility for the technical aspects of their care are insufficient. Helping them to find social supports and to become involved in groups that actively work toward community improvement will go a long way to develop their sense of coherence about their environment and their ability to deal constructively with it.

Ultimately, however, health professionals have no less of an obligation, as citizens, to act on their concerns about social and environmental threats to health. The burden is, perhaps, even greater for physicians and other health professionals, because problems that relate to illness are more readily apparent to them than they are to nonprofessionals. Involvement in social affairs that have an impact on health has a long tradition within medicine, and particularly within pediatrics. Virchow, the eminent cellular pathologist, said that "improvement of medicine would eventually prolong human life but improvement of social conditions could achieve this result more rapidly and successfully."

REFERENCES

Antonovsky, A.: Health, Stress, and Coping. San Francisco, Jossey-Bass, 1979.

Berkman, L.: Physical health and the social environment: A social-epidemiological perspective. *In* Eisenberg, L., and Kleinman, A.: The Relevance of Social Science for Medicine. Dordrecht, Holland, D. Reidel, 1981.

Black, D.: Inequalities in Health. Report of a Working Group. Great Britain, Department of Health and Social Security, 1980.

Cassel, J.: The contribution of the social environment to host resistance. Am. J. Epidemiol., *164*:107–123, 1976.

Dubos, R.: Mirage of Health: Utopias, Progress, and Biological Change. New York, Harper and Row, 1959.

Eisenberg, L., and Kleinman, A.: The Relevance of Social Science for Medicine. Dordrecht, Holland, D. Reidel, 1981.

Haggerty, R. J., Roghmann, K., and Pless, I. B.: Child Health in the Community. New York, John Wiley and Sons, 1975.

Haggerty, R. J.: Life stress, illness, and social support. Dev. Med. Child. Neurol., 22:391–400, 1980.

Hinkle, L. E., Jr., and Wolff, H. G.: The nature of man's adaptation to his total environment and the relation of this to illness. Arch. Intern. Med., 99:442–460, 1957.

Hinkle, L. E., Jr.: Measurement of the effects of the environment upon the health and behavior of people. *In* Hinkle, L. E., Jr., and Loring, W. C., (Eds.): The Effect of the Man-Made Environment on Health and Behavior. Atlanta, Center for Disease Control, 1977 (DHEW Publication No. (CDC) 77-8318).

McWhinney, I.: An Introduction to Family Medicine. New York, Oxford University Press, 1981.

Norwood, C.: At Highest Risk: Environmental Hazards to Young and Unborn Children. New York, McGraw-Hill, 1980.

Starfield, B.: Family income, ill health, and medical care of U.S. children. J. Pub. Health Policy, 3:244–259, 1982.

2

COMPLIANCE

Barbara M. Korsch, M.D.

The extent to which patients fail to comply with medical advice has been a surprise to most observers. On the average, one third of medical advice, even when it is perceived and comprehended, is not acted upon by the patient (Fox, 1962; Marston, 1970; Mitchell, 1974). Thus, assuming that medical prescriptions are usually beneficial (an assumption that will not be evaluated critically, but which may also be open to question), it becomes clear that noncompliance is not a trivial problem. In many instances the cost of noncompliance to patient and community is very high in dollars and in pain and suffering. Moreover, there are a significant number of patients who lose their lives unnecessarily because they are unable to or unwilling to follow important medical advice.

Noncompliance is a complex phenomenon influenced by a host of known variables, yet in many respects poorly understood. Explanations for noncompliance have been found in the following categories:

1. Attributes of the patient
2. Attributes of the physician
3. The setting in which the advice is given
4. The characteristics of the illness (diagnosis, seriousness, prognosis)
5. The nature of the medical advice given
6. The doctor-patient relationship
7. Doctor-patient communication

Factors in follow-through on medical advice which have practical implications for the clinician, which are based upon objective evidence, and which may be subject to modification by the aware practitioner are emphasized in the discussion.

ATTRIBUTES OF THE PATIENT

There is an unfortunate but understandable tendency for the practitioner to blame the patient for things that go wrong in the process of medical care. Placing the blame for failure on the patient, while it exonerates the physician, is not very constructive. Occasionally a practitioner may decide appropriately that, since he is unable to elicit any cooperation from a particular patient, there is little value in continuing a nontherapeutic association. More often, by blaming the patient, the physician erects additional barriers to future productive cooperation with a patient for whom he continues to have responsibility.

Demographic Variables. Patients' age, sex, race, and socioeconomic status, especially the educational level (Charney et al., 1967; Davis, 1968a; Deuschle et al., 1960; Gordis et al., 1969; Kegeles, 1969), are only rarely found to be strong determinants in follow-through on medical advice (Caldwell et al., 1970; Glasser, 1958; Kegeles, 1963). Notable exceptions include the finding of poor cooperation with health supervision and preventive health behavior among certain ethnic and lower socioeconomic groups (Becker et al., 1974) and for certain specific treatment regimens. For instance, cooperation with dietary modification in patients at risk for hypertension have been found to be especially difficult to enforce among the poor and otherwise socially deprived (Caldwell et al., 1970; Cassell, 1958).

The female sex is documented to be less compliant than the male especially during adolescence (Gordis et al., 1969). Certain ethnic and religious groups with strongly held health beliefs at variance with modern scientific medicine will fail to comply when the advice is contrary to their convictions.

Contrary to the prejudices expressed by many practitioners, poorly educated patients are not predictably less compliant, unless the patients' reading level or comprehension is inadequate to process the information they are given (Elling et al., 1960; Gordis et al., 1969).

Attempts to correlate specific personality attributes, such as dependency or respect for authority, with compliance have been unconvincing. While patient attributes affect compliance at times, more importantly patient attributes *as perceived by the physician* influence the doctor-patient relationship and therefore have an impact on compliance. As an example, Reader and Pratt showed that physicians underestimated their patient's knowledge of medical information and, consequently, offered less health education than the patient might have wished or understood (Pratt et al., 1957).

ATTRIBUTES OF THE PHYSICIAN

Very few consistent determinants of patient compliance have been documented as due to the attributes of the physician. Many attributes of the physician's approach to the patient, especially his communication style, do have an impact on patient responses, however.

Personality factors in the physician, such as authoritarianism and self-confidence, have not been shown reliably to influence compliance; however, the way in which the patient perceives the physician's personality is very important for the level of patient cooperation (Freeman et al., 1971). Whether the physician seems old or young, competent or unsure, caring or cold have been blamed by patients for causing their lack of motivation to comply with advice. The well-known controversies over the physician's beard, white coat, tie, and conservative clothing vs. blue jeans all seem to relate more to the patient's perceptions and the responses of a particular group of patients than to any objective physician attributes or qualities related to overall compliance.

There has been no documentation that better compliance will be elicited if the physician is more similar to his patient, that is, of the same race, socioeconomic status, sex, etc. However, there may be situations in which it is desirable to have a health-care provider who is socially closer to the patient group he serves, especially from the point of view of access. A striking example of this is the well-known tendency for physicians themselves to be noncompliant with other physician's advice. Although somewhat oversimplified, it can be stated that what the physician does and how he approaches the patient seem far more important in eliciting patient cooperation than *who* he is.

THE SETTING OF MEDICAL CARE

A personal, concerned, quiet, unhurried atmosphere seems to promote doctor-patient communication and patient follow-through (Ley and Spelman, 1965). Continuity of care has also been shown to enhance cooperation (Becker et al., 1974; Charney et al., 1967). Whether a patient will cooperate better if forced to pay for medical service has not been settled. Studies in prepaid medical services tend to show compliance levels similar to those in fee-for-service settings. Access to medical care, ease of obtaining medical treatment, etc., clearly constitute practical determinants of compliance. Nurse practitioners and clinical pharmacists, have been shown to increase patients' compliance, probably because they take time to explain and listen.

CHARACTERISTICS OF THE ILLNESS

Noncompliance has been documented over the entire spectrum of diagnoses, illnesses, and health threats. Patients have interrupted their immunosuppressive treatment following kidney transplantations and have suffered reduced renal function and allograft loss in consequence (Korsch et al., 1978). Other patients ignore advice for trivial or readily treatable disorders. It is not the seriousness of the disease as perceived by the health professional, but the seriousness of the health threat as perceived by the *patient* that determines the likelihood of compliance (Becker et al., 1974; Francis et al., 1969; Gordis et al., 1969). Compliance is also influenced by the patient's perception of the likelihood that a particular treatment will help him (Rosenstock, 1966). Duration of illness, nature of illness, or organ system involved has not been shown to be a significant determinant of compliance (Francis et al., 1969; Lendrum and Kobrin, 1956; MacDonald et al., 1963).

NATURE OF THE MEDICAL ADVICE GIVEN

Medication prescribed once a day is more likely to be taken than that required two or three times daily, and simple prescriptions are more readily accepted than complex ones (Davis and Eichhorn, 1963; Francis et al., 1969; Jenkins, 1954). In some studies, undesirable side effects promote noncompliance (Korsch et al., 1978). In others, misconception about the action of the drugs prescribed has this effect.

The more a particular bit of medical advice impinges upon the patient's daily life style, the less likely it is to be accepted. Whereas specific treatments and medications may be acceptable, modifications in diet, advice to avoid smoking, and advice to change daily activities are the most likely to result in noncompliance (Berkowitz et al., 1963; Davis and Eichhorn, 1963).

THE DOCTOR-PATIENT RELATIONSHIP

It has been shown that continuity of the doctor-patient relationship enhances compliance, and a setting in which continuing comprehensive care is provided by one physician is more likely to result in patient cooperation than care that is episodic or given by a number of different caretakers (Becker et al., 1974). This is true even in group practices where better cooperation was enlisted when the patient saw the particular physician whom he considered his primary physician as compared to another member of the same practice group (Charney et al., 1967). This does not mean that because a patient has known the physician for a long time compliance will necessarily be better.

One study suggests that patients will be more compliant in the setting of a specialty clinic and when treated by a specialist than when seen by a generalist for the same illness (Johnson et al., 1962). It may be that more compliant patients are more likely to be seen by a specialist, and it cannot necessarily be inferred that the specialist's care elicited more consistent compliance.

DOCTOR-PATIENT COMMUNICATION

There is compelling evidence that the communication process very definitely influences patient responses (Becker and Maiman, 1975; Davis, 1968a and b; Francis et al., 1969; Freeman et al., 1971; Korsch et al., 1968; Ley and Spelman, 1965; Marston, 1970). Along with the patient's perceptions of the seriousness of his disease, and his general health beliefs, doctor-patient communication is one of the strongest predictors of patient compliance (Francis et al., 1969). It is not the number of minutes that the physician spends with the patient but the way they are spent that seems to influence outcome. Thus, even under the ever-present time pressures for doctors, there are ways of enhancing effective communication.

Listening to the patient's concerns, not just the chief complaint but also the underlying fears and worries, is probably the single most important thing the practitioner must do in order to gain the patient's cooperation (Korsch et al., 1968). In order to accept the advice offered, the patient must feel that his complaint is fully understood by his doctor. However, we were astonished to find that in our first survey of 800 medical visits by mothers of acutely ill children, there were more than 300 cases in which the mothers felt that the physician never really understood the main concerns for which they were consulting him! Frequently, the mother was not given the opportunity to express her concern, or if she did mention it, the physician failed to acknowledge it, so she still felt poorly understood and dissatisfied.

How, with his busy schedule, can the physician take the time to listen to the patient's concerns? It is reassuring to learn that there is no indication that listening to the patient's concerns prolongs the visit. On the contrary, an early attempt at listening to such concerns often resulted in shorter and more effective communications. Poor communications, in which the patient keeps trying to engage the doctor's interest in his or her problem while the doctor rigidly pursues a more objective, systematic, and technical agenda, are often very time-consuming.

Another effective technique in doctor-patient communication is to elicit the patient's expectations (Korsch et al., 1968). Clearly, when these expectations are unrealistic, the physician should make it clear to the patient that he does understand and accept the patient's anticipations and also explain why they cannot be fulfilled and what will be done instead. Otherwise the patient will assume that the physician failed to meet the patient's expectations because he did not understand and will be dissatisfied and noncompliant (Francis et al., 1969).

It takes but two or three short questions to get to the heart of communicating with the patient, namely getting at his concerns and expectations. Fairly simple, nonthreatening, nonjudgmental questions such as, "What especially were you concerned about when you brought your child to see me today?" "Why did that concern you?" and "What had you hoped we might be able to do for you today?" or "Were there any special things you wanted me to tend to today?" or ". . . explain to you today?" are the type of questions that quickly facilitate effective medical consultation (Korsch et al., 1968).

This approach is also time- and effort-saving. Since physicians often assume that patients have much more global and unrealistic anticipations than are actually the case, they are pleasantly surprised and relieved to find that the patient actually hopes for something that is easy to accomplish. Some patients simply want reassurance that their complaint is not due to some underlying more serious condition or that they are doing a good job in caring for themselves and nothing more needs to be done.

Most patients are more satisfied with a warm, friendly approach from the physician and will cooperate more with an accessible than with an authoritarian or business-like physician. Evidence suggests a strong association between unfriendliness, and critical and judgmental communication from the physician and poor outcome in terms of patient satisfaction and follow-through (Freeman et al., 1971).

Common courtesy is often neglected by health professionals. A surprising number of physicians do not introduce themselves, do not greet the patient, and do not call their patients by name. ("Mother," "honey," or "you there" does not really do the trick.)

Physicians, especially under the pressure of time and where the need for medical intervention seems urgent, tend to concentrate more on the task and less on the relationship with the patient. It has been shown that even a few moments of attention to the patient as a person will pay off in terms of cooperation and will also make the patient feel a great deal better (Freeman et al., 1971).

Patients respond favorably to doctors who offer them information freely, who appear concerned, and who seem supportive rather than judgmental. They are more satisfied when they get a fairly clear statement of diagnosis and etiology, or a clear statement of why such an explanation is not offered or available at that time. They appreciate doctors who listen rather than interrogate. They do better when they are given an opportunity to express their own perceptions of the illness and its severity even when it is at variance with the physician's assumption.

Even though fear arousal or threats are mostly counterproductive, they are perhaps the most widely used communication technique employed by health professionals, especially in situations in which they anticipate or have experienced noncompliance (Janis and Feshbach, 1955; Janis and Terwilliger, 1962). Almost every bit of advice given carries a threat—implicitly or explicitly: "If you don't do what I say, you will get worse, you won't get better, you won't get well, I will be angry and disapprove of you." Raising a moderate amount of anxiety in the patient, especially in situations where appropriate medical action is readily available and can be offered promptly to the patient, probably does promote compliance (Reisinger et al., 1981). However, there is also compelling evidence that escalating anxiety, especially in patients who are already anxious, which includes a high proportion of all patients, causes withdrawal and noncompliance (Hovland et al., 1963; Janis and Feshbach, 1955; Leventhal, 1965).

It is important for the practitioner to be aware of the way in which physician and patient attributes, the patient's diagnosis, and the nature of the advice offered may influence patient responses, specifically compliance. Such an awareness may lead to more astute observations, better assessment of the outcomes of treatment, and more satisfactory explanations for possible treatment failure.

REFERENCES

Becker, M. H., and Maiman, L. A.: Sociobehavioral determinants of compliance with health and medical care recommendations. Med. Care, *13*:10, 1975.

Becker, M. H., Drachman, R. H., and Kirscht, J. P.: A new approach to explaining sick-role behavior in low-income populations. Am. J. Public Health, *64*:205, 1974.

Berkowitz, N. H., et al.: Patient follow-through in outpatient department. Nurs. Res., *12*:16, 1963.

Caldwell, J. R., et al.: The dropout problem in antihypertensive treatment. J. Chron. Dis., *22*:579, 1970.

Cassell, J.: Social and cultural implications of food and food habits. *In* Jaco, E. G. (Ed.): Patients, Physicians, and Illness. Glencoe, Illinois, The Free Press, 1958.

Charney, E., et al.: How well do patients take oral penicillin? A collaborative study in private practice. Pediatrics, *40*:188, 1967.

Davis, M., and Eichhorn, R. L.: Compliance with medical regimens; a panel study. J. Health Hum. Behav., *4*:240, 1963.

Davis, M. S.: Physiologic, psychological and demographic factors in patient compliance with doctors' orders. Med. Care, *6*:115, 1968a.

Davis, M. S.: Variations in patients' compliance with doctors' advice: An empirical analysis of patterns of communication. Am. J. Public Health, *58*:274, 1968b.

Deuschle, K. W., Jordahl, C., and Hobby, G. L.: Clinical usefulness of riboflavin-tagged isoniazid for self-medication in tuberculous patients. Am. Rev. Respir. Dis., *82*:1, 1960.

Elling, R., Whittenmore, R., and Green, M.: Patient participation in a pediatric program. J. Health Hum. Behav., *1*:183, 1960.

Fox, W.: Self-administration of medications: A review of published work and study of problems. Bull. Int. Union Tuberc., *32*:307, 1962.

Francis, V., Korsch, B. M., and Morris, M. J.: Gaps in doctor-patient communication: Patients' response to medical advice. N. Engl. J. Med., *280*:535, 1969.

Freeman, B., Negrete, V. F., Davis, M., and Korsch, B. M.: Gaps in doctor-patient communication: Doctor-patient interaction analysis. Pediatr. Res., *5*:298, 1971.

Glasser, M. A.: Study of the public's acceptance of the Salk vaccine program. Am. J. Public Health, *48*:141, 1958.

Gordis, L., Markowitz, M., and Lilienfeld, A. M.: Why patients don't follow medical advice: A study of children on long-term antistreptococcal prophylaxis. J. Pediatr., *75*:957, 1969.

Hovland, C., Janis, I., and Kelly, H.: Communication and Persuasion. New Haven, Yale University Press, 1963, pp. 67ff.

Janis, I. L., and Feshbach, S.: Effects of fear arousing communication. J. Abnorm. Soc. Psychol., *48*:78, 1955.

Janis, I. L., and Terwilliger, R.: An experimental study of psychological resistance to fear arousing communications. J. Abnorm. Soc. Psychol., *65*:403, 1962.

Jenkins, B. W.: Are patients true to T.I.D. and Q.I.D. doses? GP, *9*:66, 1954.

Johnson, A. J., et al.: Epidemiology of polio vaccine acceptance: A social and psychological analysis. Jacksonville, Fla.: Florida State Board of Health, 1962 (Monograph 3).

Kegeles, S. S.: A field experiment attempt to change beliefs and behavior of women in an urban ghetto. J. Health Soc. Behav., *10*:115, 1969.

Kegeles, S. S.: Why people seek dental care: A test of a conceptual formulation. J. Health Hum. Behav., *4*:166, 1963.

Korsch, B. M., Fine, R. N., and Negrete, V. F.: Noncompliance in children with renal transplants. Pediatrics, *61*:872, 1978.

Korsch, B. M., Gozzi, E. K., and Francis, V.: Gaps in doctor-patient communication. 1. Doctor-patient interaction and patient satisfaction. Pediatrics, *42*:855, 1968.

Lendrum, B., and Kobrin, C.: Prevention of recurrent attacks of rheumatic fever; problems revealed by long-term follow-up. J.A.M.A., *162*:13, 1956.

Leventhal, H.: Fear communications in the acceptance of preventive health practices. Bull. N.Y. Acad. Med., *41*:1144, 1965.

Ley, P., and Spelman, M. S.: Communication in an outpatient setting. Br. J. Soc. Clin. Psychol., *4*:115, 1965.

MacDonald, M. E., et al.: Social factors in relation to

participation in follow-up care of rheumatic fever. J. Pediatr., *62*:503, 1963.

Marston, M. V.: Compliance with medical regimens: A review of the literature. Nurs. Res., *19*:312, 1970.

Mitchell, J. H.: Compliance with medical regimens: An annotated bibliography. Health Educ. Monogr., *2*:75, 1974.

Pratt, C., Seligman, A., and Reader, G.: Physicians' views on the level of medical information among patients. Am. J. Public Health, *47*:1277, 1957.

Reisinger, K. S., et al.: Effects of pediatricians' counseling on infant restraint use. Pediatrics, *67*:201, 1981.

Rosenstock, I. M.: Why people use health services. Milbank Mem. Fund Q., *44*:94, 1966.

3

PROVIDING HEALTH SERVICES TO THE UNDERSERVED

Margaret C. Heagarty, M.D.

Pediatrics is characterized by a common set of assumptions about children: (1) every child is important, the child from the middle class suburban family being no more or no less important than the child from a low income family in an urban ghetto; (2) all children have an intrinsic right to a protective and nurturing environment, to the food, shelter, clothing, and education necessary to have a fair chance to reach their full potential; (3) all children, no matter what their social or economic status or where they live, have a right to humane and civilized medical care; and (4) all pediatricians have a special obligation to serve as protectors and advocates of children, individually and collectively. All pediatricians at one time or another care for these underserved children in the clinics of urban hospitals, in public health department well child clinics, in emergency rooms of community hospitals, or in their offices.

HEALTH CARE FOR THE UNDERSERVED CHILD

To some extent the provision of medical care for the child from an underserved group will differ in its content and focus from that provided to a more advantaged child. Available information makes clear that the underserved or disadvantaged child is at higher risk for certain diseases and conditions. The pediatrician confronted with such a child must have an agenda that includes a recognition of these health risks.

At the outset, and perhaps most importantly, the underserved child is much more likely to begin life at a significant disadvantage (Egbuono and Starfield, 1982). Prematurity, defined as low birth weight (less than 2500 grams), is more common in disadvantaged groups. Since prematurity has long been associated with an increased incidence of major and minor central nervous system defects, one must be sensitive to the possibility that any disadvantaged child, especially one with a low birth weight, may suffer from a range of central nervous system deficits, which include moderate to mild mental retardation, specific learning disabilities, and vision or hearing problems. In addition to the increased incidence of these chronic conditions, disadvantaged children are also more vulnerable to certain acute diseases. Lead poisoning, iron-deficiency anemia, rheumatic fever, purulent otitis media, *Hemophilus influenzae* meningitis, gastroenteritis, and parasitic infections have all been reported as more common in disadvantaged children.

The delivery of medical care is based upon a transaction between a physician and a patient, upon the development of a working relationship or contract between the professional and the afflicted. It is this aspect of the delivery of health services for the underserved which presents the pediatrician with the greatest challenge. Since pediatricians tend to come from middle or upper class families, they cannot use their own life experiences to understand the life stresses of disadvantaged children and parents; therefore, the pediatrician must, as a first step, admit the presence of the experiential distance between himself and the disadvantaged child and parent.

Second, the pediatrician committed to providing effective care for the underserved must invest some time in an investigation of the life styles, customs, norms, problems, and concerns of this group of children and their parents. Those who listen carefully to their disadvantaged patients and their parents can learn a great deal about their lives and problems. The novels and plays written by those who have emerged from this group also offer insights into the lives of the underserved. Indeed, Dicken's description of London slum children in the mid-nineteenth century remains germane to an understanding of the contemporary child living in similar areas of this country. Within the past decade, several studies by psychiatrists and cultural anthropologists provide fascinating and useful information about the lives of disadvantaged children and their families (Coles, 1964, 1967, 1971; Lewis, 1965).

Confronted by underserved children with major social and/or environmental problems, the practicing pediatrician may be tempted to try to change that environment; however, the limitations of any one practitioner's ability to change the life situation of the underserved child must be recognized. Failure to accept such realities leads to frustration, anger, and fatigue, which too often turn into eventual abandonment of efforts to serve such children and families. The pediatrician must achieve realistic and modest appreciation of his role in the life of any patient. Without it, the pediatrician will not achieve a sense of the delicate balance between the possible and the impossible which will allow him to help the underserved cope with or change their situation.

HEALTH CARE PROGRAMS FOR THE UNDERSERVED CHILD

For some pediatricians the frustrations of trying to provide direct services for underserved children cause them to become involved in the development of programs specifically designed to serve this population. Characteristically, personal health services for underserved children are fragmented, episodic, crisis-oriented, and underfinanced. Disadvantaged children traditionally receive pediatric care in hospital emergency rooms and clinics, in health department well child clinics, and in school health programs. Coordination of clinical care among these various sites, usually sponsored by separate agencies, is virtually impossible. More importantly, the disadvantaged child and family are denied the opportunity to establish a relationship with a single physician who assumes responsibility and accountability for the child's health.

In the past 20 years a variety of government-financed programs have been developed to provide coordinated and comprehensive health services for disadvantaged children (Davis and Schoen, 1978). The Medicaid program, enacted in 1965, is the largest government health program for the disadvantaged. Whatever its failures, there is, at this time, sufficient evidence to conclude that this federal-state program has removed financial barriers to and thus has increased access to medical care for a significant proportion of disadvantaged children. In 1964, the year prior to the passage of the Medicaid legislation, poor children on the average saw a physician 2.7 times each year, compared to 3.8 visits for all children annually. By 1974, disadvantaged children had on the average as many visits to a physician as children from high-income families. Although there has been considerable public debate over the cost of the Medicaid program, in 1975 the average annual payment for services for children enrolled in the program was slightly lower than that for all other children in this country. While Medicaid has provided some financial underpinning to the provision of health services to the underserved, it has not, in itself, changed the structure of the health care system for this population. Indeed, in some areas Medicaid's low reimbursement rates for the pediatrician in private practice has discouraged the entry of disadvantaged children into the private sector of the health care delivery system and has perpetuated the fragmented system.

In addition to Medicaid, other programs for disadvantaged children were developed and funded as part of the social legislation of the sixties, e.g., neighborhood health, children and youth, and maternal and infant care programs. All of these programs were based on the premise that the delivery of continuous primary care by an identified physician would improve the health status of disadvantaged children. The existing evaluations of these primary care programs for the disadvantaged suggest that they have been successful in reducing infant mortality rates, reducing morbidity rates for certain diseases, increasing immunization rates, reducing hospitalization and emergency room use, and reducing the cost of care for the population they serve.

"I've been rich and I've been poor. Rich is better." Any pediatrician tempted to try to develop health programs for underserved children must thoroughly understand this simple precept. The health care programs developed in the 1960s and 1970s reached, at best, a minority of disadvantaged children. In times of economic recession and dislocation, health programs for these children are in constant jeopardy.

The pediatrician who seeks to develop or maintain health care programs for underserved children must bring to the task a set of traits and skills not learned in medical school or residency training. First, the pediatrician must be extraordinarily persistent, that is, absolutely determined to do what is required to ensure that these children receive adequate health care. Anything less than iron resolve will melt quickly in the fire of general disinterest and/or active opposition. But such determination must be tempered with enough flexibility to make accurate judgments about what is possible at any one time. A sense of humor, the brother of flexibility, is also a useful if not essential strength. There must be a fair tolerance for ambiguity and for risk taking. In short, the development of programs for disadvantaged children is never a tidy process. Most such programs are put together with the proverbial cellophane tape and bailing wire; many, if not most, lead a hand-to-mouth existence.

Such a pediatrician must also develop political skills. Since the underserved patients themselves are relatively powerless and since the pediatrician is not likely to have personal power, he must be able to analyze where he can find allies in the community who possess or have access to the power required to supply the resources needed for the health care program. The astute pediatrician can find these allies in local business, in politicians running for office, and in middle class service organizations looking for a cause to support.

Finally, the pediatrician must develop the general organizational skills necessary to recruit and develop personnel for the program, to establish patterns for the care delivered, and to develop the information systems necessary for its evaluation. In the enthusiasm required to establish a new health care program, time for and consideration of the need for evaluation is often overlooked. Since programs for the underserved are always under critical if not hostile scrutiny, careful attention to the development of data systems designed to establish the value of the program is essential. Without quantitative data showing that the program has made a difference and is less costly than alternatives, the pediatrician in a program for the underserved will find himself or herself without an adequate defense when the inevitable attack on the program begins.

While this description of a model pediatrician working in programs for the underserved suggests the need for the virtues and vices of Francis of Assisi, Machiavelli, and Theodore Roosevelt, in fact, there are many pediatricians in this country who have successfully devised new programs for the care of underserved children (Parker et al., 1976; San Agustin et al., 1976).

HEALTH POLICY FOR THE UNDERSERVED

The dictionary defines "policy" as "a definite course or method chosen from among alternatives and in light of given conditions to guide and determine present and future decisions." While an extended description of the health policy apparatus at the local, regional, or national level exceeds the boundaries of this chapter, no discussion of health services for the underserved would be complete without a comment on this aspect of the issue.

In general, policy decisions are made in this country in small incremental steps which reflect the opinions and desires of its citizens as interpreted by those given the power by the public to make those decisions. It is a complex process in which small bits of information or misinformation can often make large differences in the outcome of the decision. Fortunately, perhaps, it is also an extremely human process in which personal influence and persuasion can, at times, sway the decision. The intervention of an individual at the right time and place can make an enormous difference.

Pediatricians, like all physicians, are accorded high status by society. With that privilege come the duty and the opportunity to participate in making the community's policy decisions. The pediatrician in his office talking with the wife of a local legislator, the pediatrician at a local PTA meeting, and the pediatrician testifying before Congress all have opportunities to inform and when necessary persuade the public and its representatives about the needs of disadvantaged children.

REFERENCES

Coles, R.: Children of Crisis. A Study of Courage and Fear. Boston, Little, Brown and Company, 1964.

Coles, R.: Migrants, Sharecroppers, Mountaineers. Volume II of Children of Crisis. Boston, Little, Brown and Company, 1967.

Coles, R.: The South Goes North. Volume III of Children of Crisis. Boston, Little, Brown and Company, 1971.

Davis, K., and Schoen, C.: Health and the War on Poverty: A Ten Year Apprasial. Washington, D.C., The Brookings Institution, 1978.

Egbuonu, L., and Starfield, B.: Child health and social status. Pediatrics, *69*:550–557, 1982.

Lewis, O.: La Vida. A Puerto Rican Family in the Culture of Poverty. New York, Random House, 1965.

Porter, P. J., et al.: Municipal child health services. A ten year reorganization. Pediatrics, *58*:704–712, 1976.

San Agustin, M., et al.: Reorganization of ambulatory health care in an urban municipal hospital. Arch. Intern. Med., *136*:1262–1266, 1976.

SECTION II

HEALTH PROMOTION

Health promotion, a term that encompasses active prevention of disease as well as maintenance of health, has been chosen as the most appropriate title for this section. *Health maintenance* implies a more static situation than exists in childhood, while *preventive pediatrics* is too limiting. But whatever name is used, the activities covered in this section are those in which the pediatrician today spends from one third to one half of his time.

The first step in health promotion is to know the diseases and impairments one wants to prevent. In the past, and even today in some parts of the world, half the live-born children die by five years of age. In these situations, illnesses likely to result in death are the main concern of medicine. But today in the United States less than one in 500 children will die during childhood, once the newborn period is safely passed. This marked reduction in childhood mortality during the last century makes it more important and possible to concentrate our efforts on those illnesses, disabilities, and discomforts which, while not likely to result in death, do have the capacity to cause considerable suffering and dysfunction.

In the past, medical care was mainly for the purpose of making suffering less intense. Only in the last century, with the rise of scientific medicine, has medical care been thought to improve health. Today, this attitude has mushroomed to the point where poor health is thought by many, and in our view, largely erroneously, to be due entirely to poor or absent medical care. Society's expectations of medical care have been too limited in the past and are too expansive in the present. Many factors, apart from health care, contribute significantly to health: housing, nutrition, environment, heredity, stress, and health habits. Much of the clinician's work in health promotion is to educate children and their families about the multiple causes of illness, the importance of healthy life styles, and the limitations of curative medicine.

Prevention of adult illness starts in childhood. Childhood should be an entryway to healthy adult life. The goal of pediatrics is to keep an individual healthy during his adult life as well as during childhood. Therefore, the pediatrician should be well aware of the major health problems in adult life. Four conditions—heart disease, cancer, stroke, and accidents—make up 70 per cent of all deaths among American adults. Heart disease, arthritis, rheumatism, back and hip problems, mental and nervous disorders, and hypertension are responsible for 40 per cent of all nonfatal adult disability. Behavior problems, school and job failure, marital discord, unwanted pregnancies, venereal disease, and violence are major causes of dysfunction in adolescents and adults. The pediatrician should, therefore, give high priority to what can be done during childhood to prevent these conditions.

The major factors contributing to some of them have been reasonably well defined: for cardiovascular disease—overnutrition (especially fat and cholesterol), hypertension, cigarette smoking, and low physical activity; for cancer—excessive tobacco use and nutritional deficiencies and excesses; and for highway accidents—alcoholism, drug abuse, impulsive personality, and poor highway and automobile designs.

Many of these factors are habits that have

their origin in childhood. Several nonfatal, but prevalent, problems of adults also have their origin in childhood, such as obesity (which is correlated with several ills of adult life). Our success in educating children to prevent such problems has not been clearly demonstrated, but this is an exciting frontier for the child health clinician.

The risk of adult disease is also due, in part, to heredity. In the future, the identification of individuals who have a genetic risk of disease, especially with exposure to certain environmental hazards, will be the major task of pediatrics. For example, if we could identify the individual at high risk for cancer of the lung from among those not at high risk, it is likely that the high-risk group could be persuaded not too smoke with greater success than the efforts of present nondiscriminating antismoking programs that are aimed at everyone.

The role and effectiveness of the personal physician in preventing these problems in adult life are obviously limited, but education should start during childhood and be reinforced whenever possible. For the effective control of many of these problems, we may have to accept a certain amount of external control, such as enforcement of drunken driving and automobile and highway safety laws in order to prevent disability and death. It seems likely that a combination of education and legislation will be most successful in changing unhealthy lifestyles.

These are but a few of the childhood events that have consequences on health years later, long after the individual is no longer a patient of the pediatrician. A much longer time frame is therefore necessary for today's child health physician than only the first 21 years of life. "We can no longer divide life into segments, such as fetal, neonatal, childhood, adulthood, and senescence. Rather, it is a dynamic equilibrium with the status at any one time being influenced by all that went before and, in turn, having an effect on all that follows" (Robbins, 1982). The task is to accomplish those things during childhood that promote and maintain health throughout life. This is more difficult in conditions with a long time lag between the cause and effect than with proven preventive services such as polio or measles vaccination, which can be more directly and simply demonstrated to be effective to physicians and parents alike. Because success of many of today's health promotion services, aimed as they are at the health problems our patients develop once they become adults, is not so immediately apparent to the child or his parents, our preventive goals are more difficult to achieve.

Even as we stress these difficult-to-achieve and not-yet-proven services, we must also remember that short-term goals such as immunizations, although much easier to achieve, are too often not fully accomplished for many children. In the pursuit of long-term goals, the proven short-term ones cannot be neglected.

HEALTH PROMOTION SERVICES

In the United States around the turn of the century, preventive services were separate from curative services—a practice still followed in much of the world today. Health departments provided well child care, while illness was cared for by the general practitioner or in the hospital. In the past 50 years in the United States, curative services have been joined to preventive for the private patient, while for the poor they remained largely separate until the 1960s, when neighborhood health centers, child and youth programs, and other comprehensive health programs were developed.

There is much to be said for integration of curative and preventive services on an individual basis, but there are also problems. In a system that is not population-based, no one knows who is missed, whereas preventive services separately organized by geographical area allow personnel to develop outreach programs for those who do not voluntarily use the services. As is so often the case, there are trade-offs in each system. No one arrangement maximizes every attribute.

In this section we are assuming that one clinician, or his team, provides to a known group of children both curative and preventive services in the same location. In the chapter on school health, however, there is also emphasis upon how the child health clinician can work in a school setting to promote health.

A list of patients registered with a practice, with a simple recording system of immunizations and screening tests completed, is useful to determine who in this defined population has not received preventive services, to identify the high-risk or vulnerable patient for special attention, and to initiate contact with these patients. Concern over unethical pursuit of patients should not be a deterrent. Regular reminders of the need for dental prophylaxis are a long-established part of dental practice, and most families are very grateful for the interest expressed in their child by such "patient pursuit."

We believe that, in the future, one of the functions of a health department will be to identify who is not getting care in the entire population and to encourage them to do so. This would remove the onus from the individual clinician who might otherwise be accused of "chasing" patients. As mentioned, however, this is rarely perceived as a problem by families.

GENERAL PRINCIPLES

The major thrust of child health care is the development of potential by determination and reduction of vulnerabilities and the wise use of strengths of children and their families. We believe with Miller et al. (1974) that "the central question for medicine today is how to make the prevention of disease as professionally satisfying as its treatment."

Health assessment and prospective evaluations in children differ from those in adults in the following ways: (1) In adults, because so much potential has already been used up, the goals for prevention have to be more short-term than in children, and many potential options for prevention have been closed by the passage of time. (2) Health appraisals and prospective pediatric evaluations of a child require that this be coupled or paired with some assessment of the parents, who are at a much different developmental level.

Good physical health is not necessarily the highest value for children or, to put it another way, the price of physical health may be too high in some instances. For example, obsessive attention to what is perceived as nutritious diet, or attempted avoidance of all infections or all risk-taking behavior may diminish some of the zest or fun of life—an equally important goal. Balance, as in most things in life, should be the goal. The clinician, the family, and the child when old enough should discuss their health goals. These will vary from family to family and physician to physician. It is wise for the clinician to determine what values and expectations each family has and to develop a "contract"(not necessarily written) with them regarding what they consider to be the proper balance for them. He should avoid pressing his own beliefs upon his patients.

We are impressed by the self-corrective resources of children, believing that more harm than good has often been done by active treatment of such normal variations in the process of growth as bowlegs and preschool dependency. We prefer to be available to help while restraining our impulses to jump in too soon.

Humility should be practiced. We have to recognize the great limitations in our knowledge about how to guide a child to health. Compared with all the other forces in society, clinicians have relatively few options available to maintain and promote health. This is partly because of unchangeable biological factors, partly from lack of knowledge of what works, and partly because of the enormously powerful social forces outside of health care. Credibility demands that we not claim more than we can deliver.

Physical and psychological health are equally important. Today more effort is expended by many pediatricians in counseling about behavior, development, play, school, television, and sex education than in treating physical illness. This is as it should be, since these are the major problems of children today. Since anything that interferes with the physical or mental well-being of a child is of concern to the physician, he and his nonphysician colleagues should be skilled in helping (or know where the child can obtain necessary help), while acknowledging that there is not yet much evidence of how to accomplish these tasks with optimal success. The physician should not try to deal with these problems alone. However, a study from Australia suggests that the interested and experienced clinician can prevent behavior problems by conducting short counseling sessions of 20 to 30 minutes twice a year during the preschool years. In this controlled study, the experimental group of children had fewer fears, sleep disturbances, and eating problems, and less aggression (Collen, 1976).

Development of constructive doctor-patient relations is a major goal of routine visits, for such relations are the primary tool used for diagnosis and management of children's problems, whether they be physical or psychosocial. Continuity and coordination of care, as well as availability during acute illness, will help to develop such a relationship.

Health promotion visits should build self-esteem of parents and child by honest praise and reassurance. Parents want and need attention, recognition, and interest for themselves as well as their children. They do better with praise and develop greater ego strength.

Depression and other emotional problems in parents and their children are common. These problems should be looked for by the pediatrician because children are often the "ticket of admission" to medical services for such disturbed parents. There are individual differences in children's temperaments, and parents are helped by understanding this.

Any therapy of change in family life style, at least for younger children, has to be achieved largely through the parents, not the physician.

Therefore, understanding of the mother's and father's feelings, background values, and wishes is essential to the success of most interventions by clinicians.

Children need to be educated to take more responsibility for their own health and to learn to use health services appropriately. Each visit is an opportunity to teach attitudes of self-help, to diminish dependency, and to foster rational use of health services. Experiments with children as young as six to eight years initiating their own visits to the clinician and with parents and children being given a copy of the full medical record are new ways that some clinicians have found useful to promote more patient responsibility in health care.

Payment for health promotion services is a central issue in determining how services are delivered. Such services need to become barrier-free at the time of their use, although we recognize that in this situation there will be a few who will overuse the services when we think they are unnecessary. In the Canadian experience with a national health service, this group is only about 1 per cent of the population. Since fees, or even co-payments at the time of service, have been shown to reduce use, especially for preventive services, a system of no fee at the time of such services seems a worthwhile trade-off for children's services in order to achieve needed access to the 15 to 20 per cent who now do not use preventive services because of fees.

We believe that "packages" of preventive care would be a helpful way to organize prepayment. A "basic" package might consist of those precedures proven to be useful, e.g., immunizations and certain screening programs. Some "enriched" packages consisting of procedures thought prudent, but not yet proven, could then be purchased by families, groups, or insurers if they wished. We should discourage procedures deemed of questionable or no value (Better Health, 1981).

Special studies should be designed to evaluate new procedures or those of questioned value. Most pediatricians will want to ensure that their patients receive both proven and prudent services. We have to make choices because of limited resources, and first priority must be given to ensuring that all children receive the "proven" procedures, rather than having some get all services (including those of questionable value) while others receive none.

We feel less secure about recommending financially barrier-free services for all illness care than for preventive services, because it can be occasionally abused by both doctor and patient. However, experience has shown that children are not excessive users of illness services, even when these services are made easily accessible at time of use. We must recognize that a minority of the population uses disproportionately large amounts of service, but not necessarily needlessly. In one study, 15 per cent of children used 50 per cent of the services. In our own studies (Robertson et al., 1974), however, making preventive services readily available resulted in a decrease in illness visits, as well as hospital and laboratory services, a worthwhile trade-off in our opinion.

In addition to financing of services, many other organizational factors determine the services given. Clinicians need to analyze the organization of their practice and their own personality and style and try to evaluate the effect it has on their efforts in health promotion.

There is no single package of care suitable to all children. While we will outline schedules for the frequency of visits at different ages and procedures to be done, these should be used only as guides to be modified on the basis of need. A first child born prematurely to an unwed teenager has need for much more service than the second child born at term to an intact family who has successfully reared their first child. Screening should seek only problems not previously known and for which efficacious treatment is available.

Prospective pediatrics should prepare the child and family both for certainty, e.g., developmental landmarks, and for uncertainty, e.g., crises and other stresses.

The pediatric clinician is person-oriented as well as problem-oriented. The pediatric clinician "cones" down on persons (children and families) rather than problems alone and assesses strengths and invulnerability resources as well as vulnerabilities and illnesses.

Health promotion for children is straightforward but difficult to achieve for all children. Such a "basic" package has been well described:

> Their mothers need a good diet during pregnancy and simple but adequate prenatal and obstetric care; children need a minimum but adequate diet—preferably human milk in the early months of life—with careful attention to their nutritional needs in the weaning and post-weaning period. They need a reasonably clean environment with plenty of clean water; they need basic immunizations against the common contagious diseases of childhood, and these must be administered properly with potent vaccines; they need simple but prompt, inexpensive and easily accessible treatment when they are ill, and the

realistic possibility of rapid referral to more sophisticated facilities and personnel when necessary. They need a family that is warm and loving, and it helps if the family enjoys at least minimal economic security. They are better off if the family is small, with a generous time interval between the children (Wray, 1975).

To this we would add that children need a continuing relationship with a health care clinician who has the ability to form a bond with parent and child, and a society that seeks to promote health.

Children present quite different problems and require different health promotion approaches at different ages. This developmental approach is one of the key differences between pediatrics and other branches of medicine. Consequently, this section is divided into traditional age groups for the convenience of the practitioner. Summary tables are included to cue the clinician when to do certain tasks.

Certain guiding principles to health promotion cut across age and stage needs. Information should be obtained about three levels of social organization—the child, the family, and the community of environment. For each of these three areas, four types of information should be sought—strengths, resources, vulnerabilities, illnesses. A final section discusses actions taken for each of the three social units. This need not be completed at each visit but can serve as a summary to be completed periodically.

SOCIAL AND BEHAVIOR FACTORS IN FUNCTION

The longitudinal study of children in Kauai (Werner, 1981), as well as several other studies completed in the past decade, has demonstrated the importance of behavior problems. One of every three youngsters in childhood, and one of every five in adolescence, developed serious behavior or learning problems. *Combinations* of social, biological, and psychological variables are the *best* predictors of later problems, emphasizing the need for a holistic health appraisal. Significantly, however, in the Kauai study, one of three high-risk children did not develop significant problems. The characteristics of these resilient children are especially important to the child health clinician. Clearly, biological differences are important: such resilient children are active, good-natured, and easy to deal with from the beginning, emphasizing the need to assess temperament. Later, other personality differences are apparent among the resilient children. They have a more positive self-concept and internal locus of control. Children who do well generally come from smaller families (four or fewer children) and have two years or greater spacing between children, have alternative caretakers and sources of support for the family in times of trouble, and have structure and rules during adolescence. Peers, friends, and elders, in addition to parents, are important contacts for resilient youth. Clinicians often wonder how they can help to change families without these characteristics. It is admittedly difficult, but referral to social agencies, including family walk-in centers (Pillai et al., 1982), have been demonstrated to be effective in preventing some forms of family disorganization, such as child abuse. In many situations, it makes more sense to strengthen available kinship and neighborhood ties than to introduce additional services.

THE CONTENT OF THE WELL CHILD VISIT

It is useful to think of preventive services at different levels: the first consists of efforts to promote health (i.e., diet, counseling, teaching healthy life styles); the second consists of specific preventive measures such as immunizations; level three is the detection of asymptomatic disease by such screening tests as vision, hearing, phenylketonuria, and tuberculin testing. Although generally not considered preventive services, level four (the early detection and treatment of symptomatic acute illness to prevent complications) and level five (the prevention of disability in chronic disease) complete the spectrum.

At each health promotion visit of a well child, tasks from the first three stages will be performed: health promotion, specific prevention, and screening to detect asymptomatic illness. To accomplish these services, a few simple tasks are indicated at each visit.

History. The history should include the following inquiries: Have there been any illnesses or injuries since the last visit? Have any concerns or problems developed? What about problems in the family or community?

Health Appraisal. Physical examination is generally limited to growth and development such as height (plus head circumference in infants) and weight, and to organ systems specifically vulnerable in each child. While a full physical examination at each visit has been shown to yield few new diagnoses once the initial complete evaluation has been made, it is reassuring to parents and child alike. Screening tests may be performed at this time.

Anticipatory Guidance. This procedure should include discussion of expected development with health implications (e.g., normal decrease in growth and appetite around one year of age, with consequent decrease in expectation of intake).

Counseling. The physician should pose questions about problems brought up or discovered since the last visit. Genetic counseling about possible future children and biological vulnerabilities is an important new area for the properly prepared child health clinician.

At first it is difficult for some physicians to find the right phrase to initiate the interview for health visits, for there is no chief complaint. A few openers we find useful are: "How have things been going?" "How is Johnny/Jane?" Sometime during opening remarks it is helpful to turn to the mother and ask, "How are *you* feeling?" With experience and expectant pauses, a far richer flow of significant information follows such open-ended queries than can be elicited with a barrage of specific questions. It is usually necessary during the course of the visit to supplement these general questions with more specific ones regarding diet, sleep, exercise, elimination, and especially specific questions on development. But it is more effective and efficient to determine first the areas that bother the mother or child rather than to compulsively go through a list of questions, only to neglect and not have sufficient time to obtain the content and feeling that come with spontaneous questions.

Many find that a review of systems and specific screening tests and procedures are best done by the nonphysician staff. With the development of skillful pediatric nurse practitioners in the last decade, the question of how much of the health promotion visit is to be done by the physician and how much by the nurse practitioner will vary in different practices. Several studies have demonstrated that nurse practitioners can do nearly all of the well child visit (as well as much of an illness visit).

Screening. Screening deserves special mention. Screening is performing some test in asymptomatic people to rule in or out illness. We prefer the term "health assessment," since it includes measurement of health status, function, resilience, resources, and strengths. Such assessment can best be done over time by a health professional who has an ongoing relationship with a patient, whereas screening has assumed, although it is not necessarily so, a mass procedure in such places as newborn nurseries, schools, or workplaces.

The site and relation to an ongoing provider make a major difference as to what is an effective assessment procedure. For instance, in the chapter on school health, screening for scoliosis in schools is questioned because of large numbers of over-referrals, lack of knowledge about the natural history of mild scoliosis so detected, and the high cost. This situation is quite different in the clinician's office. Here an ongoing relation means that a minimal deviation from normal can often be followed before referral, and any specific screening test is only one among many done in the course of a health promotion visit. Such differences in setting make universal recommendations on screening tests inappropriate.

There are, however, several general conditions that should be present before one uses a screening test or assesses a particular aspect of a patient.

1. The potential problem must be important—either of fairly high frequency (visual problems) or great severity even if infrequent (hypothyroidism).
2. There must be agreed-upon criteria for diagnosis of the condition.
3. The potential problem being assessed must be more effectively treated in the asymptomatic phase, and there must be effective treatment.
4. There must be treatment facilities available, and some connection between screening program and treatment facility to ensure referral and follow-up.
5. The cost must be known and acceptable, i.e., generally cost-effective treatment.
6. Parental consent must be obtained.

No discussion of screening can avoid using the concepts of sensitivity, specificity, and predictive positives. The ideal test, which would have 100 per cent sensitivity and specificity, does not exist. In general, we seek high sensitivity (ability to detect *all* who have the problem) without sacrificing too much specificity (ability to detect *only* those with the problem). We do not want to miss positives. But if false positives are too high, the cost of referral and follow-up (anxiety costs as well as dollars) make the test less useful (the situation with scoliosis screening). With rare diseases, even high specificity will result in a large number of over-referrals. A 1 per cent error (if 99 per cent specificity—a rare phenomenon) with disease with a 1/3000 prevalence will result in only 3 per cent of patients with positive tests actually turning out to have the disease (predictive positive).

The concept of proven and prudent packages (Breslow and Somers, 1977) of preventive services holds especially well for screening procedures. A British working party determined that the only proven screening tests were hematocrit for iron-deficiency anemia, a tuberculin test, and, for adults, Rh determination in pregnant women and a urine sugar test. Clearly, in practice, a prudent approach would include more than this very parsimonious list, but it does make us pause in our sometimes overenthusiastic promotion of screening tests.

In pediatrics, most physical problems have low frequencies. Hearing and visual problems and asthma are the only ones present in more than one in every one hundred children. This is quite different than in adults. But developmental and behavioral problems are present, as noted, in as many as one in five children. For most of these conditions, there is no simple test available, although the development of the Denver Development Screening Test is a major attempt to develop a standard assessment procedure. More research is necessary to determine reliable methods to accurately assess development within the practical realities of the limited time available in practice. Recently efforts have been made to assess development at the time of testing of other procedures, such as the reaction of the child to vision screening as a measure of developmental status (Sturner et al., 1980). At the other extreme, a complex assessment instrument has been developed to determine children at high risk of academic failure or behavior problems during school (Levine and Schneider, 1982). This test, the PEER (Pediatric Examination of Educational Readiness), has been shown to be reliable and predictive, but whether it is practical in office practice is not clear. Tools to assess development, vulnerabilities, strengths, and resources are needed in pediatric practice. In the meantime, history will have to suffice for many of these areas. Specific screening tests for the various age groups are discussed in subsequent chapters.

USE OF GROWTH CHARTS

The plotting of simple growth on some standard chart has become a standard screening test in health promotion. Whether it meets all the criteria above is now questioned, but we still advocate its use as an effective way to educate parents (and later the child) concerning normal growth. There are several variations of growth charts available. Clinicians should become familiar with one standard form and use it consistently. Needless to say, measurements should be made accurately and plotted carefully. Data from the large-scale Health Examination Survey now provide growth charts based upon large numbers of children from a broad socioeconomic range, and cover the teen-age years (Hamill et al., 1976).

Single measurements at any point in time are not helpful unless they are exceedingly deviant or unless there is marked discrepancy between height, weight, or head circumference percentiles. Much more important are the repeated measurement and recording of such data. Children do not follow "channels" (stay at one percentile over long periods of time), but they are generally reasonably consistent from month to month (in infancy) and year to year (in older children). When a marked change occurs (two or more percentile lines, e.g., from 90th to 50th), some explanation must be sought.

PATIENT AND PARENT EDUCATION

Part of the clinician's job is to teach parents and children to lead healthy lives. Health education is being given increasing emphasis as we recognize the importance of health habits to health and the limitations of curative medicine on many health problems. Most child health clinicians already spend a large part of their time teaching their patients health habits. The question is, how effective is this teaching and how can it be improved?

It is clear from the few carefully conducted studies that telling people what to do to lead healthier lives is not very effective. Even if knowledge is transmitted, behavior is rarely changed. But there is a new enthusiasm being generated that better results can be achieved with new methods of health education. The clinician is not the only one to teach health. Indeed, the importance of reinforcing health education through many channels is now recognized to be a key point. Several principles of successful behavior change are now recognized (Haggerty, 1977).

Use of Clinical Setting

Patient education by the child's personal clinician is more likely to result in behavior change than traditional health education in schools. The clinical setting is an especially good place to teach healthy behavior because patients are more highly motivated then.

In one study, pediatricians were quite successful in influencing their patients to use seat belts (Bass and Wilson, 1964). The power of a respected personal physician and doctor-patient relationship should not be minimized. Many pediatricians use printed material, posters in the office, and slide shows in the waiting room, as well as one-to-one teaching, to help patients to learn health habits, but most such efforts have not been as carefully evaluated as the Bass and Wilson study. The condition of being a patient seems more likely to be associated with motivation and to result in behavior change than does passive learning by nonpatients in other settings, and this fact should be utilized. The developmental approach also is essential, with the presentation tailored to the age and stage of the child and family. For example, children under the age of 7 to 10 years have difficulty with logical concepts (Bibace and Walsh, 1980). Such an optimistic view of the potential of health education does not diminish the reality that most encounters in pediatric practice are too short to effect behavior change (Reisinger et al., 1980). With other personnel doing much of the education, better reimbursement, and adherence to proven methods, we remain optimistic that the future of health education is bright.

Active Learning

Active learning is far more effective than passive. Studies during World War II demonstrated that behavior changes in diet were more likely when people learned diet changes for themselves and publicly affirmed their intention to change their diet than when they merely listened to a lecture. This principle of the need for active learning has been understood but rarely used in clinical practice.

Discovery learning in schools (projects in which children actively discover the relationship between health practices and health) and self-help movements (as seen in the many health books—*Our Bodies, Our Selves; The Well Body Book; Take Care of Yourself;* and of course the well-accepted Spock book, *Baby and Child Care*) have shown the great interest most people have in health.

In the past, physicians have often generated too great a dependence on themselves and discouraged active, responsible roles for their patients. The practice of giving patients their own records (or at least a problem list and medication and immunization records) has become increasingly common as one way to stimulate an active role in health by the patient. Other studies have shown that people changed their health habits more when they taught others than when they were passive recipients of health education.

A recent program in which elementary school children were given the right to seek health care in a school when they wanted to, rather than only when their parents so decided, was shown to help children develop a sense of self-control and responsibility which seems to be essential for the development of healthy life styles. Parents and children need to develop more independence and more security and skill in their own ability to manage common illnesses and carry out preventive measures, if health education is to be successful. Other active learning can be accomplished by role-playing in psychodrama exercises and peer counseling in school.

Table 1. HEALTH HABITS

Recommended Behavior
Nutrition
Caloric balance between intake and output, end result to be not more than 10 per cent over or under mean weight for height. Start in childhood to prevent early obesity.
Content balance: at least minimal vitamins, fat, carbohydrates, protein. Protein content to shift more to plant than animal sources.
Physical Exercise
Maintenance of caloric balance and vigorous muscular activity.
*Accident Prevention Behavior
Seat belt use, safe driving, elimination of household poisons (or safe storage), fire precautions at home, firearm control, etc.
*Smoking Control
*Alcohol Consumption: moderate.
Other Drugs Limited: both prescribed and nonprescribed.
Mental Health
Role of life stress in illness taught—crisis intervention.
Child rearing: developmental tasks fostered, e.g., "trust" in first year, autonomy in second and third, caring for others as major trait of adulthood.
*Illness Behavior
How to choose and then use medical care appropriately.
Consumer information about disease, causes, diagnoses, and treatment—limits and hazards as well as effectiveness.
*Sex Education: venereal disease, intimacy, contraception.
*Dental Health: limitation of carbohydrates in diet, flossing, dental hygiene.

*Behavior convincingly linked to disease.

Table 2

GUIDELINES FOR HEALTH SUPERVISION

Each child and family is unique; therefore these **Guidelines for Health Supervision of Children and Youth**[1] are designed for the care of children who are receiving competent parenting, have no manifestations of any important health problems, and are growing and developing in satisfactory fashion. **Additional visits may become necessary** if circumstances suggest variations from normal. These guidelines represent a consensus by the Committee on Practice and Ambulatory Medicine, in consultation with the membership of the American Academy of Pediatrics through the Chapter Chairmen.

The Committee emphasizes the great importance of **continuity of care** in comprehensive health supervision[2] and the need to avoid **fragmentation of care**[3].

A **prenatal visit** by the parents for anticipatory guidance and pertinent medical history is strongly recommended.

Health supervision should begin with medical care of the newborn in the hospital.

	INFANCY						EARLY CHILDHOOD					LATE CHILDHOOD					ADOLESCENCE			
AGE[4]	By 1 mo.	2 mos.	4 mos.	6 mos.	9 mos.	12 mos.	15 mos.	18 mos.	24 mos.	3 yrs.	4 yrs.	5 yrs.	6 yrs.	8 yrs.	10 yrs.	12 yrs.	14 yrs.	16 yrs.	18 yrs.	20+ yrs.
HISTORY																				
Initial/Interval	●	●	●	●	●	●	●	●	●	●	●	●	●	●	●	●	●	●	●	●
MEASUREMENTS																				
Height and Weight	●	●	●	●	●	●	●	●	●	●	●	●	●	●	●	●	●	●	●	●
Head Circumference	●	●	●	●	●	●														
Blood Pressure										●	●	●	●	●	●	●	●	●	●	●
SENSORY SCREENING																				
Vision	S	S	S	S	S	S	S	S	S	O	O	O	O	O	S	O	O	S	O	O
Hearing	S	S	S	S	S	S	S	S	S	S	O	O	S[5]	S[5]	S[5]	O	S	S	O	S
DEVEL./BEHAV. ASSESSMENT[6]	●	●	●	●	●	●	●	●	●	●	●	●	●	●	●	●	●	●	●	●
PHYSICAL EXAMINATION[7]	●	●	●	●	●	●	●	●	●	●	●	●	●	●	●	●	●	●	●	●
PROCEDURES[8]																				
Hered./Metabolic Screening[9]	●																			
Immunization[10]		●	●	●			●	●				●					●			
Tuberculin Test						●	←	←	●[11]	→	→	←	←	●[11]	→	→	←	←	●[11]	→
Hematocrit or Hemoglobin[12]	←	←	←	←	●	→	←	←	●	→	→	←	←	●	→	→	←	←	●	→
Urinalysis[13]	←	←	←	●	→	→	←	←	●	→	→	←	←	●	→	→	←	←	●	→
ANTICIPATORY GUIDANCE[14]	●	●	●	●	●	●	●	●	●	●	●	●	●	●	●	●	●	●	●	●
INITIAL DENTAL REFERRAL[15]										●										

1. Committee on Practice and Ambulatory Medicine, 1981.
2. Statement on Continuity of Pediatric Care, Committee on Standards of Child Health Care, 1978.
3. Statement on Fragmentation of Pediatric Care, Committee on Standards of Child Health Care, 1978.
4. If a child comes under care for the first time at any point on the Schedule, or if any items are not accomplished at the suggested age, the Schedule should be brought up to date at the earliest possible time.
5. At these points, history may suffice; if problem suggested, a standard testing method should be employed.
6. By history and appropriate physical examination; if suspicious, by specific objective developmental testing.
7. At each visit, a complete physical examination is essential, with infant totally unclothed, older child undressed and suitably draped.
8. These may be modified, depending upon entry point into schedule and individual need.
9. PKU and thyroid testing should be done at about 2 wks. Infants initially screened before 24 hours of age should be rescreened.
10. Schedule(s) per Report of Committee on Infectious Disease, ed. 18, 1982.
11. The Committee on Infectious Diseases recommends tuberculin testing at 12 months of age and every 1-2 years thereafter. In some areas, tuberculosis is of exceedingly low occurrence and the physician may elect not to retest routinely or to use longer intervals.
12. Present medical evidence suggests the need for reevaluation of the frequency and timing of hemoglobin or hematocrit tests. One determination is therefore suggested during each time period. Performance of additional tests is left to the individual practice experience.
13. Present medical evidence suggests the need for reevaluation of the frequency and timing of urinalyses. One determination is therefore suggested during each time period. Performance of additional tests is left to the individual practice experience.
14. Appropriate discussion and counselling should be an integral part of each visit for care.
15. Subsequent examinations as prescribed by dentist.

N.B.: **Special chemical, immunologic, and endocrine testing** are usually carried out upon specific indications. Testing other than newborn (e.g., inborn errors of metabolism, sickle disease, lead) are discretionary with the physician.

Key: ● = to be performed; **S** = subjective, by history; **O** = objective, by a standard testing method.

Promoting Healthy Behavior

Behavior is influenced by repeated reinforcement rather than by knowledge transfer alone. The failure of most antismoking education programs results, in part, because there is so little reinforcement of nonsmoking behavior after the program ends. Indeed, most unhealthy habits in children (accident-prone behavior, risk-taking, smoking, overeating, etc.) are reinforced as desirable by peers rather than the more healthy behavior taught by physicians and parents. Finding ways to develop effective peer group reinforcement of healthy behavior presents one of the challenges for the health professional. Working with schools, social groups, storefront teen-age clinics, church groups, and the women's movement are ways in which socially reinforcing units might be enlisted in health education and result in greater change in behavior than the usual one-to-one type of education.

Better presentation of health information by interesting audiovisual means is important to change behavior. By itself, no passive medium seems very successful. Use of pamphlets or slide shows in the office should be coupled with reinforcing discussion between parent and child and the health professional. The nurse practitioner has proved to be especially effective in the educational role.

The behaviors one seeks to change should be reasonably well established as important to health. Much of the lack of effect of health education has been due to the "mixed messages" given to the public, with one source advocating one approach and another often the opposite. Table 1 lists behaviors or health habits reasonably agreed upon as being highly related to health.

It is wise to concentrate health education on fewer habits, but ones upon which there is generally wide agreement of importance and which will make a significant difference to health. This should also lead to reinforcement of the desired behavior by other messages saying the same thing.

Part of the clinician's job, which he must share with others, is to help teach parents and children a healthy attitude toward their bodies and minds and to help them develop healthy habits.

THE FREQUENCY OF HEALTH PROMOTION VISITS

Rigid schedules of visits are less important than determining risk factors and vulnerabilities and then scheduling visits to meet the needs of the individual. There is, of course, a minimal number of visits necessary to assess health at key periods in a child's life and to accomplish needed immunizations. For children with low risk and high strengths, and where immunizations are done by personnel other than the physician, relatively few visits with the doctor are needed. For other children at high risk, frequent visits may be needed. Guidelines for health supervision (Table 2) developed by the American Academy of Pediatrics, show suggested age-specific frequency and content of health promotion visits. For children with low risk, reduced frequency is advocated by some (Hoekelman, 1975). For most children, the total number of visits for health promotion will be somewhere between, but the difference in these recommendations has large implications for cost and manpower needs.

REFERENCES

Bass, L.W., and Wilson, T.R.: The pediatrician's influence in private practice, measured by a controlled seat belt study. Pediatrics, 33:700, 1964.

Better Health for Our Children: A National Strategy. The Report of the Select Panel on Child Health to The United States Congress and the Secretary of Health and Human Services. U.S. Department of Health and Human Services. (PHS) Publication #79-55071, 1981.

Bibace, R., and Walsh, N.E.: Development of children's concepts of illness. Pediatrics, 66:912, 1980.

Breslow, L., and Somers, A.: The lifetime health monitoring program. N. Engl. J. Med., 296:601, 1977.

Collen, K.J.: A six year controlled trial of prevention of children's behavior disorders. J. Pediatr. 88:662, 1976.

Haggerty, R.J.: Changing lifestyles to improve health. Prevent. Med., 6:276, 1977.

Hamill, P.V.V., Drizd, T.A., Johnson, C.L., Reed, R.B., and Roche, A.F.: NCHS Growth Charts. 1976 Monthly Vital Statistics Report, 26:June 22, 1976 (HRA) 76-1120, Supplement HEW.

Health Promotion and Consumer Health Education Task Force Report, Sponsored by the John E. Fogarty International Center for the Advanced Study in the Health Sciences and The American College of Preventive Medicine. Prodist, N.Y., 1976.

Hoekelman, R.A.: What constitutes well baby care. Pediatrics, 55:313, 1975.

Levine, M., and Schneider, E.: PEER, Pediatric Examination of Educational Readiness, Children's Hospital Medical Center. Boston, Educators Publishing Service, 1982.

Miller, F.J.W., Court, S.D.M., Knox, E.G., and Brandon, S.: The school years in Newcastle-Upon-Tyne. London, Oxford University Press, 1974.

Pillai, V., Collins, A., and Morgan, R.: Family walk in centre—Eaton Socon: Evaluation of a project on preventive intervention based in the community. Child Abuse and Neglect, 6:71, 1982.

Reisinger, M.D., et al.: Anticipatory guidance in pediatric practice. Pediatrics, 66:889, 1980.

Robbins, F.C.: The long view. Am. J. Dis. Child., *104*:499, 1982.

Robertson, L.S., Kosa, J., Heagarty, M.C., Haggerty, R.J., and Alpert, J.A.: Changing the medical care system: A controlled experiment in comprehensive care. New York, Prager, 1974.

Sturner, R.A., Funk, S.G., Barton, J., Sparrow, S., and Frothingham, T.E.: Simultaneous screening for child health and development: A study of visual developmental screening of preschool children. Pediatrics, *65*:614, 1980.

Vickery, D.M., and Fries, J.F.: Take Care of Yourself. A Consumer's Guide to Medical Care. Menlo Park, Cal., Addison-Wesley, 1976.

Werner, E. E., and Smith, R. S.: Vulnerable, but Invincible: A Longitudinal study of Resilient Children and Youth. New York, McGraw-Hill, 1981.

Wray, J.D.: Child care in the People's Republic of China. Pediatrics, *55*:734, 1975.

Robert J. Haggerty

4

IMMUNIZATION

Martin B. Kleiman, M.D.

The results of few areas of health promotion compare to the dramatic success achieved worldwide by the routine immunization of children against selected infectious diseases. The practitioner should develop an orderly system for the administration of effective vaccines, maintaining accurate records, and continuing to place a high priority on immunization in the care of children, adolescents, and adults in his practice.

The current edition of the Report of the Committee on Infectious Diseases (American Academy of Pediatrics, 1982), usually referred to as the "Red Book," is the most authoritative source for the answers to questions pertaining to childhood immunization and an indispensable resource for the practitioner. Tables 4–1 and 4–2 present the currently recommended schedules of active immunization for normal infants and children (Table 4–1) and for infants and children not initially immunized at usual recommended times in early infancy (Table 4–2). It should be understood that the recommendations are suggestions which in many instances, make immunological, epidemiological, and cultural compromises designed to permit the safest, most efficient, and least costly means for immunizing the majority of children. Individual circumstances occasionally may dictate the need for deviation from the schedules, e.g., the need to protect children against measles earlier than one year of age if measles is prevalent in the community. In general, adherence to the recommendations is desirable.

No vaccine is completely safe. The patient or parent should be reasonably informed of the risks of the vaccine product and consent should be obtained. Live viral vaccines should be avoided in patients with impaired immune mechanisms and in patients who are pregnant. Records of site of administration, vaccine, manufacturer, lot number, and expiration date should be kept by the physician and copies given to the patient for his permanent health records. These records become especially important later in childhood and adolescence when school or employment requirements necessitate documentation of immunization. The practitioner should develop a procedure that permits the periodic assessment of the immunization records of patients in his care. The early adolescent years are an excellent time to review the adequacy of immunization against rubella. Outbreaks of rubella are most common in the high school and college-age populations and adequate protection in the pre-adolescent age period should eliminate the risk of congenital rubella syndrome.

In addition to the routine immunizations, active or passive immunization may be available for a variety of other illnesses (Table 4–3). The practitioner may need to take into account conditions or illnesses that alter the type and schedule of immunizations (Table 4–4). The "Red Book" and other sources should be consulted for detailed discussions of these topics.

IMMUNIZATION

A schedule for routine immunization should be developed.
A schedule for the ongoing, periodic assessment of immunization records should be developed.
No vaccine is completely safe; informed consent should be obtained.
The report of the Committee on Infectious Diseases, American Academy of Pediatrics, should serve as the major reference for immunization practices.
Live attenuated vaccine products should be withheld in children with immunodeficiency.
Patients should receive records of immunizations for their personal health records.

Table 4–1. RECOMMENDED SCHEDULE FOR ACTIVE IMMUNIZATION OF NORMAL INFANTS AND CHILDREN

Recommended Age	Vaccine(s)	Comments
2 mo	DTP[1], OPV[2]	Can be initiated earlier in areas of high endemicity
4 mo	DTP, OPV	2-mo interval desired for OPV to avoid interference
6 mo	DTP (OPV)	OPV optional for areas where polio might be imported (e.g., some areas of southwestern United States)
12 mo	Tuberculin test[3]	May be given simultaneously with MMR at 15 mo (see text)
15 mo	Measles, Mumps, Rubella (MMR)[4]	MMR preferred
18 mo	DTP, OPV	Consider as part of primary series—DTP essential
4–6 yr[5]	DTP, OPV	
14–16 yr	Td[6]	Repeat every 10 years for lifetime

[1]DTP—Diphtheria and tetanus toxoids with pertussis vaccine.
[2]OPV—Oral, attenuated poliovirus vaccine contains poliovirus types 1, 2, and 3.
[3]Tuberculin test—Mantoux (intradermal PPD) preferred. Frequency of tests depends on local epidemiology. The Committee recommends annual or biennial testing unless local circumstances dictate less frequent or no testing.
[4]MMR—Live measles, mumps, and rubella viruses in a combined vaccine (see text for discussion of single vaccines versus combination).
[5]Up to seventh birthday.
[6]Td—Adult tetanus toxoid (full dose) and diphtheria toxoid (reduced dose) in combination.
For all products used, consult manufacturer's brochure for instructions for storage, handling, and administration. Biologics prepared by different manufacturers may vary, and those of the same manufacturer may change from time to time. The package insert should be followed for a specific product. (From the Report of the Committee on Infectious Diseases. American Academy of Pediatrics. Copyright American Academy of Pediatrics, 1982.)

Table 4–2. RECOMMENDED IMMUNIZATION SCHEDULES FOR INFANTS AND CHILDREN NOT INITIALLY IMMUNIZED AT USUAL RECOMMENDED TIMES IN EARLY INFANCY

		Alternatives			
Timing	*Preferred Schedule*	*#1*	*#2*	*#3*	**Comments**
First visit	DTP #1, OPV #1 Tuberculin test (PPD)	MMR, PPD	DTP #1, OPV #1, PPD	DTP #1, OPV #1, MMR, PPD	MMR should be given no younger than 15 mo old.
1 mo after first visit	MMR	DTP #1, OPV #1	MMR, DTP #2	DTP #2	
2 mo after first visit	DTP #2, OPV #2		DTP #3, OPV #2	DTP #3, OPV #2	
3 mo after first visit	(DTP #3)	DTP #2, OPV #2			In preferred schedule, DTP #3 can be given if OPV #3 is not to be given until 10–16 mo.
4 mo after first visit	DTP #3 (OPV #3)		(OPV #3)	(OPV #3)	OPV #3 optional for areas for likely importation of polio (e.g., some southwestern states).
5 mo after first visit		DTP #3 (OPV #3)			
10–16 mo after last dose	DTP #4, OPV #3 or OPV #4	DTP #4, OPV #3 or OPV #4	DTP #4, OPV #3 or OPV #4	DTP #4, OPV #3 or OPV #4	
Preschool	DTP #5, OPV #4 or OPV #5	DTP #5, OPV #4 or OPV #5	DTP #5, OPV #4 or OPV #5	DTP #5, OPV #4 or OPV #5	Preschool dose not necessary if DTP #4 or #5 given after fourth birthday.
14–16 yr old	Td	Td	Td	Td	Repeat every 10 yr.

Alternative #1 can be used in those more than 15 months old if measles is occurring in the community.

Alternative #2 allows for more rapid DTP immunization.

Alternative #3 should be reserved for those whose access to medical care is compromised by poor compliance.

DTP = Diphtheria and tetanus toxoids with pertussive vaccine.

OPV = Oral, attenuated poliovirus vaccine contains types 1, 2, and 3.

Tuberculin test = Mantoux (intradermal PPD) preferred. Frequency of tests depends on local epidemiology. The Committee recommends annual or biennial testing unless local circumstances dictate less frequent or no testing.

MMR = Live measles, mumps, and rubella viruses in a combined vaccine (see text for discussion of single vaccines).

Td = Adult tetanus toxoid (full dose) and diphtheria toxoid (reduced dose) in combination.

For all products used, consult manufacturer's brochure for instructions for storage, handling, and administration. Biologics prepared by different manufacturers may vary, and those of the same manufacturer may change from time to time. The package insert should be followed for a specific product. (From the Report of the Committee on Infectious Diseases, American Academy of Pediatrics, Copyright American Academy of Pediatrics, 1982.)

Table 4–3. ILLNESSES FOR WHICH ACTIVE OR PASSIVE IMMUNIZATION MAY BE INDICATED

Bacterial Infections	
Neisseria meningitidis serogroups A, C, Y, W-135	A
Streptococcus pneumoniae (14 types)	A
Clostridium tetani	A,P
Viral Infections	
Hepatitis A	P
Hepatitis B	A,P
Varicella	P
Rabies	A,P
Influenza A	A
Influenza B	A
Measles	A,P

A = Active immunization; P = Passive immunization.

Table 4–4. ILLNESSES OR CONDITIONS THAT MAY REQUIRE SPECIAL CONSIDERATION FOR IMMUNIZATION

Asplenia
Primary or acquired immunodeficiency
Prematurity
Immunosuppressive therapy
Sibling of a child with impaired host defenses
Disseminated malignancy
Household contacts with undetermined susceptibility to poliovirus infection
Previous CNS or other severe reaction to a vaccine product
Progressive neurological disorders
Children in military populations
Pregnancy

5

PRENATAL/INFANCY—THE FIRST 24 MONTHS

Ernest E. Smith, M.D.

The prenatal period and first several years of life are sensitive and formative times for children and their families. With the present realities of limited extended family contacts, lack of education for parenting, the barrage of opinions from friends, relatives, and media about child health and development, and stresses such as single parenthood and working mothers, young families have limited options for reliable, consistent information and guidance regarding their child's health, growth, and development. The pediatrician's early and frequent contacts with children and their families through the prenatal and early childhood periods provide unique opportunities to prevent, detect, and manage both the biomedical and biosocial aspects of child health. The cumulative effects of well child care during this period allow for (1) development of a supportive and therapeutic relationship, (2) establishment of a family data base, (3) education and counseling regarding child health, (4) building of parental self-esteem and confidence, (5) detection of asymptomatic disease, and (6) early recognition and treatment of symptomatic acute illness to prevent complications.

PEDIATRIC PRENATAL CARE

The opportunity for pediatrician and expectant parents to meet prior to a child's birth offers counseling and intervention advantages at a very strategic time. The prenatal visit is timely in establishing a supportive relationship between the pediatrician and the parents, obtaining a data base of medical, social, and emotional history about the family and pregnancy, providing education and counseling concerning aspects of child care that would be moot after delivery, and offering helpful information about the arrangements of a pediatric practice. See Table 5–1 for detailed guidelines for a prenatal visit.

A single prenatal visit should be routinely planned in the last trimester of pregnancy at six to eight months' gestation. With special circumstances such as maternal depression, excessive parental anxiety, or a medically high-risk pregnancy, the initial visit might be scheduled earlier and subsequent visits arranged as needed.

While parents and referring physicians are becoming more aware of its value, prenatal

Table 5–1. SUGGESTED GUIDELINES FOR PRENATAL VISIT

A. Scheduling:
   Last trimester of pregnancy. Earlier and additional visits if needed for emotionally and medically high-risk pregnancy.

B. For Whom:
   Parents in first pregnancy, new to practice, or with special concerns. Should be offered with later pregnancies. Mother accompanied by father.

C. Purpose:
   To establish a supportive relationship, to obtain data base about family and pregnancy, to counsel concerning aspects of infant care, to stress availability, and to acquaint parents with one's practice.

D. Common Concerns and Questions:
   Breast/bottle feeding; circumcision; normality of baby; perinatal contingencies; baby care.

E. Obstetrical History:
   Previous pregnancies and outcome, difficulties with conceiving, infections, nutrition, drugs, bleeding, alcohol, smoking, hypertension, glycosuria, rubella titer, Rh factor, attendance at prenatal classes.

F. Family Genetic and Medical Histories

G. Psychological Adjustment to Pregnancy:
   How has your pregnancy been?
   Are you expecting a boy or a girl?
   Names?
   Was this a convenient time for you to be pregnant?
   Parents' affect and degree of concerns.

H. Assessment of Parenting Abilities:
   How were you reared and how do you expect to rear your child?
   Personal data about parents, support systems, stressful life events such as divorce, recent moves, family illness.
   Preparation for infant at home.
   Previous experience with children.

I. Other:
   Preparation of siblings, arrangements for help with housework and other siblings when mother comes home, car safety restraint, review of the office policies.

J. Reassure appropriately and stress availability.

visits are still more the exception rather than the routine. The interested pediatrician needs to inform referring obstetricians about his or her preference in seeing parents prenatally, especially those expecting their first infant and those with high-risk pregnancies. Pediatric office staff can communicate the prenatal visit policy when parents call prior to delivery to arrange for pediatric care. Prenatal classes also offer opportunities for parents to understand the importance of a prenatal pediatric visit. Self- and word-of-mouth referrals should increase as prenatal visits become recognized by parents as a helpful and practical aspect of child health care.

As each pregnancy is a unique experience for the family, a prenatal visit should also be considered for subsequent pregnancies. At times, issues such as parental expectations and concerns about a subsequent pregnancy and the preparation of siblings for the birth might be managed during the health care visits of the siblings; however, a prenatal visit with each pregnancy provides the opportunity for both parents to focus on the novelty and unique concerns of the current pregnancy.

The visit should start with the pediatrician briefly reviewing the purpose of the session. "I find that meeting with parents before the birth is helpful in getting to know one another and in reviewing how things are going with the pregnancy. I also will try to answer whatever questions you have and review some things you might find helpful in preparing for your baby."

After the purpose of the visit is reviewed, the pediatrician might summarize briefly for the family his training, background, interests, and experience. Whether they ask or not, most parents are interested in the physician's qualifications, and this helps ease the tension of a first visit while allowing the parents to get to know the pediatrician. As parents' awareness of the pediatrician's interests and knowledge might be narrowly focused on biomedical issues, this is a good time for the physician to state that as a pediatrician he or she is concerned not only with children's physical well-being but also with their growth and development and how they get along with family and friends. As effectiveness in counseling is largely dependent on the parents' perception of the pediatrician's interest and knowledge, such a statement identifies that the pediatrician is interested in all aspects of the child's life.

The content of the visit should include review of parents' questions and concerns, obstetrical history, family genetic and medical histories, psychological adjustment to pregnancy, and assessment of parenting abilities, including the father's role.

Parental Concerns and Questions

Frequently, questions arise about issues of breast or bottle feeding, circumcision, and normality of the baby. Whether questions are asked or not, these issues should be discussed with the parents.

Breast milk is the optimal nutrition for infants. There are biomedical/nutritional, immunological, preventive (infection, allergies), and economic advantages to breast milk. Successful breast feeding can elicit intense positive feelings in the mother, and these may reinforce other positive maternal-infant interactions. Unfortunately, psychosocial factors frequently influence the parents against breast feeding. The pediatrician must be sensitive to these issues in counseling parents about the importance of breast feeding. A prudent approach would be to outline the advantages and disadvantages of breast and formula feeding for those parents who are undecided or who "have decided to bottle feed," so that their decision is an informed one. Those women who show some motivation to breast feed should receive informed assistance and support; on the other hand, those who elect not to breast feed should not be coerced or criticized. The mother who elects to formula feed needs the equivalent support and guidance regarding infant feeding as does the breast feeding mother. Areas that should be covered for the mother who plans to breast feed include problems that might make breast feeding difficult, e.g., retracted nipples, nipple preparation, and identification of someone to help the mother with breast feeding in the hospital (Hill, 1981). For the mother who plans to formula feed, important information includes the different infant formulas and forms available and supplies needed.

The parents' questions or decision regarding circumcision should also be explored. They should be informed that circumcision is a procedure that has some risk and that there are no medical indications for the procedure. Religious and strong social reasons for parents wanting their infant circumcised should be respected. Frequently, parents are concerned that the uncircumcised child will suffer psychologically, since the majority of children are still being circumcised. They should be assured that there is no evidence to support this concern. The child's "adjustment" is most likely influenced by how comfortable the parents are with their decision.

The Obstetrical History

The mother's pregnancy history should be reviewed, including previous pregnancies and outcome, difficulties in conceiving, infections, nutrition, drugs, bleeding, alcohol, smoking, rubella titer, and Rh factor. Much of this information can be gathered by forms.

Family Genetic and Medical Histories

The family history should be explored for genetically determined diseases and congenital anomalies. Inquiry should be made about the general health of the parents and any significant systemic or organ system difficulty. The importance of such information about the mother is obvious; however, medical information about the father and immediate family members is helpful, as acute and chronic illness in the family can cause much stress and limit family support.

Psychological Adjustment to Pregnancy

A careful history of the parents' psychological adjustment to the pregnancy can be as important as a detailed biomedical data base. A statement such as "How have you been feeling?" directed to both parents can often elicit information regarding psychological as well as biological factors. Other questions that might give insight into the parents' feelings include "Have you decided on names for the baby?" "Any preference for a boy or girl?" and "Was this a convenient time for you to be pregnant?" Observation of the parents' affect and the degree of anxiety related to concerns raised also helps the pediatrician in determining their adaptation to the pregnancy.

Assessment of Parenting Abilities

Personal data concerning the parents which are important in an assessment of their parenting abilities include educational level, occupation, and family experiences. Especially important is a history of the mother's relationship with her own mother. A facilitative question is "Recalling how you were raised, in what ways do you plan to rear your baby the same way and in what ways differently?" Important life events that might affect the family should be reviewed, e.g., marital separation, divorce, recent moves, illness in other family members, previous pregnancies, abortions, fears, mother's plans to return to work, unemployment, and financial concerns. The parents' previous experience with infants and children should be explored. Since support available to the family is an important parenting resource, they should be asked about the availability of extended family and friends.

The pediatrician should explore the parents'

plans and preparation regarding the nursery, sleeping arrangements, equipment, and infant clothes. Preparations the family has made or is planning to make for the infant at home reflect their knowledge regarding infants. Also, this information identifies for the pediatrician practical issues that need further discussion with the family.

Other areas that should be covered during the prenatal visit include finding ways to involve older children in preparation of arrangements for care of the siblings during the lying-in period, preparation for separation of mother from the siblings during the hospitalization, arrangements for the siblings to visit during the hospitalization, and the possibility of regression in toileting in a toddler. In addition, plans for help with housework and other siblings when the mother comes home should be discussed. Very importantly, the use of approved car safety restraints starting with the infant's first ride home from the hospital should be stressed and the parents provided with a brochure about car safety.

A brief review of the policies of the pediatric practice should be provided either verbally or in written form. This formation could include fee schedules, night call and emergency coverage, office hours, and guidelines for use of the telephone.

The session can be ended by reviewing the significant concerns, if any, of the family and offering appropriate reassurance. High-risk factors are best managed by assuring the parents that everything possible is being done and stressing the availability of the pediatrician or his/her associate at birth or in the immediate newborn period.

The information obtained and the supportive relationship established during the prenatal visit is invaluable, especially if the infant is born prematurely, becomes ill immediately after birth, or has a congenital anomaly. Every effort should be made to establish pediatric prenatal visits as an imperative aspect of child health care.

THE NEWBORN PERIOD

The postpartum period is a time when parents are in need of and receptive to factual information and support concerning the well-being and health care of their infant. It is a time for furthering the physician-parent supportive relationship through meticulous attention to mother, father, and infant. Specific parental concerns identified during the prenatal visit can be further addressed, along with the exploration of other areas that may be of more immediate concern now that the baby is born.

The pediatrician should examine the newborn and talk with the parents within the first 12 to 24 hours after delivery. If the parents have expressed significant anxiety about their child's well-being, the infant should be seen as soon as possible, even if the child is healthy and without problems. Subsequent hospital visits can be arranged depending on the needs of the infant and family and the availability of other health care providers such as nurses or PNAs who can provide support and counseling. Prior to discharge, the pediatrician should again do a complete assessment of the child and have a relaxed, unhurried counseling session with the family to provide additional information and answer questions.

Since the health of their infant is their highest priority, parents are particularly interested in discussing and observing the examination of their baby. Assessment of the infant in the presence of the parents offers the pediatrician the opportunity to point out and discuss common findings such as toxic erythema and hemangiomas, which the parents might view as abnormalities, demonstrate the unique competencies of the newborn infant, and observe the parents' interaction with their new baby.

Table 5–2 outlines the health promotion and

Table 5–2. SUGGESTED GUIDELINES FOR NEWBORN VISIT

A. Interview and physical examination in first 24 hours and repeat before discharge.
   Discuss and demonstrate physical examination with parents.
   Identify congenital anomalies, assess gestational age, measure head circumference.
   Observe parent-child and parent-parent interactions.
B. Discuss and demonstrate infant's organized/disorganized behavior and sensory/social responsiveness to parents.
C. Discuss breast/bottle feeding and ensure the help of nurses in feeding. Discuss schedules, vitamin/fluoride/iron supplementation, common problems and their management.
D. Prepare mothers for procedures on infant such as Dextrostix and metabolic screen.
E. Provide anticipatory guidance regarding common concerns, parentcraft, accident prevention, indicators of illness, parent/family needs.
F. Promote participation of father.
G. Compliment mother, mention availability, and call primiparous family two to three days after discharge.

counseling issues to be covered during the newborn period. In addition to attention to the infant, the pediatrician is interested in how the mother is feeling and is alert to both physical and emotional issues, e.g., fatigue and postpartum blues, that might cause difficulties for the mother in caring for her infant. Most mothers find the first weeks difficult. They are involved and preoccupied with their new role and new baby and often feel inadequate. The demands may seem overwhelming to them, and they need to know that this reaction is normal.

The physical and neurodevelopmental assessment should include special attention to the presence of congenital anomalies, no matter how minor. The parents are certain to note them and have concerns if they have not been prospectively addressed. A gestational age assessment should be performed routinely on every newborn because of the unique problems of small-for-gestational-age, premature, and large-for-gestational-age infants. On physical examination, particular attention should be directed to jaundice, cloudiness of cornea, cleft palate, auscultation of the heart, palpation of peripheral pulses, abnormalities of the genitalia including hypospadias and hydrocele, and examination of the hips for dislocation.

Owing to the physiological depression that usually occurs during the first 24 hours after birth, the neurodevelopmental evaluation of the newborn is best done on the second or third day of life. The neurological examination should go beyond the routine examination of movement of extremities, cry, muscle tone, and the presence of certain primitive reflexes. The infant's organized/disorganized behavior and various state changes should be noted. Such observations as ability to be comforted, length of alertness, and irritability reveal much about the newborn's neurological organization as well as the characteristics of the infant that might facilitate or inhibit social interaction and care-giving behavior. The ability of the infant to respond to auditory and visual stimulation, such as visually fixing and following the human face and turning toward the human voice, should be assessed. Discussion of the infant's sensory and organizational capabilities with the parents promotes their ability to view the baby as an individual and to understand and respond appropriately to the infant's behaviors. Observation of the parents' handling of their infant is extremely helpful in gaining impressions of the parents' capabilities, anxiety, and knowledge regarding newborns. Eye-to-eye contact, the way in which the infant is held, and the manner in which the mother attempts to alert or comfort the infant are all important observations that give evidence of the ease or difficulty with which reciprocity will be established.

Initial screening for phenylketonuria (PKU) and congenital hypothyroidism and, in some states, other inborn errors of metabolism should be done on every infant before he/she leaves the nursery. If there are doubts about adequacy of the screen and amount of protein intake or the infant is sick, the baby should be rescreened within a week or two of discharge.

The postpartum period represents a time when families are very receptive to information and support that will facilitate care of their infant. Since the parents' comfort with their infant is, in part, due to their ability to understand and respond to the baby's physical, temperamental, and developmental needs, it is helpful to discuss the following topics during the lying-in period. This information can be supplemented and reinforced by means of written material or tape cassettes personally dictated by the pediatrician.

Neurological Organization. The variability of the organizational state of the newborn should be discussed. During the early weeks of life, predictable wake-sleep cycles should not be expected. Infants are extremely variable in the number of the hours they sleep and in their sleep schedules. Normal newborns sleep between 14 and 20 hours per day. Parents should understand that (1) crying is normal behavior for newborns, and (2) the amount of crying generally increases during the first 2 to 3 months of life. Frequently, inconsolable crying occurring in the early to late evening appears to represent immature neurological development rather than adverse external stimuli.

Sensory and Social Responses. Discussion and demonstration of the sensory and social competencies of their infant facilitates parent-infant interactions. The abilities of the newborn to alert, to fix and follow to face and voice, to quiet himself/herself when upset, to cuddle, and to shut out stimuli from the environment should be discussed with the parents. Offering the parents techniques to enhance their infant's responsiveness, i.e., gentle rocking in a semireclining position to facilitate alerting and holding objects at the appropriate focal length of 19 cm, takes only minutes of the pediatrician's time.

Feeding. Nurses should be prepared and available to help mothers establish breast feeding successfully. The let-down reflex, breast engorgement, sore nipples, manual expression of breast milk for supplemental feedings, milk storage, and the use of a breast-milk pump should be discussed. Sore nipples may be treated by decreasing length of feedings, use of a breast shield, washing the nipples with cotton balls, and exposure of the nipples to warmth from a light bulb several times a day. A supplement of 400 I.U. vitamin D may be prescribed for breast-fed infants. Fluoride supplementation in a dosage of 0.25 mg/day from birth to 24 months should be recommended if the infant is breast fed or if the formula is being mixed with unfluoridated water. Iron supplementation in the form of iron-fortified milk, cereal, or iron drops should be introduced no later than 4 months of age in term infants and 2 months in preterm infants and continued through the first year of life. Parents should be instructed that introduction of solid foods should be delayed for 4 to 6 months.

Skin Care. In general, the less manipulation of the skin the better. The major objective is cleanliness while preventing excessive irritation. Most infants can tolerate a daily bath with mild soap and warm water; however, baths can be given as infrequently as 2 to 3 times per week if excessive drying is a problem. The infant should not be immersed in water until after the umbilical cord has healed properly. Baby oils and lotions should be avoided, as they often contain perfume substances that tend to result in hypersensitivity reactions or irritations. Protection of the skin in the diaper area can be accomplished with some type of water repellent such as petroleum jelly, corn starch, or zinc oxide.

Umbilicus. It is important to keep the umbilical cord area clean, either with soap and water or with alcohol. The skin should be retracted from around the cord during this cleansing process to allow the cord to dry better. After the cord has fallen off, the area can be cleansed with alcohol twice a day until complete healing occurs.

Circumcision Care. A thin layer of vaseline can be applied to the end of the penis until the circumcision heals. This protects the penis from moisture and from sticking to the diaper. If a plastic apparatus is used for the circumcision, parents should be instructed not to remove it prematurely. Retracting the foreskin in uncircumcised infants and that remaining in those who are circumcised should not be done due to possible tearing apart of partially healed skin edges or causing more difficulty with adhesions. Gentle retraction of the foreskin in cleansing is all that is needed. In some children, the foreskin cannot be completely retracted until age 3 or 4.

Stool Patterns. The number and consistency of the stools depend on the child's diet and individuality. The breast-fed infant is expected to have 1 to 6 salve-like yellow or golden colored stools containing seed-like particles. The formula-fed infant's stools are slightly firmer, yellow to light brown in color, and more rancid in odor and occur with a frequency of 1 to 2 per day. The number of stools per day can be quite variable, ranging from a frequency of 1 to 7 per day to once every several days. Owing to undeveloped abdominal musculature, newborn infants demonstrate mild difficulty passing bowel movements and frequently seem to be straining at stool. Since the infant's straining and color change is sometimes a concern to the parents, they should be informed that this is normal and that mechanical or pharmaceutical agents are not needed to decrease the "constipation."

Exposure to Crowds. During the early weeks, it is best to caution the parents about exposure of the infant to crowds.

Indicators of Illness. Parents should be instructed in how to take the infant's temperature and read the thermometer. They should also be told what temperature indicates a fever and be instructed to notify the physician if the infant does not look good, will not eat, is unusually irritable, or has excessive regurgitation, vomiting, or diarrhea.

Safety and Accident Prevention. The use of an approved car seat must be stressed. Parents should be instructed to examine the crib to make sure it is sturdy, the crib bars are no further than 2⅜ inches apart, the mattress fits snugly against all sides, and there is a bumper guard. In order to avoid the danger of strangulation the parents should be discouraged from hanging objects within the crib. Parents should be made aware that even the youngest infant can roll off a changing table or bed if left unattended.

Pacifiers. If the parents are interested in utilizing a pacifier, they should be instructed to find one that is of one-piece construction and never to tie it around the infant's neck. Parents should be encouraged to stop the pacifier before 4 to 5 months of age, as the older child might have difficulty giving it up, especially if the pacifier becomes a transitional object.

Parent/Family Needs. The mother should be instructed to take it easy and not become involved in many activities outside of infant care. The possibility of maternal blues or let-down and its signs and symptoms should be discussed with the family. The possibility of "sibling rivalry" should be reviewed, noting that it is a normal response and providing strategies for management.

Prior to discharge of mother and child, the pediatrician should emphasize his/her availability if needed. There should be plans made for telephone contact, especially for the primiparous family, within 48 to 72 hours after returning home. An initial office visit at two weeks should be scheduled prior to the infant's discharge.

THE FIRST TWO YEARS

Tables 5–3 through 5–11 are health promotion guidelines for office pediatrics during the child's first two years of life. These general guidelines, which incorporate biomedical, developmental, and psychosocial issues in health supervision, are intended for the care of children who are thought to be receiving competent parenting and who have no important health problems. The scheduling of appointments and suggested activities follow the guidelines for health supervision established by the American Academy of Pediatrics. Flexibility of schedules and modification of issues are obviously indicated to accommodate a practitioner's individual style or special circumstances that arise with any particular family and child, e.g., single-parent families, children with long-term illness or handicaps, and families of various socioeconomic and cultural backgrounds.

Each visit includes the following five areas: (1) interview, (2) assessment of physical, developmental, and affective status, (3) immunizations and procedures, (4) anticipatory guidance, and (5) closing the visit. A visit should not entail a reflex checking off of items in each area. Rather, a solid knowledge base of particular items to cover at each age provides the structure that allows for flexibility as needed.

The Interview

The interview should include questions exploring parental concerns, with particular attention directed to common age-related concerns such as crying and sleeping in the first several months, stranger and separation anxiety at 6 to 8 months, and temper tantrums and discipline at 12 months. Questions that focus on family adaptation, parent-child mutuality, and individ-

Table 5–3. SUGGESTED FORMAT FOR HEALTH PROMOTION 2–4 WEEK VISIT

A. Interview
1. How are you? How are things going?
2. What problems/concerns have you had? Sleeping? Vomiting? Colic and irritability? Crying? Feeding? Bowel movements?
3. How is your husband? How is he at helping out? How are the other children doing?
4. How would you describe ________'s personality? When ______ gets fussy or upset, how do you soothe him/her?
5. Support systems? Help caring for baby?
6. Return to work? Plans for infant care?
7. Family crises? Illness, death, separation?

B. Physical/Developmental/Affective Assessment
1. Plot weight, length, head circumference.
2. Physical exam with particular attention to red reflex, heart, abdomen, and hips.
3. Observe parent-infant mutuality and attachment: Holding, comforting, eye-to-eye contact.
4. Observe infant's temperament: Irritable, passive, alert, placid.
5. Developmental assessment: Raises head slightly when prone; hands open or partially fisted; fixes and follows with eyes; makes quiet throaty noises; responsive smile; responds to sound with alerting, quieting, directional head turn.
6. Review neonatal screening: PKU, thyroid and repeat if needed.

C. Immunizations: next month.

D. Anticipatory Guidance:
1. Nutrition: Breast/formula only, adequacy, schedule, vitamin/fluoride/iron needs, expected weight gain in next month. May drop a formula feeding over next 6 weeks. Hold for night bottle.
2. Accident prevention: Car safety restraint; rolling off dressing table or bed; burns, hot liquids, water temperature less than 125°F; crib bars and bumpers.
3. Sleep: Predictable sleep-wake cycles should not be expected; regularity should improve over next month; might be sleeping through night by next visit.
4. Elimination: Patterns, straining, urinary stream.
5. Development: Discuss accomplishments parents might look for over next month.
6. Other: Irregular respirations; startle; sneezing; hiccoughs; needless fears regarding "spoiling"; skin care; naval care; birth control.

E. Closing the Visit: Other questions? Compliment. Stress availability and set return appointment.

Table 5–4. SUGGESTED FORMAT FOR HEALTH PROMOTION 2 MONTH VISIT

A. Interview
   1. How are you? How are things going?
   2. Have there been any problems or concerns? Excessive crying? Sleep? Unpredictability of schedule? Unresponsiveness?
   3. How is your husband? The other children?
   4. What do you and your husband enjoy most about ________? What do you find most difficult about ________'s care?
   5. What changes have you seen in development? Social smile? Cooing verbalizations?
   6. Return to work? Child care?
   7. Any unusual or unexpected family stresses/crises?

B. Physical/Developmental/Affective Assessment
   1. Plot weight, length, and head circumference. Share with parents.
   2. Physical exam with particular attention to strabismus, heart, abdomen, and hips.
   3. Parent-infant mutuality and attachment: Cuddling, comforting, verbal communication, infant's responsiveness.
   4. Infant's temperament: Fussy, irritable, complacent, passive, actively engaging.
   5. Developmental assessment: Direct regard of people; retains objects in hand briefly; social smile; beginning vowel sounds (ah, eh); raises head recurrently when prone; holds head erect when held upright; stops crying when spoken to.

C. Immunizations: counsel regarding purpose, contraindications, common side effects; DPT #1, OPV #1

D. Anticipatory Guidance:
   1. Nutrition: Stress adequacy of breast and/or formula feedings only, until 4–6 months of age; expectation of more consistent feeding schedule with increasing intervals, especially at night; "spitting-up" common.
   2. Accident prevention: Car safety restraint; rolling off elevated surfaces; toys should be soft, washable without removable parts or sharp edges and large enough not to fit into mouth.
   3. Sleep: Schedule becoming established; may sleep uninterrupted for a 12-hour span or awaken every 3–4 hours; stress sleeping in own room and bed.
   4. Development: Discuss expected accomplishments over next 2 months; toy suggestions include soft toys that make music, rattles to place in hand, mobile.
   5. Other: Ask parents to consult pediatrician regarding use of any proprietary medications; encourage parents to find competent babysitter so they might have an evening out.

E. Closing the Visit: Other questions? Compliment. Set return appointment.

Table 5–5. SUGGESTED FORMAT FOR HEALTH PROMOTION 4 MONTH VISIT

A. Interview
   1. How are you? How are things going?
   2. What problems/concerns have you had since your last visit? Night crying? Resistance when put down to sleep? Crying on separation? Worry about spoiling? Sibling rivalry? Thumb sucking?
   3. How is your husband?
   4. Have you been out with your husband?
   5. What are some of ________'s new achievements? Reaching and feeling with open hand? Laughing out loud? Hand play, mutual fingering? Vocal-social response?
   6. Any unusual or unexpected family stresses/crises?

B. Physical/Developmental/Affective Assessment
   1. Plot weight, length, head circumference. Share with family.
   2. Physical exam. Check for strabismus.
   3. Observe parent-infant interaction. Evidence of reciprocal vocal and social responses.
   4. Observe infant's temperament. Best if defined by parents through interview. Parent's perceptions should regularly be positive even if infant is trying at times.
   5. Developmental assessment: Sitting with support; steady head control when upright; rolls prone to supine; hands open at rest; grasps objects near head; takes objects to mouth; several consistent noncrying sounds.

C. Immunizations: Again review benefits and risks. Ask about any previous reaction. DPT #2, OPV #2.

D. Anticipatory Guidance
   1. Nutrition: Stress adequacy of breast and/or bottle. For parents who are adamant about starting solids, rice cereal mixed with formula and fed by small spoon can be added to 1–2 feedings each day. Infant should have a predictable schedule of 4–5 feedings per day.
   2. Accident prevention: With increasing motor skills, prevention becomes more important. Playpen convenient and usually accepted at this age; gates for stairways; begin accident-proofing house, i.e., poisons and small objects that might be swallowed. Review management of choking.
   3. Sleep: Part-time predictable schedule. Stress own bed and room.
   4. Development: Discuss stranger awareness. Encourage play alone in playpen as well as with parents and siblings. Toys to suggest include rattles, spoons, cups, plastic containers and lids, ball to clutch. All should be too large to be placed entirely in infant's mouth.
   5. Other: Teething.

E. Closing the Visit: Other questions? Compliment. Set return appointment.

uality of the child are important. The following questions should be asked in some form at each visit:

1. How are you?
2. How are things going?
3. Are things going as you had hoped?
4. Have there been any problems or concerns since your last visit?
5. How would you describe ________'s personality these days?
6. How do you tell what ________ needs?
7. Can you tell what ________ wants by his/her crying?
8. When ________ gets upset, how do you soothe him/her?
9. Do you have someone you can ask when you have questions about the baby?
10. What does your husband most enjoy about ________ ?
11. How is he at helping out?
12. Is he able to spend enough time with you and the baby?
13. How are your other children doing?
14. Have there been any unusual or unexpected stresses (illness, death, separation) in the family since I last saw you?
15. Have you gone out socially since the baby was born?

Questions related to developmental progress should be asked at each visit. History regarding the child's developmental achievements is an important addition to in-office observation and formal developmental assessment. The developmental history helps the pediatrician evaluate the parents' awareness and perception of their infant's abilities.

Physical, Developmental, and Affective Assessment

The growth parameters of length, weight, and head circumference should be obtained and plotted on appropriate graphs at each visit. A complete physical examination should be done during each visit. Developmental and affective assessment should include observation of parent-child interaction, mutuality, and attachment; evaluation of the child's gross motor, fine motor, problem-solving, receptive/expressive language, self-help, social, and play skills; and the child's individuality and temperament patterns.

Table 5–6. SUGGESTED FORMAT FOR HEALTH PROMOTION 6 MONTH VISIT

A. Interview
   1. How are you? How are things going?
   2. Have there been any problems or concerns since your last visit? Sleeping through the night? Feeding problems?
   3. Do you get enough help in taking care of ________?
   4. Who takes care of ________ when you work?
   5. How do you and your husband share in taking care of ________?
   6. Is it easy for you to know what ________ wants?
   7. Would you describe one of ________'s typical days? How does ________ spend his/her time?
   8. Does ________ turn to sounds that originate from out of immediate sight? Play at making sounds alone or with others?
   9. Any unusual or unexpected family stresses/crises?

B. Physical/Developmental/Affective Assessment
   1. Plot weight, length, and head circumference. Share with family.
   2. Physical examination. Check for first tooth; observe for evidence of adequate vision and hearing.
   3. Observe parent-infant mutuality and attachment. Mutal gazing and vocal interaction; play games with each other; discrimination of strangers.
   4. Developmental assessment: Rolls both ways; pulls to sit without head lag; sits with support or leaning forward on hands when placed; bears some weight on lower extremities; transfers objects hand to hand by end of sixth month; indicates feelings of pleasure or eagerness; shows displeasure at loss of toy.

C. Immunizations: Ask about any previous reaction. DPT #3, OPV #3. Optional in geographical areas in which polio might be imported, e.g., some areas of southwest United States.

D. Anticipatory Guidance
   1. Nutrition: Stress continuation of breast milk and/or formula. Instruct regarding introduction of solids, beginning use of cup, allowing to finger feed as adequate reach and pincer grasp is gained, scheduling of four feedings per day.
   2. Accident prevention: Car restraints; check house for accident hazards and household poisons; hot liquids; falls off elevated surfaces; danger of walkers; gates on stairs and open windows; vulnerability of extremities to jerking; dangers of shaking; plastic plugs in outlets; tablecloths and electrical cords out of reach; supervise bath.

Table continued on opposite page.

Table 5–6. SUGGESTED FORMAT FOR HEALTH PROMOTION 6 MONTH VISIT *(Continued)*

3. Sleep: Counsel regarding management of night wakening.
4. Development: Stress developmental enrichment; toy suggestions and activities include bath toys, squeaky toys, string and paper to handle, play in front of mirror, nested plastic cups.
5. Other: Teething, encourage firm objects on which the infant may chew rather than use of over-the-counter topical anesthetics.

E. Closing the Visit: Other questions? Compliment. Set return appointment.

Anticipatory Guidance

Anticipatory guidance, which composes a large portion of the pediatric health promotion visit, involves discussion and counseling regarding aspects of child care and development so that parents might better manage common developmental and child-rearing issues. Timing of such guidance is important, as information must be presented prior to the age at which such issues might arise. Items that should be discussed include nutrition and feeding behavior, accident prevention, developmental stages and enrichment, sleep behavior, toilet training, discipline, and a variety of other general child care issues.

Nutrition and Feeding Behavior. There should be active encouragement of breast feeding as the optimal nutrition for infants. A commercially prepared formula is an acceptable alternative. During the newborn period a flexible rather than rigid schedule should be suggested. After 6 weeks to 2 months of age, a more consistent schedule can be expected. At 4 months most infants should have a predictable schedule of 4 to 5 feedings per day; at 6 months, 4 feedings per day; and at 9 months, 3 meals per day. Owing to different energy requirements among infants, the quantity of formula consumed per 24 hours is variable; however, 6 oz/kg/day serves as a guideline. An infant should be allowed to stop eating at the earliest signs of satiety and the habit of finishing each bottle discouraged.

Breast-fed infants should receive supplements of iron (7 mg/day), vitamin D (400 I.U./day), and fluoride (0.25 mg/day) even if the family lives in a community with fluoridated water. Infants fed commercially prepared, iron-fortified formulas require no supplements ex-

Table 5–7. SUGGESTED FORMAT FOR HEALTH PROMOTION 9 MONTH VISIT

A. Interview
1. How are things going? Problems/concerns? Breathholding, sleep problems?
2. Explore parents' adaptation to child's beginning autonomy and mobility. Does ___ keep you busy? How do you and your husband manage now that ______ is on the go? Does ______'s messiness with eating and the desire to feed himself cause any difficulties at mealtime?
3. What are some of ______'s new achievements?
4. Any unusual or unexpected family stresses/crises since your last visit?

B. Physical/Developmental/Affective Assessment
1. Plot weight, length, head circumference. Share with parents.
2. Physical exam.
3. Observe parent-infant interaction. Appropriate monitoring of motor activity with reasonable freedom to explore and anticipation of dangerous situations.
4. Observe infant's response to limit-setting, frustration level, persistence.
5. Developmental assessment: Sits steady indefinitely; creeps on hands and knees; crude purposeful release of toys; beginning pincer grasp; uncovers toys hidden by cloth (object permanence); "dada" and "mama" may be specific; comprehends "Bye Bye," "So big"; imitates tapping with hand.

C. Immunizations: Current?

D. Anticipatory Guidance
1. Nutrition: Warn about foods such as nuts and popcorn that might be aspirated. No added salt to foods fed infant. Discuss infant's normal decrease in appetite at this time. Encourage self-feeding skills, cup, spoon, finger foods. Three meals per day; no bottle to bed.
2. Accident prevention: Infant now extremely mobile and active. Review items covered last visit. Give syrup of Ipecac with instructions for its use if necessary. Provide phone number of poison control center. Discuss need for new toddler car restraint seat.
3. Sleep: Need for bedtime routine and constant bedtime. Anticipate night awakening, use of transitional objects (favorite toy or possession).
4. Development: Encourage parents to reinforce vocalizations and communication; play social games to develop interaction and imitation, encourage self-exploration by infant. Toys and activities include naming body parts, cloth books, stacking toys, blocks and container for in and out activity, containers that fit into each other, toy on a string.

Table continued on following page.

Table 5–7. SUGGESTED FORMAT FOR HEALTH PROMOTION 9 MONTH VISIT *(Continued)*

5. Other: Discuss discipline. Advise about limit setting through verbal "No" and physical controls.

E. Closing the Visit: Other questions? Compliment. Set return appointment.

cept fluoride (0.25 mg/day if fluoride content in local drinking water is less than 0.3 ppm). Solids should not be introduced until 4 to 6 months of age. Not more than one or two new foods should be introduced in the same week. After 6 months, when intake of foods other than formula amounts to 200 gm (1½ jars strained baby food), formula may be replaced by homogenized, vitamin D–fortified whole milk. A source of vitamin C is required when whole milk is fed. Milks of reduced fat content are not recommended (Forman et al., 1979).

At each visit the establishment of good eating behavior should be discussed with the parents. These include allowing the infant to stop feeding at the earliest signs of satiety, discouragement of taking a bottle to bed, consistent feeding schedule for the older infant and toddler, and allowing the child to develop feeding skills, e.g., cup at 6 months, finger foods at 8 to 9 months, spoon at 10 to 12 months.

Accident Prevention. Safety guidance discussion with parents should be reinforced with written information. In the early infancy period, the focus should be on crib safety, car safety, and prevention of falls and drownings.

Before the child becomes more mobile, parents must be aware of and limit the accident potentials in the house. These include electric outlets covered and electric cords in good repair and out of reach; use of mesh type gates on stairways and open windows; avoidance of small objects that might be aspirated; use of toys that have no small or detachable parts; breakable and sharp objects placed out of reach; use of a harness on highchairs; use of a playpen as a safe and convenient place to put the child when parents are busy; cleanser and other toxic products placed in locked cabinets; child-proof latches on cabinet doors; availability of syrup of Ipecac and poison control phone number; water temperature adjusted to less than 125°F, and turning pot handles to the center of the stove. No matter how much "accident proofing" is

Table 5–8. SUGGESTED FORMAT FOR HEALTH PROMOTION 12 MONTH VISIT

A. Interview
   1. How are you? How are things going?
   2. What problems/concerns have you had? Sleep problems? Separation problems? Temper tantrums? Breathholding spells? Developmental delay? Feeding problems?
   3. What are some of the new things your baby is doing? Cruising? Walking? New words? Feeding self?
   4. Who takes care of ________ when you are at work or when you and your husband go out?
   5. What do you and your husband enjoy most about ________ now?
   6. Does ________ enjoy other people?
   7. Any unusual or unexpected family stresses/crises since your last visit?

B. Physical/Developmental/Affective Assessment
   1. Plot weight, length, head circumference.
   2. Physical exam.
   3. Observe mother-infant mutuality and attachment. Note variety of maternal responses to infant.
   4. Developmental assessment: Cruising or walking alone; tries to build cube tower; 2–3 specific words; imitates words; puts one object inside another, precise pincer grasp.

C. Immunizations: Make sure they are up to date. Tuberculin skin test (if indicated in your practice).

D. Anticipatory Guidance
   1. Nutrition: Switch from formula to whole cow's milk and discourage use of 2% or skim milk. Vitamins no longer needed if eating good variety of solids. Continue to encourage use of cup and spoon. Discuss how little and how whimsically child may eat at this age.
   2. Accident prevention: Syrup of Ipecac on hand; telephone number of poison control center; poison-proofing of house; car seat restraint; containers of hot liquids kept out of reach.
   3. Sleep: Own bed and own room if possible. Consistent bedtime routine. Discourage reinforcing night wakening with play, feeding, taking into parents' bed.
   4. Development: Encourage speech development through naming objects and use of picture books. Encourage play alone and with parents and siblings. Discuss major spurt in autonomy and the need to allow child independence and exploration within safe environment. Toys and activities include blocks for stacking and building, naming body parts, smelling things, beginning imitation of adult activities, toy telephone, ball to roll back and forth.

Table continued on opposite page.

Table 5–8. SUGGESTED FORMAT FOR HEALTH PROMOTION 12 MONTH VISIT *(Continued)*

5. Other: Discuss parents' ideas about discipline. Stress positive reinforcement for good behavior; prohibitions few but firm; consistency. Discuss child's developing autonomy and independence with resultant normal oppositional behavior.

E. Closing the Visit: Other questions? Compliment. Set return appointment.

done, parents should be reminded that infants and toddlers need close supervision and at times of upset or change in routine of the family the risk is highest.

Sleep Behavior and Problems. The unpredictable sleep-wake cycles in the first several months of life can be very fatiguing for parents, and they should try to nap whenever the infant sleeps. By two months of age, the infant may be sleeping through the night and have better-defined wake-sleep cycles during the day. By four months of age, if possible, infants should be in their own bedroom so that parents are not disturbed by early morning awakening or night crying. Starting from four to six months of age infants might have night awakening and resistance to being put down to sleep. Parents should check on their baby's safety and comfort and then put the child back to bed. Parents should not develop the habits of taking the infant into their bed, offering nighttime feedings, and playing with the baby. As the infant gets older, parents should be encouraged to establish a regular bedtime and a standard bedtime routine. Parents should be warned about the problems an infant might have in settling down if overtired or overstimulated.

Toilet Training. A developmental approach to teaching toileting skills should be emphasized. Most children demonstrate readiness for learning toileting between 18 and 24 months of age, although it may be into the third and fourth year of life before training for bowel and bladder control is successful. At the fifteenth-month visit, the pediatrician should talk with parents about psychological and physiological readiness signs such as child's desire to please parents and imitate adults, adequate motor skills of sitting and walking well, and willingness and ability to communicate toileting urge and/or uncomfortableness with wet and soiled diapers. At the 18 month visit, steps for training can be outlined, such as introducing the potty chair, encouraging the child to sit on the potty chair

Table 5–9. SUGGESTED FORMAT FOR HEALTH PROMOTION 15 MONTH VISIT

A. Interview
1. How are things going? Any problems or concerns? Temper tantrums? Breathholding? Sleep difficulties? Concerns about managing activity and demanding behavior?
2. Support systems? Help caring for baby?
3. Do you and your husband generally agree on how to manage ________'s behavior?
4. What changes have you seen in development? Walking? Additional words? Jargon?
5. Return to work? Child care?
6. Any unusual or unexpected family stresses/crises?

B. Physical/Developmental/Affective Assessment
1. Plot weight, length, head circumference.
2. Physical exam. Discuss toeing-in, toeing-out with parents.
3. Parent-child mutuality and attachment. Is parent affectionate or distant; overindulgent or overstrict; gives contradictory messages ("Do it," "Don't do it")? Does parent exhibit confidence in ability to care for child and express reasonable pleasure in parenthood.
4. Infant overactive or underactive, easily excited or overstimulated, shy or fearful?
5. Developmental assessment: Walks well alone; builds tower of 2 cubes; scribbles spontaneously and demonstrates incipient imitation stroke; 4–6 word vocabulary; uses jargon; shows shoe on request; pats pictures in book and definitely attends; indicates wants by pointing or vocalizing.

C. Immunizations: Review results of tuberculin skin test. Give MMR.

D. Anticipatory Guidance
1. Nutrition: Continue to stress self-feeding and use of a cup and spoon. Review that nutritional requirements are quite minimal and children this age are typically picky eaters. Stress discontinuation of bottle. Remind parents of dangers of certain foods such as nuts, popcorn, and chewing gum, which might be aspirated.
2. Accident prevention: Instructions provided during previous visit should again be reviewed.
3. Toilet training: Discuss with parents that most infants are not developmentally prepared to begin toilet training until 18–24 months. Discuss indicators of readiness for toilet training and encourage parents to defer at this time.
4. Development: Increase in imitative behaviors such as sweeping, dusting, play with dishes and dolls. Toys might include stuffed animals, small cars, pull toys, books. Activities include teaching body parts; drawing and imitating strokes; chasing and "roughhouse" play.

E. Closing the Visit: Other questions? Compliment. Set return appointment.

Table 5–10. SUGGESTED FORMAT FOR HEALTH PROMOTION 18 MONTH VISIT

A. Interview
   1. How are things going? Problems or concerns? "Negativitism"? Temper tantrums? Hitting behavior? Activity level? Development?
   2. How are you managing his behavior? Do you and your husband agree on expectations and management?
   3. How does ________ spend his day?
   4. Return to work? Child care?
   5. Any unusual or unexpected family stresses/crises?

B. Physical/Developmental/Affective Assessment
   1. Plot weight, length, head circumference.
   2. Physical exam.
   3. Parent-infant mutuality and attachment. Increase in stranger anxiety at this age signifies continued importance of attachment.
   4. Assess parents' view of child's behavioral style and the predictability of child's responses to certain situations.
   5. Developmental assessment: Hurls ball; climbs into adult chair; builds tower of 3–4 cubes; looks selectively at pictures in book and identifies one; vocabulary of 10 words but it is not abnormal if only mothers can understand them; names several body parts; turns pages in book.

C. Immunizations: Ask about any previous reactions. DPT #4, OPV #4. Review common side effects.

D. Anticipatory Guidance
   1. Nutrition: Minimal nutritional requirements at this age. Parents should not get into battles with their child over eating. Continue to encourage self-feeding skills.
   2. Accident prevention: Car safety restraints should always be used. This includes adults as well, as they provide good models for the child. Warn regarding unsupervised play by child around street or driveway.
   3. Toilet training: Discuss developmental approach to toilet training.
   4. Development: Toys and activities might include small jars and screw caps; a case for carrying things in; popbeads; rough and tumble play; reading stores to; assigning little chores to do; toys which the child can take apart and build with.
   5. Other: Discuss the child's use of a favorite toy as a security blanket and thumbsucking as age-appropriate behavior and a manner in which the child handles developmental tensions at this age of development.

E. Closing the Visit: Other questions? Compliment. Set return appointment.

Table 5–11. SUGGESTED FORMAT FOR HEALTH PROMOTION 24 MONTH VISIT

A. Interview
   1. How are you? How are things going?
   2. Have there been any problems or concerns? Negativism? Resistive behavior? Temper tantrums? Separation anxiety? Development?
   3. How is your husband? Do both of you agree in your management of ________'s discipline? How are the siblings doing?
   4. What is a typical day like for ________? (Review activities and interactions in 24-hour period.)
   5. What do you and your husband enjoy most about ________? What do you find most difficult about ________'s care?
   6. Return to work? Child care?
   7. Any unusual or unexpected family stresses/crises?

B. Physical/Developmental/Affective Assessment
   1. Plot weight, length, head circumference.
   2. Physical exam.
   3. Parent-child interactions.
   4. Child's temperament: Stress wide variation among normal children in the achievement of impulse control.
   5. Developmental assessment: Mastery of language a major objective. "What's this" or "What's that" labeling questions frequent. Walks up and down stairs alone or holding rail; jumps off floor with both feet; stands on one foot momentarily; executes circular strokes; uses 3-word sentence with pronouns such as I, me, you.

C. Immunizations: Review to be sure they are up to date.

D. Anticipatory Guidance
   1. Nutrition: Should be handling spoon and cup well. Remind parents not to get into battles or struggles surrounding mealtime.
   2. Accident prevention: Review previous visit discussion.
   3. Toilet training: Discuss progress with parents and advise regarding any problems encountered.
   4. Development: Parallel play predominates, with child engaging mainly in solitary play. Discuss development of capacity for interactive play that will emerge over next year. Stress importance of child's learning through both structured and imaginative play. Encourage parents to limit TV.
   5. Other: Touching genitalia is often a concern at this age and its normalcy should be stressed. Instruction to child in the use of toothbrush and need to schedule dental appointment.

E. Closing the Visit: Other questions? Compliment. Set return appointment.

fully clothed and later with diapers off, changing diapers on the potty chair and dropping them into the pot, and the use of training pants. Parents should be encouraged to have a flexible and relaxed approach while communicating a consistent and positive attitude that this is a skill they expect the child to gain. Parents should not force the child to sit on the pot or punish the child for accidents. The parents should be informed that the child may not be trained until 2½ to 3½ years of age. If a child is not trained by 4 to 5 years of age, there may be significant parent-child interaction problems, and the parents may be having difficulty encouraging and supporting limit-setting in other areas of the child's life.

Discipline. The pediatrician should help parents understand that discipline is a form of teaching and guidance with the goal of helping children gain self-control, respect the rights of others, learn the rules by which society operates, and choose behaviors appropriate to particular situations. At the nine-month visit the pediatrician should begin discussing discipline with the parents. Limit-setting, restriction of movement, and saying "No" are necessary to protect infants and young children. Parents should not expect their child to accept such limitations without protest and resentment. The importance of consistency, limited but definite rules, parent models of self-control and appropriate behavior, and praising correct behavior should be stressed. Parents should be reminded that young children might need many trials to learn appropriate behavior. Parents should learn to anticipate and avoid unnecessary conflict situations, i.e., put valuable and breakable articles out of toddler's reach for a while rather than constantly saying "No." Corporal punishment should be discouraged.

Closing the Visit

As each visit comes to a close, the pediatrician should inquire if the parents have anything else they would like to ask about. Sometimes the discussion during the visit will bring additional questions or concerns to mind; however, if major issues are expressed, then additional time should be scheduled rather than responding hurriedly and inadequately. The parents should be appropriately complimented regarding their child care. The pediatrician should reinforce his/her availability if needed and a time should be set for the next appointment.

REFERENCES

Brazelton, T.B., Parker, W. B., and Zuckerman, B.: Importance of behavioral assessment of the neonate. Curr. Prob. Pediatr., Vol. 7, 1976.

Canny, C. R., and Leventhal, J. M.: The pediatric prenatal visit: A questionnaire survey. J. Devel. Behav. Pediatr., 3:29, 1982.

Committee on Genetics, American Academy of Pediatrics: New issues in newborn screening for phenylketonuria and congenital hypothyroidism. Pediatrics, 69:104, 1982.

Dworkin, P. H. (Ed.): Pediatric Group Practice Manual of Anticipatory Guidance. Department of Pediatrics, West Virginia University School of Medicine.

Fazen, L. E., and Felizberto, P. I.: Baby walker inquiries. Pediatrics, 70:106, 1982.

Fomon, S. J., Filer, L. J., Anderson, T. A., and Ziegler, E. E.: Recommendations for feeding normal infants. Pediatrics, 63:52, 1979.

Greenberg, J. W., Rice, H. W., and Rice, R.: Postpartum education: A pilot study of pediatric and maternal perceptions. J. Devel. Behav. Pediatr., 2:44, 1981.

Greensher, J., and Mofenson, H.: Emergency treatment of the choking child. Pediatrics, 70:110, 1982.

Growing Child. Lafayette, Ind., Dunn and Hargitt, Inc., 1978.

Guidelines for Health Supervision of Children and Youth: American Academy of Pediatrics. Committee on Practice and Ambulatory Medicine. News and Comments (AAP), Vol. 33, No. 6, June, 1982.

Health Supervision Packages: American Academy of Pediatrics Committee on the Psychological Aspects of Child and Family Health. In press.

Hill, R. M.: Breast Feeding. Evanston, Ill., American Academy of Pediatrics, 1981.

Lawrence, R. A.: Breast Feeding: A guide for the Medical Profession. St. Louis, The C. V. Mosby Company, 1980.

Mondell, M. D., and Yoyman, M. W.: Developmental aspects of well child office visits. J. Devel. Behav. Pediatr., 3:118, 1982.

Osborn, L. M., Metcalf, T. J., and Mariani, E. M.: Hygienic care in uncircumcised infants. Pediatrics, 67:365, 1981.

Reinhart, J. B.: The physician's approach to bowel training. J. Devel. Behav. Pediatr., 2:61–63, 1981.

Report of the Committee on Infectious Diseases (The Red Book). Evanston, Ill., American Academy of Pediatrics, 1982.

Schmitt, B. D.: Infants who do not sleep through the night. J. Devel. Behav. Pediatr., 2:20, 1981.

Weiss, J., DeJong, A., Packer, E., and Bonanni, L.: Purchasing infant shoes: Attitudes of parents, pediatricians, and store managers. Pediatrics, 76:718, 1981.

Wessel, M. A.: The pediatrician and corporal punishment. Pediatrics, 66:639, 1980.

6

HEALTH PROMOTION IN PRESCHOOL AGE CHILDREN

Patrick H. Casey, M.D.

The preschool period, between 18 and 60 months of age, is marked by striking maturation in physical, cognitive, emotional, and social skills. Table 6–1 lists the major achievements for toddlers and preschool age children and the goals for parents of children in this age group. The goals of health promotion visits are to assess children's physical and developmental health, to prevent problems in these areas, and to promote future well-being with counseling and anticipatory guidance. Because evidence has accumulated that positive outcomes in most developmental spheres are related to constructive parent-child interactions in the early years of life, the clinical focus for health promotion in this chapter is the enhancement of the quality of parent-child interactions, accommodating for individual differences. Pediatricians' awareness of the temperamental style of their patients; the parents' style, emotional status, and living situation; and how these factors affect the parent-child interaction is useful during health promotion visits.

Table 6–2 presents the clinical content areas that will be discussed in this chapter. Two separate schedules for age and content of health promotion visits are presented. The basic health promotion schedule is designed for children considered to be at low risk for health, developmental, or behavioral problems. Such children have normal past medical histories and parents who have demonstrated the ability to meet their children's needs in the first 18 months of life. The supplemented schedule is suggested for children and/or families who are considered at increased risk for health, developmental, or behavioral difficulties. This group includes children who have had a significant or a potentially significant medical event such as premature birth, meningitis, or hyperbilirubinemia. Also included in this group are families who have experienced problems meeting their children's needs in the early months of life or who have a higher risk of such problems in the future. Such families include single parents, families of limited economic means, families of divorce, parents with a psychoemotional need or habit disorder, etc. However defined, this group may have problems in parent-child interactions resulting from vulnerabilities in either the parent or child, or both, which may ultimately result in problems in child health, development, or behavior.

An important question for clinicians is how to utilize their personal time most effectively to motivate parents to change their own health behavior. Since physician counseling in specific areas such as accident prevention and nutrition has been shown to be more effective than other types of health education, it is important that the physician provide personal counseling in the areas of greatest age relevance. Alternative educational approaches must be utilized in other clinical areas owing to time constraints. These approaches may include group sessions with parents, distribution of written materials, and audiovisual instructional resources such as videotapes for viewing in the clinical setting. Parent group sessions for interested parents may be a useful way to provide detailed information regarding specific clinical areas as a follow-up to audiovisual educational efforts.

Table 6–1. MAJOR ACHIEVEMENTS OF PRESCHOOL AGE

Children

1. Achieve developmentally appropriate activities of daily living, e.g., toilet training, dressing
2. Achieve normal language maturity
3. Tolerate separations and develop a sense of control of their world
4. Begin to acquire socialization skills, ethical values, and impulse control

Parents

1. Promote appropriate training and practices
2. Encourage speech and other learning
3. Assist development of appropriate socialization
4. Set standards for acceptable conduct
5. Respect child's sense of individuality and identity

Table 6–2. CLINICAL CONTENT AREAS OF PRESCHOOL HEALTH SUPERVISION

Health Assessment
1. Areas of historical concern
2. Physical examination

Problem Prevention
1. Screening for problems not clinically obvious
2. Active prevention with immunization

Health Promotion
1. Parent-child interaction
2. Accident
3. Nutrition
4. Dental care
5. Development and behavior
6. Life style

This chapter provides suggestions regarding health education efforts in the different clinical areas.

The following recommendations are based primarily on recommendations developed by the American Academy of Pediatrics.

RECOMMENDED SCHEDULES

The suggested basic and supplemented health promotion schedules for preschool children between 18 and 60 months of age are presented in Table 6–3. Although the American Academy of Pediatrics currently recommends visits at 18, 24, 36, 48, and 60 months for all children, the following recommendations modify these slightly in order to allow flexibility in health supervision planning according to the individual status of the child and the child's family. Visits are recommended at 18 or 24, 42, and 60 months in the basic schedule for children in families considered at minimal risk for problems of health, development, and behavior. For children and/or families considered at "increased" risk for such problems, visits are recommended at 18, 24, 30, 36, 48, and 60 months in the supplemented schedule, or more often if necessary. The table suggests how clinicians might expend their personal efforts to cover the clinical areas of concern. In the supplemented health promotion schedule, for example, a brief history and physical examination are recommended at the 18- and 30-month visits, along with personal counseling regarding parent-child interaction, accident prevention, and nutrition and dental health. At the 24- and 36-month visits a more thorough history and physical evaluation are recommended, along with personal counseling on normal developmental expectations and problems. The shortened physical examination provides the extra clinical time as well as the hands-on-the-child entrée into conversation regarding the child's interactional style.

CLINICAL CONTENT

Health Assessment

Identifying Areas of Concern in the History

Most toddlers have had a baseline complete medical history performed by the age of 18 to 24 months. The health promotion interview in this period is thus an effort to assess interval problems and progress and to identify current concerns. Information regarding the child's health status and concerns regarding development and behavior are best obtained by first asking several open-ended questions. The quality of the parent-physician communication established in these open-ended conversations may determine the adequacy of the history and the success of the over-all management plan.

Table 6–4 lists questions that may be asked during a brief history. Interval illness history, current living situation, eating patterns, the child's behavior with adults and peers, and particular developmental or behavioral concerns are elicited by the health clinician. This initial aspect of the health promotion visit should require no more than six to eight minutes. These specific questions overlap with the physical examination and save clinical time.

Physical Examination

Studies demonstrate that pediatricians still devote a majority of their time in child health supervision to the physical examination; however, multiple clinical reports have documented that routine yearly complete physical examinations have an extremely low yield. Still, benefits may be derived from the physical examination in terms of family expectations and satisfaction. In the basic schedule brief physical examinations at the 18- or 24-month and 42-month visit, and a "complete" physical examination at the 60-month visit are adequate. The supplemented schedule suggests a "complete" physical examination at 24, 36, 48, and 60 months, and a shortened examination at 18 and 30 months of age. The actual content of the examination will vary depending upon the history.

A child's growth over time, monitored by uniformly obtained height and weight measurements plotted on standardized growth charts,

Table 6–3. CLINICIAN EFFORT IN CHILD HEALTH SUPERVISION

Supplemental Schedule	Basic Schedule
18 Months Brief history and physical exam Personal counseling Parent-child interaction Nutrition Dental health Accident prevention	*18 to 24 months* Complete history and brief physical exam Personal counseling Parent-child interaction Nutrition Accident prevention Development and behavior
24 Months Complete history and physical exam Personal counseling Development and behavior	*42 Months* Complete history and brief physical exam Personal counseling Parent-child interaction Nutrition Accident prevention Development and behavior
30 Months Brief history and physical exam Personal counseling Parent-child interaction Nutrition Dental health Accident prevention	*60 Months* Complete history and complete physical exam Personal counseling Parent-child interaction Nutrition Accident prevention Development and behavior
36 Months Complete history and physical exam Personal counseling Development and behavior	
48 Months Complete history and physical exam Personal counseling Parent-child interaction Nutrition Development and behavior	
60 Months Complete history and physical exam Personal counseling Nutrition Accident prevention Development and behavior	

is the best screening assessment for the child's overall physical well-being. These data can be collected at all visits by health assistants. Other specific aspects of a brief examination include visualization of both tympanic membranes for serous otitis media and assessment of vision, hearing, eye alignment, teeth, and genitalia. Minor orthopedic deformities are commonly found on routine evaluations. Although these deformities are usually of little clinical importance and require no specific therapy, they create parental concern that can often be alleviated by discussion. Neurodevelopmental assessment includes neurological examination and awareness of the quality of gross motor and fine motor style such as clumsiness, the quality of the child's language, and the child's behavioral style, activity level, and ability to follow directions. Frequent routine examination of the heart and lungs with stethoscope is more of an expected ritual than a useful assessment device if there have been no abnormalities found during the first year of life. The situational context of the physical examination allows clinical assessment of the quality of the parent-child interaction. The relationship between the parents and child, the way they react to the examination, the parental presence during the examination, the warmth of interaction and age appropriateness of language used by the parent, and the hygiene and dress of the child are assessed by the child health clinician.

The physical examination should require only a few minutes of the child health clinician's time for a partial examination and no more than five minutes for the complete evaluation. The examination should usually overlap with history interview, anticipatory guidance, and counseling.

Problem Prevention

Screening

Vision. Visual problems are the most common abnormality detected in routine physical exams of preschool age children. Careful screening by the clinician is required prior to the age of three using fixation patterns. After this age, a health assistant can utilize a Snellen Illiterate E chart or a Titmus tester at each scheduled visit. Any significant difference in acuity between eyes or vision less than 20-40 requires an ophthalmological evaluation. Color vision may be evaluated at the 60-month visit using the Titmus tester.

Hearing. Hearing problems are commonly detected in routine examinations of preschool children. Screening pure tone audiometry should be performed by office personnel at scheduled visits beginning at age three to four, depending on the maturity of the child. Tympanometry should be performed in the presence of mild conductive hearing loss.

Laboratory Evaluation. Few routine laboratory screening tests are required in the preschool child. Hemoglobin determinations and sickle cell tests are necessary only if not done prior to 18 months.

Lead poisoning occurs most commonly in children aged 18 months through five years. Because of the accumulating evidence that subclinical elevations in blood lead levels may be associated with developmental and behavioral problems, children who live in homes with pre–World War II paint or near lead smelters should be screened at least yearly using the free erythrocyte protoporphyrin (FEP) test.

Routine urinalysis, although frequently performed, has been found to yield very little new or treatable disease. Routine screening recommendations for tuberculosis detection vary according to the prevalence in the community.

Developmental Assessment. Many experienced clinicians assess development by direct observation of the child's behavior. Examples of developmental skills are provided in the clinical tables. A step-wise screening procedure utilizing standardized developmental screening tests objectifies the screening approach to identify as many children as possible who suffer from developmental problems while avoiding the false labeling of those who are normal. This approach is preferable for most clinicians. The Denver Pre-Screening Developmental Questionnaire (PDQ) is recommended for developmental screening in the basic health promotion schedule at 18 or 24 months and at 42 months. In the PDQ the parent answers ten "yes-no" questions at each age. If a child has six or fewer passes, a more complete developmental screening test should be performed. In the supplemented health promotion schedule, the PDQ is recommended at 18 and 30 months of age. The Denver Developmental Screening Test (DDST) is recommended at 24, 36, 48, and 60 months for this higher-risk group. These well-standardized screening tools provide reasonably valid results, and they offer a clear course for the clinician when abnormalities are detected. Although this DDST can be performed by office personnel, approximately 20 minutes is normally required for its completion. A shortened, revised version of the DDST is currently under study, and developmental screening may be even simpler if this DDST-R is found to be acceptable. Other screening approaches, like the recently published successful simultaneous use of visual assessment and developmental observations, may require modification of screening recommendation in the future.

Some precautions need to be emphasized regarding these developmental screening procedures. First, clinicians must not overinterpret their results and utilize diagnostic labels on the basis of these screening instruments alone. Children identified as abnormal on these tests require further diagnostic assessments. Second, some children may demonstrate marked discrepancies in different aspects of development. Children who show significant delays in a single area of development, such as language, should have further assessment promptly.

Speech-Articulation. Overall language development is monitored with the developmental screening test described above. Particular note should be made of the child's ability to formulate words correctly. Articulation problems are commonly seen in children with other minor developmental difficulties. Eighty to 90 per cent of the speech of a three-year-old child should be intelligible, and 100 per cent of a four-year-old child's speech should be understood by a stranger. Any child over three years of age whose daily speech is not easily understood should be evaluated by a speech pathologist. Although screening instruments like the Denver Articulation Screening Exam and the Physicians' Developmental Quick Screening for Speech Disorders (a second PDQ) are available, they are not as well validated as the DDST.

School Readiness. The decision as to whether a five-year-old child is "ready" for school is best made with an awareness of the child's and family's progress over the preceding years. Children of low medical and social risk who have demonstrated normal developmental progress in the past, whose families have met their needs, and who are age-appropriate on the DDST at age five should be expected to perform adequately at school.

Children at "increased" risk for developmental problems require careful review at five years of age. Subtle developmental deviations often can be detected at this time. The child's and the family's developmental and behavioral history should be reviewed in the context of current functioning as documented by the DDST. Social skills such as self-care, separation from parents, and peer interaction are assessed. Fine motor skills measured by copying a square and drawing a man of at least six parts are documented. Gross motor and language skills are likewise assessed utilizing the DDST. Adequate short-term memory, selective attention, and the ability to handle instructions efficiently are other areas important to school success that can be assessed in an office visit.

Although several "readiness" tests are available, none has been adequately validated. The new Pediatric Examination of Education Readiness (PEER) evaluates developmental attainment, processing efficiency, and neurological maturation along with behavioral adaptation, patterns of activity level, and attention control. Although preliminary validation studies of the PEER are encouraging, the time required to complete this instrument will limit its routine clinical utility. Most health clinicians will judge "school readiness" based on current overall developmental functioning in the context of past medical history and developmental progress. Combinations of subtle developmental deviations, such as problems in articulation, fine motor skill, and behavioral control can result in performance problems in school. Severe problems in any of these areas may require specific therapeutic approaches, such as speech or occupational therapy. It is uncommon that "waiting another year" is the most appropriate approach in children with such problems. Often the extra supports available with school entry justify the initiation of schooling at the age-appropriate time.

Immunization

Diphtheria-pertussis-tetanus (DPT) toxoid with trivalent oral polio virus (TOPV) vaccine should be administered at 18 months and four to six years of age. The measles-mumps-rubella (MMR) vaccine may be administered concomitantly with the DPT and TOPV boosters to children who are out of step with the recommended immunization schedule (see Chap. 4).

Health Promotion: Anticipatory Guidance and Counseling

Parent-Child Interaction

Counseling and guidance during health promotion visits focus primarily on improving the appropriateness and the responsive quality and quantity of the parent-child interaction. This approach is particularly relevant in the preschool age group, since there is no set of "parenting" instructions or rules that is appropriate for all parents and children as they deal with discipline, autonomous behavior of two-year-olds, toilet training, and numerous other age-related tasks. This approach does not attempt to enforce a narrow set of beliefs or a collection of rules on parents. Rather, an attempt is made to accommodate the individuality of the child, the parents, and their living situation while providing guidelines regarding behavioral interactions. A competent parent-child pair provide each other with specific behaviors that are consistent, readable, and mutually responsive. A responsive interaction is exemplified by a situation in which a child offers a comment and the parent hears and responds in an appropriate way. If such experiences occur consistently over time, both the child and parent become comfortable with their ability to signal and interpret the other effectively. In general, this clinical approach attempts to improve parental skills in reading their child's behavior and to foster sensitivity and appropriate responsiveness to this behavior.

Counseling regarding parent-child interaction in this age group is guided by the general principles of child development that parents need to provide love with emotional and physical support, responsiveness, restriction when necessary, and stimulation. The following are the specific goals that the clinician can use for each parent-child pair to improve the parent-child interaction: (1) ensure that the parents understand normal childhood development and normal variations of development for each age; (2) help the parents understand the individuality of their toddler; (3) promote the parents' awareness of the child's social skills; (4) encourage parental responsiveness to the positive social behaviors, and support their responsibility to control and eliminate negative behaviors; (5) enhance the parents' feelings of confidence and competence to promote their children's health and development.

The first goal is met by describing age-related expectations for development and behavior. For example, at the 24-month visit a major developmental transition is the confrontational style with which toddlers explore their autonomy and the limits of control of their environment. The stubbornness, whining, temper tantrums, and other similar behavior of this age are explained in the context of their developmental meaning. The notion of childhood "temperament" can be used here to describe variations of these expected behaviors. The next goals are achieved by exploring the occurrence of positive social behaviors like smiling, talking, social interaction with adults and peers, and cooperativeness and by encouraging direct social responsiveness to these behaviors when they occur. This direct response increases the likelihood that these positive behaviors will occur more frequently, which in turn increases the parents' positive feelings and responsiveness toward the child. This creates a cycle of positive feedback and reward between parent and child. Although parents and families vary in determining what is not acceptable, all families need skills to manage negative behaviors typical of preschool children. Skills in managing children's behavior may be learned from written materials but in many cases will require clinical counseling. Whatever the method used, management of these negative behaviors should occur in the context of the ongoing positive emotional and physical support described earlier. The final clinical goal is to promote the parents' feelings of confidence in interacting with their child and their sense of ability to have a positive effect on their child's health and behavior. This is achieved by direct counseling from the health clinician and by positive feedback regarding the positive health and developmental course of the child. This counseling approach is modified according to the child's age and the developmental expectations of that age.

Counseling regarding parent-child interaction generally requires some degree of continuity of physician-family contact over time in order to accommodate successfully to the individuality of the pair. This effort requires personal physician time but overlaps with the physical examination and guidance in other clinical areas. Related information such as normal age-related development and behavioral control can be conveyed with books and pamphlets. Parent groups have been shown to improve parent-child interaction when interested parents are involved.

Nutrition and Dental Health

The goals of normal nutrition are to produce an adequately, not excessively, nourished child whose diet contains all the essential nutrients provided in a reasonable distribution of fat, carbohydrate, and protein. Topics of age-appropriate clinical relevance for nutrition and dental care are listed in the clinical tables. For children followed in the basic health promotion schedule with no demonstrated clinical problems, the clinician may spend only moments emphasizing the importance of adequate nutrition and dental care and urging parents to follow diet recommendations and dental care advice provided in written materials or audiovisual presentations.

Audiovisual presentations may be particularly useful for education in appropriate dental care.

A different approach is suggested for children followed in the supplemented health promotion schedule. At the 18-, 30-, and 48-month visits, after the discussion regarding parent-child interaction, the health clinician should personally counsel the family regarding issues listed in the clinical tables when appropriate for the individual child and parent. For example, the association of childhood obesity and adult obesity is fairly well documented. Discussions regarding obesity prevention at 18 and 30 months are necessary for children with excess weight gain or for families in which obesity is prevalent. Presentations about the normal balanced diet and the importance of meals at regularly scheduled times as social events, as opposed to unsupervised snacking throughout the day, are provided personally when necessary. Discussions about the use of fluoride and proper dental care are presented at 18, 30, 48, and 60 months when necessary. Appropriate written material should be available for distribution at the 24- and 36-month visit when personal clinician time is not expended.

The decision to utilize personal time and counseling in these areas must be individualized according to the child's and family's needs. Problems such as children's behaviors and appetite, mealtime behavior, and the normal loss of appetite are handled with counseling similar to that of the parent-child interaction.

Accident Prevention

Accident prevention is an important clinical area in contemporary health promotion. A carefully planned effort to educate parents regarding the importance of this problem and to motivate them to change their behavior in accident prevention is required. In the preschool age child, motor vehicle accidents are the most common cause of mortality, followed by burns, water-related accidents, falls, and poisonings. By the age of five, pedestrian accidents, bicycle accidents, and firearm injuries increase in incidence. Boys are more often victims of accidents. Toddlers who are very active, curious, and daring are at increased risk. Families stressed by divorce, job tension, interadult pressures, lack of environmental organization, poverty, and other problems are also at increased risk for childhood accidents.

The clinical tables provide suggestions for anticipatory guidance regarding accident prevention at age-related visits. In the basic schedule, the clinician educates the parents regarding the importance of accidents to overall childhood mortality and about specific age-related accidents. Encouragement is provided to alter health behaviors according to the detailed information provided in written handouts.

Clinicians should spend more personal time describing the details of age-related accident prevention at 18, 30, and 48 months for children followed in the supplemented health promotion schedule. Details of appropriate automobile restraint use should be reviewed at 18 and 30 months. Information regarding different brands of automobile seats, their cost, and where they may be obtained should be available. A review of household accidents such as kitchen scaldings and poisonings should occur, accompanied by recommendations for their prevention. At 48 months accident counseling focuses on the use of standard car seat belts and the increased incidence of pedestrian, bicycle, and drowning deaths. Appropriate written materials and/or audiovisual aids are used at the 24-month and 36-month visit.

Counseling regarding the parent-child interaction provides important background to accident prevention. An effective parent-child interaction decreases the environmental risk for accidents as a result of better parental awareness of the child's developmental and temperamental status and better responsivity to the child. Problems that arise in accident prevention efforts (like keeping a child buckled in a car restraint or special alertness to accidents during times of family illness or stress) can often be dealt with in the discussion of the parent-child interaction and personal temperament.

Development and Behavior

The clinician's task is to promote wellness and prevent problems. The clinical approach that attempts to foster the mutually adapted parent-child interaction over time is probably the most effective approach for clinicians to promote wellness and prevent problems in the areas of development and behavior. Central to this approach is the need for parents to understand normal development in order to maintain appropriate expectations for their preschool children. This has been presented in the discussion on parent-child interaction. Two related general areas regarding parents' effect on development and behavior are important and should be dealt with. First, the developmental psychology literature has unequivocally documented that the quality of stimulation provided personally by parents and the structure of their physical environment has an impact on children's developmental outcomes. Parents need to be made aware of this fact. Secondly, several surveys have documented that 15 to 40 per cent of parents of preschool age children have concerns regarding behavior problems. In contrast, only a small percentage of these are typically brought to the attention of clinicians. Caution is urged for clinicians in these areas. Since no "parenting approach" to discipline and child-rearing is known which inevitably results in more optimal behavioral outcomes, general guidance in this regard should be cautious and should be based on characteristics of the child, the parents, and their living situation. Also, there is little indication that minor behavioral deviations in preschool age children increase the likelihood of later behavior problems.

Parents of children followed in the basic health promotion schedule receive personal counseling regarding normal developmental expectations at each visit. This occurs during the counseling aimed at improving parent-child interaction. The need for information regarding developmental stimulation should be emphasized and provided in written materials. Examples of parent play activities for developmental stimulation are provided in the clinical tables. Several books are available for parents, and age-related handouts can be synthesized from these if necessary. A list of several of the most common age-related behavioral concerns is provided in the clinical tables. If behavior problems are a matter of parental concern, they should have been identified during the initial open-ended interview or counseling regarding parent-child interaction. The appropriate management of these problems should take into account the quality of the parent-child interaction and the family situation. If there are no significant problems in these areas, personal counseling and/or books for parents regarding behavior modification techniques and simple parenting approaches to minor behavioral concerns should be provided.

Parents of children followed in the supplemented health promotion schedule receive personal counseling regarding normal developmental expectations, developmental stimulation, and common behavioral concerns at the 24-, 36-, 48-, and 60-month visits. Because children followed in this schedule are at "increased" risk for developmental and behavioral problems, more time is allotted at the 24- and 36-month visits for counseling in these areas, while the 18- and 30-month visits focus specifically on other health promotion topics. While the general approach to these areas is the same as that described for the basic health promotion schedule, more time is used describing normal developmental stages, the importance of the parents "teaching" style and the quality of the physical environment to children's development, and the management of minor behavioral problems.

Guidance with this approach, overlapping with counseling regarding parent-child interaction, should require only a few minutes in the basic health promotion schedule and perhaps a few minutes more in the supplemented schedule. This time framework will be adequate to identify those problem situations that may require separate appointment time for more in-depth management or referral.

Life Style

The importance of life-style habits to current mortality and morbidity is striking. Improper health habits such as overnutrition leading to obesity and excess dietary salt and lipids, excessive cigarette and alcohol use, and lack of exercise are known to increase significantly the risk of the four major causes of adult deaths—heart disease, cancer, stroke, and accidents. Some life-style problems, such as exposure to environmental toxins and smoking, can impact directly on childhood mortality and morbidity.

Approaches available to effect changes in life style involve educating children regarding these risks in order to encourage them to take greater control of their own health and similarly educating their parents. Because parents are the primary means of access to preschool age children for health education, parents should be made aware of the importance of the role model they provide for their children and how that model may impact on their children's current and long-term physical health. Owing to the lack of adequate knowledge regarding health education in these areas, each child health clinician must determine the approach in this clinical area based on his or her personal medical philosophy and practice style. One aspect of life style is the appropriate use of medical providers. Some families overutilize health care, making clinic visits for minor ailments or medicalizing nonphysical problems, while others inappropriately underutilize medical care. Education regarding life style includes instructions regarding how and when to use medical providers with minor and major acute disease and how to benefit from scheduled child health supervision visits. Parental attitudes and beliefs about health care and their child's illness susceptibility affect the frequency of medical visits.

Table 6–4. HEALTH SUPERVISION: 18 TO 24 MONTHS

Interview
- A. How are things going for you? How is your family?
- B. Have there been any problems with __________'s health?
- C. Have there been any problems with __________'s development or behavior?
- D. How is __________ eating? How often? How much?
- E. Have there been any major stresses or crises in the family?
- F. What are some of __________'s new achievements?
- G. How does __________ spend his day?
- H. Is __________ willing to be separated from you? Can __________ play alone for several minutes when you are out of sight?
- I. Are you working? Who takes care of __________ while you are at work?
- J. Do you get out by yourself occasionally?

Physical Examination and DPT and OPV Booster

Screening
- A. Hematocrit and sickle screen if not done earlier
- B. Lead (FEP) and TB (PPD) in endemic areas
- C. Development
  - PDQ: Basic schedule
  - DDST: Supplemented schedule at 24 months

Developmental Assessment
- A. Parent-infant interaction based on interview, observation, or both
  1. The competent parent is affectionate, consistent, confident in ability to care for child, excited about and supportive of child's emerging abilities and skills, expresses reasonable pleasure in parenthood, is able to read the needs of the child as expressed through his behavior, makes complimentary statements about the child, admires and encourages his autonomy and initiative, copes well with stress and frustration, and can set limits effectively. Parents to be concerned about are those who are distant, overindulgent, overcritical, overcontrolling, intrusive, overwhelming, give contradictory messages, are insecure, anxious, unavailable, unencouraging, withdrawn from the child, and disorganized by stress.
  2. The competent child demonstrates a variety of affects and behaviors such as pleasure, anger, protest, joy, warmth, assertiveness, interest in exploration, loving, interest in new experiences, and ability to be separate from parents. The competent child plays alone in the waiting room, explores away from parent, goes to parent if threatened, and initiates move for affection. Toddlers to be concerned about are those who seem "out of control," noncommunicative, very passive or withdrawn, highly negativistic, demanding, stubborn, and fail to initiate activities.
  3. Evaluate physician-child interaction. Child independent or clinging; pleasant or irritating; quiet or active; cooperative or uncooperative; self-assured or fearful; behavior appropriate or inappropriate?
- B. Developmental skills of child based on interview, observation, or both (see text for explanation)
  1. Stacks three or four cubes.
  2. Throws ball.
  3. Walks fast, may run stiffly. Walks up stairs with one hand held. Walks backwards. Sits in small chair. Climbs into an adult chair. Kicks ball.
  4. Vocabulary of 4 to 10 words with specificity. May combine two-word phrases. Understands and follows two simple directions. May tell two or more wants. Imitation vocabulary is greater than spontaneous vocabulary. Identifies (points to) several body parts. Names pictures.
  5. Feeds self. Uses spoon appropriately. Holds and drinks from cup accurately.
  6. Imitates crayon stroke on paper.

Parents with an active, interventionist orientation toward health care and parents who attribute good health and low illness susceptibility to their children are high users of health promotion visits and have fewer illness and accident visits. On the other hand, more passive parents and those who attribute poor health to their children account for fewer health promotion visits and more acute disease visits. The earlier discussion of parent-child interaction overlaps in this clinical area. Parents engaged in an effective parent-child interaction may be better able to interpret behaviors and symptoms in ways other than illness or disease.

AGE-RELATED VISIT CONTENTS

18 to 24 Months

Tables 6–4 and 6–5 illustrate the suggested contents of health supervision visits at 18 and 24 months. Developmental screening is performed utilizing the Prescreening Developmental Questionnaire (PDQ) or the complete Denver Developmental Screening Test (DDST), depending on the health supervision schedule by which the child is being followed. Table 6–4 lists developmental skills typical of this age for clinicians who assess and discuss

Table 6–5. ANTICIPATORY GUIDANCE FOR 18 TO 24 MONTHS

Nutrition and Dental Health
- A. Encourage regular family meals. Discourage snacks.
- B. Food likes and dislikes changing. Food requirement not large. Recognize child's emerging autonomy and avoid fruitless struggles.
- C. No bottles.
- D. Fluoride supplementation in the absence of natural or artificial fluoridation of water supply.
- E. Routine dental care practices.

Accident Prevention
- A. Stair and window safety.
- B. Car restraint system.
- C. Warn parents regarding unsupervised play by child around street or driveway. Child does not understand danger or remember "no."
- D. Never leave child unattended in car.
- E. Guard against falls.

Development and Behavior
- A. Activities with Parents
  1. Encourage playmates; expect difficulty in sharing.
  2. Recommend toys that child can take apart and use to build. Toy phone. Interested in drawers and waste baskets.
  3. Read to child regularly, especially at bedtime.
  4. Play games, both quiet and active, such as chase.
  5. Beginning to help with household chores, e.g., pick up toys.
  6. Give child a toothbrush. Imitative activity.
  7. Provide place to climb and outlet for physical activity.
  8. Encourage parents to limit television viewing. Watch children's programs with child when possible.
- B. Behavior Concerns
  1. Sleep Practices
     - a. Night fears.
     - b. Regular bedtime.
     - c. Changing nap patterns. Takes from none to two naps.
  2. Toilet Training
     - a. Most children show readiness for toilet training between 18 and 24 months.
     - b. Bowel training usually precedes training for urination.
  3. Discipline
     - a. Need for autonomy and independence.
     - b. Do you and your spouse agree on expectations and management? Do you have a set of rules? Is one of you said to be too strict? Too easy? Do you spank? For what?
     - c. Advice about limit-setting, verbal followed if necessary by physical reinforcement.
     - d. Reinforce good behavior. Emphasize that child is pleased by parental approval.
  4. Thumb sucking and other soothing, self-stimulating activities and use of a favorite toy, teddy bear, or security blanket are age-appropriate behaviors for handling tensions.

Life Style: Effect of inhalation of cigarette smoke on children's respiratory health.

development based on history and observation. Screening for lead poisoning with an FEP and for tuberculosis is performed at this age for children living in endemic areas.

Topics for anticipatory guidance at these ages are presented in Table 6–5. The amount of effort expended here is individualized according to need. Children who live in areas that lack natural or artificial fluoridation of water supply should receive 0.5 mg of fluoride daily. Parents are reminded of the use of car restraint systems. Home accidents such as burns, poisoning, drowning, and falls are reviewed and preventive measures are discussed. The normal toddler phase of increased independence and autonomy-seeking and the related problems of discipline, temper tantrums, and toilet training are discussed as outlined in the table.

30 Months

A clinical visit at 30 months of age is recommended for toddlers followed in the supplemented schedule. This visit is used as an opportunity for the clinician to devote more personal time to counseling parents about nutrition, dental care, accident prevention, and parent-child interaction after a brief history and shortened physical examination, as noted in Table 6–6.

36 to 42 Months

Tables 6–7 and 6–8 illustrate the suggested contents for health supervision at 36 and 42 months (3 and 3½ years) of age. Screening for visual and auditory acuity is first performed at this age, if possible. Developmental screening should be performed with the complete DDST in the supplemented health supervision schedule or with the PDQ in the basic schedule. Screening for speech articulation should be performed by clinically assessing how understandable the child's language is. During the 36-month visit of the supplemented schedule, personal counseling is devoted to the topics of normal development and behavior described in Table 6–8.

Personal guidance during the 42-month visit of the basic schedule is focused on the areas of

Table 6–6. HEALTH SUPERVISION: ADDITIONAL ASPECTS FOR 30-MONTH VISIT

Interview: Other possible questions to ask parent
- A. How is toilet training going?
- B. What do you and your spouse enjoy most about ____________ now?
- C. What do you find most difficult about ____________'s care now?
- D. How are your other children doing?

Physical Examination

Screening: Development: PDQ in supplemented schedule

Developmental Assessment
- A. Parent-infant interaction (same as 18 months)
  1. Parent should be aware of social cues and communication.
  2. Parents should attempt to respond rapidly to these social cues.
- B. Developmental skills of child based on interview or observation (see text for explanation)
  1. Climbs and descends steps alone, one step at a time, while holding stair rail or parent's hand.
  2. Kicks a ball. Throws overhand.
  3. Jumps off floor with both feet. Stands on one foot momentarily, runs well.
  4. Makes two short sentences with pronouns such as "I," "me," "you." Refers to self by name. Uses some plurals.
  5. Asks frequent questions: "What's that?"
  6. If speech is not intelligible to parents or is delayed, child should be referred for diagnostic speech and hearing evaluation.
  7. Responds to two-part verbal command.
  8. Imitates horizontal and circular stroke with a crayon.
  9. Interest in bowel and bladder control.
  10. Imitates domestic adult activities and work.
  11. Shows interest in helping to get dressed; washes and dries hands.
  12. Should use spoon and cup well.

Anticipatory Guidance
- A. Nutrition and dental health } as at 18- to 24-month visit
- B. Accident prevention }

Table 6–7. HEALTH SUPERVISION: ADDITIONAL ASPECTS FOR 36- TO 42-MONTH-OLD CHILD

Interview: Same as 18- to 24-month visit plus:
  Possible concerns of this age group: Fears and fantasies, sexual curiosity, getting along with siblings and other children, speech, advisability of nursery school, destructiveness

Physical Examination

Screening
- A. Vision and hearing screen
- B. Lead: FEP (endemic area)
- C. Development
  - PDQ: Basic schedule
  - DDST: Supplemented schedule
- D. Speech articulation

Developmental Assessment
- A. Parent-child interaction: Same as 18- to 24-month visit
- B. Developmental skills of child based on observation and interview
  1. Gives full name, knows age and sex. Counts to three.
  2. Comprehends "cold," "tired," "hungry," "bigger," and "smaller." Imitates cross, copies circle, recognizes some colors.
  3. Jumps in place, kicks ball, balances, and stands on one foot briefly.
  4. Puts on clothes, feeds self, builds tower of nine cubes, imitates bridge of three blocks.
  5. Alternates feet on stairs, opens doors.
  6. At least half of speech intelligible.

Table 6–8. ANTICIPATORY GUIDANCE FOR 36- TO 42-MONTH-OLD CHILD

Nutrition and Dental Health
- A. Balanced diet. Avoidance of junk drinks and foods. Child feeds self entirely.
- B. Fluoride supplementation in the absence of natural or artificial fluoridation of water supply.
- C. Home dental care. First visit to the dentist.

Accident Prevention
- A. Car safety restraint. Regular automobile safety belt may be used between three and four years of age or at weight of 40 pounds.
- B. Keep door locked if there is a danger that the child may fall down steps, or place gate at the top of the stairs.
- C. Keep knives out of reach. Watch for boiling water.
- D. Teach danger of following a ball thrown or dog darting into street, but do not depend on this. Child has to be closely supervised when near a street.

Development and Behavior
- A. Activites with parents
  1. Provide child with opportunities to talk about his day.
  2. Allow to explore, make choices, and communicate.
  3. Out-of-home experiences such as nursery school, other peer-age play groups. Comprehends taking turns. Beginning to share.
  4. Importance of regular bedtime. Bedtime ritual. May have occasional night fears.
  5. Plays with blocks, simple puzzles, beads, and pegs. Pretend play is well developed, using both toys and household objects.
- B. Behavior concerns
  1. Discipline
     - a. Allow the child to experience and understand the consequences of unacceptable behavior.
     - b. Encourage self-discipline and positive sibling relationships.
  2. At this age or earlier, children will be curious about where babies come from and about the differences between boys and girls. The parents should be prepared to answer these questions honestly, at a level appropriate to the child's understanding and within the boundaries of the question. Advise parents to use correct terms for the genitals and to understand that the child's sexual curiosity and explorations are normal.
  3. Most children have reached adequate bowel control. May not achieve full day or night bladder control until age four.

Life Style: Importance of regular physical exercise to children's general health.

parent-child interaction, nutrition, accident prevention, and development and behavior as described in the table. The dose of fluoride for children three years old or older who live in areas with nonfluoridated water supplies is 1 mg/daily.

48 to 60 Months

A health supervision visit is recommended at 48 months of age for children followed in the supplemented schedule. This visit includes an interval history and physical evaluation. Among other screening assessments, developmental screening is performed using the full DDST. Table 6–9 lists developmental skills for clinicians who prefer to devote personal time to assessing development by history and observation. Personal guidance is focused on parent-child issues, accident prevention, and development and behavior using the issues presented in Tables 6–9 and 6–10.

A visit at 60 months of age is recommended for both the basic and supplemented schedules. As presented in Table 6–9, along with the complete history and physical examination, selected screening procedures are recommended. Speech articulation and school readiness are assessed clinically in the context of the child's development and behavioral progress, along with the DDST screening instrument. Areas that may require personal counseling are listed in the table. The decision to devote personal time to these areas is based on the child's and family's prior history in the various clinical areas. For many families, written instructional material may be adequate at this age.

These guidelines provide for a clinical approach focused on parent-child interaction, with separate schedules for children at minimal as well as increased risk for problems in health, development, or behavior. Suggestions are made regarding the areas to which health clinicians should devote their personal time and effort in each visit. A visit that follows these guidelines should require 15 to 25 minutes. The initial part of the visit consists of collection by a health assistant of the screening data appropriate for the child's age. Next occurs the history-gathering interview (6 to 8 minutes). The physical examination follows next (2 to 5 minutes), with overlap with history taking and

Table 6–9. HEALTH SUPERVISION: ADDITIONAL ASPECTS FOR 48 TO 60 MONTHS

Interview: Same as 18- to 24-month visit plus:

- A. Is ____________ in nursery school?
- B. Possible concerns of this age group: Sexual curiosity, separation, tantrums, talking back, destructiveness, recklessness, developmental delay, peer problems, shyness, night terrors, jealousy, disobedience, masturbation, bad words, speech, enuresis, limb pains.

Physical Examination and DPT and OPV (at age five)

Screening

- A. Vision and hearing
- B. Lead (FEP) and TB (PPD) in endemic areas
- C. Development: DDST
- D. Speech articulation
- E. School readiness (at age five)

Developmental Assessment

- A. Parent-child interaction
    1. Evidence of affection and mutuality
    2. Ability of child to demonstrate some independence and coping in parent's presence
- B. Developmental skills of child based on observation and interview
    1. Alternates feet descending stairs, hops, jumps forward, stands on one foot three to five seconds, rides tricycle
    2. Names and matches three of four primary colors
    3. Increased skill in counting; learning ABCs
    4. Conversational give and take
    5. Dries hands
    6. Dresses and undresses except laces
    7. Plays cooperatively, sex play normal
    8. Gender identification formed
    9. Copies cross, circle, square
    10. Builds tower of 10 cubes

Table 6–10. ANTICIPATORY GUIDANCE FOR 48- TO 60-MONTH-OLD CHILD

Nutritional and Dental Health
- A. Balanced diet with pleasant, stable mealtime atmosphere.
- B. Avoidance of excess sucrose, partly for snacks.
- C. Need for increased responsibility for dental care.

Accident Prevention
- A. Supervision; safe toys; electrical tools, firearms, matches, and poisons out of reach.
- B. No unsupervised access to streets on bicycle or on foot.
- C. Proper car restraints.
- D. Supervision near water.
- E. Teach child's name, address, phone if lost.

Development and Behavior
- A. Activities with parents
  1. Encourage child to sleep in own bed.
  2. Answer questions about sex naturally.
  3. Encourage duties in house.
- B. Behavior concerns
  1. Discipline
     - a. Reprimands given privately
     - b. Simple explanation should be provided for rules if broken
     - c. Consequences should promptly follow act
     - d. Continuing threats not effective
     - e. Balance between limits and independence
     - f. Normal for four-year-old to "make up a story"
  2. Toilet training
     By age four, 95% of children are bowel trained; 70% are bladder trained and dry during daytime; and 75% are dry at night.

Life Style: Importance of the role model of the parents on multiple behaviors such as health-related (e.g., smoking), ethical, and others.

counseling regarding parent-infant interaction. Counseling on parent-child interaction occurs next (5 minutes), and finally, guidance for nutrition, dental health, accident prevention, and development and behavior follows last (3 to 5 minutes). These recommendations represent an amalgamation of information from pediatrics, developmental psychology, health education, and health care research, tempered with clinical experience. Since conclusive clinical research is not available, experience and educated opinions are the major guidance available until health-care studies assess the efficacy of such a clinical approach.

Clinicians have limited ability to impact on children's health and developmental well-being. The ecology of a family's living situation (income, household crowdedness and organization, stability and stress, etc.) often has such restrictive impact on the family and child's functioning that health promotion visits in isolation may be only moderately effective. Unfortunately, children in such situations are less likely to be brought for child health supervision visits. Outreach nurses, social workers, and community-based education and social programs often need to be used with such families to promote as optimal a home environment as possible. In spite of these difficulties, clinicians can affect child health and development. They have easy and accepted access to children prior to birth and throughout childhood years. Only clinicians have the ability to focus on the whole child, including medical, social, developmental, and behavioral aspects, in the context of the child's family. Finally, the clinicians' traditional role as an authority on children's well-being makes them the one professional, outside of the family, from whom parents are most willing to accept advice. The clinician is thus clearly in a position to achieve the broad goals of health promotion in preschool age children by focusing on strengthening the parents role in fostering child health and development.

REFERENCES

Becker, M. H., Nathanson, C. A., Drachman, R. H., and Dirscht, J. P.: Mother's health beliefs and children's clinic visits: A prospective study. J. Commun. Health, 3:125–135, 1977.

Beckwith, L.: Caregiver-infant interaction as a focus for therapeutic intervention with human infants. *In* Walsh, R. N., and Greenough, W. T. (eds.): Environment as Therapy for Brain Dysfunction. New York, Plenum Press, 1976.

Casey, P. H., and Bradley, R. H.: The impact of the home environment on children's development: Clinical relevance for the pediatrician. J. Devel. Behav. Pediatr., *3*:146–152, 1982.

Casey, P. H., and Whitt, J. K.: Effect of the pediatrician on the mother-infant relationship. Pediatrics, *65*:815–820, 1980.

Casey, P., Sharp, M., and Loda, F.: Child health supervision for children under two years of age: A review of its content and effectiveness. J. Pediatr., *95*:1–9, 1979.

Childhood accidents: Prevention and treatment. Pediatr. Ann., *6*:No. 11, 1977.

Clarke-Stewart, K. A.: The family drama of child development. *In* Brazelton, T. B., and Vaughn, V. C. (eds.): The Family: Setting Priorities. New York, Science & Medicine Publishing Co., 1979.

Fandal, A. W., Kemper, M. G., Frankenburg, W. K., et al.: Needed: Routine developmental screening in all children. Gerber Publications, 1979, Vol. 24 pp. 4–15.

Levine, M. D., Oberklaid, F., Ferb, T. E., et al.: The pediatric examination of education readiness: Validation of an extended observation procedure. Pediatrics, *66*:341–349, 1980.

Newbrun, E.: Dietary fluoride supplementation for the prevention of caries. Pediatrics, *62*:733–737, 1978.

Osburn, L. M., and Woolley, F. R.: Use of groups in well child care. Pediatrics, *67*:701–706, 1981.

Osofsky, J. D., and Conners, K.: Mother-infant interaction: An integrative view of a complex system. *In* Osofsky, J. S. (ed.): Handbook of Infant Development. New York, John Wiley & Sons, 1979.

Palfrey, J. S., Levine, M. D., Oberklaid, F., et al.: An analysis of observed attention and activity patterns in pre-school children. J. Pediatr., *98*:1006–1011, 1981.

Paradise, J. L.: Otitis media during early life: How hazardous to development? A critical review of the literature. Pediatrics, *68*:869–873, 1981.

Rutter, M.: Raised lead and impaired cognitive/behavioral functioning: A review of the evidence. Devel. Med. Child Neurol., *22*(Suppl. 42):1–26, 1980.

Starfield, B.: Behavioral pediatrics and primary health care. Pediatr. Clin. North Am., *29*:377–390, 1982.

Sturner, R. A., Funk, S. G., Barton, J., et al.: Simultaneous screening for child health and development: A study of visual developmental screening of pre-school children. Pediatrics, *65*:614–621, 1980.

Welch, N. M., Saulsbury, F. T., and Kesler, R. W.: The value of the pre-school examination in screening for health problems. J. Pediatr., *100*:232–234, 1982.

7

HEALTH CARE FOR THE ELEMENTARY SCHOOL AGE CHILD

Catherine De Angelis, M.D.

CHARACTERISTICS OF THIS AGE

To provide appropriate health care for the school age child, as in all other age groups, it is important to understand the normal physical and psychosocial growth and development associated with this age.

PHYSICAL CHARACTERISTICS

During this period, physical growth, like psychological development, is relatively slow but steady, with an average annual gain of about 7 pounds in weight and 2 to 3 inches in height. Growth of head circumference is much slower than in earlier years, with an increase of only one inch (2 to 3 cm) between the ages of 5 and 12 years. By the time the youngster reaches the pre-adolescent growth spurt, his brain has virtually reached adult size. The general habitus of the youngster is more erect and stockier than that of the lordotic, pot-bellied toddler and preschooler. The relatively mild degree of pes planus and genu valgum often found in the preschooler tends to disappear in the first few years of elementary school. Development of the facial bones continues with enlargement of the sinuses, the frontal sinus developing by the seventh year of life.

The rate of growth is faster for girls than for boys during this period. One need only attend a sixth grade dance to understand the implications of this difference. These years are marked by a great increase in physical strength and coordination. Running, jumping, and climbing that predominate in the preschool years become more directed and skilled, and sports activities play a large role in the lives of most of these youngsters.

The primary canines and molars are lost, and overbite is reduced during this time. The eight permanent incisors and four permanent molars usually have erupted by 9 years of age and the premolars by 11 or 12 years. The lymphatic tissues reach their peak size, which is about twice that of an adult, and usually begin to decrease around the time of puberty.

PSYCHOLOGICAL CHARACTERISTICS

Although known as the latency period, this is really not a dormant or quiescent time. The youngster becomes more independent, acquires greater self-control and inner direction, and develops moral reasoning.

Sex games and discussions occur frequently but almost never in the presence of adults. Immature heterosexual love relationships, although developed by some school children, usually occur only in fantasy. Most youngsters play almost exclusively with children of their own sex. Masturbation increases, especially in boys, and some homosexual play also occurs, primarily in the form of genital manipulation.

Erikson (1963) refers to this time as the stage of industry, because the child develops a mastery of his environment. Piaget (1962) regards the early school years as the time of transition from pre-operational to operational thinking. Prior to this time, children give reasons for what they do and develop concepts mostly based on intuition. They function primarily by what they can see rather than by a set of basic principles.

With the onset of operational thinking, children learn to use concepts of what should be. This process, which takes time, begins at different times for different children; however, around seven or eight years of age most children have developed the basic understanding of serial relationships necessary to learning mathematics. Also, simple riddles become an integral part of their language play.

Many variables are involved in the development of mental skills. Experience plays a significant role in the successful accomplishment of tasks, and generally a familiar environment, such as one classroom, also helps. Memory is also essential, and some children appear to be unable to perform simply because they are confused. Language competence is also very important in learning, and some children are hampered by poor language skills.

With increasing mental development, the child can better understand right from wrong. Unlike the preschooler, whose behavior depends on immediate instructions and consequences, the school age child acts according to learned rules. At first these rules are based on the approval of an adult, but eventually a morality develops based on the child's own perceptions of right and wrong.

Some of these personal standards are based on identification with family members and other influential persons. Generally, what these individuals do is more inportant to the youngster than what they say. Consistency is essential. At this point, our knowledge about conscience development and the influence of childrearing is meager. However, the important factors are probably a strong parent-child relationship, modeling behavior of the parents and other influential adults, and encouragement of certain behaviors of the child.

An important experience of the school age years is making friends with a variety of children. Social skills have to be learned. The need to try out new social skills and the fluctuations that occur in interests and activities contribute greatly to the changing patterns of friendship. These tend to be intense but often transitory relationships. Popularity is based on a number of factors, including physical maturity, a pleasing physical appearance, and sports ability. High intelligence can lead to unpopularity if other characteristics are not positive. Identification with the same-sex peer group increases during the later school years, and children are more influenced by peer group than by adult norms.

School attendance exerts a great influence on these children in the development of intellectual and social skills. Teachers can become very influential role models as the child works his way toward independence from his family.

MORTALITY AND MORBIDITY

Early school age years are a physically healthy period of life. Mortality rates, which are at their lowest level during the school years, have been decreasing steadily, in the United States at least, over the last 40 years or so. In 1977, the mortality rate was 34 per 100,000 in the 5- to 9-year and 35.1 per 100,000 in the 10- to 14-year age groups. This compares with 68.8 per 100,000 for the 1- to 4-year and 101.6 per 100,000 for the 15- to 19-year age groups. The leading cause of death for school age children is accidents.

Unless he has a chronic illness, a serious injury, or parents who adhere to an annual health maintenance visit schedule, a school age child might not be seen by a physician for several years. This is in stark contrast to his earlier years, since the average child has been examined some 14 times prior to beginning school (Bailey, 1974; Casey et al., 1979). These frequent examinations, immunizations, and environmental strengths contribute to the relative good health of children entering schools. Only a small percentage of abnormalities found on examination of children entering school had been previously undetected (Yankauer and Lawrence, 1955; Grant et al., 1973).

According to the American Academy of Pediatrics' School Health Guide (Rogers, 1981), approximately 3 per cent of elementary school age children have some type of hearing problem; about 25 per cent have visual defects, most of which are correctable with lenses; about 1 per cent have a major speech disorder, which is usually correctable; about 10 to 20 per cent have a reading disorder; about 3 per cent are educationally handicapped; and about 1 per cent have epilepsy.

The most common physical ailments are trauma and its consequences; allergies; and respiratory, gastrointestinal, and dermatological problems, most of which are infectious. Behavioral problems, learning difficulties, and emotional problems are common. In one study, 5 to 15 per cent of the children seen in seven nonteaching primary care facilities were diagnosed as having such "new morbidity" problems (Starfield et al., 1980).

SCREENING (SEE PAGE 32 TO 33 IN SECTION II)

The primary purpose of screening is to identify disabilities sufficiently early to intervene before serious or irremediable consequences occur. In the best sense, screening also includes early identification of potential vulnerabilities that might interfere with the child's healthy functioning and of positive resources that will assist recovery if needed. Almost every state requires screening of school age children for all or some of the following: vision, hearing, scoliosis, blood pressure, height, and weight.

Although the concept of screening is a good one, there are some inherent limitations:

1. All screening tests have some degree of error resulting in false positive and false negative findings.

2. The person administering the test may do so inconsistently and/or incorrectly, leading to more than the expected number of erroneous results.

3. The environment in which the test is administered may be inappropriate, e.g., audiometric evaluations performed in a noisy room.

4. The test or tester may be too sensitive, resulting in many costly and anxiety-provoking referrals of normal children.

5. Facilities or finances for correcting the problem may not be available in the community and anxieties may be raised unnecessarily.

6. No follow-up is provided. In this event the chance for quality control, i.e., the examiner finding out that he is over-referring, is missed. In addition, reinforcing instruction or therapy that might have been prescribed by the consultant does not occur. For example, if a child found to have a visual defect in school screening is referred to an ophthalmologist and receives corrective lenses but then does not wear them in school, the potential contribution of the screening test is lost. If follow-up had occurred, the person responsible for the referral, having informed the child that he should wear glasses, could request the teachers to exert their influence.

7. The periodicity, i.e., the timing and frequency, of screening tests does not always maximize the utility of these efforts; for example, it is probably not as cost effective to screen in schools for scoliosis in children under the age of eight years as it is in the prepubertal years, when the incidence is higher and the ability to correct the defect without surgery is still possible. On the other hand, screening for scoliosis, as part of a physical examination for all school age children, by a primary care practitioner may be effective for health education purposes.

Vision Screening. The American Academy of Pediatrics suggests that every child have a test for visual acuity by four years of age. If conducted in the schools, it should begin at school entry, including transfer students, and continue annually throughout elementary school and high school. Most visual defects are errors of refraction. Approximately 5 per cent of first graders have such problems, but almost 50 per cent of children develop them by the end of high school. Strabismus and anisometropia are present in 1 to 5 per cent of school age children.

Children with corrective lenses should be tested while wearing them. Testing should include making sure the lenses fit properly and reinforcing the importance of wearing them.

The Snellen test identifies most children with vision problems. Young children may be better tested with the E form of the Snellen test or by Sheridan's Test for Young Children and Retardates (STYCAR). Cards using picture symbols are not valid for testing the vision of preliterate children.

Strabismus should also be tested by means of the Cover-Uncover Test. The child is asked to look at a small light source at eye level about 20 feet away when one eye has been covered. If the child has esotropia or exotropia, when the cover is removed, the eye that has wandered will immediately resume its straight ahead position. The Titmus Tester can be used for children over five years of age.

Hearing Screening. The American Academy of Pediatrics recommends that every child have a hearing test by four years of age. Pure tone audiometry is the test of choice. The audiometer produces tones of a specified intensity and different frequencies ranging from 250 to 6000 Hertz (Hz). The human ear can respond to frequencies of 20 to 20,000 Hz, but normal speech sounds fall in the range of 250 to 4000 Hz, with 70 per cent falling between 500 and 2000 Hz.

In audiometry, the ear is exposed to a series of pure tones of calibrated loudness (decibels) occurring at different frequencies. Zero decibels is designated as the "loudness" at which a normal child can hear the sound 50 per cent of the time. If the child cannot hear this level, the loudness is increased until he can hear the louder sound 50 per cent of the time. The additional loudness in decibels is the measure of hearing loss. A loss of more than 15 decibels at any given frequency is significant. Each ear is measured for both bone and air conduction, and the results are recorded on special grids.

The use of tympanometry in the diagnosis of hearing problems has become popular over the past few years. Whether it has resulted in overdiagnosis or has improved outcome is not yet clear.

Approximately 5 per cent of elementary school age children do not pass hearing screening tests. When retesting is done several weeks later, about half of those who had previously failed will pass. This pattern is probably the result of upper respiratory infections, fluid in the middle ear, misunderstood instructions, or disinterest in the tests.

The American Academy of Pediatrics School Health Committee recommends that hearing testing be performed in kindergarten, first grade, and grades 3, 6, 9, and 12. Children with known hearing impairment should be retested annually. This testing is best done in areas designed to minimize noise. Most offices and clinics are not so equipped.

Hypertension Screening. Screening children for hypertension is based on the assumption that early detection and treatment will provide a more favorable prognosis. There is some evidence now that most young school age children whose first systolic and diastolic blood pressure readings were above the 95 per cent range for age reverted to normal on second testing. Only a few of the children with sustained hypertension had readings sufficiently high to meet the criteria of the American Academy of Pediatrics Task Force on Blood Pressure Control in Children for drug therapy. Therefore the American Academy of Pediatrics School Health Committee does not recommend screening school children for hypertension because of its low yield of cases requiring treatment. However, it is a good idea to include blood pressure measurement as part of the routine physical examination after age three in order to (1) establish baseline values, (2) allow the child to become accustomed to the procedure, (3) teach the child and parent that it is an important part of the routine physical examination, especially as the child gets older, and (4) discover the occasional child with hypertension resulting from organic etiology.

Scoliosis Screening. Scoliosis occurs in 0.5 to 2 per cent of the population, more frequently in females. Screening for scoliosis is most appropriate in the prepubertal or early pubertal years when skeletal trunk growth is rapid. Children who have a relative with scoliosis are at higher-than-normal risk.

Scoliosis screening is best done with the child barefooted and stripped to the waist, with girls wearing brassieres. The youngster stands erect with shoulders back, head up and looking straight ahead, hands hanging loosely at the sides, knees straight, and feet together. The youngster then flexes forward slowly, forming a right angle at the hips with head hanging in a dependent, relaxed position, arms dangling with the palms pressed together, and the knees straight. The observer should note the symmetry of shoulder height, scapulae, arm hang, flanks, and hips; the alignment of occiput over the intergluteal cleft; and the alignment of the spinous processes (Fig. 7–1). Other spinal deviations, such as kyphosis and lordosis, are noted by viewing the child from the side (Kane et al., 1978).

Any asymmetry or prominence of the back in the flexed position may be a sign of scoliosis. If the screening is conducted in the school, youngsters who do not pass the screening test should be evaluated by a physician (Asher, 1975; Drummond et al., 1979).

Screening for scoliosis has become somewhat controversial in the past few years. Undetected scoliosis can progress to unsightly physical appearance and even significant cardiopulmonary difficulties. A long, difficult treatment program, often including surgery, may be required. However, there are very few data upon which to conclude whether early intervention reduces long-term morbidity and the need for surgery.

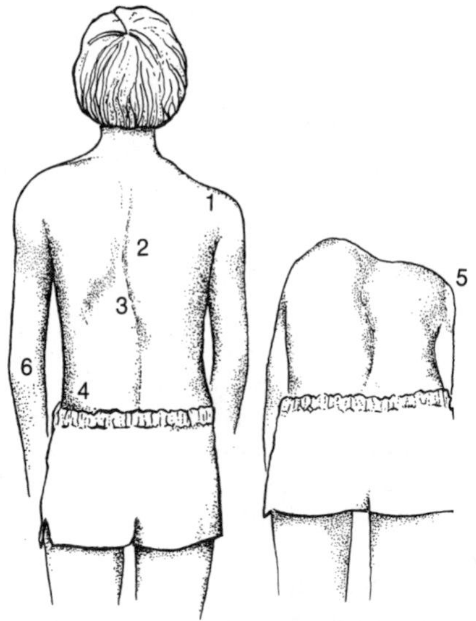

Figure 7–1. Scoliosis checklist: (1) shoulder level; (2) symmetry of scapulae; (3) alignment of spinous processes; (4) symmetry of flanks; (5) symmetry of thorax; (6) evenness of hang of the arms. (From Rogers, K. (ed.): School Health: A Guide for Health Professionals, 1981. Evanston, Ill., American Academy of Pediatrics, 1981, p. 253. With permission.)

The natural history of the disease is not well-understood, uncertainties exist concerning the characteristics of surgical and brace candidates, the possibility exists that many of the radiographic tests may be unwarranted, and reliable cost-effectiveness data are nonexistent (Joffe, 1982). All of these factors must be considered when routine screening for scoliosis is evaluated. It is useful for practitioners to perform the screening as part of the routine physical examination. If a problem is found, the physician can monitor the child's progress and consult an orthopedic specialist, if necessary, to provide the most effective care for the child.

Dental Screening. The school age child should be under the care of a dentist for supervision of dental development and consultation. If this is not possible, and the consultative and referral services of a dentist are available, an annual dental screening in the school for caries, soft tissue disease, and oral hygiene instruction is important.

Laboratory Screening. Very little, if any, laboratory screening is indicated for the elementary school age child. The prevalence of iron deficiency, commonly found in some preschoolers and menstruating adolescent females, is low in school age children.

Routine screening for hyperlipidemia is not indicated in these children because of its low predictive value for later coronary artery disease. Certain high-risk children (primarily those with a family history of a close relative with early coronary artery disease) may benefit from hyperlipidemia screening.

Urinalysis screening is not recommended as part of routine screening because it seldom identifies previously undetected disease (Gutgesel, 1978). Although screening school girls for bacteriuria is moderately productive in identifying urinary tract infections, the benefit from treatment is uncertain. Although bacteriuria is fairly common in girls and women, adult renal failure secondary to infection is rare and the spontaneous "cure" of asymptomatic bacteria is high.

Height and Weight Screening. In the school age child, these determinations are not effective in identifying obesity, undernutrition, or shortness of stature that is not obvious by simple inspection. However, periodic measures of height and weight are valuable to determine velocity of growth. In the child with short stature, more frequent measurements may be necessary for diagnostic purposes and to monitor changes with therapy.

PHYSICAL EXAMINATION

The minimal frequency of periodic physical examinations for school attendance is set by law in many states, with most states now requiring only a pre-entrance medical examination.

Recent attention has focused on the shortcoming of traditional, routine physical examinations for school age children in light of the cost of these evaluations for parents, the disaffection with the procedure on the part of many students, parents, school personnel, and administering physicians, and the questionable effectiveness of these examinations in identifying health needs in the population (Yankauer and Lawrence, 1955; Kohler, 1972; Welch et al., 1982). They have been seen as relatively unsuccessful in identifying previously undiagnosed, significant health problems (Welch et al., 1982; Grant et al., 1973; Kohler, 1977). Less expensive mass screenings have been compared favorably to physical examinations in their ability to detect a range of health needs that could impact upon school performance (Welch et al., 1982; Grant et al., 1973; Torrell et al., 1981).

On the other hand, physical examinations result in the identification of a broader range of problems than do screenings, and other investigations have found them to be effective in identifying previously undiagnosed, significant health problems that could not have been found on screenings (De Angelis, 1982).

IMMUNIZATION AND TUBERCULOSIS SURVEY

The American Academy of Pediatrics Committee on Infectious Diseases recommends that every child be immunized fully against diphtheria, pertussis, tetanus, polio, measles, mumps, and rubella prior to school entry. In addition, boosters for diphtheria and tetanus should be given (see page 38).

The frequency of tuberculosis screening, either by old tuberculin or preferably by intradermal purified protein derivative, depends on the customary practice of the region and the risk of the population under care. The American Academy of Pediatrics Infectious Disease Committee recommends annual or biennial testing unless local circumstances dictate less frequent or no testing.

HEALTH MAINTENANCE VISITS

Table 7–1 provides a guideline for the history to be included in health maintenance visits for the elementary school age child. The American Academy of Pediatrics Committee on Practice and Ambulatory Medicine has recommended that the pre-teen school age child have a health maintenance visit at ages 5, 6, 8, 10, and 12 years for those who are receiving competent parenting, have no important health problems, and are growing and developing in a satisfactory manner. The excellent opportunities provided by these visits for the clinician to influence the child's health behavior can have significant effects on future physical and emotional health. Table 7–2 outlines the timing and content of the typical health maintenance visit for the school age child.

Figure 7–2 is a sample of a problem-oriented form that can be used to record these visits. Time should be spent discussing at least some of the following issues with the child and his parents, especially since the clinician may not see the child more frequently than every two years. If good counseling is to be done, the

Table 7–1. HEALTH SUPERVISION, 6 TO 10 YEARS

I. Interview: Questions are to be directed both to the parents and to the child. In addition, the child should be seen alone for a few minutes.
   A. Some possible questions for the parent(s)
      1. How are you? How are things going in your family?
      2. Have there been any problems or concerns about ________? Possible concerns at this age include activity level ("hyperactivity"), no friends, inability to get along with peers and siblings, poor school progress, learning disability, reluctance to separate from parent, school avoidance, frequent school absence, disobedience, talking back, uncooperativeness, short attention span, enuresis, encopresis, recurrent nightmares, shyness, low self-esteem, nervousness, fears, effeminate behavior, depressive symptoms, masturbation, tics, and acting-out or aggressive behavior (fighting, destructiveness, fire-setting, stealing, or lying).
      3. Have there been any unexpected or unusual stresses in your family (illness, death, separation, divorce) since your last visit?
      4. How is school going for ________ this year?
      5. What is ________'s usual mood and attitude toward life? Is it easy or hard for him to express his feelings?
      6. Does ________ get along with you (mother/father)? Siblings? Peers?
      7. What do you do individually or together with ________?
      8. How is communication in your family? Good? Fair? Could be improved?
      9. What are your arrangements for ________'s out-of-school supervision when you are away?
      10. How have you planned to provide ________ with sex education?
      11. What are some of the things about ________ that you are especially proud of?
      12. How are things going for you at work?
   B. Some possible questions for the child
      1. How do you like school? How are the teachers? How are the other children?
      2. What do you like to do for fun? What is your favorite thing to do?
      3. Do you have a friend?
      4. Do you have a pet?
      5. Do you want to ask me a question?

Table 7–2. HEALTH MAINTENANCE FOR ELEMENTARY SCHOOL AGE CHILDREN

Category	Procedure	Timing
History	Complete data base	On initial visit
	Interval history:	Annually
	Parental concerns	
	Living situation	
	School adjustment	
	Extracurricular activities	
	Temperament	
	Physical status	
	Emotional status	
	Diet	
Physical Examination	All systems including neurological	On initial visit; as indicated thereafter
School Readiness	General Screening:	Prior to school entry
	Denver Developmental	
	Goodenough-Harris Draw-a-Person	
	Ammon's Quick Test	
	PRESS Test	
	More extensive:	As indicated
	PEER Test	
Screening	Vision	Annually
	Hearing	Ages 5, 6, 9, 12, and 15
	Blood Pressure	As part of physical examination
	Dental	Annually
	Scoliosis	Initially during prepubertal growth spurt and thereafter as indicated
	Hemoglobin/Hematocrit	On initial visit
	Tuberculosis	Annually in endemic areas; as indicated in others
Immunizations	Diphtheria	Preschool booster
	Pertussis	Preschool booster
	Tetanus	Preschool booster
	Polio	Preschool booster
	Diphtheria, tetanus	Every 10 years thereafter
Anticipatory Guidance	Consistency of approach	
	Need for praise	
	Independence	
	Allowance	
	Modeling of behavior	
	Responsibilities and role in family	
	Honesty and ownership	
	Fears and fantasies	
	Television	
	School responsibilities	
	Punctuality	
	Sex education	
	Safety	
	Friends	
	Anger	
	Lying	
	Stealing	
	Enuresis	
	Encopresis	

Date of Visit:

S. Parental Concerns:

Living Situation:

School & Grade: Adjustment

Extracurricular Activities: Hobbies, Sports

Eating Habits:

General Health:

Parents' Description of Child's Temperament
- Adjustments to Home, Environment
- Attention Span
- Distractibility
- Peer Relationships

Problems Identified & Reviewed (S.O.A.P., Use History Sheet P.R.N.)

A. Physical & Emotional Status:

P. Diet: Obesity Prevention, Dietary Needs, Habits, Snacks

Anticipatory Guidance: Consistency of approach, guidance, need for praise, independence, allowance, modeling of behavior, responsibilities & role in family, honesty & ownership, fears & fantasties, T.V., school responsibilities, punctuality, homework, sex education, literature for parents & child.
Safety: cars, bikes, guns, water, mini bikes. dental care.

Accompanied By: ______

O. Age ______ Wt ______ Ht ______
BP ______/______ Pulse ______

Vision: Ⓡ ______/______ Ⓛ ______/______ Color ______
Hearing: Gross ______ Audiogram ______

Urinalysis ______ Urine Culture ______
Adjustment to Clinic Visit:

Mood:

Intensity of Reactions:

Speech & Language

Note—Present (+) or Absent (−) as Appropriate
(Cross Off Parts Not Examined or Not Applicable)

	N	ABN
Skin: Color, Texture		
Head: Symmetry, Scalp, Hair		
Eyes: EOM, Pupils, Cornea, Conjunctivae, Fundi		
Ears: Pinnae, Canals, Tympanic Membranes		
Nose: Nares, Turbinates		
Mouth: Tongue, Gums, Number of Teeth ( )		
Throat: Pharynx, Tonsils		
Neck: Movements, Thyroid		
Nodes: Axillary, Cervical, Inguinal, Submandibular		
Chest: Expansion, Breast Tissue		
Lungs:		
Heart: Rhythm, S1, S2, Murmur		
Abdomen: Contour, LSK, Mass		
Genitourinary: Vagina, Testes, Urethral Orifice, Hernia		
Neuromuscular: Equilibrium, Motor Strength, Sensory, Coordination, Cranial Nerves, DTRs, Babinski		
Spine: Posture, Hip & Shoulder Levels		
Extremities: Gait, Range of Motion of Joints		
Anus: Rectal		
Sexual Development: (Describe)		

Describe Abnormal Findings:

Parents' Interactions with Child NO* = Not Observed Here

O.	NO*	M = Mother F = Father
		Makes Eye Contact
		Touches Child
		Hovers Over Child
		Spontaneously Identifies Positive Qualities
		Reassures Child Who is Unsure of Situation
		Limits Activity by Verbal Command
		Limits Activity by Physical Command
		Voice Calm When Talking to Child
		Reinforces Behavior Through Approval & Attention
		Terminates Activity With Some Forewarning
		Allows Child to Answer for Self
		Interrupts Child's Conversation
		Limits Child's Exuberance

Other Observations:

A. Parent-Child Interactions:

______ P.N.P.

______ M.D. Return to Clinic in ______ Months

Figure 7–2. Health maintenance for elementary school age children. (From Chun, M.: 1981. University of Wisconsin–Madison School of Medicine. Used with permission.)

visit needs to be at least 20 to 30 minutes in length and charges made appropriately.

Changes in family constellation, health, jobs, and housing can affect the child's behavior. As the child grows older, his need for privacy becomes extremely important. If possible, he should have his own special space in the house.

The child who is older or younger than most of his classmates and playmates may have special problems. Any physical or emotional difference from the norm that is obvious to other children may cause ridicule. Minority children and those who are socially aggressive, extremely bright, obviously physically different, handicapped, or intellectually and physically slow are at special risk. These children need to know how and, if possible, why they are different. It may be possible to teach them to counter harsh remarks with positive statements about their differences.

It is important to assess the parents' expectations of the child's academic and other achievements. Information about the child's performances should be obtained. If he is having problems, he may need further evaluations. The parents may have unrealistic expectations, or the child may need extra assistance to achieve his potential.

The school age child spends many hours each day doing homework; playing with friends; taking part in organized sports, music, and crafts; and watching television. Time allowed for various activities (e.g., homework vs. playing) should be negotiated between parents and child, making sure there is variety and free time to allow the child to use his imagination and initiative. Teaching the child how to organize his time can begin in the early school age years, and the responsibility for school work and chores can be shifted gradually from parent to child as the child matures.

The early school age child begins to think abstractly, and explanations of choices and consequences can be understood. Independence and responsibilities need to be nurtured according to the capabilities of the child, but some firm limits still need to be set. The child may have fears and fantasies that may not have been resolved, and they should be distinguished from the rational fear of real danger. The younger school age child may mix fantasy and truth, and explanations rather than punishment are probably more appropriate at this stage of development.

Sex education may be offered in school, but the parents should know what is taught and what the child understands. Depending on the child, more complete explanations may be necessary. If the parents are uncomfortable with teaching the child about sex, the clinician can suggest ways of approaching the subject and books that can help the parents.

The parents' main nutritional concern should be offering a balanced diet and allowing special treats at home so as to decrease buying and eating "junk food" outside the home.

Injury control should be stressed. Safety bicycle checks and rules of the road should be reinforced by the clinician. The potential hazards of activities such as swimming, sledding, skating, and contact sports should be discussed. The older school age child can be taught first aid and encouraged to promote safety.

Whenever possible, the father should accompany the child to the physician's office or clinic. Changes in American society, including mothers' working, have stimulated many fathers to become more aware of the rewards involved in direct child care. All suggestions for health care should include the father. The exception to this is, of course, the mother-based, single-parent family. As the child begins adolescence, the physician should begin to see him/her alone as well as with the parents and help the child prepare for adolescence (see Chapter 8).

Approximately one of every six pediatricians and many other physicians in the United States are involved in some form of school health services. Many serve as the official athletic team physician, perform routine athletic physicals, precept or consult with school nurses, assist in establishing health and safety guidelines for school personnel, or are members of the school board. Schools play a vital role in the lives of children, and health professionals can exert much influence on health curricula and attitudes by devoting a relatively small amount of time to this community service.

In 45 states, local boards of education have primary responsibility for conducting school health programs; in only 5 does it rest with local health departments. At the state level, 24 departments of education and 12 departments of health have the principal regulatory responsibility for school health services. In the other states, more than one agency is usually involved (Kohn, 1979).

School districts spend at least one billion dollars annually on health activities. They employ approximately 30,000 school nurses. In addition, as stated above, almost one of every six pediatricians and an unknown number of other physicians participate in school health services.

School Readiness. Developmental screening tests, such as the Goodenough-Harris Draw-a-Person Test (Harris, 1963), Ammon's Quick Test (Pless et al., 1965), the Denver Developmental Screening Test (Frankenburg and Dodds, 1967; Frankenburg et al., 1981), and the PRESS Test (Rogers and Rogers, 1972), can be effective in alerting the health professional to conditions that may prevent a child from reaching his full potential in school.

The Goodenough-Harris Draw-a-Person Test, a simple screening test that takes very little professional time, can be administered by an assistant while the child is in the waiting room. Given a pencil and a sheet of blank paper, the child is instructed to "draw a person" or "draw the best person you can." No additional directions are necessary unless the child draws a stick person, whereupon he is requested to draw the best person he can. The child receives one point for each detail present on the drawing according to a scoring guide, and norms are provided to determine age-appropriateness as follows:

DRAWING OF A PERSON

1. Head present
2. Neck present
3. Neck, two dimensions
4. Eyes present
5. Eye detail: brow or lashes
6. Eye detail: pupil
7. Nose present
8. Nose, two dimensions (not round ball)
9. Mouth present
10. Lips, two dimensions
11. Both nose and lips in two dimensions
12. Both chin and forehead shown
13. Bridge of nose (straight to eyes; narrower than base)
14. Hair I (any scribble)
15. Hair II (more detail)
16. Ears present
17. Fingers present
18. Correct number of fingers
19. Opposition of thumb shown (must include fingers)
20. Hands present
21. Arms present
22. Arms at side or engaged in activity
23. Feet: any indication
24. Attachment of arms and legs I (to trunk anywhere)
25. Attachment of arms and legs II (at correct point of trunk)
26. Trunk present
27. Trunk in proportion, two dimensions (length greater than breadth)
28. Clothing I (anything)
29. Clothing II (2 articles of clothing)

Drawing of a Person—Score

Age	*Boys*	*Girls*
3	4	5
4	7	7
5	11	12
6	13	14
7	16	17
8	18	20

Ammon's Quick Test can also be administered by an assistant. The test consists of three cards, each containing four line drawings. The child holds one card at at time, and the examiner reads a list of words of increasing subtlety. The child points to the picture on the card that is the best response for each word. Scoring is performed by counting the number of correct answers and comparing the total with given standards.

The Denver Developmental Screening Test, perhaps the best known and most widely used test at this time, can also be administered by an assistant. The complete test takes approximately 15 to 20 minutes per child, but a new, abbreviated form takes less time to administer and is especially useful in a setting where the child is seen on a continuing basis. Both forms are appropriate up to the age of six. Kits for administering the test can be purchased through the Ladoca Project and Publishing Foundation, Inc., East 51st Avenue and Lincoln Street, Denver, Colorado 80216.

The PRESS Test can be performed while the child is receiving his preschool physical examination. The child is requested to tell the examiner the colors of grass and of the sky, to repeat a sequence of four numbers, to say whether Christmas comes in winter or summer, to show where his heel is, and to draw a square. The answers are combined with a general assessment of personal-social maturity. A low score should alert the examiner that the child may not be ready to enter school and that further evaluations are indicated.

Investigators have also identified specific signs that are thought to be associated with later school failure. These include finger agnosia (Levine et al., 1980a), poor impulse control and attention span (Becker, 1976; Fesbach et al., 1974), difficulty with using a pencil (Eaves et al., 1974), inability to recognize letters and numbers (Colligan, 1973), and poorly established eye or hand dominance and delayed laterality (Denhoff et al., 1968).

Attempts at early recognition of potential deviations raise the problem of labeling. If care is not taken to explain to the parents that no single test or sign can predict achievement and potential with certainty, the child may perform as the parents expect, i.e., poorly. In an attempt to circumvent this problem and to provide a broader perspective on the individual child, the PEER Test has been designed and field-tested (Levine et al., 1980b).

The PEER Test encompasses six basic features: (1) a standardized observation procedure integrated with a physical examination, sensory assessment, and comprehensive historical review between the ages of four and six years; (2) a multilevel observation of function, including developmental attainment, processing efficiency, and neurological maturation; (3) documentation of activity and attention control at three strategic points during the evaluation; (4) prediction of school performance in the earliest grades and the need for further evaluations or special services when particular problems are discovered; (5) provision of a narrative description of a child rather than giving him a score; and (6) avoidance of specific labels and identification of syndromes.

The total evaluation, including a structured examination, dressing activities, attention activity, behavioral adaptation (performed three times), and neurodevelopmental assessment of function, takes about 45 minutes to perform. Obviously it is not practical to use this test routinely, and Levine and his associates do not at this time recommend universal application of the PEER Test. However, the results thus far have demonstrated the need for health professionals to be sensitive to a broader range of developmental issues than is traditionally pursued. This test provides the practitioner with a method of further assessing a child who has some signs of problems. A kit for administering the test is available from The Educators Publishing Service, Cambridge, Massachusetts.

School Underachievement. A common reason for parents to seek the counsel of their physician is their child's underachievement in school. In many cases, the parents have been encouraged by the school personnel to have the child evaluated.

Reasons for a child's underachievement include unrealistic expectations by the parents or teachers, mismanagement of education, family problems causing stress, lack of motivation, chronic or acute physical illness, sensory deficits, subnormal intelligence or other handicapping problems, and psychological problems. Some of these etiologies can be assessed by a complete history and physical examination, including screening for hearing and vision, all of which may have been performed already. If these are normal, psychometric evaluation may be indicated to evaluate the child's intellectual capacity and functioning. (See also Chapter 81 on Learning Problems.)

SPORTS MEDICINE (see also Chapter 25)

School athletic programs, Little League, and other organized programs are an important part of the life of a school age child. At the elementary school level, intramural programs provide valuable opportunities to develop and maintain coordination and physical fitness and to interact with peers as a team. In the best sense, sports build self-esteem and morale if students are provided with a broad-based program that maximizes participation by allowing unskilled and skilled athletes to participate at levels commensurate with their abilities.

The Education Amendments Act of 1972, Public Law 92–318, Section 901, states that women be given the right to participate equally with men in sports. Therefore, opportunities and facilities must be equally available to girls and boys. Since the enactment of the law, a seven-fold increase has occurred in the number of girls participating in school sports.

In prepubescent youngsters, there are no significant differences in physical abilities or susceptibility to injuries between boys and girls. Therefore it is not necessary to separate these children in sports activities.

Physicians who volunteer or are employed to advise about content, philosophy, or management of school sports programs require special skills and knowledge to do so effectively: Professional organizations, such as The American Academy of Pediatrics Committee on School Health, have developed valuable guidelines about school athletic programs which are available on request (Rogers, 1981).

CLOSING THE VISIT

A few moments should be reserved at the end of the visit to allow final and often significant questions to be raised. The physician can ask, "Is there anything else you (parent and child) would like to ask about?" If a problem is raised at this point or earlier which requires more time than has been scheduled, arrange a special appointment. Mention the physician's interest and availability for psychosocial, developmental, and educational as well as physical problems. Compliment the parents and child. Mention their strengths. Finally, set a time for the next appointment.

REFERENCES

Asher, M., Adler, F., and Jacobs, R.: Idiopathic adolescent scoliosis: Rationale and techniques of early detection. J. Kan. Med., *761*:285, 1975.

Bailey, E.: Screening in pediatric practice. Pediatr. Clin. North Am., *21*:123, 1974.

Becker, L.: Conceptual tempo and the early detection of learning problems. J. Learn. Disabil., 9:433, 1976.

Casey, P., Sharp, M., and Loda, F.: Child health supervision for children under two years of age: A review of its content and effectiveness. J. Pediatr., 95:1, 1979.

Colligan, R., and O'Connell, E.: Should psychometric screening be made an adjunct to the pediatric preschool examination? Clin. Pediatr., *13*:29, 1973.

De Angelis, C., Oda, D., Berman, B., et al.: The comparative values of school physical examinations and mass screening tests. J. Pediatr., *102*:477–481, 1983.

Denhoff, E. S., Queland, M., Komich, M., et al.: Developmental and predictive characteristics of items from the Meeting Street School Screening Test. Dev. Med. Child Neurol., *10*:220, 1968.

Diagnostic and Statistical Manual of Mental Disorders, 3rd ed. (DSM-III). Washington, D.C., American Psychiatric Association, 1980.

Drummond, D., Rogala, E., and Gurr, J.: Spinal deformity: Natural history and the role of school screening. Orthoped. Clin. North Am., *10*:751, 1979.

Eaves, L., Kendall, D., and Crichton, J.: The early identification of learning difficulties: A follow-up study. J. Learn. Disabil., 7:632, 1974.

Erikson, E.: Childhood and Society, 2nd ed. New York, Norton, 1963.

Fesbach, S., Adelman, H., and Fuller, W.: Early identification of children with high risk of reading failure. J. Learn. Disabil., 7:639, 1974.

Frankenburg, W., and Dodds, J.: The Denver Developmental Screening Test. J. Pediatr., *71*:181, 1967.

Frankenburg, W., Fandal, A., Sciarillo, W., et al.: The newly abbreviated and revised Denver Developmental Screening Test. J. Pediatr., 99:995, 1981.

Gillenwater, J., Harrison, R., and Kunin, C.: Natural history of bacteriuria in schoolgirls. N. Engl. J. Med., *301*:396, 1979.

Glueck, C.: Detection of risk factors for coronary artery disease in children: Semmelweis revisited? Pediatrics, *66*:834, 1980.

Grant, W., Fearnow, R., Heberston, L., et al.: Health screening in school-age children. Am. J. Dis. Child., *125*:520, 1973.

Gutgesell, M.: Practicality of screening urinalysis in asymptomatic children in a primary care setting. Pediatrics, *62*:103, 1978.

Harris, D.: Goodenough-Harris Drawing Test Manual. New York, Harcourt Brace and World, 1963.

Health United States, 1979. U.S. Department of Health, Education and Welfare Office of Health Research, Statistics and Technology. DHEW Pub. No. (PHS)80-1232.

Joffe, A.: Screening in pediatrics. *In* Barness, L. (ed.): Advances in Pediatrics. Chicago, Year Book Medical Publishers, 1982.

Kane, W., Brown, J., Hensinger, R., et al.: Scoliosis and school screening for spinal deformity. Am. Family Phys., *17*:123, 1978.

Kohler, L.: Health control of four-year-old children: An epidemiological study of child health. Acta Paediatr. Scand., *235*:4, 1972.

Kohler, L.: Physical mass examinations in the school health service. Acta Paediatr. Scand., *66*:307, 1977.

Kohn, M.: School Health Services and Nurse Practitioners: A survey of State Laws. Washington, D.C., Center for Law and Social Policy, 1979.

Levine, M., Oberklaid, F., Ferb, T., et al.: The pediatric examination of educational readiness: Validation of an extended observation procedure. Pediatrics, *66*:341, 1980a.

Levine, M., Brooks, R., and Shonkoff, J.: A Pediatric Approach to Learning Disabilities. New York, John Wiley and Sons, 1980b.

Nora, J.: Identifying the child at risk for coronary disease as an adult: A strategy for prevention. J. Pediatr., *10*:220, 1968.

Piaget, J.: Stages of intellectual development of the child. Bull. Menninger Clin., *26*:120, 1962.

Pless, E., Snider, M., Eaton, A., and Kearsley, R.: A rapid screening test for intelligence in children. Am. J. Dis. Child., *109*:533, 1965.

Rogers, K. (ed.): School Health: A Guide for Health Professionals, 1981. Evanston, IL, American Academy of Pediatrics, 1981.

Rogers, W., and Rogers, R.: A new simplified pre-school readiness experimental screening scale (the PRESS). Clin. Pediatr., *11*:448, 1972.

Rutter, M. (ed.): Helping Troubled Children. New York, Plenum Publishing Corp., 1976.

Starfield, B., Gross, E., Wood, M., et al.: Psychosocial and psychosomatic diagnoses in primary care of children. Pediatrics, *66*:159, 1980.

Thompson, H. (ed.): Standard of Child Health Care, 3rd ed. Evanston, IL, American Academy of Pediatrics, 1977.

Torrell, G., Nordwall, A., and Nachemson, A.: The changing pattern of scoliosis treatment due to effective screening. J. Bone Joint Surg., *63A*:337, 1981.

Welch, N., Saulsbury, F., and Kesler, R.: The value of the preschool examination in screening for health problems. J. Pediatr., *100*:232, 1982.

West, C.: Asymptomatic hematuria and proteinuria in children: Causes and appropriate diagnostic studies. J. Pediatr., *89*:172, 1976.

Yankauer, A., and Lawrence, R.: A study of periodic school medical examinations: I. Methodology and initial findings. Am. J. Public Health, *45*:71, 1955.

8

ADOLESCENT HEALTH CARE

Iris F. Litt, M.D.

The paucity and type of health care services available to adolescents reflect our society's perception of the health needs of this age group. With a prevailing attitude that adolescence is the healthiest time of life, little attention has been paid to providing health care, training pediatricians in adolescent medicine, or encouraging parents or teenagers themselves to seek periodic health-promoting types of care. The resulting limitation on contact between the pediatrician and adolescent has reinforced this impression that their health needs are minimal. Services created for this age group exist primarily in response to the stereotypes of the adolescent as a drug abuser or a promiscuous person at risk for venereal disease and pregnancy. National studies of adolescents over the past two decades have demonstrated the existence of a broad range of health problems, as well as the potential for prevention of later morbidity by intervention during adolescence.

Adolescent health problems result from the rapid growth that characterizes puberty and the special behavioral characteristics of this age group or may be forerunners of adult disease. Some problems are the result of improved life expectancy of congenitally disabled or chronically ill infants and children. The majority of these may be managed on an ambulatory basis. The additional challenge is that of bringing the adolescent and the physician together. Although the traditional approach has been to expect patients to seek out their doctors, there may be some rationale for reversing this approach during adolescence. Programs have been developed which bring health care to adolescents, rather than vice versa. Accordingly, the "exportation" of physicians to schools, detention facilities, mobile vans, and athletic and amusement events is no longer a rarity. Combining health care with other services (vocational, educational, and recreational) for youth (e.g., "The Door") provides another attractive model.

Although the content may vary somewhat according to the setting, the goals of ambulatory health care for adolescents remain (1) to identify the adolescent with a health program, (2) to identify the adolescent at risk for future dysfunction—social, psychological or physical, (3) to prevent physical or psychological dysfunction through education, immunization, and prophylactic treatment of the adolescent, his/her family, and peers when appropriate, (4) to treat identified health problems, and (5) to train adolescents to become informed future consumers of health care.

CONTENT OF THE HEALTH VISIT

The History

The following are some possible questions that have proved useful in interviewing adolescents:

How have things been going for you? Are you having difficulties at home?

How is school going? How are the teachers? The subjects?

What sports do you enjoy the most?

What kind of things do you do for fun when you're not in school?

Who is your best friend? What do you do together? Do you find it hard to make friends?

What are the rules at home? Do you think they're fair?

How do you rate your own health? Most teenagers have some questions or concerns about their development. How about you? What else?

Is there anyone in the family whose health worries you?

What are some of the things you worry about? Who can you talk to when you're worried?

What are some of the things that make you sad? What are some of the things that make you mad? What do you do when you're angry about something?

What do you and your mother/father do together?

Tell me about those things that you're best at...proudest of. What would you like to do even better? What kind of change(s) would you like to see in yourself? What would you like to change about your life?

Screening

Identification of existing health problems (many of which are subclinical) or of risk factors for future development of dysfunction is based on use of appropriate screening techniques (see Section II, page 32). No screening tests should be performed on an adolescent unless corresponding normative data are available for this age group. Physicians should avoid detection of trivial conditions, the discovery of which may further the adolescents' natural propensity to feel flawed and "imperfect." Other principles of available effective therapy and frequency are the same as for other age groups.

Laboratory Tests

The rationale for choice of screening tests is similar to that applied elsewhere in pediatric practice, but during adolescence additional dimensions of the cost-benefit ratio arise. The potential psychological impact of discovery of an asymptomatic condition, particularly if the therapeutic implications of early intervention are unclear, during that time in life when one is in the process of developing a healthy self-image, must be considered. On the other hand, knowledge of one's potential for transmission of genetic defects may be important during adolescence, when the individual is planning for the future. These counterbalancing considerations should be weighed in deciding which tests are to be performed, as well as the timing of their performance. Laboratory tests shown to have a high yield for this age group should be performed as part of the well adolescent examination (Tables 8–1 and 8–2). Differentiation is made on the basis of gender and stage of adolescence. Accordingly, the early adolescent female should undergo a screening urinalysis and urine culture. The finding of white cells in the urinary sediment may indicate cervicitis, vaginitis, or urethritis, as well as an asymptomatic urinary tract infection. A hematocrit is indicated due to the frequency of iron-deficiency anemia among female adolescents. The reference standard for evaluating hematocrits is different for adolescent males, owing to the stimulatory effect of increasing levels of androgens on erythropoietin as puberty progresses. Accordingly, the mean hematocrit for males prior to onset of puberty (Tanner 1) is 39 per cent and rises to 43 per cent by the completion of pubertal development (Tanner 5). Conversely, in females progression of puberty is associated with a lowering of hematocrit, not only because of the advent of menstrual blood loss but also because estrogen tends to inhibit erythropoietin. A rubella titer should be obtained in all females and those found to lack protective levels immunized regardless of history of previous infection or immunizations (see Immunizations, p. 38). These tests, with the exception of the rubella titer, should be repeated in mid and late adolescence. The yield on these examinations for asymptomatic male adolescents is sufficiently low to preclude their routine inclusion. In sexually active adolescents of any age, screening for common sexually transmitted diseases (STD) is indicated (see Chapter 26, Sexually Transmitted Diseases).

Hein et al. (1977) described a prevalence rate of early neoplastic changes in the Papanicolaou's smear of 35/1000 of 12- to 16-year olds from the inner city. That this observation is not unique to a low socioeconomic population is supported by a study of youngsters from middle and upper socioeconomic groups, in whom the rate of positive Pap smears was 5/1000. Sampling problems may influence the outcome of this screening procedure, as indicated by a study showing that the addition of a second cervical scrape to the standard cervical and vaginal pool sample, at the same visit, will increase the detection rate of suspicious cytology by 26.3 per cent.

The timing of performance of screening tests for genetic disease (sickle cell trait, Tay-Sachs, etc.) remains controversial. On the one hand, this information should be available to the young person sufficiently early to be useful in making decisions about future reproduction. On the other hand, it is unlikely that many adolescents, particularly those not at the stage of formal operational thinking, will choose to utilize the information in what is often an emotional, rather than rational, decision. Moreover, the impact on the developing self-image of learning that one is "flawed" has not been examined. Whenever these tests are performed, they should be accompanied by an age-appropriate counseling program to ensure an opportunity for the youngster to have questions answered and unspoken fears allayed. We were recently reminded of the importance of such a "debriefing" session when one of our patients, upon learning that she had sickle cell trait and that it could be passed on to an offspring should sexual intercourse result in a pregnancy, assumed that it was a kind of venereal disease.

Hearing Evaluation

A longitudinal study of British youngsters from 7 through 16 years showed an appreciable elevation of audiometric thresholds in adoles-

Table 8–1. PACKAGE OF CARE THE WELL ADOLESCENT VISIT I EARLY ADOLESCENCE (TANNER 1 and 2)

	Females	Males
Screening		
Physical	Hematocrit	—
	Urine culture screen	—
	Rubella titer (once)	—
	Tuberculin	
Psychosocial	Self-image	Self-image
	Depression	Depression
	Peer interaction (including sexuality)	Peer interaction (including sexuality)
	School performance	School performance
	Substance abuse	Substance abuse
Health Promotion	Self-examination of breasts	Self-examination of scrotum
	Nutrition counseling	Nutrition counseling
Prevention	Smoking	Smoking
	Cycle safety	Cycle safety
	Automotive passenger safety	Automotive passenger safety
	Immunization update (see Table 8–3)	Immunization update (see Table 8–3)
Anticipatory Guidance	Developing independence	Developing independence
	Dealing with peer pressure	Dealing with peer pressure
	Confidentiality	Confidentiality
	Variations in growth and development	Variations in growth and development
	Dating	Dating
	Preparation for menarche	—
Physical Examination Special attention to:	Blood pressure	Blood pressure
	Height, weight	Height, weight
	Skinfold thickness	Skinfold thickness
	—	Grip strength
	Stage of sexual development	Stage of sexual development
	Scoliosis	—
	Goiter	—
	Acne	Acne
	—	Gynecomastia
	Tibial tubercle	Tibial tubercle
	Gait	Gait
Symptomatic Treatment (anything revealed by the above +)	Acne	Acne
	Dysmenorrhea	—

cence. Prolonged exposure to highly amplified music is known to adversely affect hearing acuity, although long-term effects are not proven. For these reasons, it is advisable to perform an audiogram during routine evaluations of the well adolescent by the pediatrician.

Scoliosis Detection

Mild curvature of the spine is common among adolescents, with a prevalence of approximately 5 to 6 per cent in males and 10 to 14 per cent in females, compared with a rate of less than 3 per cent in 4- to 10-year-olds of both sexes. Scoliosis appears to be most prevalent at the time of peak growth velocity (12 years for females and 14 years for males). Approximately half of curves discovered at this time are "structural," the remainder being "postural," often associated with leg-length inequality. It is unlikely that curvatures measuring less than 10 degrees at puberty will progress appreciably, but structural curves in prepubertal children and those greater than 10 degrees in adolescents should be followed until growth is complete. Scoliosis mass screening in schools is another

Table 8–2. PACKAGE OF CARE THE WELL ADOLESCENT VISIT II MID–LATE ADOLESCENCE (TANNER 3–5)*

	Females	Males
Screening		
Physical	Vision testing	Vision testing
	Hearing testing	Hearing testing
	Genetically transmitted diseases	Genetically transmitted diseases
If sexually active	Pap smear	—
	VDRL	VDRL
	Gonorrhea culture	Gonorrhea culture
Prevention	Automotive safety	Automotive safety
	Venereal disease prevention	Venereal disease prevention
	Prevention of pregnancy	Prevention of pregnancy
Anticipatory Guidance	Planning for marriage	Planning for marriage
	Vocational/educational planning	Vocation/educational planning
	Cults	Cults
	Becoming a health-care consumer	Becoming a health-care consumer
Physical Examination	Breast masses	Gynecomastia
	—	Testicular tumor
	Vaginal discharge	Urethral discharge
	Pregnancy	—
Treatment	Corrective surgery (after growth complete)	Corrective surgery (after growth complete)

*Incremental with items listed for Early Adolescence.

matter and yields high false positive rates (see Chapter 7, page 71).

Hypertension Detection

Most pediatricians view sphygmomanometric assessment as part of the routine physical examination, but since it may be performed in isolation in settings other than the doctor's office or by personnel other than physicians, it may be considered a screening test. In contrast to criteria for hypertension in adults, which are clear-cut (greater than 140/90 mm Hg), those for children and adolescents are based on age-specific norms that reflect the knowledge that blood pressure increases with pubertal maturation. In this context, any individual whose blood pressure exceeds two standard deviations for age may be considered to have an elevated blood pressure. This conclusion is valid when blood pressure is measured in the sitting position with a cuff that covers two thirds of the upper arm and the second and third consecutive readings are averaged, using change rather than disappearance as the diastolic pressure. The prognostic significance of hypertension, so defined, remains to be established. Most adolescents with elevated readings are noted to have normal readings at other times and, on that basis, are usually diagnosed as having labile hypertension. A finding of labile hypertension should not be an indication for extensive evaluation. Approximately 50 per cent of teenagers with labile hypertension progress to sustained hypertension, typically those who have a family history of essential hypertension, who have hypercholesterolemia, or who are obese. Even with these risk factors, there is no evidence that early therapeutic intervention (i.e., when hypertension is still labile) alters the ultimate prognosis. Limitation of dietary salt is a prudent measure but one unlikely to be followed by most adolescents. Blood pressure should be checked twice a year in those with labile hypertension. The finding of persistent elevation of blood pressure, on the other hand, should be followed by an evaluation to determine its etiology. Sustained hypertension in the adolescent is most likely to be of renal origin, when an etiology can be determined. Less often, endocrinopathies may manifest themselves as hypertension in adolescence.

Self-Screening

Breast Examination

Teen-age females are routinely taught the procedure for self-examination of the breast. This may be done by the nurse or physician and if the latter is male, incorporation of this educational process into the performance of the physical examination often serves to reduce embarrassment. The patient is instructed to "Pay attention to what I am about to do, so that you may be able to examine yourself in the future," thus distracting her from thinking about the potentially sexual implications of her breasts being touched. Most masses discovered during adolescence will be benign cysts or fibroadenomas, and only rarely will a low-grade malignancy (cystosarcoma filloides) be found. Hein et al. (1982) have found that breast masses are often first discovered by teenagers themlves, but the long-term impact of providing this education at this early age has not yet been evaluated.

Scrotum Examination

Teaching self-examination of the scrotum during adolescence serves as a means of diverting the patient's attention from the sexual aspects of the examination, but its major value rests in the fact that it may result in early detection of a malignant testicular tumor. Germ cell tumors account for 95 per cent of testicular tumors in this age group, and their peak incidence is reached in late adolescence and early adulthood.

Prevention

The pediatrician's role in prevention of physical and psychological illness and accidents continues into the second decade of the patient's life. Updating of immunizations, anticipatory guidance, and accident prevention continue to be an important part of the agenda for the well adolescent visit. A major difference is that this counseling is done primarily with the patient himself or herself rather than with the parent(s). In addition, the scope of conditions amenable to prophylaxis or early detection becomes broader (pregnancy, sexually transmitted diseases, malignancy). Immunization in adolescents is covered on page 38.

Toxic shock syndrome has emerged in the past few years as a disease that affects adolescent females out of proportion to their representation in the population, with 42 per cent of cases occurring in this group. Case control studies suggest that the risk of contracting this disease may be reduced by avoiding use of high-absorbency tampons, by washing hands before insertion of a tampon with an applicator, and possibly by wearing tampons intermittantly, rather than continuously, during menses.

Prevention of Sexually Transmitted Diseases (STDs)

In Sorensen's study, adolescents appear "willing to assume the risks of catching V.D., largely because of their considerable distaste for asking their sex partners whether they might have it and partly because they cannot tolerate the idea that they would have sex with a person who would have a venereal disease" (Sorensen, 1973). In addition, he found that girls view boys as being at lower risk for V.D. than boys do girls. Accordingly, physicians need to discuss not only mechanisms for preventing contraction of STDs (e.g., condoms or spermicidal foams and jellies containing nonoxynol-9) but also issues of vulnerability. Inclusion of screening for STDs reinforces this concept (see Chapter 26).

Pregnancy Prevention

The pediatrician may be called upon to prevent pregnancy in the crisis atmosphere that follows a rape (one third to one half of rape victims are teenagers), following an episode of consensual unprotected intercourse, or by the sexually active teenager who requests contraception. Equally often, the fact that an adolescent is sexually active without protection arises during the course of an evaluation for an unrelated medical problem, adding the problem of creating motivation for using contraception as well as that of providing it.

POSTCOITAL CONTRACEPTION

In the first two instances, involving single episodes of coitus, pregnancy may be prevented by hormonal or mechanical means. Administration of ethinyl estradiol (2.5 mg P.O. twice daily for 5 days) is effective in preventing pregnancy, if initiated within 72 hours of the episode of unprotected intercourse. More recently, a one-day course of Ovral (2 pills immediately and 2, 12 hours later) has been shown to be efficacious. Insertion of a copper intrauterine device postcoitally may accomplish the same goal and has the advantage of providing long-term contraception for the patient who will continue to be sexually active. Its major drawback relates to the discomfort of insertion, which is particularly undesirable following a rape.

ONGOING CONTRACEPTION

For the sexually active teenager who requests contraception, a number of alternatives exist. The older concept that the adolescent is an unsuitable candidate for some contraceptive methods by virtue of her age alone is no longer valid, nor is it appropriate to assume that the pediatrician's advice for abstinence will be heeded. On the other hand, initiating a discussion of the adolescent's feeling about her sexual activity may reveal that she is ambivalent or being pressured. The pediatrician may help the patient examine the reasons for her sexual activity, and, if it is not pleasurable or growth-promoting, assist her in recognizing that her needs may be met in some other way. Poor self-image and fear of losing a boyfriend are not uncommon findings. Even if she elects to continue sexual activity, frequent follow-up, preferably every three months, is indicated to monitor compliance as well as her feelings about the relationship. Before prescribing any contraceptive method, it is important to recognize that a request for birth control does not always mean that contraception is the true agenda. Often a young woman who is worried about sterility (because she has been sexually active without becoming pregnant, because she has had V.D., or because of prior abortion) or has missed a period and now worries about pregnancy may request birth control as a means of having a pelvic examination which she assumes will address these concerns. To prescribe contraception without attempting to uncover these often unspoken concerns will often result in noncompliance.

In our clinic population, for example, only 55 per cent of adolescents who had received an effective contraceptive method were found to be still using it four months later, despite continued sexual activity. Among this group, compliance was best among those who had themselves requested contraception and abysmally poor for the group in whom inquiries about the need for contraception have been initiated by the pediatrician. This finding underscores the importance of working with the sexually active teenager to increase her own motivation for birth control. In deciding on a specific method, risks of that method must be weighed not only against its effectiveness (Table 8–3) but also against the risk of pregnancy, which for adolescents, particularly those under 15 years of age, is formidable. Pregnancy in this age group is associated with an increased rate of toxemia, postpartum hemorrhage and infection, and small-for-gestational-age or stillborn infants. The emotional, educational, and economic toll of adolescent pregnancy is often even greater than the physical.

Table 8–3. FIRST-YEAR FAILURE RATES OF BIRTH CONTROL METHODS

Method	Failure Rate in Typical Users (%)
Medroxyprogesterone	0.25
Combined birth control pills	2
Progestin-only pill	2.5
IUD	4
Condom	10
Diaphragm (with spermicide)	10
Cervical cap	13
Foam, creams, jellies, and vaginal suppositories	15
Coitus interruptus	23
Fertility awareness techniques (basal body temperature, mucous method, calendar and "rhythm")	20–30
Douche	40
Chance (no method of birth control)	90

Adapted from Hatcher, R. A., Stewart, G. K., Stewart, F., et al.: Contraceptive Technology 1982–1983. New York, Irvington Publishers, Inc., 1982.

Contraception may be accomplished by preventing ovulation (hormonal methods), preventing spermatogenesis (hormonal methods), preventing fertilization of the ovum (barrier methods), destroying the sperm (spermicidal foams and jellies), preventing implantation of a fertilized ovum (IUD, progestin), or interrupting early implantation of a fertilized ovum (menstrual extraction, dilatation and curettage).

Hormonal Methods. By interfering with gonadotropin production, administration of estrogens and/or progestins will prevent ovulation or adversely influence spermatogenesis. The prototype of this method of birth control for the female is "the Pill," an oral contraceptive containing a combination of an estrogen and progestins. There are currently marketed 16 different preparations, composed of either menstranol or ethinyl estradiol as the estrogen and norethindrone or norgestrel as the progestin. The original oral contraceptives contained much higher doses of estrogens (150 μg) compared to those currently available, which contain either 35 μg, 50 μg, or 80 μg. Knowledge of long-term effects of oral contraceptives containing estrogens based on a 20-year follow-up of patients using higher dose preparations may not be applicable to patients using oral contraceptives today. Moreover, these follow-up studies have been based entirely on adult populations.

These caveats notwithstanding, much is now known about long-term effects of estrogen-containing oral contraceptives. Initial concerns that such agents may predispose to cervical and breast cancer and diabetes have not been supported. In fact, it has been demonstrated that the incidence of breast disease is less in women on "the Pill." The only malignancy that appears to occur with greater frequency in this group is hepatocarcinoma, but this remains rare. Cardiovascular disease, specifically myocardial infarction, stroke, and thrombophlebitis, is clearly increased, but only in women over 35 years of age, with the incidence even higher in women on "the Pill" who also smoke more that 15 cigarettes daily. This risk persists even after discontinuation of pill use. Thus far, cardiovascular complications have not been reported during the adolescent period. Our review of 30 adolescent patients with thrombophlebitis failed to reveal any who were taking oral contraceptives. Cholestatic jaundice and elevations of hepatic enzymes are rare complications of use of estrogen-containing pills. Pill use is associated with a decreased incidence of anemia, cystic ovarian disease, and gallstones.

Because estrogens have a growth-retardant effect when administered to females in early puberty, it is appropriate to question the advisability of oral contraceptive use prior to completion of the pubertal growth spurt. Although one study demonstrated decreased levels of somatomedin in adolescents on "the Pill," others have failed to document any actual effect on growth. One of the few other studies of adolescent oral contraceptive use have shown an unexplained elevation of high density lipoproteins, in contrast with adult women, whose low density lipoproteins are known to be elevated by these agents. Another study has failed to confirm the finding in adult women of a decrease in antithrombin III levels which presumably contributed to hypercoagulability. Lowering of serum folate, pyridoxine, riboflavin, and vitamin B_{12} levels has been found in users of estrogen-containing preparations of all ages, while vitamin A levels are increased by these agents. During the first few months on estrogen-containing oral contraceptives, many patients experience transient nausea, breast fullness, and weight gain (in the range of 2 pounds). Breakthrough bleeding is seen somewhat more often in patients receiving the 35 μg estrogen preparation, but our studies fail to demonstrate any significant difference in other side effects based on estrogen dose.

In response to concern about estrogen effects, contraceptives containing progestins alone have been developed. The so-called mini pill, typically contains either 35 μg norethindrone or 7.5 μg norgestrel and the injectable form, medroxyprogesterone, given in a dose of 150 mg every three months. Progestin-only preparations have been implicated as possibly responsible for producing hypertension in adult women, as well as acne and depression. Medroxyprogesterone is not approved by the FDA currently for use as a contraceptive agent because of the finding of an increased incidence of benign breast neoplasia in laboratory animals. It is, nonetheless, the most widely used contraceptive agent worldwide. Medroxyprogesterone may cause irregular bleeding with the first one or two cycles, after which menses cease completely. The effect of this agent on both menses and ovulation is reversible within four months after the last dose.

Besides differences in complications and side effects, the various hormonal preparations have different levels of effectiveness. The most effective is medroxyprogesterone (Depo-Provera) given intramuscularly in a 150-mg dose every three months. The pregnancy rate associated with its use by adult women is 0.008 to 0.25 per 100 woman-years. The least effective of hormonal methods are the all-progestin preparations, for which the pregnancy rate is 2.5 per 100 woman-years, again in adults.

Based on these data about effectiveness and complications, "the Pill," with a combination of estrogen and progestin, is the contraceptive agent of choice for the adolescent having regular sexual intercourse, unless she has liver disease or any condition that might be worsened by hypercoagulability (e.g., replaced cardiac valve, sickle cell anemia). A patient with diabetes, a seizure disorder, or hypertension may be begun on this preparation, but, she must be carefully observed for signs of worsening of these problems. Smokers should be informed of the possible risk of later cardiovascular disease, and an attempt made to have smoking discontinued or reduced. In our experience, some teenagers are sufficiently motivated to use "the Pill" and to demonstrate their maturity by improving health habits that they may be willing to stop smoking. For those not so inclined or those whose underlying disease worsens with use of estrogen-containing preparations, the all-progestin pill is appropriate.

The possibility of noncompliance with any

pill-taking regimen should be considered before the prescription is written, as well as periodically thereafter. Patients should be asked if they have had difficulty remembering to take pills of any kind when prescribed in the past, as well as whether or not they anticipate any problems with taking these specific pills. Particularly if parents are unaware of their daughter's sexual activity, the pressure to conceal the fact may interfere with the patient's ability to comply. In our experience, teenagers who continue to use oral contraceptives correctly are those who have a positive self-image, who act autonomously and responsibly (e.g., pay for their medical care, make their own medical appointments, come on time for visits or call when necessary to break appointments, and have a steady sexual partner). Because teenagers may not continue to use contraceptives despite continued sexual activity and, recognizing that these decisions are often based on peer pressure, adolescents felt to be at risk for future noncompliance may benefit from more frequent visits and, if available, contact with a peer counseling program to provide skills for resisting negative pressures. For those who have demonstrated noncompliance, as well as for the mentally retarded, use of injectable medroxyprogesterone (or IUD) should be considered. Hormonal methods for male contraception are not yet available.

Barrier Methods. These methods exert their contraceptive effect by providing a physical barrier to unions of gametes. The prototype of this approach is the condom; although devices such as the diaphragm and cervical cap will also be included in this section, it is felt that they may actually serve primarily as containers for spermicidal jellies and creams.

Condoms are among the most popular birth control devices in other countries (e.g., Japan). Condom use among partners of 15- to 19-year-old females has increased in the United States from 15 per cent in 1976 to 20 per cent in 1979 (Zelnik and Kantner, 1980). Except for rare cases of contact dermatitis there are no complications associated with condom use. Its availability without prescription and its relatively low cost are also desirable. If the condom is not removed immediately after ejaculation and the penis remains in situ, however, sperm may leak into the vagina, increasing the risk of pregnancy. As a result, the pregnancy rate associated with condom use is quite high (~10 to 15 per 100 woman-years). When used in conjunction with a spermicidal vaginal foam, however, the pregnancy rate is significantly reduced and approaches that of the most effective means.

The diaphragm must be filled with spermicidal jelly and positioned before intercourse and must be left in place for at least eight hours after intercourse. Teenagers often dislike this method because its use implies the expectation of intercourse or because it is "messy" or requires them to touch their genitals for insertion and removal. On the other hand, diaphragm use has increased among older adolescents, particularly college students, who are concerned about potential complications of use of other methods. Its effectiveness varies from 2 to 20 pregnancies per 100 woman years.

The cervical cap is a thimble-shaped device made of firm thick rubber which must be expertly fitted to cover the cervix, to which it adheres by suction. Its advantage over the diaphragm is that it may be left in place for up to three days. It, too, must be filled with spermicidal jelly. Reported studies are of small populations in which pregnancy rates have been unacceptably high (e.g., 7 of 24 college students became pregnant within an average of 11 months after onset of use of the cap).

Spermicides containing nonoxynol-9 are available as "over-the-counter" creams, foams, jellies, effervescent tablets, and recently as impregnated sponges. These agents have the advantage of being easily available but may produce a contact vaginitis and are in the lower range of efficacy in terms of pregnancy prevention (10 to 15 per 100 woman-years). Used in conjunction with condoms, however, the pregnancy rate is significantly reduced (2 to 20 per 100 woman-years) and approaches that of oral contraceptives and the IUD. Recent case control studies suggest that this chemical may be absorbed, as its use is associated with an increased risk of chromosomal anomalies, including Down's syndrome.

Agents That Prevent Implantation of a Fertilized Ovum. Intrauterine devices (IUDs) are believed to exert their contraceptive effect by rendering the endometrium unfavorable to implantation. The findings of an inflammatory response in the endometrium, of increased endometrial prostaglandins, and of increased myometrial contractility in association with the presence of an IUD have been cited as possible mechanisms by which IUDs act. IUDs are small plastic devices tagged with a fine string. The device itself is introduced into the uterine cavity with an applicator by a trained individual, and the string is allowed to protrude through the cervical os into the vagina. The patient is trained to palpate the string after completion of each menstrual period to be sure that the IUD has not been expelled. IUDs were initially proscribed for nulliparous adolescents because of mechanical difficulties with insertion and a high incidence of cramping, bleeding, and expulsion. The smaller size of the newer varieties (Copper 7 or T) has eliminated these problems. Copper wire wound around the plastic core appears to increase the endometrial inflammatory response and the small amount of copper that leaches out has been shown to be gonococcocidal in vitro. One manufacturer has incorporated a well that releases progesterone as part of the IUD. These devices reportedly decrease menstrual cramping. The copper-containing IUDs must be replaced every three years and those containing progesterone, every year. The pregnancy rate associated with IUDs ranges from 2 to 4 per 100 woman-years. A slightly increased risk of ectopic pregnancy exists for users of the progesterone-containing IUD. The other major complication of IUDs is that of infection. The risk of salpingitis is highest among adolescents and those with multiple sex partners. The obvious advantage of an IUD is freedom from worries about compliance.

Prevention of Malnutrition

Adolescents are at high risk for poor nutrition. The reasons for increased adolescent vulnerability are threefold. On the one hand, developing the capacity for formal operational thinking often leads to involvement in religious activities, some of which include dietary restrictions. Desire for involvement in athletic competition or ballet dancing often arises during adolescence and, lastly, most adolescent females view themselves as being fat with the advent of puberty and its effect of increasing adiposity and widening of the hip girdle. Self-imposed dietary restrictions that follow come at the very time when the increase in height, weight, and muscle mass and development of secondary sex characteristics demand that an adequate supply of calories and nutrients become available to the growing teenager.

Caloric requirements appear to parallel growth velocity curves. Accordingly, girls at the peak of their growth velocity curve, at about 12 to 13 years, consume approximately 2550 kilocalories daily, whereas the average energy intake for boys peaks at 3470 kilocalories by age 16. Corresponding values for protein intake at these times are 80 gm/day for girls and 100 gm/day for boys (11 to 12.5 per cent of calories). When caloric intake is restricted, as is often the case when adult diet guidelines are inappropriately applied to adolescents, protein will be diverted from its important anabolic function to that of supplying energy.

Calcium requirements for the rapidly growing skeletal system of adolescents consist of 1200 mg daily, rarely met by the average American diet without the addition of a liter of milk.

Menstrual iron loss in females approximates 0.5 mg daily. This is comparable to the additional iron required for expansion of blood and muscle mass in adolescent males. Accordingly, both sexes require 18 mg of iron daily. Unfortunately, a nationwide dietary survey revealed that foods high in iron are among those most disliked by adolescents. Iron-rich snacks, especially in combination with citrus fruits, such as peanuts, dried fruits, and burritos, are excellent supplements to the traditional iron sources: liver, muscle meats, green vegetables, and iron-fortified cereal products.

Zinc deficiency has been implicated as a cause of sexual maturational delay, as well as of acne. Fifteen mg of zinc is the recommended daily allowance in order to provide the 400 μg needed by the male during the adolescent growth spurt. For adolescents on traditional diets, every 10 gm of protein corresponds to 1.5 mg of zinc. For other than animal protein sources, the amount of available zinc is generally lower, placing adolescents on vegetarian diets potentially at risk for a zinc deficiency. The zinc-lowering effect of oral contraceptives has not yet been shown to have clinical sequelae.

The energy and growth needs of adolescents create a greater need for vitamins at this age than at any time since infancy. Recommended daily allowances for each are listed in Table 8–4. Most nutritional surveys conclude that American adolescents have inadequate intakes of vitamins A, B_6, and C and folacin. Oral contraceptive use has been shown to decrease levels of the latter, as well as pyridoxine, riboflavin, and vitamin B_{12}, while increasing vitamin A levels.

Dieting

Weight Reduction. Dieting for the purpose of losing weight is a common interest of adolescent females, particularly those who mature in advance of their peer group. In addition, adolescents interested in participation in certain sports that value leanness often undertake dieting to accomplish their goal.

Determination of skinfold thickness will permit accurate assessment of body fat composition, a more realistic measurement than absolute weight for counseling adolescents about weight reduction. For females, it is important to take into consideration the observation that menses may become irregular or cease when

Table 8–4. RECOMMENDED DIETARY ALLOWANCES OF NUTRIENTS FOR ADOLESCENT MALES, FEMALES, AND PREGNANT ADOLESCENTS

		Males		Females		Pregnant Females	
		11–14 yr	*15–18 yr*	*11–14 yr*	*15–18 yr*	*11–14 yr*	*15–18 yr*
Weight	(kg)	45	66	46	55	46	55
Energy	(kcal)	2700	2800	2200	2100	2500	2400
Protein	(g)	45	56	46	46	76	76
Vitamin A	(μg R.E.)	1000	1000	800	800	1000	1000
Vitamin A	(IU)	5000	5000	4000	4000	5000	5000
Vitamin D	(μg)	10	10	10	10	15	15
Vitamin D	(IU)	400	400	400	400	600	600
Vitamin E	(mg α T.E.)	8	10	8	8	10	10
Vitamin C	(mg)	50	60	50	60	70	80
Folacin	(μg)	400	400	400	400	800	800
Niacin	(mg)	18	18	15	14	17	16
Riboflavin	(mg)	1.6	1.7	1.3	1.3	1.6	1.6
Thiamine	(mg)	1.4	1.4	1.1	1.1	1.5	1.5
Vitamin B_6	(mg)	1.8	2.0	1.8	2.0	2.4	2.6
Vitamin B_{12}	(μg)	3.0	3.0	3.0	3.0	4.0	4.3
Calcium	(mg)	1200	1200	1200	1200	1600	1600
Phosphorus	(mg)	1200	1200	1200	1200	1600	1600
Iodine	(μg)	150	150	150	150	175	175
Iron	(mg)	18	18	18	18	18+	18+
Magnesium	(mg)	350	400	300	300	450	450
Zinc	(mg)	15	15	15	15	20	20

Adapted from Marino, D. D., and King, J. C.: Nutritional concerns during adolescence. Pediatr. Clin. North Am., 27:126, 1980.

body fat falls below 20 per cent (3/4 inch of skinfold thickness).

Loss of one pound of body fat requires expenditure of 3500 calories in excess of those consumed. In planning a diet for an active adolescent, it is important to recall that athletic participation requires a minimum of 2000 calories daily. Losing calories through dieting alone demands food restriction intolerable to most teenagers. Accordingly, a combination of exercise and dieting is desirable. An ideal weight-loss program for a growing adolescent would aim for a two-pound reduction each week. This could be accomplished by a reduction in calorie intake of 500 calories daily coupled with an hour of bike-riding, 20 minutes of running, or 15 minutes of swimming each day. In no case should a loss in excess of four pounds weekly be permitted (see Chapter 65, Obesity).

Weight Gain. The demands of athletic competition (or of self-image in the case of some later-maturing males) occasionally are such as to cause teenagers to desire to gain weight. In order to gain one pound in the form of muscle mass (lean body weight), it is necessary to consume 3500 calories in excess of usual intake, and active exercise should accompany the diet in order to avoid accumulation of excess fat. Synthetic anabolic steroids and testosterone have been used to increase muscle mass and strength. Their adverse effects on bone growth, spermatogenesis, and/or liver histology should serve to proscribe use for this purpose in any adolescent.

Vegetarianism. The idealism of adolescence, the awakening of religious faith, and/or an interest in achieving a healthier body often lead teenagers to espouse vegetarianism. Common to all vegetarians is the refusal to consume meat. Differences exist, however, among the various types of vegetarians. The vegans, for example, will eat no animal foods whatsoever. If this diet is followed for more than three years, vegans may suffer a vitamin B_{12} deficiency, which may be prevented by use of fortified soybean milk. This diet is also low in vitamin B_6, riboflavin, calcium, iron, and zinc, a situation worsened when spinach, parsley, and chard are eaten regularly, as the oxalate they contain may bind the zinc. The lactovegetarians will eat milk and cheese in addition to fruits and vegetables. They, and the ovolactovegetarians, who eat eggs as well, need suffer no dietary deficiencies. A vegetarian diet that meets the minimum daily requirements for adolescents is listed in Table 8–5.

Table 8–5. FOOD GUIDE FOR THE ADOLESCENT CONSUMING A MIXED PROTEIN, OVOLACTOVEGETARIAN, OR VEGAN DIET

	Number of Servings for Type of Diet		
	Mixed	*Ovolactovegetarian*	*Vegan*
Milk and Milk Products	4	4	0
Protein Foods			
Animal sources	2	0	0
Legumes	1	2	3
Nuts	1	1	2
Fruits and Vegetables			
Vitamin C–rich	1	2	2
Dark green	1	1	3
Other	2	3	1
Whole Grain Cereal Products	4	6	6
Fats and Oils	2	2	2

Adapted from Marino, D. D., and King, J. C.: Nutritional concerns during adolescence. Pediatr. Clin. North Am., 27:130, 1980.

The Zen macrobiotic diet in which the ultimate state consists of ingestion of rices is the most dangerous of those diets espoused by adolescents. Scurvy, hypoproteinemia, anemia, hypocalcemia, kwashiorkor, and impaired renal function have been demonstrated to result from adherence to this diet.

Pregnancy. The continuing growth requirements for the adolescent herself, as well as those of her baby, place the pregnant teenager at nutritional risk. There are data linking preeclampsia in gravid adolescents with low protein and caloric intake and low circulating levels of vitamin B_6. These notwithstanding, the actual requirements for the pregnant adolescent have not been established. Supplementation with elemental iron (30 to 60 mg daily) is suggested. (see Table 8–4).

Prevention of Accidents

The importance of continuing to focus on accident prevention during the adolescent years is underscored by the knowledge that automotive accidents are the leading cause of death during adolescence, responsible for approximately 70 deaths per 100,000 in the 12- to 17-year-old age group. Despite the known effectiveness of helmets and seatbelts in reducing morbidity and mortality from motor vehicle accidents, we have found that only 18 per cent of the adolescents in our clinic population use these safety devices regularly. Automotive accidents are more common among young drivers and those who use alcohol or marijuana while driving. In our clinic population, 12 per cent admitted to using these substances before operating a motor vehicle. In a study by Hingson et al. (1982), teenagers who drove after smoking marijuana on at least 6 occasions each month were 2.4 times more likely to be involved in traffic accidents than a comparison group who did not drive after marijuana use. When marijuana was used on 15 or more occasions monthly, the risk of accidents rose to 2.9 times that of the comparison group. Anticipatory guidance should, therefore, include discussions about these factors, including the possibility of beginning a dialogue between parent and teenager on contingency plans in the event that either he or she or a friend who is driving becomes drunk at a party or becomes involved in some other potentially hazardous situation.

In addition to automotive accidents, participation in athletics is often associated with serious injuries. (See Chapter 25 for a more complete discussion of sports injuries).

Although one does not worry about accidental ingestions among adolescents as one does with younger children, it is important to remember that teenagers may inadvertently ingest a toxic substance offered as a known mind-altering drug or naturally occurring substance. Often P.C.P. is marketed as marijuana, and a poisonous mushroom may accidentally be eaten by the teenager who expects it to be a "safe" hallucinogen.

Prevention of Psychosocial Problems—Anticipatory Guidance

Growth and Development

An integral part of the health supervision examination is the assessment of physical growth and development and comparison of the individual with group norms. This component of the well adolescent visit is perhaps the most important, as the patient and his or her family will undoubtedly have made their own informal comparative assessment before actually seeing the doctor. Rather than simply recording height and weight on the traditional growth curve, the pediatrician should routinely chart these findings on a velocity curve such as that designed by Tanner and Whitehouse (1976) because of the importance of *rate* of growth as well as *absolute* growth for assessment of normal growth in this age group. The recognized relationship between timing of the peak of the growth velocity curves and pubertal events such as menarche make it desirable to have these data available in the counseling situation as well. In addition, the well adolescent visit includes measurement of additional growth variables. Determination of skinfold thickness as a reflection of body fat is valuable in assessing nutritional status and, accordingly, in counseling athletes and others interested in weight control. Grip strength is measured in males, as this parameter also reflects pubertal growth. Staging of pubertal development is best accomplished with the guidance of established standards for assessment of secondary sex characteristics, such as pubic hair in both sexes, breasts in females, and genitalia in males. Both Greulich and later Tanner categorized puberty into five stages based on these characteristics. Because same-sex teenagers have much more in common (anatomically, physiologically, and probably psychologically) with others at their same stage of development of secondary sex characteristics than at their same chronological age, "Tanner" staging, as it is often called, provides a useful basis for assessing pubertal growth and development. Pediatricians should become comfortable with its routine use.

Any perceived deviation from the growth pattern of a teenager's peer group is typically interpreted by the adolescent to reflect an abnormality rather than the actuality of his or her falling within the range of normal. Male adolescents (or their parents) tend to worry if they are short or thin or they notice breast development, while females (or more rarely their parents) in general worry about being thin and about lack of menarche or breast asymmetry. A recent trend, which represents an apparent departure from the past, is the desire on the part of some teen-age females to be taller and more muscular, most likely reflecting the increasing female participation in athletics. These body-image concerns may be the avowed agenda for the visit, may be revealed only by the physician's probing, or may be disguised in the form of a request for an excuse from gym class for a seemingly minor problem. Thirty to 40 per cent of normal teenagers in our clinic admit to worrying about some aspect of their physical growth when given an opportunity to do so using a checklist administered in the waiting room (Fig. 8–1). In a survey of seventh-grade public school students, Duke has found that 26 per cent of males and 65 per cent females wish to be thinner, 82 per cent of males and 47 per cent of females wanted to be more muscular, and 53 per cent of males and 37 per cent of females wanted to be taller, suggesting the widespread nature of these concerns.

Certain groups of adolescents appear to be at greater risk for certain of these body-image problems, particularly those whose onset of pubertal maturation differs from that of their peer group. Analysis of data collected by the Center for Health Statistics indicated that desire to change one's body was more prevalent among males who were late maturers, although well within the range of normal (Gross and Duke, 1980). Not only are these males more likely to have a poor self-image, but they also appear to be at a disadvantage socially and educationally and are less likely to be school leaders. These young people, as well as their parents and teachers, have lower educational aspirations and expectations than do early-maturing males. Among females, the timing of puberty does not have as consistent an effect. In a longitudinal study of a small sample of females (Jones et al., 1971), early-maturing females were found to be at a disadvantage socially if they were from the lower socioeconomic groups. In their study of adolescent females, Simmons et al. (1978) found that the impact of timing of puberty was significantly modified by environmental events. Accordingly, early-maturing females who moved from elementary to junior high school (rather than staying at a K–8th school) and those who began to date early had lower self-image, as well as poorer school performance, when compared to later-maturing females. Regardless of timing of puberty, the onset of puberty itself is associated with the desire to be thinner among females in the data analyzed by Gross and Duke.

The male adolescent concerned about his height should be evaluated from the perspective of his previous growth pattern and that of his family. If he has consistently been growing at the lower end of this growth curve, it is not

Figure 8–1. Medical history for adolescent patient. *Stanford Adolescent Clinic Questionaire*

Name:
Birthdate:
Today's Date:

I. Past Medical History
  A. Birth
    1. Medications during pregnancy? ______ (what?) ______
    2. Was pregnancy full term (9 months?) ______
    3. Did patient stay in hospital after mother went home? ______ (why?) ______
  B. Past Illnesses

	Date		
1. Rheumatic Fever	____________	Chickenpox	____________
2. Tuberculosis	____________	Measles	____________
3. Hepatitis	____________	Mumps	____________
4. V.D. (Syphilis, Gonorrhea, etc.)	____________	German measles (Rubella)	____________
		Other	____________

  C. Immunizations

	Date of Last
1. DPT (Diphtheria, Pertussis, Tetanus)	____________
2. Polio (by mouth)	____________
3. Measles	____________
4. Mumps	____________
5. German measles (Rubella)	____________
6. Smallpox	____________
7. B.C.G.	____________
8. Tine test for T.B.	____________
9. Others	____________

  D. Hospitalization
    1. Overnight stay in hospital— Date: ____________ Reason: ____________
    2. Surgery: Date: ____________ Reason: ____________

  E. Allergies
    1. Medication (which one?) ____________ Type of Reaction ____________
    2. Food ____________ Type of Reaction ____________
    3. Other ____________ Type of Reaction ____________

II. Personal Information
  A. Present Medications or Drugs (include vitamins, nonprescription and street drugs, etc.)

Name	Dose	How Often	Reason	Prescribed by M.D.?

  B. Diet
    1. Regular Yes ________ No ________
    2. Special—Type: ____________
      For How Long: ____________
      For What Reason: ____________

Figure continued on opposite page

Figure 8–1. Medical history for adolescent patient. *Stanford Adolescent Clinic Questionaire* (Continued)

C. Habits
1. Any habits you would like to break?
   List ____
   ____
   ____
2. Do you drink alcohol-containing beverages: Yes ________ No ________
   If yes—How much each day ____________________ or each week ____________________
   What type? Beer; Wine; Whiskey
   How old were you when you first began to drink? ____________________
   Do you drink when you are: happy; sad; alone; worried; in a group (circle all that fit)
3. Do you smoke? Yes ________ No ________
   If yes—How many each day? ____________________
   What type cigarettes; joints; other ____________________ (circle)
   How old were you when you first began to smoke? ____________________
   Do you want to quit? ____________________

D. Below are listed a number of common problems reported to us by other teenagers. Check yes or no for each, so that we may be in a better position to help you.

	Yes	No
1. Trouble falling asleep	______	______
2. Awakening during the night	______	______
3. Being very tired during the day	______	______
4. Occasionally wetting the bed	______	______
5. Pain with menstrual period	______	______
6. Bothered by headaches	______	______
7. Bothered by stomach aches	______	______
8. Bothered by dizzy spells	______	______
9. Bothered by leg pains	______	______
10. Worrying about health	______	______
11. Concerned that I am too short	______	______
12. Concerned that I am too tall	______	______
13. Concerned that I am too thin	______	______
14. Concerned that I am too fat	______	______
15. Concerned that my breasts are too small	______	______
16. Concerned that my penis is too small	______	______
17. Worried that I might become pregnant before I am ready	______	______
18. Worried that I might make someone pregnant	______	______
19. Worried that I might not be able to get pregnant	______	______

Figure continued on following page

Figure 8–1. Medical history for adolescent patient. *Stanford Adolescent Clinic Questionaire* (Continued)

20. Not yet ready for sex, but feel pressured ________ ________
21. Worried about my parents' relationship ________ ________
22. Would you like to change something in your relationship with your parents? ________ ________
23. Do you have a friend you can talk to about anything at all? ________ ________
24. Trouble getting to school ________ ________
25. Worried about school ________ ________
26. Troubled about future plans ________ ________
27. Sometimes I'm so sad that I think about dying. ________ ________
28. Have other personal problems which I would like to discuss with the doctor, but rather not write down ________ ________

E. Family History
   1. Is there any one in the family whose health worries you?

   ____

   2. List family members:

	Name	Age	Living at home?	Any health problems?
Mother				
Father				
Sisters				
Brothers				

F. When was the last time:
   1. You had a checkup by a doctor? ________________
   2. You had a checkup by a dentist? ________________
   3. You had your vision checked? ________________
   4. You had your hearing checked? ________________
   5. You had a pelvic—Pap smear? ________________

G. Safety
   1. Do you drive a car? Yes ________ No ________
      If yes, do you: always use a seat belt?
      sometimes use a seat belt? (circle one)
      never use a seat belt?
   2. Do you drive a motorcycle, bike, car? (circle)
      If yes, do you: always wear a helmet?
      sometimes wear a helmet? (circle one)
      never wear a helmet?
   3. If yes, do you sometimes: drink alcohol before driving? Yes ________ No ________
      smoke a joint before driving? Yes ________ No ________

unusual that he will have his growth spurt later than his larger peers. This phenomenon should result in somewhat greater ultimate height than if the growth spurt occurred earlier, because of the resultant increase in length of growing time prior to epiphyseal closure, an observation that may provide some solace to the patient. The other information that should be elicited relates to the timing of onset of the growth spurt of parents. There appears to be continuity between the mother's pattern of growth and that of her offspring of either sex, such that children of heavier and earlier-maturing mothers will tend to develop earlier. Obtaining a history of a late growth spurt from a 6-foot-tall father is often the perfect solution to the self-doubt and worry of the late-developing teenager. If physical examination and history are otherwise negative, a diagnosis of constitutionally delayed puberty may be considered in the male. If he is 14 years old or older, without the characteristics of puberty and a serum testosterone level of less than 100 μg, it is unlikely that he will have his growth spurt within the ensuing 18 months. Accordingly, we would offer him the option of receiving testosterone therapy in order to accelerate the onset of puberty. Initial concerns of reducing ultimate height by this intervention have not been substantiated, and side effects have been absent in our experience. The rare complications of testosterone therapy such as hepatocarcinoma must, however, be shared with the patient and family before decision to treat is made.

Gynecomastia occurs in 30 to 50 per cent of normal adolescent males and is unilateral in 25 per cent. Stimulated by metabolites of testosterone, or possibly by failure of metabolism of dehydroepiandrosterone to testosterone, breast tissue tends to hypertrophy during early puberty (Stages 3 to 4), with regression noted within two years of onset in the majority. Embarrassment is the typical response to noting its presence and avoidance of public undressing (such as in the school locker room) a common response. Reassurance and education about etiology and prognosis are indicated upon discovery by the pediatrician, regardless of whether the teenager mentions it himself.

Concern about penile size often exists among young male adolescents. They should be informed about the lack of relationship between the size of the flaccid and the erect penis, as well as the fact that there is a visual artifact that tends to diminish the appearance of their own penis when viewed from above, compared with their lateral view of that of another male. They should also be reassured that ultimate penile size is not achieved until Tanner Stage V.

The female adolescent who is concerned about lack of menarche should first be evaluated to determine if she actually has primary amenorrhea (see p. 97). This possibility should be considered if she is older than 16 years, if she is more than one year older than was her mother or sister at their menarche, or if she has failed to develop signs of puberty by the age of 13 years. If she does not fulfill one of these criteria, she should be reassured and arrangements for a 6-month follow-up made.

It has, in our experience, been helpful to teenagers with concerns about their development to see where they fall in the spectrum of normal physical development, using photographs of the five stages of pubertal maturation which indicate the normal age range for each.

Depression and *suicide* are major problems in adolescence. As part of the routine health promotion examination, symptoms and signs should be elicited (Fig. 8–1). Further discussion is found in Chapter 36.

The Role of Peers

In anticipation of adolescence, parents often fear that their authority will be undermined and family principles and morals supplanted by those of the peer group once this age is reached. This fear does not appear to be supported by available information, with two exceptions. It is typical for adolescents to use the peer group rather than the family setting for experimentation with sexuality and aggression. It is well recognized, for example, that teenagers will curse and swear among their peers but not among family members. Similarly, mutual masturbation among young males is less often a forerunner of homosexuality than it is a safe testing ground for sexual prowess. Peers serve as the major source of information, often erroneous, about sex. Although, in most surveys, teenagers profess to prefer that this role be assumed by their parents, the latter commonly feel inadequate to the task. Indeed, in many matters, it may be that gravitation toward the peer group is the result of bidirectional forces, as much a pushing-out by parents as a pulling-in by peers.

Regardless of the cause, it is apparent that the peer group is more important during adolescence than at any other time. Its potentially positive influence has been marshalled in a number of projects designed to provide teenagers with skills necessary to resist negative peer pressure. Recognizing that peer pressure is often responsible for adolescents' initiation of smoking, drug use, and sexual activity, these programs have focused on utilization of peer support for prevention of these behaviors. One of the most carefully designed and evaluated of these is the Smoking Prevention Program of McAlister et al. (1979), in which seventh graders were found to have a significantly lower rate of initiation of smoking after participation in a peer group intervention program. We have preliminary data to suggest that utilization of peer counselors who teach skills necessary to communicate with sexual partners may enhance self-esteem, reduce stress, avoid exploitation, and increase contraceptive utilization by sexually active adolescents as well. In summary, peers may be involved to provide positive behavioral models, to teach, to counsel and facilitate, and to provide meaningful links with adult institutions.

Some potentially negative outcomes of peer influence are manifested in the apparently growing involvement of adolescents in cults. Predominantly a phenomenon of the older, well-educated Caucasian adolescent, there are currently 2500 to 3000 such groups. It is not surprising that this age group would be particularly vulnerable, not only because of susceptibility to peer pressure, but also because of their arrival at the cognitive level of formal operational thought, which often arouses interest in the spiritual and religious. Recent studies have undertaken exploration of possible antecedent factors associated with adolescent cult membership. Although research in this area is still in its infancy, certain situational and family factors are emerging as correlates, if not causes, of this phenomenon. Situational stress (e.g., examination time, a broken romance) and periods of transition (e.g., graduation) appear to be times of increased vulnerability. Family factors delineated by Zerin (1982) in a study comparing selected families of offspring who joined versus resisted cult membership include "(1) Chronic undercurrent of often-unacknowledged marital disharmony. (2) The 'absent father' syndrome—father may be physically present and still 'not there,' so that there was a missing Father Rescuer in the individual's childhood, leading them to look for 'True Father' later in a cult. (3) Lack of preparation . . . for independence—kids were allowed to 'decide for themselves' before they learned how to make choices and decisions. They were given a prescription . . . but not the pattern . . . for making it happen. The cult gives them a way out of this script dilemma. (4) Lack of unconditional positive strokes—too much stroking for performance, not enough for just being. (5) Double binds (injunctions) like think/don't think, feel/don't feel (especially anger), grow up/don't grow up, hurry up/take your time. (6) A big switch in family style at the time of high school graduation—from centripetal (binding) to centrifugal (expelling), instead of fine-tuning the style to the developmental needs of the individual child. (7) Lack of meaningful religiosity, membership in a church or synagogue notwithstanding (a shallowness. . . of values and goals in the family interaction). (8) Lack of training in values clarification. (9) Lack of boundaries." It is obvious that many families with similar characteristics do not produce offspring who are cult members, and many families of cult members do not fit this description. Nonetheless, it may be prudent to counsel families about appropriate parenting during adolescence, as well as to alert older teenagers about potential stresses and vulnerabilities.

Menstrual Problems of Adolescents

Dysmenorrhea

The most common menstrual problem of this age group is dysmenorrhea or menstrual cramps occurring in nearly two thirds of postmenarcheal adolescents. Fourteen per cent are incapacitated by dysmenorrhea, resulting in its being the leading cause of short-term absence from school among female teenagers. Dysmenorrhea is classified as being primary—that is, without any underlying structural or infectious abnormality—or secondary—when a congenital abnormality of the uterus, cervix, or vagina, a foreign body, or endometriosis or endometritis is responsible. Primary dysmenorrhea, the more common form, was, in the absence of obvious pathology, long regarded as a psychosomatic symptom. It is now recognized that painful menses result from the myometrial stimulation by prostaglandins E_2 and $F_{2\alpha}$ produced in the endometrium. Understanding of the pathogenesis of dysmenorrhea facilitates its prevention and treatment by interfering with prostaglandin production, by destroying already formed prostaglandins, or by eliminating endogenous production of progesterone, thought to sensitize the myometrium to the prostaglandin effect. The former is accomplished by treatment with antiprostaglandin drugs, of which naproxen sodium appears to be most effective. We recommend a regimen of two 275-mg tablets at the onset of menses, followed by one tablet every 6 hours that first day. It is rare that therapy is needed longer than one day. In order to avoid severe gastric irritation, the patient should be cautioned not to take this medication on an empty stomach. This short-term intermittent regimen is unassociated with other known side effects or complications. Patients with dysmenorrhea who are also in need of contraception may be considered candidates for combination (estrogen-progesterone) oral contraceptives. These agents are thought to prevent painful menses by inhibiting ovulation and the resultant production of progesterone by the corpus luteum. Another possible mechanism of its antidysmenorrheic action is the inhibitory effect on endometrial proliferation, perhaps secondarily resulting in a decrease in prostaglandin production. Adolescents who fail to respond to either pharmacological approach should undergo laparoscopy, assuming that the initial routine pelvic examination was entirely normal, for the purpose of identifying a structural anomaly or, more commonly, evidence of endometriosis.

Amenorrhea

Primary amenorrhea is defined as failure to reach menarche by 16 years of age (more than two standard deviations from the national mean of 12.4 years), within two years of the onset of development of secondary sex characteristics, or by one year later than the age of the patient's mother or sister at their menarche. Secondary amenorrhea refers to absence of menses for four or more months in a previously menstruating individual.

Delay in menarche may be physiological or pathological, the former suggested by observations correlating menstrual function with body fat composition. Obese individuals have menarche earlier than lean, and those involved in strenuous training for athletics or dance are still later than otherwise lean females. Generational continuity in patterns of menarche indicates the importance of genetic factors in determining age of menarche. True primary amenorrhea results from functional or anatomical disruption along the cerebral-hypothalamic-pituitary-ovarian/uterine axis.

The differential diagnosis of amenorrhea is given in Table 8–6. All conditions that cause secondary amenorrhea may also cause primary amenorrhea, whereas the reverse is obviously not true, considering that congenital anomalies may be responsible for the latter in 20 to 40 per cent of cases. The recent availability of synthetic hormones and laparoscopy has greatly enhanced our ability to understand and diagnose the etiology of amenorrhea. A scheme for the work-up of the patient with amenorrhea is presented in Figure 8–2.

Weight loss, chronic illness, psychiatric illness, and emotional stress may be responsible for amenorrhea. Amenorrhea results when the ovary is rendered unresponsive to circulatory gonadotropins because of congenital or acquired problems. The prototype of a congenital anomaly associated with primary amenorrhea is Turner syndrome, in which the absence of one X chromosome results in an undifferentiated gonad. The inability of the gonad to produce estrogens or progestins and the consequent failure of a negative feedback loop results in pituitary hypersection of gonadotropins (more than 100 times normal). Destruction of ovarian tissue by radioisotopes, chemotherapeutic agents, certain viruses, or autoimmune disease may cause anovulation with resultant amenorrhea. In addition, ovarian tumors may secrete hormones that suppress pituitary gonadotropin secretion and thus inhibit ovulation. When work-up suggests these problems, the patient should be evaluated with ultrasonography and referred to a gynecologist for further study, which may include laparoscopy.

As menstrual flow originates in the uterus, it is obvious that any condition that interferes with growth or shedding of its endometrial lining or access to the exterior will also appear as amenorrhea. Accordingly, irradiation or multiple or excessive curettage may result in irreversible endometrial hypoplasia, while that resulting from the adolescent's use of combination oral contraceptives is typically reversible within 18 months after discontinuation of the medication. Any anomaly resulting from failure of normal differentiation of the Mullerian duct, ranging from absence of the uterus to cervical stenosis, may prevent menses. Pelvic or rectal examination may reveal absence of the cervix or a uterus enlarged by retained menstrual blood. Similarly, an imperforate hymen will cause a midline mass (hematocolpos) as well as abdominal pain and the simulation of primary amenorrhea.

Pregnancy, the most common cause of secondary amenorrhea, may rarely occur in a female before she has had her first menstrual period. Performance of a serum β-subunit HCG test should therefore be mandatory to evaluate the possibility of pregnancy, as well as the rare tumors such as choriocarcinoma or pituitary teratoma that will also secrete this hormone.

In addition to the drugs listed in Table 8–6

Table 8–6. DIFFERENTIAL DIAGNOSIS OF AMENORRHEA

	Primary	Secondary
Congenital Anomalies		
Mullerian duct system	+	
Gonads (secondary to chromosomal abnormalities)	+	
Cyanotic heart disease	+	+
Chronic Illness		
Endocrinopathies	+	+
Pituitary insufficiency (complete/isolated LH)	+	
Hyperthyroidism (rarely hypothyroidism)	+	+
Adrenal insufficiency/hypersecretion	+	+
Diabetes mellitus (poor control)	+	+
Neoplasms (hypothalamus, pituitary)	+	+
Hematological		
Sickle cell anemia	+	+
Thalassemia major	+	+
Gastrointestinal		
Inflammatory bowel disease	+	+
Cystic fibrosis	+	+
Cardiac		
Cyanotic	+	+
Congestive heart failure	+	+
Psychiatric Illness		
Anorexia nervosa	Rare	+
"Boarding school" syndrome		+
Weight loss	+	+
Gynecological		
Ovarian		+
Polycystic	Rare	
Viral disease	+	+
Autoimmune disease	+	+
Infiltrative disease	+	+
Drugs (see below)	+	+
Neoplasm	Rare	+
Uterine		+
Pregnancy	Rare	
Endometrial hypoplasia	+	+
Mullerian duct system anomalies (see above)	+	+
Drugs		
Suppress ovulation by inhibiting LH/FSH	Rare	+
Estrogens		
Progestogens		
Testosterone		
Heroin		
Stimulate prolactin	Rare	+
Methyldopa		
Phenothiazines		
Destroy ova	+	+
Radioisotopes (^{32}P, ^{131}I, ^{198}Au)		
Chemotherapeutic agents (cyclophosphamide, chlorambucil, vincaleukoblastin, methylhydrazines)		

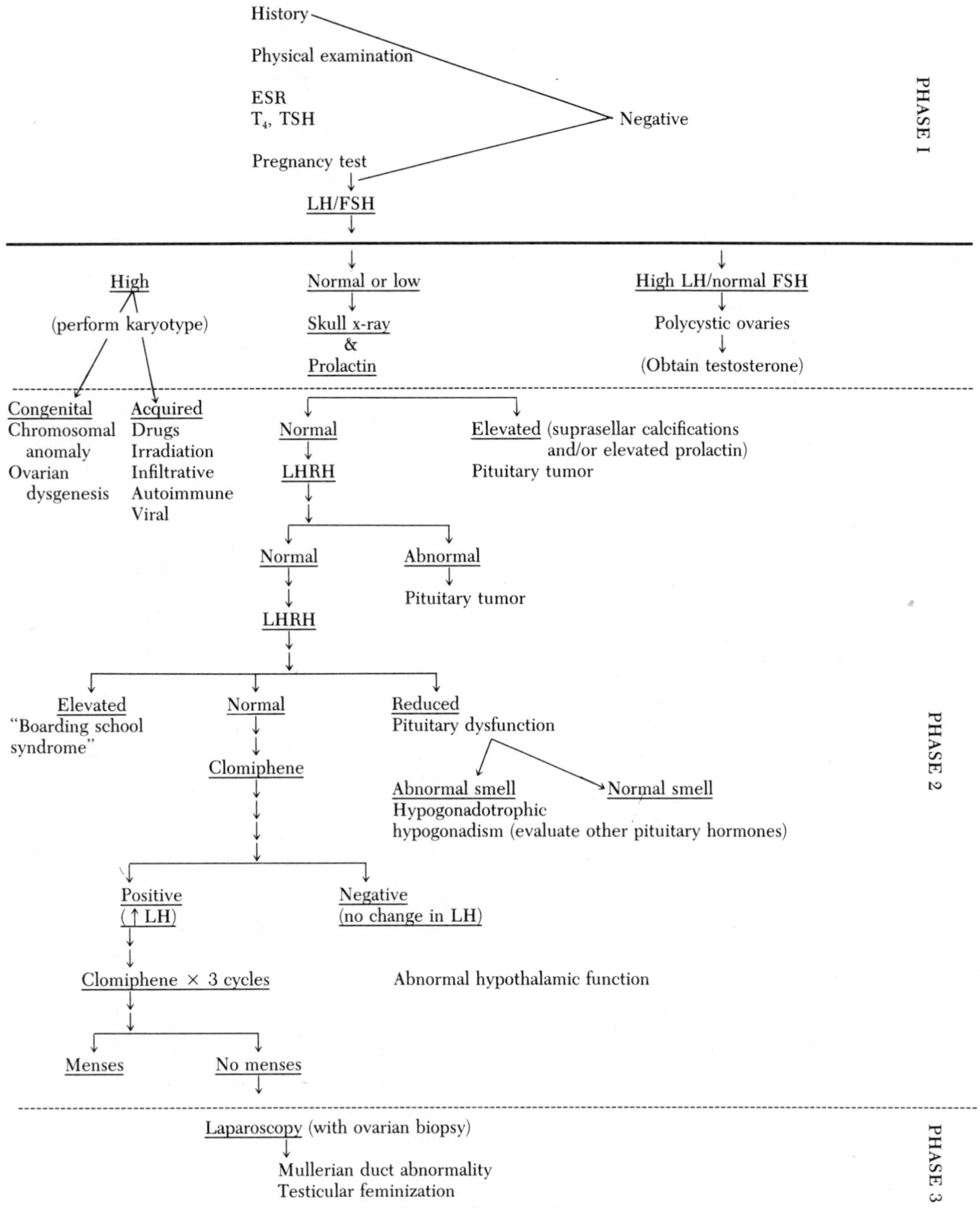

Figure 8–2. Evaluation of adolescent amenorrhea. (Adapted from Litt, I. F.: Menstrual disorders. Pediatr. Rev., *4*:203–212, 1983.)

and their presumed mechanisms for producing amenorrhea, it should be noted that interpretation of some tests employed in the evaluation of the amenorrheic patient may be confused by use of certain medications or drugs; for example, use of opiate drugs or phenothiazines may result in a false-positive urine pregnancy test based on the hemagglutination inhibition technique.

Menometrorrhagia

Excessive and frequent menstrual bleeding, among the few gynecological emergencies of the adolescent, often results in anemia and, occasionally, in shock. Its potential seriousness notwithstanding, this disorder can be well managed by the primary care physician once the underlying mechanisms are understood.

This problem arises (1) when clotting is impaired, (2) when constant endometrial stimulation by estrogen, unopposed by progesterone, causes its proliferation and ultimate excessive shedding, (3) as a result of traumatic injury to blood vessels, (4) from a tumor, or (5) from interruption of a pregnancy.

Impaired clotting may be congenital or acquired. In the congenital category, Von Willebrand disease often remains asymptomatic and hence undiagnosed until menarche, when the combination of low levels of Factor VIII and a defect in platelet adhesiveness results in massive bleeding. Acquired coagulopathies may result from the effect of the acetyl moiety on platelet adhesiveness in sensitive individuals who have ingested therapeutic doses of aspirin within 14 days of menses or from any condition that decreases platelet number, such as lupus erythematosus, idiopathic thrombocytopenic purpura, or aplastic anemia.

Most commonly, menometrorrhagia is the result of continuous endometrial hyperplasia from estrogen stimulation. This most often results from the anovulatory cycles characteristic of the first year to 18 months following menarche, so-called dysfunctional uterine bleeding. Less commonly, this phenomenon results from the polycystic ovary syndrome. Hypothyroidism is also associated with this type of menometrorrhagia.

Traumatic first intercourse or that associated with rape may cause excessive vaginal bleeding. Sensitivity on the part of the physician and privacy necessary to facilitate obtaining the history are necessary for diagnosis and subsequent treatment.

Tumors are the leading cause of excessive bleeding in the adult woman, resulting in a tendency to consider a diagnostic (and therapeutic) dilatation and curettage part of the management of this problem. In the adolescent, however, endometrial tumors are exceedingly rare, eliminating the necessity (or advisability) to perform this procedure in this age group in most circumstances. Although still relatively rare, adenocarcinoma of the vagina has been increasing in frequency, usually secondary to in utero exposure to diethylstilbestrol. When bleeding occurs as a result of this tumor, it is rarely of the massive variety and more typically consists of spotting. Imminent abortion typically presents with heavy bleeding, as well as crampy pain. An ectopic pregnancy may be accompanied by unilateral pain (bilateral and generalized if it has ruptured) and vaginal spotting. The history of unprotected intercourse requires sensitivity and assurance of confidentiality and may not always be easy to obtain. A serum β-HCG, which will remain positive up to two weeks after interruption of pregnancy, is one appropriate diagnostic test. A dilatation and curettage by a competent gynecologist is the appropriate treatment once this diagnosis is made.

With this differential diagnosis in mind, determination of the specific etiology of menometrorrhagia is dependent upon history taking, physical examination, and laboratory testing. The latter should include a CBC with platelet count, bleeding time, T_4 and TSH, and serum β-HCG. When bleeding is massive, a specimen for typing and cross-matching should obviously be obtained during the process of providing cardiovascular support, as these patients often need to be transfused. When trauma or pregnancy is determined to be the cause of the bleeding, gynecological consultation should be obtained immediately. For the other conditions described, hemostasis may be accomplished by pharmacological means through the use of compounds containing estrogens and progesterones. In our experience, the oral administration of Enovid 25 mg will usually cause bleeding of any other etiology to cease within two hours of administration. If not, an additional dose of 5 to 10 mg may be given at that time. Because nausea and vomiting may result, use of an antiemetic may be necessary. Once the bleeding has stopped, its recurrence will be prevented by careful tapering. An effective regimen is outlined in Figure 8–3 and consists of reducing the daily dose by one 5 mg tablet until a total daily dose of 5 mg is achieved. The patient is then maintained on this dose for the duration of a 21-day cycle, counting the day of

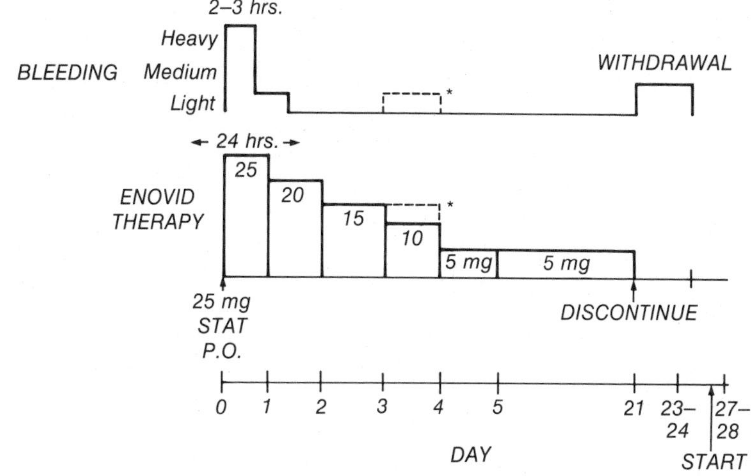

Figure 8–3. Therapeutic plan for dysfunctional uterine bleeding. (From Litt, I. F.: Menstrual disorders. Pediatr. Rev. *4*:203–212, 1983.

initiation of therapy as Day 1. If bleeding recurs at any point within this tapering period, the previous day's dose should be given. After 21 days, all medication is discontinued, and bleeding is allowed to occur. On the fifth day of bleeding, a 21-day course of conventional combination oral contraceptives is begun. Patients with underlying systemic illness often require additional specific therapy, including platelet transfusions, but in the emergency phase this regimen is effective even in them.

REFERENCES

Duke, P. M.: Adolescent sexuality. Pediatr. Rev., *4*:44–52, 1982.

Duke, P. M.: Unpublished data.

Greulich, W. W., Dorfman, R. I., Catchpole, H. R., et al.: Somatic and Endocrine Studies of Puberal and Adolescent Boys. Monograph of the Society for Research in Child Development, *7*:3. Washington, D.C., National Research Council, 1942.

Gross, R. T., and Duke, P. M.: The effect of early versus late physical maturation on adolescent behavior. Pediatr. Clin. North Am., *27*:71–77, 1980.

Hatcher, R. A., Stewart, G. K., Stewart, F., et al.: Contraceptive Technology 1982–1983. New York, Irvington Publishers, Inc., 1982.

Hein, K., Dell, R., and Cohen, M. I.: Self-detection of a breast mass in adolescent females. J. Adol. Health Care, *3*:15–17, 1982.

Hein, K., Schreiber, K., Cohen, M. I., et al.: Cervical etiology: The need for routine screening in the sexually active adolescent. J. Pediatr., *91*:123–126, 1977.

Hingson, R., Heeren, T., Mangione, T., et al.: Teenage driving after using marijuana or drinking and traffic accident involvement. J. Safety Res., *13*:33–38, 1982.

Jones, M. Bayley, N., Macfarlane, J., et al. (Eds.): The Course of Human Development. Toronto, John Wiley and Sons, 1971.

Litt, I. F.: Menstrual problems during adolescence. Pediatr. Rev., *4*:203–212, 1983.

Marino, D. D., and King, J. C.: Nutritional concerns during adolescence. Pediatr. Clin. North Am., *27*:125–139, 1980.

McAlister, A. L., Perry, C., and Maccoby, N.: Adolescent smoking: Onset and prevention. Pediatrics., *63*:650–658, 1979.

Ory, H. W., Rosenfeld, A., and Landman, L. C.: The Pill at 20: An assessment. Fam. Plann. Perspect., *12*:278–282, 1980.

Simmons, R. G., Blyth, D. A., VanClease, E. F., et al.: The impact of school structure and puberty upon the self-esteem of early adolescence. Am. Soc. Rev., 1978.

Sorensen, R. C.: Adolescent Sexuality in Contemporary America. New York, World Publishing, 1973.

Tanner, J. M., and Whitehouse, R. H.: Clinical longitudinal standards for height, weight, height velocity, weight velocity, and stages of puberty. Arch. Dis. Child., *51*:170–179, 1976.

Zelnik, M., and Kantner, J. F.: Sexual activity, contraceptive use and pregnancy among metropolitan-area teenagers: 1971–1979. Fam. Plann. Perspect., *12*:230, 1980.

Zerin, M.: The Pied Piper phenomenon: Family systems and vulnerability to cults. The Script, *12*:1–2, 1982.

SECTION

III

EPISODIC DISORDERS

The chief criterion for inclusion of a specific disease in this section has been its frequency in children seen by the office practitioner. Acute disorders are usually of short duration, although they may recur. If they are part of a recurrent episode of asthma or other long-term illness, we call them chronic illness; if they are not part of such a continuum, e.g., upper respiratory infections or repeated lacerations, we do not. Three of the acute illnesses (upper respiratory infection, otitis media, and diarrhea) account for a large proportion of all illness visits to pediatricians. We have given prominent place to discussion of these illnesses in this section. In this edition, we have also added chapters on the acute scrotum, sexually transmitted diseases, sports medicine, and the care of children with serious emergencies to reflect the increasing importance of these problems.

It is not as easy as one might suppose to document the frequency of different types of children's illnesses, nor precisely how they are changing. Mortality data are by far the most accurate we have, but deaths occur rarely in a pediatric practice. Among approximately 2000 children in an average pediatric practice, one may expect only two or three deaths per year among newborns and one or two deaths per year among all other age groups (except where referrals concentrate more seriously ill patients). The cause of these deaths should be known to the child health clinician in order to guide his continuing education and to reinforce his concern for accident prevention, accidents being the most common cause of death after the newborn period. Clinicians should be able to diagnose and manage, or refer appropriately, children with rare but potentially fatal illnesses.

The precise frequency of different causes of morbidity is more difficult to define. The frequency varies depending on whether one uses data derived from reasons for office visits, from household interview surveys, or from daily diaries of symptoms. This variation arises, in part, because so many acute infections produce only mild symptoms and because there is great variation in the degree to which people report such symptoms or consult the doctor. Although the number of more common illnesses reported by these different methods varies at least tenfold, the relative frequencies of the items on the list remain fairly constant. Household diaries yield the highest number of episodes of illness. The Cleveland Family Study reported over 10 episodes of illness per preschool child per year (Dingle et al., 1964), and the Rochester Child Health diary study, which asked mothers to record any symptoms of ill health, yielded nearly 20 per year in young children, but only one in 10 of these (or two per year per child) was thought serious enough to require a doctor's attention (Roghmann and Pless, 1975).

The data most often used on the incidence of acute illness, defined as symptoms severe enough to limit activity or require a doctor's attention, are from the National Health Survey based on household interviews. By this definition, children under five have about 3.5 acute illnesses per year, with 8.8 days of restricted activity, whereas children ages five through fourteen have 2.9 episodes and 9.4 days of disability. Acute illnesses are less frequent in the first six months of life, increase thereafter until age three or four, and then decline with increasing age, although usually a small peak occurs during the first year or two in school. In the total volume of acute illness, respiratory infections occur two or three times as often as all other illnesses combined! Accidents account for only 3 per cent of all acute illness but are more often the cause of calling the doctor because of their seriousness. Acute illness takes up nearly half of the time and accounts for more than half of the patient volume of pediatricians. Most of these acute illnesses, even those brought to the doctor, are mild and self-limited.

Table 1 lists illnesses, largely acute, that cause children to be brought to a pediatrician as compared to a family physician.

Another way to look at the work of the doctor in dealing with acute illness is to examine the number of children who are hospitalized. After the newborn period, well over half of all hospitalizations of children in the United States today are for surgical procedures. About 150 children will be hospitalized per year from among the average-sized pediatric practice of 2000 children. Since only 75 of these will be for medical reasons, the average pediatrician will have only one or two of his patients in the hospital in any week.

Whatever the organization of child health services, it is clear that the management of acute illness must be planned for, whether by physicians, nurses, or parents. The way in which acute illnesses are handled will determine to a large degree the total utilization and cost of any service. Visits can easily be increased if the physician sees all "fevers," has all children with sore throats return for a follow-up culture, or uses laboratory studies frequently; they can be decreased by more reassurance and by teaching parents more about caring for acute illness. Obviously a major way to control costs is to teach patients to use health services more parsimoniously for acute illness yet to be alert to the few serious but treatable conditions: otitis media, dehydration, pneumonia, sepsis, and meningitis.

Child health care is becoming increasingly concerned with the care of children with chronic disorders, defined as conditions that persist for more than three months. These are the subject of Section V.

MANAGEMENT OF ILLNESS

In recent years, as more controlled clinical trials have been completed, it has become apparent that traditional methods of treatment often do little to change the course of a significant number of diseases. It would be useful if we could neatly list those diseases for which medical management has no demonstrable beneficial effect (or even a detrimental effect), those which are self-limited, with or without treatment, and those for which we have data on the proven efficacy of treatment.

Unfortunately, in the present state of knowledge, such a task is beyond us. But we believe that the successful clinician can always provide

Table 1. DIAGNOSTIC GROUPING OF DOCTOR VISITS (EXPRESSED AS PER CENT OF ALL VISITS)

Reason for Visit	Pediatrician	Family Physician, Generalist
Newborn—well child care	36.4	24.9
Respiratory illness	22.3	29.7
Diseases of central nervous system, senses	8.3	6.7
Miscellaneous symptoms	6.2	4.4
Digestive disorders	4.4	3.9
Allergic—metabolic	4.4	4.5
Infection	4.3	4.4
Accidents—poisoning	4.2	11.0
Skin	3.5	5.0
Neonatal complications	1.2	0.4
Genitourinary	1.1	1.4
Behavioral	1.0	0.6
All other	2.5	2.8

Study includes 1971 figures on newborns and children up to age 15 years. From Rosenbloom, A. C.: Chronic Illness in Children and Adolescents seen in Private Practice. 67th Ross Conference on Chronic Physical Disease in Children. June, 1974.

services that are of value to the sick patient, whether in the form of reassurance that the disease is self-limited, or comfort and caring and symptomatic relief even for those afflicted with diseases for which there is no drug or surgical treatment of proven value.

Of the types of treatment available to the clinician—drugs, counseling, interviewing, bed rest, physical therapy, surgery, behavior modification, and environmental change—it is striking how predominant drug prescribing has become in the United States. In nearly two thirds of all physician contacts, a prescription is given. Parents, reflecting the popular belief in a "magic bullet" for every ill, often expect a drug, even when the doctor knows the agent to be ineffective. This inappropriate practice, costly in terms of dollars and side effects, also deprives the clinician of the opportunity to develop his other therapeutic skills and the family of the benefit of other and more effective therapeutic methods, especially counseling.

One reason why physicians prescribe so much is that the quickest way to end an office visit to the apparent satisfaction of the patient is to write a prescription. As much as we think unwise, overburdened clinicians have limited options unless they can incorporate the help of other professionals such as social workers, developmental technicians, and nurse practitioners for some health care and can learn skills of efficient counseling. The use of pediatric protocols has been shown to decrease use of laboratory and drugs without changing outcome and may become more widespread in the future.

"Caring" is the therapy most missed by patients. It is a powerful agent with few side effects. The problem is how best to administer it. In addition to the personal interest of the doctor and conscious development of such skills, nurse practitioners can often provide more caring by having time for patients to talk, simultaneously reducing the need for tests, drugs, or other therapy.

The danger of overuse of drugs is great. There is, however, the other side of the coin—failure to use or to take medicines when needed. Compliance is discussed in Chapter 2.

Bed rest, a time-honored treatment, is nearly useless for children (Illingworth, 1968). If the child is sick enough to benefit, he will voluntarily go to bed. If not, nothing but increased metabolism of child and parent will result from the attempt. Its continued popularity derives, in part, from the same reason that drugs are too widely used—it is readily accepted, terminates the interview, and is "doing something." We believe strongly that doing nothing is often the best but most difficult task. Doing nothing should not preclude listening and counseling; these are methods that rank among the most potent therapy we have.

SYMPTOMATIC MANAGEMENT

In medical schools most physicians learn to look askance at those who treat symptoms without probing into the pathophysiology of the disease in order to understand and to base treatment on the cause. While it may seem retrogressive to talk about symptomatic management in this book, there is a dilemma. For only a few conditions (usually fairly rare ones) has the development of detailed knowledge of the pathophysiology resulted in dramatic improvement in management. We hope that more and more problems and symptoms can be subjected to in-depth study.

Meanwhile, patients present with problems that defy such approaches. We believe that it is useful for two reasons to present in this part of the book some of the problems (e.g., fever) that bear these "superficial" labels. First, that is the way in which patients present to the practitioner, and second, for most of these problems or symptoms we do not have clear pathophysiological information at the time decisions on treatment need to be made. In other instances, there is no specific treatment. For example, in the Dingle et al. (1964) study in Cleveland, of all patients, only 3 per cent had a respiratory illness that would respond to specific drug treatment. In addition, for most problems there is no single cause of the illness; more often multiple factors (social, psychological, environmental, genetic, and physiological) are involved. Since the great majority of symptoms are cared for by the parent, the reason for seeking medical care is often based on anxiety and other stresses.

The overemphasis on pathophysiology may lead to ignoring or downplaying problems in which biological dysfunction has not yet been defined, a disregard for other causes that may be more amenable to therapy, and denial to the patient and his family of relief of troublesome symptoms provided by personal care, as well as by drug therapy. Treating all problems symptomatically without thinking clearly about pathophysiology and thereby missing a more effective approach to management is obviously to be deplored; equally to be avoided is the danger of minimizing and not attempting to relieve the patient's symptoms where cause may not yet be known. The effective physician now chooses a prudent balance.

REFERENCES

Dingle, J. H., Badger, G. F., and Jordan, W. S.: Illness in the Home, A Study of 25,000 Illnesses in a Group of Cleveland Families. Cleveland, Western Reserve University Press, 1964.

Illingworth, R.: Indications for bed rest. *In* Green, M., and Haggerty, R. J. (eds.): Ambulatory Pediatrics. Philadelphia, W. B. Saunders Co., 1968.

Miller, F. J. W., Court, S. D. M., Walton, W. S., and Knox, E. G.: The School Years in Newcastle-upon-Tyne. London, Oxford University Press, 1974.

Roghmann, K. J., and Pless, I. B.: Health and illness. *In* Haggerty, R. J., Roghman, K. J., and Pless, I. B. (eds.): Child Health and the Community. New York, Wiley Interscience, 1975.

Rosenbloom, A. L.: Chronic Illness in Children and Adolescents Seen in Private Practice. 67th Ross Conference on Chronic Physical Disease in Children, June, 1974.

Rosenbloom, A. L., and Ongley, J. P.: Who provides what services to children in private medical practice. Am. J. Dis. Child., 127:357, 1974.

Werner, E. E., Bierman, J. M., and French, F. E.: The Children of Kauai. Honolulu, University of Hawaii Press, 1971.

Werner, E. E.: Sources of Support for High Risk Children. *In* Fandal, A. W., Anastasiou, N. J., and Frankenburg, W. K. (eds.): Proceedings of the 3rd International Conference, Early Identification of At-Risk Children. J. F. Kennedy Child Development Center, University of Colorado, Denver.

Robert J. Haggerty, M.D.

9

FEVER

Martin B. Kleiman, M.D.

Fever has been recognized as a sign of illness for many centuries, long before normal and disease-related effects on thermoregulatory function became subjects of scientific scrutiny. Routine measurement of body temperature has been practiced for fewer than 150 years. During the past 50 years there has been an explosion of knowledge concerning the pathophysiology of disordered thermoregulation. Similarly, an enormous variety of simple or complex, self-limited or life-threatening, benign or malignant conditions that may present with fever have been recognized. The evaluation of the febrile child thus often presents a considerable challenge and responsibility for a physician, albeit among the most common.

Fever has always been the complaint that most frequently leads to a "nonroutine" office visit. In order to evaluate its cause, the physician must have at his disposal a large body of factual knowledge, clinical experience, and a familiarity with the patient and with those parental concerns that commonly accompany febrile illnesses. Through a carefully reasoned, orderly approach the physician's role will be to (1) recognize and treat progressive, life-threatening conditions, (2) explain to parents and older patients the most probable diagnosis and the reasons for arriving at this judgment, (3) emphasize that fever is a nonspecific sign that has been caused by and therefore accompanies the disorder but is *not* an illness of itself, (4) offer reasonable expectations for the course of the illness and the anticipated course of the diagnostic evaluation, (5) explain the principles of the therapy used for control of fever and, if indicated, for treatment of the inciting illness, (6) carefully advise the parents of signs and symptoms about which the physician wishes to be informed and the means by which this should be done (telephone, office visit, etc.), (7) reassure parents and patients and emphasize that the diagnostic evaluation does not end with the initial visit but will continue by phone, future visits, or other means until the child has returned to good health. An invitation to call even if the child is better or unchanged always serves to reassure the parent of the physician's sincere concern.

DEFINITION

A circadian temperature rhythm is present in normal humans. The "normal" body temperature, 37°C (98.6°F), is an average that occurs for a short period of time during the day. Body temperature peaks in late afternoon and is lowest in early morning; the difference between high and low extremes is larger in young children than in adults. A child is considered febrile when temperature exceeds 38.3°C (101°F) rectally or 37.9°C (100.2°F) orally. High ambient temperature and strenuous activity may elevate the body temperature in nondisease states. Infrequently, temperature elevations in an abnormal range may occur without obvious cause or symptoms. These "fevers" are *not* indicative of illness and do not require diagnostic evaluation.

PATHOPHYSIOLOGY

The anterior hypothalamus contains thermosensitive neurons that control the constancy of body temperature and are important in the initiation of fever. There appears to be strong resistance to fever in excess of 41°C, an effect that has been postulated to result from a second regulatory center.

The initiation of fever in man involves the manufacture of endogenous pyrogens by monocytes that are responding to exogenous pyrogens (Dinarello and Wolff, 1982) (Fig. 9–1). These exogenous pyrogens may result from a variety of causes, including toxins, immunological reactions, and infectious agents. Endogenous pyrogen is a protein that is released and enters the circulation after new messenger RNA and protein are synthesized. Fever results from a complex interaction of endogenous pyrogen with specialized receptors near the thermosensitive neurons in the anterior hypothalamus. Possible mediators in these reactions include prostaglandins, monoamines, and cyclic AMP. Information is relayed to the posterior hypothalamus and to vasomotor centers, which act to constrict peripheral vessels and thereby decrease dissipation of heat and increase core temperature. The antipyretic effect of salicylates is thought to occur through interference with prostaglandin synthesis (Dinarello and Wolff, 1978), whereas the antipyretic properties of acetaminophen result from its effect on hypothalamic heat-regulating centers, leading to increased dissipation of body heat (Koch-Weser, 1976).

ILLNESSES OR CONDITIONS ASSOCIATED WITH FEVER

Virtually every type of illness—infectious, collagen-vascular, and neoplastic—may cause fever in humans. Granulomatous diseases of unclear etiology, inflammatory bowel disease, drug fever, and factitious fever must also be included in the broad differential diagnosis. The practitioner's job is made easier when one considers the statistical likelihood of the occurrence

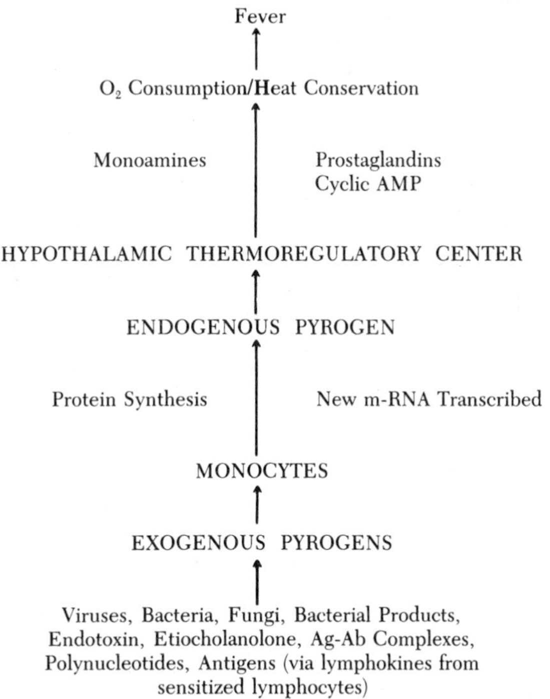

Figure 9–1. Causes of fever in man. (From Dinarello, C. A., and Wolff, S. M.: Pathogenesis of fever in man. N. Engl. J. Med., 298:607, 1978.)

of the diseases enumerated above. Self-limited viral, mycoplasmal, and mild bacterial infections account for the overwhelming majority of febrile illnesses that occur during childhood. Infrequently, severe bacterial or viral infections of short duration occur and threaten major organ systems. Differentiation of the latter illnesses from self-limited or easily treated conditions is the challenge that will be dealt with in the remainder of this chapter. Rarely, children with fevers of short duration (less than 2 weeks) will be found to have collagen-vascular, neoplastic, or malignant disorders. Fevers lasting longer than two weeks which defy simple diagnostic efforts will be discussed under "true" fever of unknown etiology (p. 109).

DATA COLLECTION: THE INTERVIEW

The careful, ordered, concise interview provides important information on which to base diagnostic decisions. It should be conducted *before* examining the apprehensive, irritable, febrile child. The physician should develop a list of specific questions and request that these be answered objectively (e.g., not accept "abdominal pain" in a 9-month-old child), while permitting the patient or parent the opportunity to offer any additional facts not uncovered in the replies to the initial questions. Major areas of inquiry should include questions pertaining to (1) persistence of significant, abnormal irritability, (2) change in level of consciousness, (3) signs of respiratory dysfunction, (4) persistent or evanescent rashes, (5) abnormalities of movement of back or extremities, (6) complaints of headache or pain in the posterior neck, (7) passive movements that elicit discomfort, (8) height and duration of fever, (9) parental estimate of progression—improving, unchanged, or worsening, (10) fluid intake and urine output, (11) persistence of vomiting or diarrhea, (12) presence of any localized complaint, and (13) exposure to illness (Table 9–1).

DATA COLLECTION: THE PHYSICAL EXAMINATION

The interview may be performed in person or by telephone. Clearly, especially in retrospect after the illness has run its course, not all children require an office visit. Mild fever of short duration in a 5-year-old child whose general activity, play, appetite, and, most important, good humor are only minimally affected and who has no other focal signs may safely be watched at home by a responsible parent. Conversely, the febrile newborn should always be seen promptly. The physician's judgment as to whether a physical examination is needed depends upon his knowledge of the family and patient, the past medical history of the child, epidemiological and environmental factors, and the data gathered from the telephone interview.

A careful, methodical physical examination is essential. A special skill, one that is difficult to describe and still more difficult to teach, accrues to the careful clinician and often permits the recognition of a "toxic" child through careful observation of the child's general behavior and appearance (McCarthy et al., 1980). Although one may be tempted to characterize this judgment as a "subjective impression," the frequency with which the expert clinician can differentiate those children with serious illnesses who require further attention from those with self-limited illnesses suggests that this is a learned skill developed through the accumulated experience of evaluating many febrile children (Waskerwitz and Berkelhamer, 1981).

The objective results of the physical examination will now identify (a) a "toxic" child who, irrespective of other history or findings, is thought to be at risk for serious infection, (b) localized signs of infection such as pharyngitis, otitis media, arthritis, nuchal rigidity, abnormal sensorium, etc., (c) nonspecific findings such as jaundice, lymphadenopathy, enanthems and exanthems, etc., (d) signs strongly indicative of specific illness, such as the characteristic exanthems of varicella, measles, meningococcemia, etc., or (e) fever in the absence of specific or nonspecific abnormalities.

Table 9–1. AREAS OF INQUIRY IN EVALUATING THE FEBRILE CHILD

1. Persistence of significant, abnormal irritability
2. Change in level of consciousness
3. Signs of respiratory dysfunction
4. Persistent or evanescent rashes
5. Abnormalities of movement of back or extremities
6. Complaints of headache or pain in the posterior neck
7. Passive movements that elicit discomfort
8. Height and duration of fever
9. Parental estimate of progression: improving, unchanged, or worsening
10. Fluid intake and urine output
11. Persistence of vomiting or diarrhea
12. Presence of any localized complaint
13. Exposure to illness

Table 9–2. CLASSIFICATION OF FEVER SYNDROMES

Patient Group	Characteristics
Fever without localizing signs	Does not appear seriously ill No abnormalities on physical exam Normal urinalysis Duration less than two weeks
Fever with nonspecific signs	Signs such as hepatosplenomegaly or abdominal mass are present, but not diagnostic Duration less than two weeks
Fever of unknown origin (prolonged unexplained fever)	Signs may be present but are not diagnostic
Fever complicating chronic disease	Patient has chronic disease with expected complication to be excluded
Fever due to a specific localized infection	Diagnosis of a specific localized infection can be made by initial physical examination
Other Special Groups	
Neonatal fever	Suspect septicemia; hypothermia equally important
High fever in infant	If <2 years old, higher risk of serious infection
Suspected septicemia	Appears seriously ill or hypotensive

From Moffett, H. M.: Pediatric Infectious Disease: A Problem Oriented Approach. Philadelphia, J. B. Lippincott, 1981, p. 244.

COLLATION OF DATA, DIAGNOSIS, AND PLAN

Next, a provisional diagnosis(es) must be formulated, and a plan selected. Should the child appear mildly ill, with signs suggesting a self-limited or easily treated condition, continued outpatient observation is appropriate. The option of acquiring additional data such as CBC, urinalysis, urine culture, chest radiograph, and blood culture may be selected. Several excellent prospective studies of febrile patients have defined parameters (such as age less than 2 years, fever in excess of 102°F, white blood cell counts in excess of 20,000/cu mm) that permit a reasonably accurate basis for prediction of bacteremia in the absence of an identifiable source of infection (Teele et al., 1979). Unfortunately, no single test or combination of clinical and laboratory abnormalities can with unfailing accuracy predict the presence of serious illness (Waskerwitz and Berkelhamer, 1981). If serious illness is a consideration or there is an identifiable source of infection that requires more detailed evaluation, hospitalization is indicated. Otherwise, continued outpatient observation with or without specific therapy may be selected.

A convenient classification of febrile illnesses has been developed by Moffett (1981), and the information collected thus far permits classification of the illness within this schema (Table 9–2). With continued observation the child will either (1) defervesce spontaneously or with the aid of specific (antibiotic) therapy, (2) develop focal signs not present at the initial evaluation, (3) develop nonspecific signs such as hepatomegaly, generalized lymphadenopathy, rash, etc., which narrow the diagnostic possibilities, or (4) remain febrile for an extended period of time (two weeks) and enter the diagnostic category of true fever of unknown origin (FUO). True FUO merits a complex evaluation, since carefully documented fevers lasting extended periods of time result from chronic or serious illness far more often than those of short duration.

TRUE FEVER OF UNKNOWN ETIOLOGY

True fever of unknown etiology is defined as one that continues for two weeks or longer. Published studies of febrile children in whom the primary physician was unable to determine the cause show that approximately 50 per cent are ultimately found to have an infection. Approximately 20 per cent are found to have collagen-inflammatory disease such as rheumatoid arthritis or regional enteritis. Ten per cent have malignancy, usually leukemia or lymphoma. Another 10 per cent fall into a variety of more unusual diagnostic categories (Pizzo et al., 1975).

MANAGEMENT OF FEVER

Children and adults feel ill when febrile, irrespective of its cause. It is the impression of most parents and practitioners that efforts to reduce fever result in subjective improvement. There is, however, little scientific evidence that antipyresis favorably affects the course of the illness. Indeed, there is some suggestion that fever may be a beneficial host defense against some infections. The overzealous application of several regimens of fever control have themselves resulted in toxicity or even death. Methods to be deplored include ice water enemas, immersion in cold water, and alcohol sponge baths.

The physician may elect to treat fever to alleviate symptoms, to help allay parental anxiety, or to evaluate the child when temperature is more closely normal. There is no evidence that the ease with which body temperature can be reduced is correlated with the etiology of the fever (viral vs. bacterial).

Aspirin, in a dosage schedule as suggested by Done et al. (1979) (Table 9–3), is an effective antipyretic. The association of salicylate usage with the development of Reye's syndrome has led to caution in the recommendation of salicylates for febrile children; however, unequivocal evidence for cause-effect relationship between aspirin and Reye's syndrome is still lacking. Acetaminophen (5–10 mg/kg) every four hours as required for temperature in excess of 102°F is also an effective antipyretic. No benefit has been demonstrated by alternating dosages of aspirin and acetaminophen. Each agent in excessive dosages, especially in the presence of limited fluid intake, can be toxic and even fatal. Parents should be cautioned to adhere strictly to the recommended dosage schedules.

Table 9–3. REVISED ASPIRIN DOSAGE SCHEDULE BASED ON AGE

Age (yr)	No. of 81-mg Tablets (every 3 hr)
Under 3	As directed by physician
3	1 (81 mg)
4–5	2 (162 mg)
6–9	3 (243 mg)
10–14	4 (324 mg)

From Done, A. K., Yaffe, S. J., and Clayton, J. M.: Aspirin dosage for infants and children. J. Pediatr., 95:620, 1979.

Table 9–4. FACTS OFTEN MISUNDERSTOOD BY PARENTS: POINTS FOR EMPHASIS

1. Fever itself is *not* an illness; it is a sign that accompanies a variety of illnesses.
2. There is a *normal* diurnal variation of body temperature; 98.6°F (37°C) is the mean; fever will also fluctuate throughout a 24-hour period.
3. Fever is, *by definition*, an oral temperature in excess of 100.2°F (37.9°C) or a rectal temperature in excess of 101°F (38.3°C).
4. Low body temperature is rarely of importance in a nonsymptomatic child (except in the newborn).
5. "Brain damage" resulting from fever alone will not occur unless fever exceeds 106°F; "brain damage" is, in fact, rare with fevers of less than 107°F.
6. The newborn can have an infection without fever.
7. Aspirin or acetaminophen (Tylenol) will reduce fever and often make a child more comfortable but will *not* shorten the illness causing the fever.
8. A child requires more fluid and should receive more fluids when febrile.
9. Skin temperature is an unreliable indicator of body (core) temperature; fever must be confirmed with a thermometer.
10. Bathing or sponging with cold water or alcohol mixtures makes the child uncomfortable and shivering should be avoided; ice water enemas should never be used.

Promoting heat loss by uncovering the body and gently moistening areas of the skin with *tepid* water and encouraging the drinking of cool liquids are helpful. The room should be kept in a comfortable temperature range. Table 9–4 presents a list of those concerns and misconceptions most frequently expressed by parents concerning fever. A simple typewritten explanation of body temperature and fever which the parents may read at their leisure after the office visit will often answer questions overlooked in the anxiety of the interview and examination. The parents must leave the office with a good understanding of the most likely cause of the fever, a reasonable prediction of what to expect, a good idea of what to do in the event of specified changes, and most importantly, a reassurance that the evaluation will not be completed until the child is again enjoying good health.

REFERENCES

Dinarello, C. A., and Wolff, S. M.: Molecular basis of fever in humans. Am. J. Med., 72:799, 1982.

Dinarello, C. A., and Wolff, S. M.: Pathogenesis of fever in man. N. Engl. J. Med., *298*:607, 1978.
Done, A. K., Yaffe, S. J., and Clayton, J. M.: Aspirin dosage for infants and children. J. Pediatr. *95*:617, 1979.
Koch-Weser, J.: Acetaminophen. N. Engl. J. Med., *295*:1297, 1976.
McCarthy, P. L., Jekel, J. F., Stashwick, C. A., Spiesel, S. Z., and Dolan, T. F.: History and observation variables in assessing febrile children. Pediatrics, *65*:1090, 1980.
Moffet, H. L.: Pediatric Infectious Disease: A Problem Oriented Approach. Philadelphia, J. B. Lippincott, 1981, p. 244.
Pizzo, P. A., Lovejoy, F. H., and Smith, D. H.: Prolonged fever in children: Review of 100 cases. Pediatrics, *55*:468, 1975.
Teele, D. W., Marshall, R., and Klein, J. O.: Unsuspected bacteremia in young children. Pediatr. Clin. North Am., *26*:773, 1979.
Waskerwitz, S., and Berkelhamer, J. E.: Outpatient bacteremia: Clinical findings in children under two years with initial temperatures of 39.5°C or higher. J. Pediatr. *99*:231, 1981.

10

RESPIRATORY TRACT INFECTIONS

Herman W. Lipow, M.D.,

Since infections of the respiratory tract are the most common infectious disorders encountered in the pediatric age group, pediatric clinicians need a well-organized approach to their evaluation and management. Parents are well aware that the practitioner has a potent armamentarium of antibiotics at his disposal. In choosing therapy, the clinician must try to avoid the two common pitfalls: overtreatment of self-limited viral respiratory infections, and undertreatment at the time of early signs of serious, or potentially serious, bacterial respiratory infections.

This appears so simple, yet identifying the infection that requires aggressive antibiotic therapy is one of the most challenging problems that faces a conscientious clinician on a daily basis. The easy answer is to treat with antibiotics almost all children brought to the office for care. This is obviously bad medical practice because the majority of viral infections are not helped by antimicrobial therapy; many children will sustain unnecessary allergic reactions to the antimicrobials, and the costs of medical care will be increased without justification.

No simple method is available to select successfully all the children who require antimicrobial therapy. The physician armed with a detailed knowledge of the clinical manifestations of the various childhood respiratory infections (including the expected physical findings) can, however, make this differentiation with reasonable success.

The classification of respiratory infections (Table 10–1) combines anatomical areas with the clinical presentation. The usual etiological agents causing each of these infections will be outlined as the diseases are discussed individually. Upper respiratory tract infections include all infections above the larynx. Lower respiratory tract infections include the larynx, air passages (trachea and bronchial tree), and the lung parenchyma. The division of lower respiratory tract infections into extrathoracic and intrathoracic infections is made because of the marked difference in obstruction and clinical symptoms

Table 10–1. CLASSIFICATION OF RESPIRATORY TRACT INFECTIONS

- Upper respiratory infections
  - Acute nasopharyngitis (acute rhinitis, coryza, common cold)
  - Acute sinusitis
  - Acute pharyngitis and tonsillitis (tonsillopharyngitis)
  - Acute otitis media
- Lower respiratory tract infections
  - Extrathoracic airway infection (croup syndromes)
    - Acute epiglottitis
    - Acute spasmodic croup
    - Acute laryngotracheitis
  - Intrathoracic airway infection
    - Acute tracheobronchitis
    - Pertussis (whooping cough)
    - Acute bronchiolitis
  - Acute infections of the lung parenchyma (pneumonia)
    - Infections affecting primarily the interstitium
      - Viral pneumonia
      - Mycoplasmal pneumonia
      - Chlamydial pneumonia
      - Rare infections
    - Infections affecting primarily the alveoli
      - Bacterial pneumonia
      - Fungal pneumonia

produced by disease in these two areas. Extrathoracic airway infection leads to inspiratory obstruction and stridor; intrathoracic airway infection results in expiratory obstruction and, frequently, wheezing (Tooley, 1982).

The severity of the illness presented by the child is always a combination of at least two major factors: the innate virulence of the infecting agent—virus, bacteria, mycoplasma, fungus, etc.—and the reaction of the child to that infection at that time. This reaction includes the patient's immunological ability to fight the infection, as well as his tendency to overreact (allergy) with excessive mucus and bronchospasm. The child's past medical history and proven ability to handle prior infections are the best guides to the management of the child's new infection.

A newly recognized deleterious factor promoting respiratory tract illness in children is the prolonged passive inhalation of cigarette smoke. The cigarette smoking parent or caregiver continually pollutes the home environment, forcing the child into a passive smoking exposure. This exposure has been shown to result in an increased incidence and severity of respiratory tract infections and asthma in early childhood. The long-term results of this exposure are unknown, but there is concern that this early initiation of respiratory illness may have permanent adverse affects on the respiratory tract (Bonham and Wilson, 1981).

Practice Pressures: The Physician and the Parents

Frequent respiratory tract infections during early childhood are a fact of life. In the now-famous Cleveland Family Study, in which the incidence of illness in the home was observed, children under six years of age averaged seven respiratory infections per year. The incidence ranged from 0 to 15 respiratory infections per year, with 10 per cent of the children having 12 or more infections (Dingle et al., 1964). Almost all of these infections were caused by viruses. Respiratory infections are more common in the winter, and the family with three or four young children can easily have one or more of them ill for a large part of this season. Most informed parents are intellectually aware of the propensity of young children to have recurrent viral respiratory infections and the physician's inability to prevent or dramatically alter the course of these infections. However, as the winter and respiratory infections continue, it is understandable that many parents, discouraged and impatient, expect the physician to "do something" to prevent these recurrent episodes.

A frank discussion with parents about the current state of knowledge of respiratory tract infections, including the necessity for each child to build his own immunity to viral infections, may help parents to accept the illnesses. We have found it useful to tell parents that children need to acquire 100 or more infections by the time they are 10 years old in order to have adequate immunity. Many parents feel guilty about the recurrent illnesses that seem to plague their children and are afraid that they may be failing in their responsibility. The physician needs to reassure the parents that they are doing a commendable job as parents and that infections are a natural and, at present, unavoidable part of childhood.

When the physician makes the diagnosis of a viral respiratory infection in a child brought to him for evaluation and treatment, he must be careful how he presents his findings and recommendations to the parents. Some parents come away from the physician's office with the following message: "The doctor felt my son's infection was just a bad cold, that the visit was a waste of the doctor's time (and the parents' hard-earned money), and that everyone should know there is no treatment for colds." The physician almost never intentionally gives the parents that message, but he may do it unwittingly on a nonverbal level.

The physician does himself (and the parents) an injustice if that is the message with which the parents leave his office. They were obviously anxious and concerned about their child, or they would not have brought him to the physician. After a careful evaluation based on a history and thorough physical examination, the physician will reassure himself that the child does not have an overwhelming bacterial pneumonia, empyema, acute epiglottitis, or incipient respiratory failure. He may feel that the child has a viral respiratory infection that is most likely self-limiting and that no specific antibiotic therapy is indicated at this time. However, the physician must take the time to reassure the parents, to agree that the symptoms might be frightening to them, to point out his findings, and to tell them why he feels that their child does not have a life-threatening illness at this time.

For the concerned parents, treatment begins with an adequate history and physical examination, continues with laboratory investigations, if indicated, and reaches full momentum when the physician explains his evaluation of the child's illness and his decision on treatment. *All children are treated.* In fact, they have been in the process of treatment since the moment they entered the physician's office. Treatment continues as the clinician discusses his findings and outlines the details of the management program. Recommendations for dietary modifications, changes in activity level, need for increased humidity, and medication for pain, fever, cough, nasal congestion, or wheezing are all forms of treatment. The decision to add or not to add antibiotics is an important one, but in no way does "no antibiotics" equal "no treatment."

Parents should be given information on the expected course of their child's illness and the signs and symptoms that might herald bacterial complications and require re-evaluation by the physician.

Extramedical Factors Influencing Treatment

There are some extramedical factors that may put the physician under considerable pressure to start antibiotic therapy. The experienced clinican makes an unconscious or intuitive level evaluation of these pressures in every encounter with a patient. Examining these factors at a conscious level may help in handling the pressures that can result in overuse of antibiotic therapy. Table 10–2 classifies some factors as they relate to the physician, parents, and child. The column on the left lists the factors that encourage the physician to make a realistic

Table 10–2. EXTRAMEDICAL FACTORS INFLUENCING TREATMENT

Factors Promoting Optimal Care *Encouraging a Flexible Realistic Approach to the Child's Problem*	**Factors Complicating Care** *May Result in Less Flexible Approach to the Child's Problem*
For the Physician	
Well established in the community	New physician in the community
Excellent reputation as children's doctor	Not recognized as expert with children
Physician known to family, with good rapport	Physician unknown to family; no opportunity to establish rapport
Physician's personal life tranquil at present	Physician's personal life in unsettled state
Physician likes and enjoys the child	Physician has no rapport with child
Physician has adequate time	Physician is rushed
For the Child	
No serious past illnesses	Many serious past illnesses
No chronic illness	Complicating chronic illness
Child enjoys contact with physician	Child seems to dislike or is afraid of physician
Child has had infrequent respiratory tract infections in the past	Child has recently had a large number of or prolonged respiratory tract infections
For the Parents	
Intact family unit	Single parent
One parent able to stay home and nurse ill child	Parent(s) must work unless child is critically ill
Family life emotionally tranquil at this time	Family life under stress
No serious financial problems	Family under great financial pressure and this visit is expected to solve all problems
Parents feel that physician accepts and likes them	Parents feel the physician does not like or accept them
Parents selected the physician as their first choice	Parents accept physician because he is available
Parents have had no past experience with unexpected or catastrophic illness with another child	Parents have had a past experience with a sudden, unexpected or catastrophic illness with another child
Parents plan to remain in the city	Parents about to leave on trip or vacation (with or without the child)
Parents have no major events planned for the next week	Parents involved in some major family event (wedding, party, etc.) within the next week

evaluation of the child's medical problems and allow him a flexible approach in prescribing the optimal course of treatment, based on his best medical judgment. The column on the right lists those complicating factors that might result in pressure to prescribe antibiotic therapy even if the physician feels that antibiotics are not necessary at the time of the visit.

A frank discussion between the physician and the child's parents of some of the applicable pressure factors can be the start of increased understanding and rapport.

UPPER RESPIRATORY TRACT INFECTIONS

Upper respiratory tract infections are the most frequent illnesses of infants and children. The infection of the mucous membranes of the upper respiratory tract involves, to varying degrees, the nasal cavity, paranasal sinuses, pharynx, and middle ear. Certain clinical patterns of illness are easily recognized from the anatomical areas involved and the sequence and duration of symptoms. These patterns help the physician to reassure the parents that the illness is a viral upper respiratory infection and can be expected to run its course to a rapid recovery. This arbitrary and mainly anatomical classification is admittedly inaccurate, because viral upper respiratory infections are diffuse even though one area may be more involved than another.

Common upper respiratory tract infections include (1) acute nasopharyngitis (acute rhinitis, coryza, common cold), (2) acute sinusitis, (3) acute pharyngitis and tonsillitis, and (4) otitis media. Although it has been shown consistently that most upper respiratory infections are of viral etiology (Montos and Ullman, 1974), these four anatomical areas are also susceptible to bacterial invasions. Such bacterial infections may occur de novo (as primary infection) or as a complication of an initial viral upper respiratory infection (secondary bacterial infection).

Acute Nasopharyngitis (Acute Rhinitis, Coryza, Common Cold)

In early childhood, repeated infection of the nasal passages is normal and expected, but it is still difficult for some parents to accept. The common viruses responsible for these infections include rhinoviruses, adenoviruses, enteroviruses, influenza and parainfluenza viruses, and respiratory syncytial viruses.

Clinical Pattern

After a short incubation period (averaging two days) the child will develop nasal congestion, sneezing, and a profuse, clear watery nasal discharge. The temperature is usually normal or minimally elevated, although in children between three months and three years of age, fever can reach 39 to 40°C (102 to 104°F) and may be the initial manifestation. Constitutional symptoms, such as headache, muscle aches, sore throat, and anorexia, are usually mild. Many viruses that cause respiratory tract infections can also involve the gastrointestinal tract and result in vomiting and diarrhea as well.

Physical examination will show inflamed and swollen mucous membranes of the nose, often with almost complete occlusion of the nasal passages. The pharynx, tonsils, and palpebral conjunctivae may be suffused and "watery." During the first few days of the infection, the eardrums are usually red and congested. Fluid may be visible behind the tympanic membrane, but this finding does not indicate that secondary bacterial infection has occurred. Cervical lymph glands may be mildly enlarged, and periodic coughing is common.

Clinical Course

The duration and severity of the illness is extremely variable. The acute manifestations average four to seven days, with sneezing and sore throat subsiding first. Nasal discharge will usually persist and gradually become turbid, suggesting a mucopurulent character. Since this turbidity may be the result of inflammatory cells and desquamation associated with the viral infection, it is not pathognomonic of secondary bacterial infection.

Treatment

The treatment of the infant or child with the common cold is supportive and symptomatic. The parents should be taught to expect an illness of about one week's duration, with their child being periodically irritable and querulous and often awakening at night. During the first few days of the illness, small doses of acetaminophen (5 to 10 mg/kg given every four to six hours) for fever or irritability may be given, although parents should be advised that it will not change the duration of the infection and is not needed unless there is discomfort with the fever.

Aspirin, as an alternative, was recommended in the past. Recently, however, there have been epidemiological data suggesting that aspirin ingested in the early stages of varicella or influenza infections results in an increased incidence of Reye's syndrome. The Committee on Infectious Disease of the American Academy of Pediatrics (Special Report, 1982b) recommends that aspirin not be prescribed for children with varicella or for those suspected of having influenza on the basis of clinical or epidemiological evidence. In fact, they recommend considering alternative means of fever control such as increased fluid intake and sponging with tepid water, and possibly avoiding antipyretic medication entirely.

Antibiotics given early in acute viral illness will not alter the clinical course and may, in fact, increase the rate of bacterial complications (Davis and Wedgwood, 1965). Telephone prescribing of antibiotics without examining the child with a respiratory tract infection is to be condemned as inadequate medical practice. Secondary bacterial complications are usually readily recognized and respond to appropriate antibiotic treatment. Topical decongestants, such as phenylephrine hydrochloride 0.25 per cent nose drops, every four hours for no more than two or three days, may help make the patient more comfortable and improve nasal patency during feedings. There is no evidence that antihistamines have any beneficial effect orally or topically.

Complications

Secondary bacterial infection of the middle ear and paranasal sinuses accounts for most complications, although suppurative cervical adenitis may also develop. Generally, young infants and older children who are malnourished or suffer from chronic illnesses are most susceptible to bacterial complications during bouts of acute viral nasopharyngitis (common cold). Bacterial otitis media usually occurs late in the course of illness (after three days); any persistence or return of fever after three days should arouse suspicion of a possible secondary bacterial infection.

Acute Sinusitis

The paranasal sinuses are direct extensions of the nasal cavity. The mucus produced in the sinuses drains freely into the nasal cavity. Each episode of acute viral nasopharyngitis (common cold) results in a generalized infection of the mucous membranes of the paranasal sinuses. As long as the sinuses continue to drain freely into the nasal cavity, the course of the infection in the sinuses will parallel the more observable infection within the nasal cavity. When thought of in this way, acute sinusitis is extremely common in childhood, with an incidence almost identical to that of acute nasopharyngitis. The expected clinical course of both infections is the same; i.e., most viral infections of the sinuses or nasal cavity heal rapidly and spontaneously. However, an anatomical fact increases the susceptibility of these sinus areas to secondary bacterial infection. The sinuses drain into the nose through the ostea, the communicating passage between the sinus cavities and the nasopharynx. If the swollen infected mucous membranes occlude the ostea, then the resultant stasis predisposes to bacterial growth and resulting secondary bacterial infection.

Acute bacterial sinusitis is seen fairly frequently in general pediatric practice as a complication of acute viral nasopharyngitis. It usually occurs after the acute phase of the illness (after three days), just when the child should begin to improve. Coincident with the bacterial infection in the sinus, the child may develop an increasing mucopurulent discharge, which may either drain into the anterior nares or, more commonly, be seen as a postnasal discharge. During waking hours, this purulent discharge is swallowed and causes little difficulty, but during sleep the material tends to accumulate in the hypopharynx and reflexly initiates the periodic bouts of coughing that are so disturbing to the sleep of the child and parents.

The classic symptoms of adult sinusitis, i.e., localized sinus pain, headache, and high temperature, are rarely encountered in early childhood. This is probably because the sinuses are rudimentary in young children during the period of frequently occurring upper respiratory infections. At birth, small maxillary antra and the anterior and posterior ethmoid cells are present. The sphenoidal sinuses remain rudimentary until about three years of age but grow rapidly thereafter. Frontal sinuses are not visible on x-ray until three years of age, and do not extend to the areas above the orbits until after six or seven years of age. Sinus infection as an isolated disorder without a diffuse upper respiratory infection is very rare before eight years of age; after that, bacterial infections may localize to a specific sinus or group of sinuses. Sphenoidal sinusitis may produce pain over the temples; frontal and anterior ethmoidal sinusitis tends to give referred pain to the forehead just above the orbits. Posterior ethmoiditis may produce suboccipital pain. Fever may be low-grade or absent but can be significantly elevated. For a current comprehensive review of this subject, see Rachelefsky et al. (1982).

Treatment

Acute viral sinusitis that accompanies each upper respiratory infection of viral origin ordinarily requires no specific treatment. The recognition that the paranasal sinuses are involved in all respiratory tract infections helps the clinician to interpret the symptoms. Older children who complain of pain over an occluded sinus can be helped by a short course of treatment (two or three days) of topical decongestants in the form of nose drops or nasal sprays (phenylephrine hydrochloride 0.25 per cent every four hours). After the acute phase has subsided, the clinician must be alert for signs and symptoms that suggest secondary bacterial infection of the nasal cavity or the sinuses. Major findings may be increasing mucopurulent discharge, persistent cough, and malaise.

The bacterial organisms most likely to cause this secondary infection are pneumococci, Streptococcus, Staphylococcus, and *Hemophilus influenzae*. A culture of the posterior nasal cavity taken with a nasal wire applicator (Caligesic swab) is likely to recover the offending organism. Most of these organisms are sensitive to ampicillin therapy (100 to 150 mg/kg/day), which is the therapy of choice. The blocked cavities are often slow to respond to antibiotic therapy, and 10 to 14 days of therapy may be necessary to clear the infection. Cultures and sensitivity studies are helpful in resistant cases but are not required routinely to initiate treatment. Nose drops, as recommended during the acute viral phase with localizing symptoms, may have a greater role in bacterial sinusitis to aid in the opening of the ostea, but the nose drops or nasal sprays should be used for only a few days because of rebound hyperemia.

X-rays of the sinuses in the first five years of life are difficult to interpret and rarely provide the information on which to base the decision for therapy. Interpretation is further complicated in that simple viral infections of the upper respiratory tract with the usual sinus involvement frequently will result in a "clouded sinus" for a few weeks (Maresh and Washburn, 1940).

Suction aspiration of the sinuses, usually called the Proetz treatment, is rarely indicated in children. Many physicians feel that allergic children are more likely to develop secondary bacterial sinus infection in the course of viral upper respiratory infections, possibly because the increased swelling of the mucous membranes obstructs normal osteal drainage. Physicians should follow allergic children closely and start antibiotics at the first signs of acute bacterial sinusitis.

Chronic sinusitis is rarely encountered in children with normal immune mechanisms. Sinus radiograms in children with cystic fibrosis, in over 90 per cent of cases examined, have shown "clouding," but symptomatic attacks of acute sinusitis are virtually unknown (Gharib, et al., 1964).

Complications

Acute orbital and periorbital cellulitis as complications of acute ethmoiditis (Gellady et al., 1978) deserve special mention. The ethmoidal sinuses are a paired series of spaces of variable number, located in the lateral ethmoidal masses between the upper part of the nasal cavities and the orbits. The orbits and their contents are peculiarly susceptible to extension of infection from the ethmoidal sinuses, as they are separated only by a thin and delicate bone, the lamina papyracea. The venous return from the paranasal sinuses passes partly into the orbit and through the ophthalmic veins and the cavernous sinus. The lymphatics probably follow the same course.

The child with acute ethmoiditis usually presents with unilateral periorbital swelling and fever. Occasionally, bilateral periorbital swelling is present. Almost half of the children have obvious rhinorrhea, and in many it is purulent. Children with ethmoidal sinusitis need to be divided clinically into two groups. The first group has periorbital cellulitis, with the infection confined to the preseptal space and not involving the deep intraorbital structures. The second group has orbital cellulitis with infection inside the orbit, which may include extraocular muscles, periosteum, and the optic nerve.

Serious complications may develop in either group but are more likely to occur with orbital cellulitis. Careful and complete eye examination, using a lid retractor if necessary, will allow the physician to detect the signs of orbital involvement: limitations of extraocular movements, severe chemosis, proptosis, and disturbances of visual acuity. If adequate examination is not possible, and the patient's response to therapy is not satisfactory, a computerized x-ray scan of the orbital region will often provide valuable information in localizing the extent of the infection (Goldberg et al., 1978). Complications may develop rapidly and include orbital abscess, cavernous sinus thrombosis, brain abscess, meningitis, optic neuritis, and blindness.

The causative organisms are the same as listed earlier for bacterial sinusitis, with the exception that *H. influenzae* may be responsible for a much larger percentage of the infections.

Owing to the increasing prevalence of ampicillin-resistant *H. influenzae* in many communities, therapy must cover these organisms as well as provide good central nervous system penetration to prevent meningeal spread. Examples of two acceptable intravenous regimens would be (1) nafcillin (100–200 mg/kg/day divided into four doses) and chloramphenicol (100 mg/kg/day divided into four doses), OR (2) nafcillin (100–200 mg/kg/day divided into four doses) and a third-generation cephalosporin active against *H. influenzae,* such as moxalactam (150 mg/kg/day divided into three doses).

Acute frontal osteomyelitis is a rare complication with a predilection for older adolescents, particularly after fulminating acute frontal sinusitis. Fever, pain, and edema over the frontal sinus and lids may be present. Displacement of the globe may follow cellulitis extending from the frontal floor. Destructive changes on the sinus radiograph may not be present for one to two weeks. The diagnosis should be made on a clinical basis and intravenous antibiotic therapy and local drainage instituted early.

Hemophilus influenzae type b cellulitis is a rare complication of bacterial nasopharyngitis or sinusitis in children (Green and Fousek, 1957). It usually occurs secondary to bacteremia and tends to localize in the cheeks, producing swelling with central induration surrounded peripherally by a nonindurated edematous zone without elevated or sharply demarcated borders. The involved area is tender and warm to hot and has a dusky or reddish purple color resembling a fading hematoma. Intensive treatment with intravenous ampicillin (200 to 300 mg/kg/day divided into six doses) or chloramphenicol (100 mg/kg/day divided into four doses) is indicated.

Acute Pharyngitis and Tonsillitis (Pharyngotonsillitis)

"Sore throat" is one of the most common complaints of children seen for medical treatment. The infection may involve the pharynx diffusely (acute pharyngitis) or may be localized predominantly to the palatine tonsils (acute tonsillitis).

The clinician faces the basic problem of trying to differentiate self-limiting viral infections from bacterial infections that require antibiotic therapy. The problem is further complicated by the fact that a small number of children with throat infections due to group A streptococci, if left untreated with antibiotics, will develop rheumatic fever. Acute rheumatic fever is a nonsuppurative complication limited to children over three years of age. Certain specific strains or types of streptococci, the so-called nephritogenic strains, may cause another nonsuppurative complication, acute glomerulonephritis, in susceptible children. There is no evidence that early antibiotic treatment of a child with clinical pharyngitis can prevent the onset of nephritis. Since we are currently unable to identify children who are susceptible to these complications, we are forced to treat all children with group A streptococcal infections in order to prevent rheumatic fever. Certain physical signs and symptoms are more common in children infected with streptococci than with acute viral throat infections. This allows the physician to make a clinical diagnosis of probable streptococcal pharyngitis and to begin therapy before the results of throat culture are available. The correlation with positive cultures is no better than 75 per cent.

Etiology

Eichenwald (1976) estimates that 80 to 90 per cent of attacks of acute pharyngotonsillitis are due to viral infections. Adenoviruses, parainfluenza, influenza, coxsackie A and B, ECHO, respiratory syncytial, and Epstein-Barr viruses all have been implicated in infections of pharynx and tonsils. *Mycoplasma hominis* type 1 has produced pharyngitis in experimental infections of volunteers but appears to be an extremely rare cause of pharyngitis in childhood (Moffet, 1975). Group A beta-hemolytic Streptococcus is the only common bacterial cause of acute pharyngitis. On rare occasions, group C hemolytic streptococci, pneumococci, and gonococci have been implicated as probable causes of acute pharyngitis.

Diphtheritic pharyngitis is now extremely rare in adequately immunized populations; however, it must always be considered in the differential diagnosis of any pharyngeal infection with exudate, as failure to institute early treatment may result in fatal complications.

Although *Staphylococcus aureus* may be recovered in pure culture (particularly with viral throat infections), it is unproven as a primary cause of acute pharyngitis, except in children with severe immunodeficiency.

Clinical Patterns

The clinical patterns of patients with acute streptococcal and acute viral pharyngitis are shown in Table 10–3. The child with a typical

Table 10–3. COMPARISON OF TYPICAL CLINICAL PATTERNS OF ACUTE PHARYNGOTONSILLITIS

	Infection	
	Acute Streptococcal	*Viral*
Time Course of Onset	Sudden	Gradual
Presenting Symptoms		
General toxicity and malaise	Moderate to severe	Mild to moderate
Abdominal pain	Common	Rare
Vomiting	Common	Rare
Headache	Common	Rare
Fever	102° to 105°F	101° to 103°F
Respiratory Tract		
Cough	Rare	Common
Hoarseness	Rare	Common
Nasal congestion	Rare	Common
Conjunctivitis	Rare	Common
Pharynx		
Sore throat	Very common	Common
Tonsillar erythema	Moderate to extensive	Minimal to moderate
Exudate	Small to extensive (if extensive rule out diphtheria)	None to small (except inf. mono, which may have extensive exudate)
Petechial mottling of soft palate	Common	Rare
Anterior Cervical Nodes		
Enlarged	Moderate to extensive	Minimal to moderate
Tender on palpation	Moderate to severe	Minimal to moderate
Age	Generally over 3 years	Any age

group A beta-hemolytic streptococcal infection has a rapid onset of sore throat, appears ill, and commonly complains of headache, abdominal pain, and vomiting. Temperature is often elevated to 103 to 104°F. On examination, the classic findings are reddened, swollen tonsils streaked with yellowish exudate. The soft palate and uvula are erythematous with petechial mottling. The anterior cervical lymph nodes (particularly Anson's tonsillar node at the angle of the jaw) are enlarged and tender to palpation. The typical clinical presentation of acute viral pharyngitis is apt to be more gradual, often associated with nasal congestion and conjunctival injection. The patient appears mildly to moderately ill, with a temperature between 100 and 103°F; other respiratory tract symptoms such as cough and hoarseness may be present. Tonsillar redness is usually less impressive than with streptococcal infection, and exudate is frequently absent. In children less than three years of age, a small amount of whitish exudate may be seen. Older children with infectious mononucleosis may show an extensive whitish or grayish exudate over the tonsils.

Although the typical clinical symptoms and physical findings of a child with acute streptococcal sore throat are usually sufficiently characteristic to allow the clinician to suspect the diagnosis, many of these patients present with an atypical pattern indistinguishable from viral pharyngitis. A culture of the throat at the infected site is the only reliable way of establishing the presence of streptococci with certainty. Outpatient throat cultures for beta-hemolytic streptococci are a necessary part of routine office practice. The required equipment is inexpensive and the necessary bacteriological skills for accurate identification are modest. Details of the throat culture technique and organism identification are discussed in Appendix B, The Well-Equipped Office.

Pantell (1981) has presented a detailed analysis of various strategies in selecting treatment. Considering outcome and cost effectiveness in an era of diminishing incidence of acute rheumatic fever, striking geographical differences in rheumatic fever attack rates, and the known calculated risk of penicillin allergy, our current rigid, aggressive treatment of all streptococcal infection may no longer be appropriate. Until new criteria are agreed upon, one practical scheme of management of acute tonsillopharyngitis is outlined in Table 10–4. Patients are categorized on the basis of their clinical findings into three groups: strongly suspected strepto-

Table 10–4. MANAGEMENT OF THE CHILD WITH ACUTE TONSILLITIS OR ACUTE PHARYNGITIS

Pattern of Presentation	Typical Streptococcal Pattern	Intermediate Pattern	Typical Viral Pattern
Clinical Evaluation	Strongly suspect streptococcal infection	Undecided	Strongly suspect viral infection
Throat culture for Group A, betahemolytic streptococci	Culture highly desirable to prove diagnosis and provide epidemiological information for the family	Always culture	Always culture
Antibiotic treatment	Start antibiotics Once started, make sure patient receives a complete course of antistreptococcal therapy—either 1 injection of benzathine penicillin G, or 10 days of oral penicillin V or G, or erythromycin.	Withhold antibiotics until throat culture report is available.	Withhold antibiotics until throat culture report is available.
		POSITIVE for Streptococcus START ANTIBIOTICS Ensure adequate treatment course	NEGATIVE for Streptococcus WITHHOLD ANTIBIOTICS Continue to observe for possible late secondary bacterial infection

coccal infection, undecided, and strongly suspected viral infection. Antibiotic therapy is started immediately on patients who present a typical picture of streptococcal pharyngitis, but is withheld pending the availability of culture results in the undecided and strongly suspected viral infection cases. A throat culture is highly desirable for all three groups and mandatory for the "undecided" and the classic viral pharyngitis groups, since in them antibiotics are withheld until results of culture are available. If streptococci are found, a 10-day course of oral penicillin or erythromycin is instituted, or one dose of injectable benzathine penicillin is given (see Table 10–5 for dosage schedules). Antibiotic therapy is still effective in preventing rheumatic fever, even if delayed one to three days after the onset of acute tonsillopharyngitis. In the patients whose cultures fail to grow streptococci, no antibiotic therapy is necessary. Patients with viral throat infections may occasionally develop secondary bacterial infections with local suppuration and should be observed for two weeks for any signs or symptoms that suggest bacterial complications. Secondary bacterial infection can lead to suppurative otitis media, acute sinusitis, cervical adenitis, peritonsillar abscess, or retropharyngeal abscess.

Antibiotic Therapy

The antibiotic of choice for the treatment of acute streptococcal tonsillopharyngitis is penicillin. Fortunately, no group A streptococci have been reported to have developed resistance to penicillin. The only justification for using any other antibiotic is allergy to penicillin. Erythromycin in its various forms, in a dose of 40 mg/kg/day in divided doses for 10 days, is a satisfactory substitute that is inexpensive and has a low incidence of significant side effects. Sulfonamides suppress but do not eradicate streptococcal infections or prevent rheumatic fever. Up to 40 per cent of streptococci have been found to be resistant to tetracyclines.

The choice of the route of administration of the antibiotic is based on the willingness of the child to take oral medication and his ability to retain it after ingestion. The physician's estimate of the parents' ability and willingness to follow through with a full 10-day course of oral treatment should also influence his decision. An outline of antibiotic dosage is given in Table 10–5. The oral administration of antibiotics is certainly the easiest for the child, and it allows discontinuation at the first sign of allergic manifestations. This route should be chosen unless the child is vomiting or so toxic that the physician has concern about the parents' ability to administer the medication. Physicians are probably unrealistic if they really believe that most of their patients actually receive a full 10-day course of therapy. Factors that promote patient compliance have been examined (see Chapter 2). These compliance studies show that the

Table 10–5. ANTIBIOTIC DOSAGE FOR ACUTE STREPTOCOCCAL TONSILLOPHARYNGITIS

Medication	Dose		Duration
Oral			
Penicillin V (phenoxymethyl penicillin)	25–50 mg/kg/day in 4 divided doses (maximum 250–500 mg q6h)		Full 10 days
If allergic to penicillin use erythromycin	40 mg/kg/day in 4 divided doses (maximum 250 mg q6h)		Full 10 days
Intramuscular	*Patient's Weight*	*Dose*	
IM Benzathine penicillin (LA Bicillin)	<30 lb (<14 kg)	300,000 units	1 dose only
	30–60 lb (14–27 kg)	600,000 units	
	60–90 lb (27–40 kg)	900,000 units	
	>90 lb (>40 kg)	1,200,000 units	

administration of medication is not improved by an authoritarian physician who exhorts the parents to give the medications for a full 10 days. Good rapport with parents and a detailed explanation of the necessity for a full 10-day course of therapy will increase compliance significantly. Parental perception of how well they are accepted and liked by the physician is probably a more important factor in compliance than has been recognized in the past.

Tonsillectomy and Adenoidectomy

Some knowledge of the history of adenotonsillectomy as an approach to treating recurrent tonsillitis and otitis media is helpful in understanding the various attitudes that physicians will encounter among colleagues and the parents of patients.

According to Williams and Phelan (1975), a survey in New York City in 1888 revealed that only 3 per cent of children had their tonsils and adenoids surgically removed. By 1909 the rate of removal had risen to 30 per cent, and by 1940 it was 50 per cent. They point out that this remarkable and unprecedented epidemic of modern surgery was probably due to a number of factors. First, the concept of focal infection as a cause of generalized debility developed during the latter half of the nineteenth century and was uncritically accepted by the medical profession. This theory justified the wholesale surgical removal of many hapless organs, including tonsils, adenoids, and teeth.

The great frequency of viral respiratory infections as a natural (and still unavoidable) part of early childhood was unrecognized, as was the natural tendency for children to have fewer upper respiratory infections after six to eight years of age. As the greatest number of operations were performed in the four- to eight-year age group, it was inevitable that the reduction in the number of infections and improvement in the child's health would be attributed to the surgery.

The focal infection theory of disease has long been discredited. Armed with epidemiological data on the natural incidence and course of childhood respiratory infections, we should logically expect that adenotonsillectomy should be out of fashion. In fact, however, tonsil and adenoid surgery continues to be widely practiced, although there has been some recent decline in the number of operations performed. Paradise (1981) estimated that the total annual expenditures for tonsil and adenoid surgery in the United States exceeds one-half billion dollars.

The mortality associated with the operation is low and probably should not exceed the irreducible minimum of anesthesia-related deaths, recently calculated at 1 per 14,000 patients. Even so, this totals about 75 to 100 deaths per year, an unacceptable tragedy if the operation was not necessary. Postoperative morbidity, usually bleeding, is much more frequent, and the incidence of psychological damage as a result of the emotional trauma of hospitalization and surgery, although more difficult to estimate, is significant.

What are rational indications for the surgical removal of the tonsils, the adenoids, or both the tonsils and the adenoids? This is a difficult question for which there is a plethora of testimonials and a remarkable paucity of adequately controlled observations. A long-term prospective study is currently underway at Children's Hospital in Pittsburgh. Paradise (1981) outlines the criteria for entering into their controlled randomized trial of tonsillectomy and adenoidectomy. Their data and preliminary conclusions warrant the attention of practitioners, including their caveat that benefits are not yet proven or disproven.

Our current state of knowledge can be summarized in the following statements:

Tonsillar and adenoidal tissue, as part of the lymphoid system, is known to increase gradually in size during the first 8 years of life and then to decrease in size slowly over the next ten years.

The relative importance of the lymphoid tissue of the palatine tonsils and adenoids in the development of a child's immunocompetence is not known.

All children will be subject to periodic bouts of tonsillitis and pharyngitis. Even those children who have had their tonsils removed continue to have pharyngitis.

The only common bacterial cause of tonsillitis is streptococci, and this responds rapidly to treatment with penicillin or erythromycin, which also prevents most complications.

Large or even huge tonsils in a child between 5 and 12 years of age are never an indication for surgical removal on the basis of size alone. There must be evidence of some pathological condition such as persistent difficulty in swallowing, disturbance in normal phonation, or sleep-state upper airway obstruction.

Recurrent bouts of suppurative otitis media or persistent serous otitis media are considered by many physicians as justification for adenoidectomy. The enlarged lymphoid tissue is thought to block the normal drainage of the eustachian tube. No good controlled study to prove or disprove the effectiveness of adenoidectomy in alleviating this problem is available.

Sleep-state upper airway obstruction (obstructive sleep apnea), usually due to enlarged adenoids and tonsils, has been recognized with increasing frequency over the past 10 years. The resultant hypoxemia and hypercapnia may cause reflex pulmonary hypertension, leading to cor pulmonale and congestive heart failure. The full syndrome with congestive heart failure is extremely rare but is an unequivocal indication for adenotonsillectomy.

The clinical significance of a much larger group of children who have sleep-state upper airway obstruction but no heart failure is still unknown. In this group of patients, prominent snoring is interrupted by episodes of total ventilatory obstruction (no air passing into the lungs despite continued inspiratory efforts for 3 to 15 seconds). The child rouses momentarily, changes head position, brings the tongue forward, which opens the airway, takes a deep breath or two, and falls back to sleep. The cycle is repeated frequently throughout the night. Parents will often provide detailed descriptions of this usually unrecognized syndrome if given an opportunity. Daytime examination in the office reveals no airway obstruction. A nighttime audio tape recording by the parents at home of prenasal or preoral breath sounds often gives documentation of these obstructive episodes. Unreported studies in our sleep laboratory, including continuous transcutaneous oxygen and carbon dioxide monitoring, show that a small number of these patients have hypoxemia and hypercapnia during these episodes. The significance of these observations is unknown, and more detailed studies are needed. Our impressions support the earlier work of Guilleminault et al. (1976) that many of these children show daytime behavioral improvement after adenotonsillectomy.

The most difficult problem facing the practioner is evaluating the validity of the parents' complaint that their child is suffering an abnormal number or severity of tonsillar infections.

Physicians should be skeptical of a history of recurrent or persistent episodes of acute tonsillitis, since parents frequently confuse diffuse viral respiratory infections with pharyngitis and acute tonsillitis. Before deciding on the necessity of surgery, the physician should make every effort to follow each child for a 6- to 12-month period, observing the type and location of the infections developed by the child. This single approach, so difficult to put into practice, would probably reduce precipitously the number of tonsillectomies, since in most cases there will be spontaneous improvement during this period.

Acute Otitis Media (Acute Suppurative Otitis Media)

Every child with fever or diffuse viral respiratory infection must be evaluated for possible ear infection. The otoscope, probably more than any other instrument, symbolizes the pediatrician's expertise and his dedication to finding the source of the illness in young children.

Children in the first three to six years of life have an average of six upper respiratory infections a year, each of which may involve the paranasal sinuses and the middle ear cavities to variable degrees. Otoscopic examination of the tympanic membrane during the first few days of a diffuse viral upper respiratory infection will usually show redness and injection, particularly around the periphery of the drum and, at times, small amounts of fluid behind the drum. At this stage of the illness, needle aspiration (tympanocentesis) of the middle ear fluid will yield fluid that is sterile on culture for bacteria.

There are probably multiple factors involved in the high frequency of bacterial otitis media in children. Anatomical differences in the structure of the respiratory tract as well as immaturity of the body's immune defense system may increase susceptibility.

Etiology

The child who suddenly in the middle of the night develops an earache that progresses rapidly (in a few hours) to rupture of the eardrum and a draining middle ear the next morning is usually suffering from pneumococcal otitis media. Other middle ear pathogens are usually less dramatic in their onset and clinical course.

Extensive bacteriological studies of middle ear samples obtained by tympanocentesis on patients with acute otitis media have consistently demonstrated that the two most frequent bacteria involved are *Streptococcus pneumoniae* and *Hemophilus influenzae*. *S. pneumoniae* is the most commonly encountered organism throughout childhood, with *H. influenzae* causing a significant number of cases in early childhood and becoming less common as children grow older. Other bacteria, including group A *Streptococcus pyogenes*, are found in low incidence.

Recent longitudinal epidemiological studies in a nursery school population have demonstrated a marked increase in acute otitis media following nasopharyngeal colonization with certain viruses, as compared with other viruses. Respiratory syncytial virus, influenzae virus (type A or B), and adenovirus resulted in a much greater incidence of otitis media than did colonization with parainfluenza, enterovirus, and rhinovirus. The relationship between this colonization, otitis media, and the possible invasion of the middle ear by bacteria is unclear at the present time but is under investigation (Henderson et al., 1982).

The role of *Mycoplasma pneumoniae* as a cause of suppurative otitis media remains unsettled. Current evidence would suggest that it is an extremely infrequent cause (Klein, 1980) and that therapy should cover the more common bacterial infections.

Diagnosis

The diagnosis of acute suppurative otitis media is based on the abnormal appearance of the tympanic membrane. When the membrane is red and bulging, with a loss of the normal light reflex, there is little argument as to the validity of the diagnosis.

Most investigators agree that the tympanic membrane may be reddened and show injection of the peripheral blood vessels during the acute state of diffuse viral respiratory infection. Usually there is no bulging of the drum, and antibiotic therapy is not indicated. The differentiation of secondary infection (and the decision to start antibiotics) is made on the presence of a full or bulging tympanic membrane and loss of light reflex. Tense, bulging tympanic membranes are not always red; they may be yellow or dull grey and still have pus behind the drum. Until another diagnostic method with proven reliability is available, a bulging tympanic membrane must be accepted as evidence of acute suppurative otitis media (Rowe, 1975).

A painful swollen external auditory canal filled with purulent exudate (otitis externa) is sometimes difficult to differentiate from acute suppurative otitis media with a ruptured ear drum draining through the external auditory canal. In either situation, it may be impossible to visualize the tympanic membrane adequately. A history of frequent swimming would make the clinician suspect otitis externa (swimmer's ear). This would be further substantiated by finding that movements of the pinna (causing pressure shifts in the external auditory canal) result in sharp pains in the canal. Swelling of the skin lining the canal usually makes visualization of the drum impossible, even after suctioning as much material as possible from the ear canal. Fortunately, the initial antibiotic treatment of draining suppurative otitis media and otitis externa is the same, although alleviation of pain is more likely to be necessary in otitis externa.

PNEUMATIC OTOSCOPY

A lack of mobility of the tympanic membrane to externally applied air pressure (pneumatic otoscopy) is strong evidence of middle ear abnormality but is in no way specific for acute suppurative otitis media. Performing pneumatic otoscopy on a struggling, crying infant is not always a simple undertaking. Just removing enough cerumen from the external auditory canal to obtain a reasonable look at the tympanic membrane can be difficult and time-consuming. Soaking the cerumen with a bland softening solution (hydrogen peroxide in glycerol) followed by gentle continuous suction applied through an Adson suction tube with a short pliable plastic tip attached will often remove the cerumen and obviate the need to use a blunt ear curette. Sometimes removal of cerumen requires syringing with water at body temperature. A Water-Pik irrigation unit often simplifies this procedure and is well accepted by children. Organizing optimal equipment and restraints for cerumen removal is essential to good pediatric practice. Details are outlined in the review article by Paradise (1980).

TYMPANOCENTESIS

Growth from cultures of the nasopharynx and pharynx shows very little correlation with needle aspirates of the middle ear in acute suppurative otitis media. Routine tympanocentesis in management of acute otitis media is not justified. By utilizing the bacteriological data of previous tympanocentesis studies, the clinician can choose antibiotics appropriate for the organisms known to cause otitis media in the child's age group.

Treatment

Decongestants. The objectives of decongestant medication are reasonable. Anything that will decongest the eustachian tubes and promote middle ear drainage will help to resolve the infection; unfortunately, the value of decongestants, oral or topical, in the treatment of otitis media has not yet been proven. Recent controlled studies using decongestants with or without antihistamines have shown no benefit (Olson et al., 1978).

Myringotomy. In preantibiotic times, myringotomy was performed almost routinely for bulging otitis media. Today, almost all cases of otitis media will respond to antibiotics without myringotomy. Roddey et al. (1966) have shown that myringotomy does not accelerate the resolution of the acute infection, and most pediatricians have almost abandoned myringotomy for the management of the acute phase of otitis media. However, a child with severe ear pain who cannot achieve rapid relief with antibiotics and analgesics can frequently be given dramatic relief by myringotomy. Failure to improve with antimicrobial therapy, including persistent bulging of the tympanic membrane, is another indication for myringotomy. Any suppurative complications such as meningitis or mastoiditis are considered by most ear specialists mandatory reasons to drain the middle ear. The myringotomy drains the abscess and provides material for culture and sensitivity studies.

Antibiotics. Acute suppurative otitis media is usually a self-limiting disease in most children, even without antibiotic therapy. Many children develop spontaneous rupture of the tympanic membrane and drain the middle ear; in other children it will resolve without drainage. The small group of children in whom it does not resolve spontaneously are prone to serious and long-standing complications, including chronic otitis media with perforation, mastoiditis, meningitis, and possible deafness.

Antibiotics are the mainstay of treatment for acute otitis media, although the acute phase of otitis media in children is virtually unaltered with antibiotic treatment. The major observable effect of antibiotic therapy is the decrease in the incidence of complications and prevention of chronic otitis media. Acute mastoiditis, a common problem in the preantibiotic era, has almost disappeared since the use of antibiotics has become widespread.

It was formerly thought that the choice of antibiotics was strongly influenced by the age of the child.

Beyond six weeks of age, outpatient treatment of acute suppurative otitis media is selected to cover both *S. pneumoniae* and *H. influenzae.* Ampicillin (50–100 mg/kg/day divided into three doses) is a good initial choice, except in geographical areas known to have a high incidence of ampicillin-resistant *H. influenzae.* Where β-lactamase–producing *H. influenzae* may be a problem, cefaclor (40–60 mg/kg/day divided into three doses) has proven effective against ampicillin-resistant *H. influenzae* as well as *S. pneumoniae.* Combining erythromycin with a sulfonamide (Pediazole) provides broad coverage and is a reasonable choice. Trimethoprim-sulfamethoxazole (Bactrim, Septra) appears to show promise for treatment of ampicillin-resistant *H. influenzae.*

Neonatal Period (Birth to Six Weeks). Pediatricians are well aware of the high incidence of infections due to gram-negative bacilli and staphylococci in the neonatal period. Extensive studies of otitis media in the neonatal period suggest that most cases are due to the same organisms as in older children and that therapy should initially be the same. If the infant appears critically ill or fails to improve on therapy, then gram-negative bacilli or a strain of Staphylococcus should be considered as a possible etiology. Therapy would then include hospitalization, tympanocentesis with Gram stain and culture, and initiation of intravenous antibiotic therapy with ampicillin (200 mg/kg/day divided into four doses) and gentamicin (6 mg/kg/day divided into three doses).

Follow-Up Care. All children with otitis media should be followed to make sure that the middle ear clears and that hearing returns to normal. A visit two to three weeks after initiation of treatment should be routine, but if the child does not seem greatly improved within a few days after starting antibiotics, earlier re-evaluation is indicated.

A small but significant number of children (3 to 10 per cent) will fail to resolve the infection and require retreatment. If the infection does not resolve after the second course of antibiotics, then re-evaluation is indicated. Chronic infection of the mastoid air cells may be present. Myringotomy of a full or thickened tympanic membrane will frequently aid resolution and provide material for culture and antibiotic sensitivity testing. Culture results will allow more specific antibiotic therapy for rare or resistant microorganisms. Consultation with an otologist should then be considered.

Nonsuppurative Otitis Media

Known by many synonyms, including serous otitis media, secretory otitis media, and glue ear, this condition contrasts with suppurative otitis media in that the effusion appears to be a grossly nonpurulent inflammation. The effusion fluid may be a thin, watery transudate or a thick, gelatinous material (glue ear). The principal symptom is a marked conductive hearing loss that may persist for weeks or months. The cause is probably eustachian tube dysfunction that results in inadequate aeration of the middle ear; oxygen is absorbed by the blood, resulting in negative pressure in the middle ear tending to retract the drum.

The cause of this effusion is inadequately understood and apparently can either precede or follow acute suppurative otitis media. Nonsuppurative otitis media may occur de novo in allergic children with upper respiratory symptoms. The longitudinal studies of Henderson et al. (1982) noted under etiology, suggest that certain viruses may be involved in producing nonsuppurative otitis media, which in turn may become suppurative. The excellent review by Paradise (1980) discusses our current knowledge of this entity and points out the difficulties of establishing diagnosis on physical examination alone, even when pneumatic otoscopy is utilized. Tympanometry, a form of impedence testing performed with an electrical instrument that delivers a fixed-frequency tone into the closed canal and measures the changes in the sound-pressure level through a microphone, produces a "tympanogram" that depicts eardrum compliance, roughly equivalent to eardrum mobility seen during pneumatic otoscopy. The test has the advantages of being simple, rapid, atraumatic, and objective. Its widespread use should broaden our knowledge of middle ear effusions considerably over the next few years and help improve our diagnosis and therapy of this disorder.

On physical examination, in a typical case, the tympanic membrane is usually diffusely opaque and retracted, exhibits a diminished light reflex, and shows impaired mobility with the pneumatic otoscope. Almost any of these signs may be absent. The color of the drum may be pink, amber, grey-white, or bluish. When physical examination is combined with impedence tympanometry, the ability to diagnose this condition is increased significantly.

The natural history of nonsuppurative otitis media is unknown, but this disorder appears to be more common in the winter months. Many cases subside spontaneously within a few months to two years. That many forms of treatment have been advocated is due to the lack of proven effect of any one approach on the natural course of this disease. If the child has not had a recent course of antibiotic therapy appropriate for suppurative otitis media, this may be tried. If chronic purulent-appearing rhinorrhea is present, the likelihood of improvement from antibiotic therapy seems increased. Oral decongestants may be tried, although they are of unproved efficacy. Children with a history and examination that suggest respiratory allergy should be managed with a conventional program of environmental control and antiallergic medication. Adenoidectomy to remove enlarged lymphoid tissue adjacent to the pharyngeal opening of the eustachian tube, while seemingly rational, has been disappointing in improving aeration of the middle ear. Placement of small plastic tympanostomy tubes (grommets) achieves aeration of the middle ear temporarily and improves hearing. Unfortunately, this does not affect the underlying problem, and when the tubes come out the problem may recur.

LOWER RESPIRATORY TRACT INFECTIONS

Lower respiratory tract infections include infections of the larynx, trachea, bronchi, bronchioles, and parenchymal portion of the lung. All infections of the lower respiratory tract have some potential for interfering with normal ventilation and, therefore, command careful evaluation. This section of the chapter will guide the clinician in identifying those children who need chest roentgenograms, cultures, antibiotics, or hospitalization.

Clinical Assessment

A careful clinical assessment allows the practitioner to make a reasonable decision. Not all children require chest x-rays or microbiological investigation. Initial evaluation divides children with pulmonary infection into two groups: those mildly affected who can be treated on an ambulatory basis without further investigation and those who appear moderately to severely ill and need more investigation before determining their treatment program. Many children in this second group will require hospitalization. The assessment includes three areas: the child's past medical history and family-home situation, the apparent severity of the illness, and the degree of pulmonary dysfunction. Evidence of abnormality or unusual findings in any of these three areas places the child in a high-risk group and requires that the physician obtain more information before he decides on management.

HISTORY AND FAMILY SITUATION

This information allows the clinician to place the infant in a normal or high-risk group. Examples of factors that increase the likelihood that an infant will develop a severe or complicated respiratory infection include inadequate nutrition, age, previous severe respiratory infection, and any chronic or underlying medical problem. The younger the infant, the higher the risk. Infants under six months of age must be considered unproven entities regarding immunological competence and ability to handle infection. Until they have recovered from a few respiratory infections, thus demonstrating their immunological capacity, each infant must be watched for signs and symptoms suggesting overwhelming infection.

The life circumstances of the child and his family, including their ability to follow a medical program, make the necessary observations, detect unfavorable changes in the child's condition, and return him for follow-up care, all enter into the physician's evaluation of how best to treat an individual child. A well-nourished child, older than one year, with no prior serious respiratory infections or other major medical problems, being cared for by a responsible adult who has the necessary physical, intellectual, emotional and financial resources to carry out the medical treatment program, has an ideal situation for home management of the respiratory infection, provided he is not too ill.

SEVERITY OF THE ILLNESS

How ill does the child appear? The physician's overall "gestalt" of the child's state of illness is a valuable index of the severity of the infection. The basis of this clinical judgment relates to many factors, objective and subjective, that physicians utilize in evaluating patients. Descriptions such as "toxic-looking" or "just looks ill" reflect an evaluation of objective physical findings combined with a subjective impression of the child's reaction to the illness.

A prostrate, inactive, apathetic infant or child who will not smile is likely to be severely ill, even if he does not have a high fever or respiratory distress. Anorexia, headache, and diffuse muscular pains as well as high fever are common toxic symptoms. Localized abdominal pains secondary to straining the abdominal musculature from spasms of coughing are common. Lower lobe pneumonia in contact with the diaphragmatic pleura may be responsible for referred pain to the upper abdominal quadrant. Children suspected of having acute appendicitis who have any abnormal respiratory tract symptoms should have a chest x-ray prior to surgery.

PULMONARY DYSFUNCTION

Any evidence of disturbance of the transfer of oxygen into the blood and carbon dioxide out of the blood is potentially serious and requires careful evaluation and early treatment.

Observation of the child's breathing pattern with the chest exposed and the child lying quietly in a supine position frequently gives more diagnostic information than percussion or auscultation of the chest. The rate, depth, and degree of difficulty in breathing can be assessed quickly. Rapid, shallow respirations are often early signs of marked dysfunction. Increased use of the accessory muscles of respiration (labored breathing), flaring of the alae nasi, or an expiratory grunt portend more serious disease. Uneven or delayed expansion of one side of the chest compared with the other (chest lag) always suggests significant disease.

Inspiratory stridor and expiratory wheezes are usually obvious on auscultation and demand careful evaluation. Other manifestations of severe pulmonary dysfunction, such as pleural effusion, lobar consolidation, pneumothorax, and pleural friction rubs, can often be detected with percussion and auscultation. All denote serious pulmonary disease.

If physical examination of the chest reveals any evidence of gross abnormalities or signs of pulmonary dysfunction, a chest roentgenogram is usually indicated to help identify or quantitate the disease process. Mild asthma responsive to bronchodilators is an exception and rarely is an indication for a chest radiograph. Another valid exception is the presence of a few localized inspiratory rales in a nontoxic child who shows no signs of respiratory dysfunction; e.g., mild viral pneumonia that develops in the course of diffuse respiratory infection does not need x-ray evaluation on the initial visit. If the patient fails to improve or other signs and symptoms suggest increasing pulmonary involvement, then a chest roentgenogram must be performed.

The chest roentgenogram provides a large amount of additional information, the most important aspect of which is the graphic picture of the state of lung aeration. Consolidated or atelectatic areas are obvious. Pleural effusion, empyema, and pyopneumothorax, as well as pneumatoceles within the consolidated areas, are readily apparent, as are enlarged hilar lymph glands and unsuspected masses within the parenchyma of the lung. Heart size and configuration and the vascular supply can be visualized. The additional information provided by a chest radiograph correlated with the clinical assessment permits the physician to decide either to treat the patient on an ambulatory basis or to hospitalize him for additional investigation and treatment.

Extra-Thoracic Airway Infection (Croup Syndromes)

The term *croup* is best discarded as a label for a specific disease entity and should be used generically to describe syndromes or diseases that present with inspiratory stridor. This approach, based on the way in which children are encountered in clinical practice, is the basis for the classification and management scheme shown in Table 10–6.

The hallmark of the croup syndrome is inspiratory stridor, usually associated with a "brassy" or "barking" cough (sometimes described as a "seal's bark"). Hoarseness is frequently present. The clinical course varies from a mild illness lasting three or four days (usually viral in etiology) to a fulminating acute epiglottitis (due to *H. influenzae* type b) that may lead to total airway obstruction and death within six hours unless the obstruction is relieved by endotracheal intubation or tracheostomy.

The croup syndrome is always a source of concern and worry to the pediatrician, because deceptively mild early signs and symptoms may change rapidly and become life-threatening in a few hours. For this reason, all children with the croup syndrome must be observed carefully and the potential seriousness of the disorder appreciated by the parents as well as the physician. Clinically, croup syndromes divide into four disease entities. Table 10–6 outlines the clinical patterns and stresses the signs and symptoms that allow classification and early institution of appropriate treatment. Excellent review articles by Davis et al. (1981) and Barker (1979) provide details and guidelines for management.

Acute Epiglottitis

Supraglottic obstruction of the larynx due to a rapidly progressive infection of the epiglottis with swelling and increasing inspiratory difficulty is almost always caused by *H. influenzae* type b, requires early and aggressive treatment, and is an indication for hospitalization. The child with acute epiglottitis is usually over two years of age and usually has no history of an antecedent upper respiratory infection, in contrast to a child with viral laryngotracheitis. Frequently there is an acute onset with inspiratory stridor, high fever, and other signs of systemic toxicity with progression over a period of 4 to 12 hours to almost total airway obstruction.

In patients seen early, when auscultation reveals good air exchange over the lung fields in spite of stridor, a cautious examination of the posterior pharynx (being careful not to touch the wall of the pharynx with the tongue blade) will reveal a grossly edematous epiglottis just beyond the base of the tongue. This swollen epiglottis has been described as resembling a bright red raspberry and is diagnostic of *H. influenzae* epiglottitis. Once the tip of the swollen epiglottis is visualized, the examination of the pharynx should be stopped, since any further manipulation of the inflamed epiglottis may cause complete laryngeal obstruction. Therapy should be given in a hospital and is not discussed further here.

In children with severe obstruction who are seen later in the course of the disease, auscultation will reveal decreased air exchange over the peripheral lung fields. The child tends to remain in a sitting position with chin extended and may complain of throat pain on swallowing; secretions tend to pool in the pharynx, and drooling is common. As the obstruction progresses, stridor may decrease as breathing becomes shallow and rapid. At this stage, the child is too ill to be moved for radiological investigation, but if confirmation of the epiglottal swelling is felt to be necessary for diagnosis, a lateral soft tissue film may be taken at the bedside with portable equipment. Examination of the posterior pharynx may cause total airway

Table 10–6. THE CROUP SYNDROMES—CLINICAL PATTERNS

	Epiglottitis (Acute)	Spasmodic Croup	Laryngotracheitis (Acute)	
			Viral	*Bacterial*
Synonyms	Epiglottitis Supraglottitis Obstructive supraglottic laryngitis	Acute spasmodic croup "Midnight croup" Allergic croup Spasmodic laryngitis	Laryngotracheal bronchitis (LTB) Viral croup Obstructive subglottic laryngitis	Acute bacterial tracheitis Membranous croup
Maximum obstruction	Above the vocal cords (supraglottic)	Variable glottic or subglottic	Below the vocal cords (subglottic)	Below the vocal cords (subglottic)
Age	Any age, maximum from 2 to 8 years	Usually 1 to 4 years, with tendency to recur	Usually 6 months to 3 years	1 month to 6 years
Etiology	Almost always due to *Hemophilus influenzae* type B, occasionally pneumococci or viruses	Unknown; suspected mild viral infections or allergy	Respiratory syncytial virus Parainfluenzae virus Influenzae virus	Staphylococci *H. influenzae* and others May need antecedent viral infection to trigger.
Onset	Usually rapid, over a period of 4 to 12 hours	Very sudden; typically late at night	Gradual; frequently in the course of a viral upper respiratory illness. May become progressively more severe over a 24-hour period of time	May start as viral LTB, then sudden progress with increasing obstruction.
Initial clinical picture	Rapidly increasing inspiratory stridor in toxic child with high fever. Sore throat with pain on swallowing, and muffled voice.	Severe inspiratory stridor, without fever, but with "barking" or "brassy" cough.	Gradually increasing inspiratory (and at times expiratory) stridor; frequently hoarse voice. "Barking" or "brassy" cough, and fever that may be low or absent.	Present as viral LTB, then rapidly becomes toxic with increasing obstruction.
Examination of posterior pharynx*	Grossly swollen epiglottis—fiery red color, but irregularly swollen appearance (like a raspberry)	Epiglottis normal or mildly reddened	Mildly reddened and mild to moderately swollen epiglottis	Same as LTB
X-ray of neck	Lateral neck films show swollen epiglottis, ballooning hypopharynx, but normal subglottic area.	Probably normal	Normal supraglottic area on lateral view; posteroanterior view: concave medial swelling in subglottic region.	Same as LTB
Clinical course	Tendency to rapid total airway obstruction within first 6 to 12 hours.	May last several hours if untreated; may be entirely well the following morning, with recurrence of symptoms the following night.	Persistent moderate airway obstruction (rarely complete), but may tire and then rapidly develop respiratory failure.	Rapidly progresses to respiratory failure, requiring either endotracheal tube or tracheostomy.
Treatment	Intensive intravenous antibiotic therapy for *H. influenzae;* careful management in intensive care unit; cold mist and oxygen; early passage of small endotracheal tube or tracheostomy.	Warm or cold mist; reassurance; rapid relief by racemic epinephrine delivered by IPPB machine	Cool mist and oxygen. Severe stridor may be temporarily relieved with racemic epinephrine by aerosol. Occasionally requires endotracheal tube or tracheostomy.	Aggressive antibiotic therapy: a secured patent airway with endotracheal tube or tracheostomy. Very frequent suctioning to maintain clear airway for first 24 hours of treatment.

*Caution: If a stridorous patient appears toxic or acutely ill (making one suspect acute epiglottitis) forceful examination of the posterior pharynx is extremely dangerous and may precipitate complete respiratory obstruction. Examination should be performed only in the operating room where full provision for emergency intubation or tracheostomy is readily available.

obstruction and should be performed in the operating room after all preparations for endotracheal intubation or tracheostomy are completed.

Once acute epiglottitis with severe airway obstruction is suspected, there is great urgency in establishing an airway. Sudden respiratory arrest is common and difficult to treat effectively.

Acute Spasmodic Croup

Attacks of acute inspiratory obstruction, which occur in some children without a clearly definable cause, tend to begin suddenly in the evening or night, last several hours, and then subside, only to recur during the next few nights. Characteristically, the child is between one and three years of age, awakens with a barking, metallic-sounding cough, is hoarse, and has a marked inspiratory stridor. Fever is absent and, although the child may have had a mild upper respiratory infection preceding the attack, examination of the posterior pharynx reveals minimal signs of inflammation. The exact site of the obstruction is unknown. Some cases may be due to localized subglottic edema, others possibly to acute adductor spasm of the vocal cords. An idiosyncratic response to viral illness or allergy has been suspected, and recurrent episodes over a period of a few years are not uncommon.

The degree of inspiratory obstruction can be frightening, with severe retractions of the supraclavicular and substernal areas. The inhalation of warm steam from running a hot shower with the bathroom door closed may bring dramatic relief in a few minutes. If the child fails to improve and is taken to a hospital emergency room, exposure to the cool night air en route will frequently break the attack before he reaches the hospital. Treatment with an aerosol of racemic epinephrine (as described in the next section) will usually terminate the attack.

Acute Laryngotracheitis

VIRAL CROUP

Viral croup is the most common croup syndrome encountered in pediatric practice. It usually occurs in the winter months when viral respiratory infections have their peak incidence. The child is usually between six months and three years of age and has had a diffuse upper respiratory infection for two to three days immediately preceding the development of inspiratory stridor. The infection spreads to the lower respiratory tract, with varying degrees of involvement of the larynx, trachea, and bronchi. Inspiratory stridor develops as a result of swelling in the subglottic region. Low-grade fever is usually present, but the child usually does not appear very ill. On cautious examination of the posterior pharynx, the epiglottis is found to be moderately red and generally edematous but fails to show the gross swelling of acute epiglottitis. The obstruction in acute laryngotracheobronchitis is primarily subglottic in location.

A great variety of viruses have been isolated from the airway secretion. The principal etiological agent has been respiratory syncytial virus, with fewer recoveries of parainfluenza, influenza, and adenovirus. Treatment of viral laryngotracheitis consists of the inhalation of an oxygen-enriched gas mixture presented as a light mist or at least fully humidified. Adequate fluid intake, preferably oral, to prevent dehydration is indicated, but overhydration is to be avoided. Oropharyngeal suction should be done cautiously, if at all, since stimulation of the posterior pharynx may cause reflex laryngeal or bronchial constriction.

Sedation is best avoided in all infants with severe airway obstruction. These infants need all their strength and faculties to maintain adequate gas exchange. Even without sedation, an occasional infant will gradually tire and develop respiratory failure with a rising carbon dioxide tension, necessitating endotracheal intubation and mechanical ventilation for a few days. Periodic blood gas tests using arterial or arterialized capillary samples to monitor the adequacy of ventilatory exchange are very helpful but upsetting to the infant. The newly available transcutaneous carbon dioxide monitors have proven very effective in our hands in following severely ill infants in our intensive care unit.

The role of racemic epinephrine administered as an aerosol to temporarily shrink the swollen subglottic region and improve ventilation remains controversial. We tend to use it less often than we did five years ago, and we find that transcutaneous carbon dioxide monitoring allows us early recognition of the few infants who really have impending respiratory failure. If after a few treatments with racemic epinephrine aerosol they fail to maintain the improvement in ventilation (lowering of the carbon dioxide tension) we intubate them before waiting for more life-threatening disturbances. We also have seen a few infants who required intubation after four or five days of very frequent use of racemic epinephrine aerosol and have been worried about the possible rebound swelling in the subglottic region, an entity well-recognized after the prolonged use of topical vasoconstrictors in the nose.

Antibiotic treatment is not indicated in mild viral laryngotracheitis, but this decision to withhold antibiotics has been made more complicated by the recent increased recognition of infants with bacterial laryngotracheitis (see below). The use of steroids also remains controversial, and we do not use them in viral croup.

ACUTE BACTERIAL TRACHEITIS MEMBRANOUS CROUP

Over the past five years, a new subgroup of patients having an acute bacterial tracheitis has been recognized. Their clinical presentation starts the same as viral laryngotracheitis, but they suddenly become more toxic, may develop fever, and rapidly progress to respiratory failure. Endoscopic examination of the subglottic area reveals a purulent infection associated with thickened secretions that appear to be membranous and very prone to cause obstruction. Bacterial cultures have grown Staphylococcus and other common respiratory pathogens. These infants require endotracheal tubes or tracheostomy with very frequent meticulous suctioning to keep their airway patent. With aggressive antimicrobial therapy (for example, nafcillin and chloramphenicol), many have improved dramatically in 24 to 48 hours. Membranous croup was a well-recognized entity in the preantibiotic era, and the factors that resulted in its reappearance in children ill with viral respiratory tract infections are not understood. The practical implications are clear. Infants with viral laryngotracheitis must be watched carefully for signs and symptoms that may herald the onset of bacterial tracheitis. When this occurs, appropriate antimicrobial therapy and close monitoring must be started immediately.

OTHER FORMS OF CROUP SYNDROME

Three additional entities may present as a croup syndrome: diphtheritic croup, foreign body impacted in the hypopharynx, and foreign body lodged in the esophagus. These are rare causes but must be included in the differential diagnosis of every child with a croup syndrome.

The symptoms of diphtheritic croup are due to an infectious membrane extending down the hypopharynx, partially occluding the glottic opening. The infant is febrile and toxic and almost always has an obvious severe pharyngitis with membrane formation on examination of the posterior pharynx. A documented history of adequate DPT immunization is almost enough to allow dismissal of this possibility.

Aspiration of a foreign body into the hypopharyngeal region occluding the glottal opening or aspiration into the larynx itself may produce acute inspiratory obstruction.

By contrast, slower and more subtle onset of a croup syndrome occurs after impaction of foreign objects in the upper esophagus. Coins that lodge in the esophagus are still the most common foreign body encountered in clinical practice. The impacted coins or other objects that give rise to symptoms of inspiratory stridor are always "hung up" at the narrowing of the cricopharyngeus, and the forward pressure on the larynx results in compression and inspiratory stridor. The history of sudden onset and the absence of an antecedent upper respiratory infection or fever should make the physician consider this diagnosis.

With radiopaque foreign bodies, such as coins, the diagnosis is easily made on roentgenograms of the hypopharyngeal area. When ordering chest radiographs for a child with respiratory distress, the physician must specify that the hypopharyngeal area be included, or the foreign body may be missed. Nonradiopaque foreign bodies, such as plastic and wood, present a more difficult diagnostic problem. They can be outlined by swallowed contrast media or visualized through the esophagoscope. Optimal management is probably immediate, esophagoscopic removal of the foreign object.

Intrathoracic Airway Infection

Acute Tracheobronchitis

Pathogenesis. Infection of the lower trachea and larger bronchi is often associated with a diffuse viral upper respiratory infection but occasionally may occur as an isolated infection. Infection in this area has been labeled acute tracheobronchitis or acute bronchitis. Rhinoviruses, respiratory syncytial virus, adenovirus, and coxsackieviruses are common etiological agents. Influenza and parainfluenza viruses have occasionally been implicated as causes of acute tracheobronchitis. Rubeola (measles) causes a diffuse tracheobronchitis as part of the widespread mucous membrane involvement. The most persistent bacterial infection localizing in the lower airway is due to pertussis and is discussed separately. Group A hemolytic streptococci are occasionally responsible for fulminating tracheobronchitis.

Clinical Aspects. The lower trachea and major bronchi are richly endowed with cough receptors. The hallmark of acute viral tracheobronchitis is persistent cough, which is initially dry and hacking. Early in the illness, auscultation may reveal a clear chest, as the alveoli and interstitial tissues are relatively uninvolved. The chest roentgenogram will be clear or show minimal peribronchial accentuation. As the disease progresses, the inflamed tracheobronchial mucosa produces a moderate amount of thickened mucus. Commonly, a few coarse rales and low-pitched rhonchi can be heard over the lung field, and small amounts of turbid yellow phlegm may be expectorated or swallowed. The appearance of yellow phlegm is normal in the course of the infection and is not diagnostic of secondary bacterial infection. As with other acute viral respiratory infections, the fever and constitutional symptoms present early in the illness tend to subside after three or four days. The cough usually subsides over seven to ten days.

Treatment. During the first four to seven days of illness, treatment should be supportive: acetaminophen is helpful in controlling fever and malaise. The importance of cough as a defense mechanism in removing tracheobronchial secretions should be stressed to parents. Physicians should be understanding of the need of parents to ask for help or medication for their persistently coughing child. The inhalation of cool or warm mist is soothing to the tracheobronchial tree of many children and should be encouraged. Syrups, such as flavored syrup of wild cherry or honey and lemon, or other demulcent mixtures seem to sooth the posterior pharynx and may reduce coughing. Cough syrups containing large amounts of antihistamines may have an atropine-like action that will thicken the mucus and impair its clearance from the lung. These are contraindicated. Those syrups that contain codeine or other narcotic cough suppressants should be used only at night, when necessary, to allow the persistently coughing child to obtain some sleep.

Complications. Persistence of a severe cough for longer than seven days or return of fever or malaise should alert the clinician to the possibility of secondary bacterial infection of the tracheobronchial tree. Pneumococci, streptococci, and *Hemophilus influenzae* are the organisms most frequently responsible for secondary bacterial invasion. In immunologically compromised hosts, such as children undergoing therapy for malignancy or post-transplant patients, widespread tracheal infection due to staphylococci or herpesvirus has been encountered occasionally. A sputum culture is highly desirable before starting therapy, if the child is able to provide a specimen. Treatment is usually with ampicillin, 100 to 150 mg/kg/day. Microorganisms recovered by throat culture show little correlation with bacteria growing within the lung.

Pertussis (Whooping Cough)

Pathogenesis. Pertussis is the most severe and persistent acute tracheobronchitis encountered in clinical practice. *Bordetella pertussis* is responsible for all epidemic cases, but sporadic cases may be caused by *Bordetella parapertussis* and certain adenoviruses.

The incidence of pertussis in the United States has decreased remarkably since pertussis vaccine has been widely utilized. Unfortunately, sometimes its protection is not complete, and attenuated cases are still encountered even in vaccinated children. Recent controversies over the use of pertussis vaccine and the incidence of neurological complications secondary to its administration have been reported in the public media as well as in medical publications. After careful study, the American Academy of Pediatrics and the Immunizations Practices Advisory Committee strongly recommend continued utilization of the vaccine. The protection benefits/complications ratios are reasonable. The rapid increase in clinical pertussis cases in areas of the world where pertussis immunization programs have been abandoned gives further support to this position. The intensified pertussis surveillance of the Centers for Disease Control (Morbidity and Mortality Weekly Report, 1982) continues to document the seriousness of the disease, particularly in infants under one year of age.

The prolonged clinical course of pertussis is difficult for parents to accept in this era of medical miracles and high expectations. Medical folklore has depicted pertussis as "three weeks in coming, three weeks in staying, and three weeks in going away." This remains a reasonable description of the clinical course of pertussis, and the widespread use of antibiotics has changed it little. Infants under six months of age are likely to have more difficulty with the illness and are susceptible to complications. Young infants should be hospitalized with constant observation because of the danger of apnea and suffocation.

Clinical Pattern. After an incubation period of 7 to 14 days, the infant or child develops a dry cough and often a watery nasal discharge. The disease is highly contagious during this catarrhal phase, which lasts from one to two weeks. The cough gradually becomes more severe and tends to occur in short bursts of paroxysmal coughing, which gradually increase in frequency and are likely to be more severe at night. Anything that disturbs the resting child, such as feeding, nursing procedures, medication, or cigarette smoke, may initiate a paroxysm of coughing. These paroxysms consist of short, repetitive, harsh expiratory coughs that may persist for 15 to 30 seconds. There is no time for inspiration between coughs and the infant becomes progressively more hypoxemic and cyanotic during the paroxysm. When the paroxysm finally abates, even temporarily, the air-hungry infant makes a violent inspiratory effort and produces a typical whoop. Small infants may be so exhausted at the end of these violent paroxysms that they are unable to generate the forces necessary for the rapid inspiratory maneuver of the whoop. Infants are prone to manifest apneic periods at the end of severe paroxysms.

Diagnosis. The diagnosis should be suspected on the basis of history and physical examination. Often *B. pertussis* can be grown from mucus obtained by nasopharyngeal swab and immediately plated on fresh Bordet-Gengou culture medium containing penicillin. Fluorescent antibody staining of nasopharyngeal mucus as a method of rapid diagnosis initially showed great promise. In practice it has proven to be technically difficult in most laboratories and has a high incidence of false positive results. During the first two weeks of illness, the total white blood cell count is usually between 15,000 and 30,000/cu mm, with 80 to 90 per cent lymphocytes. The white blood cell count may occasionally be elevated to over 100,000 cells/cu mm.

The disease affects primarily the airways. No rales or other evidence of parenchymal involvement is usually present during the first weeks of the disease. The paroxysmal stage lasts from four to eight weeks. The course may be shortened by treatment with erythromycin (Committee on Infectious Disease, 1982a). Gradually there is a reduction in the frequency and severity of the paroxysms and the child begins to convalesce. Subconjunctival hemorrhages due to severe coughing are common.

Secondary invasion of the lung parenchyma by bacteria (particularly staphylococci) may occur and requires intensive antibiotic therapy. Lobar or segmental atelectasis, probably secondary to plugging of the airway by inflammatory debris, has been reported in about 15 per cent of infants with pertussis. This collapse tends to resolve spontaneously as the infant recovers and is usually not secondarily infected.

Acute Bronchiolitis

Pathogenesis. This is a viral infection of the small distal bronchioles which results in marked expiratory airway obstruction and severe respiratory distress. Bronchiolitis, which occurs most frequently in the winter and spring, is the most common serious lower respiratory infection in infants. Affected infants are usually under 12 months of age, most being less than 6 months. Respiratory syncytial virus is the cause of 60 to 70 per cent of the infections, but other viruses such as parainfluenza, adenovirus, and influenza virus can cause similar illness.

Pathology. The walls of the small bronchi and bronchioles are thickened, edematous, and infiltrated with inflammatory cells. The lumina are often almost occluded with leukocytes and debris. There is marked obstruction to expiration with gas trapping. Impairment of gas exchange is striking, with marked hypoxemia being common. The greatly increased work of breathing, secondary to severe expiratory airway obstruction, frequently results in hypercapnea, particularly in infants with other problems such as congenital heart disease or cystic fibrosis.

Clinical Pattern. Because onset is gradual and progresses over a period of one or two days, the parents are frequently surprised when they realize that their infant is severely ill. Commonly, the infant has been exposed to someone with a respiratory infection within the prior week. Coryza, followed by an irritating cough, is an early symptom. The infant then gradually develops rapid breathing and a prolonged expiratory phase. Respiratory rates of 60 to 80 are the rule and, occasionally, may be over 100 times a minute. The infant is in obvious respiratory distress, and cyanosis is common. The body temperature is rarely higher than 38.5°C (101°F). The chest is barrel-shaped due to hyperinflation. The accessory muscles of respiration are active, and flaring of the alae nasi is present. Intercostal and subcostal retractions may be striking due to the increased negative intrapleural pressure during inspiration.

On auscultation, expiratory wheezing is present but because of the very rapid respiratory rate may not be impressive. Inspiratory crepitations (rales) may be absent but are frequently audible if the infant is quiet. The infant has an anxious appearance, and all his energies are concentrated on breathing. Frequently, he is unwilling or unable to attempt nursing his bottle because this further interferes with breathing. The liver is usually palpable 2 to 3 cm below the right costal margin, owing to pulmonary hyperinflation depressing the diaphragm. Cardiac failure is a very rare complication and probably occurs only with associated heart disease. Arterial blood gases, while breathing room air, show moderate to severe hypoxemia. Carbon dioxide tension is normal or elevated (Wohl, 1977). Chest radiographs show extreme hyperinflation of the lung with flattened diaphragms. Scattered areas of patchy consolidation may be present, but often the lung fields are clear.

Diagnosis. The clinical picture is distinctive and permits rapid diagnosis. The differential diagnosis should always include other causes of severe tachypnea and air hunger, such as severe metabolic acidosis from diabetic ketoacidosis, severe salicylate poisoning, and renal failure. None of these conditions is ordinarily associated with expiratory airway obstruction or hypercapnea. An arterial or arterialized capillary blood gas is extremely helpful in differentiating respiratory from metabolic acidosis. Acute bronchospasm in a young infant is rarely due to allergic asthma. Differentiating allergic asthma from acute bronchiolitis may be difficult, and giving the infant one injection of epinephrine to test reversible bronchospasm is often helpful.

Clinical Course and Treatment. The acute phase of bronchiolitis usually lasts 24 to 48 hours. If moderately or severely ill, such children should be admitted to the hospital, but many mild infections can be managed supportively at home. Particulate mist therapy confers no additional benefit and may increase bronchospasm.

For the hospitalized infant, humidified oxygen in concentrations necessary to control hypoxemia should be given, even if concentrations above 50 per cent are required. There is no evidence that the respiratory drive in these infants is on a hypoxemic basis. Intravenous fluid overload must be assiduously avoided, as even a small increase in pulmonary interstitial water can further impair pulmonary gas exchange.

Close observation and charting of vital signs to detect evidence of increasing fatigue and the onset of respiratory failure are important. Transcutaneous carbon dioxide monitoring is a most satisfactory and easy way of following the severely ill infant. If a transcutaneous monitor is not available, then periodic arterial or arterialized capillary blood gases will quantify the adequacy of the infant's ventilatory exchange. Approximately 1 or 2 per cent of infants with acute bronchiolitis will require mechanical ventilation to survive the severe respiratory failure that may develop within the first 48 hours of their acute illness (Downes et al., 1968).

Sedation of any type is contraindicated in any infant with severe respiratory distress. A series of clinical trials using corticosteroids in acute bronchiolitis has failed to demonstrate that their use results in any improvement in the clinical course. Antibiotics have no effect on the viral infection causing bronchiolitis. If signs of progressive pulmonary infection develop, or significant pulmonary infiltration appears on chest roentgenogram, the physician must assume that secondary bacterial pneumonia is present. A combination of nafcillin (100–200 mg/kg/day divided into four doses) and either ampicillin (200 mg/kg/day divided into four doses) or moxalactam (150 mg/kg/day divided into three doses) given intravenously is indicated while studies to identify the infecting organism continue.

Acute Infections of the Lung Parenchyma (Pneumonia)

Pneumonia remains one of the common serious infections of childhood, although its incidence has decreased over the past 30 years. Most childhood pneumonias either resolve spontaneously or respond satisfactorily to antimicrobial therapy. Although serious complications are not rare, they can usually be treated effectively. Many parents and grandparents still vividly remember the preantibiotic era when pneumonia was often a life-threatening illness and a diagnosis of pneumonia in their child would precipitate great anxiety. Physicians must remember this recent past, be prepared to explain the current status of childhood pneumonia, and reassure the parents of the probable satisfactory prognosis.

Hospitalization vs. Home Management of Children with Pneumonia

For children, hospitalization is always psychologically undesirable and frequently emotionally traumatic. The costs of the illness are increased and the child is exposed to other respiratory tract pathogens from fellow patients at a time when there is already demonstrated difficulty in handling an infectious organism.

The decision on where to treat the child is based on three factors: the severity of the constitutional disturbance (toxicity), the degree of pulmonary dysfunction, and the physician's estimate of the family's ability to provide treatment and supportive care needed by the child at home.

Infants in the first year of life are more likely to develop severe pneumonia and its complications. The younger the infant, the more the physician should be concerned about the infant's ability to handle the infection. Infants in the first year of life must be considered to have unknown and unproven immunocompetence.

Any signs of pulmonary distress should alert the physician to a potentially serious infection.

In children over two years of age, most pneumonias are due to pneumococci, viruses, or *Mycoplasma pneumoniae*. If the child's past history reveals no cause for concern, the family situation is satisfactory, and he does not appear seriously ill, treatment at home is usually desirable. The reasoning behind this decision should be discussed candidly with the family, as well as the small possibility that the child's pneumonia may not respond satisfactorily and may still require hospitalization. The parents can be reassured by the knowledge that the physician is willing to reconsider hospitalization at any time. The presence of modest infiltration on chest roentgenogram need not alter this approach. Cultures of the nasopharynx, blood counts, and tuberculin, coccidioidin, and histoplasmin skin tests should be available on an ambulatory basis.

Many infants in the first two years of life should be hospitalized for more complete evaluation of their illness and kept in the hospital only long enough to demonstrate definite improvement or response to treatment. It is rarely necessary to keep the mild to moderately ill infant in the hospital for the full course of antibiotic therapy, and certainly not until the radiographs show definite improvement, since the radiograph may lag behind the clinical response by many days and occasionally weeks. Hospitals are unsatisfactory and, at times, unsafe places for children. Once definite improvement has occurred and diagnostic tests have been performed, the situation should be discussed frankly with the parents, and treatment continued at home. However, the small possibility of the need for rehospitalization should be discussed with the parents before discharge, since, if rehospitalization is necessary, parents would naturally wonder if their child's course and recovery would have been improved by a longer initial hospitalization. It is much easier to discuss this problem with the parents before discharging the child than when indications for rehospitalization arise.

Classification. The lung parenchyma refers to the functional elements of the lung where gas transfer occurs; it does not include the airways. The parenchyma is divided into the interstitium (the alveolar walls and all of the structures lying within the walls, including blood vessels, lymphatics, and nerves) and the alveoli (the spaces lined by the alveolar walls).

The interstitial area was once thought to be an inert framework holding blood vessels as they came in contact with the air in the alveoli. However, recent investigations show the interstitium to be extremely active metabolically, with constant fluid flux between the pulmonary vascular bed and adjacent lymphatics.

Clinically, pulmonary infections can be classified in two groups: those primarily affecting the interstitial areas, with little tendency to "fill up" the alveoli, and those prone to fill alveoli with inflammatory debris or fluid. This second group always involves the interstitium locally but may not show widespread interstitial involvement.

Acute bacterial infections of the lung tend to produce localized disease that results in a rapid inflammatory reaction that fills (consolidates) the alveoli with exudate. Early viral infection may cause minimal inflammatory reaction in the alveolar spaces but tends to involve the interstitium diffusely. On chest roentgenogram, early changes in the interstitium are difficult to recognize. In contrast, the water-density material filling the localized alveoli (seen early with bacterial infection) is easily identified as patchy exudate and, if more widespread, lobar consolidation.

Unfortunately, these two distinct patterns of inflammation and their associated etiologies do not always hold true in clinical practice. Acute pneumococcal pneumonia occasionally may start with interstitial involvement, while mycoplasma pneumonia (closer to a virus than a bacterium) is prone to develop widespread patchy areas of consolidation on x-ray, with few findings on auscultation.

The classification in Table 10–7 is offered as a working basis for clinical diagnosis of pulmonary infections, and is an aid to treatment.

The clinical patterns of acute pneumonia in children present a broad spectrum of signs and symptoms, varying from the gradual onset of cough with no constitutional symptoms to a fulminating infection with marked toxicity and rapid progression of respiratory insufficiency leading to death.

Infections Affecting Primarily the Interstitium

Viral Pneumonia

The most common pneumonias encountered in pediatric practice are caused by respiratory tract viruses. Typically pneumonia develops in the course of diffuse viral respiratory illness that also involves the upper respiratory tract.

The spectrum of illness resulting from viral invasion of the lung parenchyma varies from a mild illness, with few symptoms beyond an

Table 10–7. ACUTE INFECTIONS OF THE LUNG PARENCHYMA

A. Infections Affecting Primarily the Interstitium	
Viral Pneumonia	
Parainfluenzae	Frequent
Influenzae	Frequent
Respiratory Syncytial	Frequent
Adenovirus	Infrequent
Coxsackievirus	Infrequent
Rhinovirus	Infrequent
Mycoplasmal Pneumonia	Frequent
Chlamydial Pneumonia	
Chlamydia trachomatis	Frequent (birth to 4 months)
Chlamydia psittaci	Rare
Pneumocystis carinii	Rare
Rickettsia—Q fever	Rare
Legionellosis	Very rare
B. Infections Affecting Primarily the Alveoli	
Bacterial Pneumonia	
Pneumococcal	Very common
Staphylococcal	Less common, but severe
Streptococcal	Uncommon
Hemophilus influenzae	Less common
Other gram-negative pneumonias	Rare
Tuberculosis	Uncommon, but important
Fungal Pneumonia	
Coccidioidomycosis	Common (regional geographical occurrence)
Histoplasmosis	Common (regional geographical occurrence)
Other Fungi	Rare

annoying cough, to an overwhelming infection, rapidly invading the entire lung and leading to respiratory failure and death within two or three days. The factors that determine the severity and course of viral pneumonia in any particular child appear to be a combination of differences in host resistance and variations in the virulence of the respiratory viruses.

Host resistance to viral infections normally improves with age. Any infant under one year of age with viral pneumonia must be considered in a high-risk category. Any evidence of immunological incompetence, inadequate nutrition, or other significant medical problems increases the likelihood of a severe infection.

Parainfluenza, influenza, respiratory syncytial virus, and adenovirus are responsible for most of these pneumonic infections in infants and young children (Williams and Phelan, 1975). Adenoviruses, particularly types 3, 7, and 21, are prone to cause a severe necrotizing pneumonia that destroys large areas of lung parenchyma. In those infants that survive, residual changes frequently lead to chronic lung disease (Kattan, 1979).

MILD VIRAL PNEUMONIA

The illness usually begins as a typical upper respiratory tract infection involving, to a variable degree, the nasal passages and the pharynx. The infant or child gradually develops a dry, hacking, usually nonproductive cough, and may manifest mild tachypnea and slightly labored respirations. The temperature can range from 100 to 104°F, and the child appears mildly to moderately ill.

On examination of the chest, inspiratory crepitant rales are audible, as well as a few coarse expiratory rhonchi. The rales may be localized in one or two lobes or may be heard diffusely throughout the chest. Air exchange in the periphery of the lung, as judged by auscultation, is usually adequate. There are no physical signs to suggest consolidation or pleural effusion.

The white blood cell count is normal or mildly elevated, and significant shifts in the percentage or maturity of the polymorphonuclear leukocytes are uncommon.

On chest roentgenogram there is fullness of the perihilar bronchovascular markings and peribronchial accentuation extending into the medial third to half of the lung field. The swelling of the interstitial areas between the alveolar spaces is not detectable on roentgenogram in the early or mildly involved patient. With more extensive pneumonia, small irregular patches or stringy areas of infiltration are visible.

The course of the pulmonary infection parallels that of the diffuse viral respiratory infection, and after three or four days most children begin to show gradual improvement. Resolution of the pulmonary congestion and disappearance of the abnormal physical findings are frequently slow and may take more than two weeks. The chest radiograph may not return to normal for three to four weeks.

This vignette covers the typical child with a mild viral pneumonia, but marked variation occurs in the clinical findings and course of viral pneumonia. Some children have impressive findings on chest roentgenogram and minimal or absent findings on physical examination. Not infrequently, the reverse is true. A normal chest roentgenogram does not rule out the diagnosis of viral pneumonia.

The mildly ill child who may have striking rales or positive x-ray findings, but no signs of respiratory dysfunction or distress, can often be managed at home with supportive therapy. No antibiotic therapy is indicated for such patients.

MODERATE TO SEVERE VIRAL PNEUMONIA

A small number of children with mild viral pneumonia will progress to more extensive pulmonary involvement that may rapidly become life-threatening.

The best index of the severity of the process is not the chest roentgenogram but the physician's evaluation of the degree of pulmonary dysfunction. If there is evidence of dyspnea, cyanosis, unexplained anxiety, or decreased air exchange over the lung periphery, the physician should be concerned and follow the child closely. Such patients should be hospitalized. Arterial blood gases will frequently reveal unsuspected significant hypoxemia in a noncyanotic patient with dyspnea. Mechanical ventilation of the critically ill infant in respiratory failure for a few days can be life-saving.

It is impossible to prove the presence or absence of bacterial infection in the child with severe viral pneumonia, and most clinicians will treat the child with the same broad antibiotic coverage they would use for extensive bacterial pneumonia. A combination of nafcillin and ampicillin, or nafcillin combined with chloramphenicol or moxalactam, may be used (see p. 140).

Hypersensitivity Pneumonitis (Noninfectious Pneumonitis)

Not all episodes of acute lung inflammation associated with fever are due to infectious causes. Some children develop a hypersensitivity response to the repeated inhalation of organic material, which results in an acute or subacute interstitial inflammation of the lung. The clinical pattern is indistinguishable from acute viral pneumonitis, but the persistence of the inflammation or the frequency of recurrence should alert the physician to consider a noninfectious cause.

The disease was originally described after the inhalation of moldy hay (farmer's lung) but also occurs after the inhalation of bird droppings (pigeon breeder's lung, bird fancier's lung) or from the inhalation of fungal spores that grow in the ducts of forced air heating systems or humidification systems (Hilman, 1980). Many other organic materials associated with farm processing and industrial exposures have been found responsible for hypersensitivity lung disease.

The acute episodes begin several hours after the exposure to the organic dust and are characterized by dyspnea, fever, and chest pain. Physical findings are minimal and consist only of a few moist rales and occasional wheezes. A roentgenogram of the chest may be normal at this stage. If exposure to the antigen continues, there is severe dyspnea, nonproductive cough, and cyanosis. Persistent basilar rales may be present as well as the gradual onset of clubbing. Chest roentgenogram may show accentuation of the interstitial markings and diffuse pulmonary infiltrates. Pulmonary function testing is consistent with restrictive lung disease.

The prolonged duration of the inflammatory response in the lungs should cause the physician to consider the diagnosis, retake the history, and search from possible exposure to organic dust. Treatment consists of removal of the patient from the dust exposure. Sometimes, short courses of steroid therapy may be needed to accelerate resolution of the inflammatory response.

Mycoplasma Pneumoniae

Pneumonia due to *Mycoplasma pneumoniae* is encountered primarily in older children, 5 to 15 years of age, and is the most common cause of pneumonia in this age group. Younger children are more likely to manifest bullous myringitis, pharyngitis, or laryngotracheitis. The incubation period varies from 7 to 35 days. The onset of symptoms is usually gradual but may be abrupt, with little to distinguish *Mycoplasma pneumoniae* infection from other viral and bacterial pneumonias. Symptoms may include malaise, anorexia, severe headache, fever, and sore throat. After a few days, a nonproductive paroxysmal cough develops, but patients are rarely severely ill. Examination of the chest may be normal early in the course of the illness, but eventually scattered, fine crepitant rales appear.

The disease is self-limited and almost never fatal, so information from histopathological study of the infected lung is limited (Denny, 1977). The infection extends throughout the trachea, bronchi, bronchioles, and interstitial areas of the parenchyma. Extension of involvement, including aseptic meningitis, encephalitis, peripheral neuropathy, myocarditis, mucocutaneous eruption, and hemolytic anemia, is being recognized with increased frequency now that serological confirmation of the diagnosis is more generally available.

The radiological findings in the chest are those of interstitial pneumonitis (increased perihilar bronchovascular markings and peribronchial accentuation) plus the presence of patchy, ill-defined areas of consolidation, particularly in the lower lobes. Classically the radiological findings are considerably more extensive than the physician anticipates on the basis of the paucity of physical findings on chest examination.

The diagnosis can be proven by culturing Mycoplasma from the sputum, but this is technically difficult and not generally available. Serological tests that will confirm the diagnosis by a rising titer to neutralizing or complement-fixing antibodies are available. A test for cold agglutinins is positive in 40 to 60 per cent of children with Mycoplasma infection but may also be positive with other viral pneumonias. The diagnosis from the practitioner's viewpoint remains one based on clinical evaluation.

The illness may last 7 to 21 days, and parents must be prepared for this slow resolution. The constitutional symptoms usually abate within a week, but cough and rales persist. In fact, the chest roentgenogram may show progression in the first two weeks at a time when the patient is beginning to improve clinically. Erythromycin and tetracycline have been shown to shorten the febrile course in adults. Antibiotic therapy in children rarely results in dramatic improvement, but may contribute to some shortening of the clinical illness (Levine and Lerner, 1978).

Rare Infections

Pneumocystis Carinii

Pneumonia due to *Pneumocystis carinii* in the United States occurs almost exclusively in very debilitated infants and immunosuppressed children. The clinical picture is that of a diffuse interstitial pneumonitis, tachypnea at rest, and occasionally low-grade fever. The diagnosis rests on identifying the organism in lung secretions or tissue sections. Bronchial brushing, lung puncture aspirate, or more usually open-lung biopsy are necessary for diagnosis. Treatment choice is trimethoprim with sulfamethoxazole. If this fails, pentamidine may be tried (Hughes, 1976).

Rickettsia (Q Fever)

Coxiella burnetii, a rickettsial organism, causes an acute pneumonitis characterized by infiltration of the perihilar and perivascular spaces with plasma cells and lymphocytes. The disease usually begins with severe headache, followed by gradual onset of chills, fever, malaise, nonproductive cough, and substernal pain. The clinical and x-ray picture is similar to that of other viral infections of the lung.

Serological testing that demonstrates a rising titer in a complement-fixing antibodies and agglutinins is the accepted method of establishing the diagnosis in most clinical situations.

The clinical course is self-limited, lasting up to three weeks, with a low mortality. *C. burnetii* is susceptible to chloramphenicol and tetracycline in vitro, but in vivo the response is not impressive.

Chlamydial Pneumonia

Two distinct types of pneumonia are now recognized as being caused by separate chlamydial species: *Chlamydia trachomatis* and *Chlamydia psittaci.*

Chlamydia trachomatis frequently causes pneumonia in young infants. Following exposure to infected genital secretions during the process of birth, infants may develop a "staccato" nonproductive cough beginning at three to eight weeks of age. This may be preceded or accompanied by a purulent conjunctivitis. The infant is afebrile; as cough increases, the infant becomes tachypneic and shows fine inspiratory crackles on physical examination and an interstitial pneumonitis on chest x-ray. Hypoxemia and respiratory distress may become severe. Mild peripheral eosinophilia is common, and elevated IgG and IgM are frequently found. Diagnosis can be made by Giemsa staining of conjunctival scrapings showing chlamydial inclusions. Culturing the organism requires special media and techniques not widely available. Diagnosis can be documented by demonstrating a rising serological titer to specific IgM antibodies.

The organism is sensitive to erythromycin, and two to three weeks of oral erythromycin (40 mg/kg/day divided into four doses) will lead to gradual resolution of the infection (Schachter, 1978).

Psittacosis-Ornithosis. *Chlamydia psittaci* produces an interstitial pneumonitis that is difficult to distinguish from viral or mycoplasma pneumonia. A history of exposure to recently imported birds or working with birds (including turkeys, pigeons, ducks, and lovebirds) should make the physician consider the diagnosis. The presenting signs, symptoms, and chest radiographs of patients with ornithosis pneumonia are indistinguishable from those of patients with viral or mycoplasma infections of the lung. Diagnosis is best confirmed by evidence of a rising titer to complement-fixing antibodies in the patient's serum. In children over eight years of age, tetracycline (50 mg/kg/day for 10 days) is the treatment of choice. *C. psittaci* organisms are variably sensitive to penicillins, erythromycin, and chloramphenicol.

Infections Affecting Primarily the Alveoli

Two groups of organisms tend to cause localized alveolar disease without widespread interstitial involvement: bacteria and fungi. The usual clinical courses of pneumonias caused by these two types of organisms are quite different. For example, bacterial pneumonia tends to progress rapidly and needs immediate and aggressive treatment; in contrast, common fungal infections of the lung may cause impressive infiltration of lung parenchyma but tend to resolve spontaneously in previously well children with normal immune defenses.

Alveolar infections of the immunodeficient or immunocompromised child are always extremely serious and will be discussed separately.

Bacterial Infections

The acute bacterial pneumonias have many common features. Pulmonary infection is usually acquired by inhalation and tends to locate in one or more of the following lobes or segments: the middle lobe, the lingula, the posterior or anterior segments of the upper lobes, or the superior segment of the lower lobes. As the infection spreads and involves a larger portion of the lung, the vital capacity decreases and the work of breathing increases. Respirations become labored and intercostal retraction is evident in young infants.

Infants and children with significant bacterial pneumonia almost always appear toxic and frequently present with signs of pulmonary dysfunction. Chest roentgenograms frequently show lobar or segmental consolidation, and pleural effusion is not uncommon. This contrasts with the large group of children with mild viral pneumonia who present with cough but few signs of toxicity or pulmonary dysfunction. Pleural effusion is infrequently seen with viral pneumonia, and consolidation is apt to be patchy.

Early diagnosis of the common types of acute bacterial pneumonia is important for two reasons: all types respond to intensive antibiotic therapy, and significant complications are frequent and can be minimized by antibiotic therapy. Complications such as pleural effusion, empyema, or pyopneumothorax may require surgical intervention, and early diagnosis will alert the physician to this possibility.

PNEUMOCOCCAL PNEUMONIA

Pneumococcal infection in the lung is characterized by a rapidly progressive inflammatory edema and the exudation of serum and red cells into the alveoli, resulting in early consolidation. The onset of pneumococcal pneumonia commonly occurs during the course of diffuse viral respiratory infection, but may occur as a primary infection.

In infants, the illness may begin with symptoms of poor feeding, vomiting, irritability, and fever. Tachypnea with grunting respirations develops rapidly, and cough is variable and, at times, minimal. Physical examination of the chest may be deceptively unremarkable. Owing to its small size and the smaller size of the consolidated area, it is usually impossible to localize the consolidated area by percussion. Decreased breath sounds or inspiratory rales are only rarely detected initially in the young infant. At this stage, the chest roentgenogram usually reveals consolidation, although occasionally this may not be visible until later in the course of the disease.

The older child will usually present with high fever, an irritating cough, and constitutional signs of systemic illness, including headache, drowsiness, and anorexia. A toxic delirium may be present. Some of the other classic adult signs of pneumococcal pneumonia (pleuritic chest pain, spiking fever, chills, and rusty sputum) are often missing in children. Abdominal pain is common, often due to soreness of the rectus abdominus muscles secondary to severe coughing. Inflammation of the pleural surface of the diaphragm may cause the pain to be referred to the epigastrium or even the lower quadrants of the abdomen. The known increased incidence of acute appendicitis associated with pneumococcal pneumonia must always be remembered.

Diagnosis. The clinical picture is sufficiently characteristic to permit diagnosis and early treatment in most children. In most cases, the chest roentgenogram will reveal a consolidated area and confirm the diagnosis. Pneumococcal pneumonia is not associated with significant hilar lymph gland enlargement; when it is present, another diagnosis is suggested, such as tuberculosis or streptococcal pneumonia.

Pneumococci can be recovered in cultures of blood taken before starting antibiotic therapy in 15 to 25 per cent of cases. Throat cultures are of no value in establishing diagnosis, as pneumococci are normal inhabitants of the posterior pharynx in many children. A total leukocyte count greater than 15,000/cu mm (particularly greater than 20,000/cu mm) is associated with a high incidence of rapid improvement after treatment with antibiotics (Shuttleworth and Charney, 1971).

As almost all children with pneumococcal pneumonia respond rapidly to antibiotic therapy with penicillin or erythromycin, bacteriological confirmation of the diagnosis is not important.

Complications. Small pleural effusions with serous fluid are relatively common but rarely develop into pneumococcal empyema, probably because antibiotic therapy is so effective. They normally resolve without drainage.

STAPHYLOCOCCAL PNEUMONIA

Rapid progression of this disease results in widespread life-threatening pneumonia. Staphylococcal pneumonia heads the list of serious diseases that must be considered in every child with suspected pneumonia. It occurs less frequently than pneumococcal pneumonia and is more common in infants than in older children. Seventy per cent of cases occur during the first year of life.

Staphylococci cause a confluent bronchopneumonia characterized by the presence of extensive areas of hemorrhagic necrosis and irregular areas of cavitation. Empyema, pyopneumothorax, and pneumatoceles occur with such regularity in staphylococcal pneumonia that they are considered part of the natural course of the illness and not a complication. All children with staphylococcal pneumonia should be hospitalized.

Clinical Pattern. The typical patient is an infant less than one year of age who has had a mild upper or lower respiratory tract infection for several days to a week and whose condition changes abruptly with the onset of high fever, increasing cough, and respiratory distress. The infant appears anxious, may be mildly cyanotic, and exhibits tachypnea, grunting respirations, and sternal and subcostal retraction. Gastrointestinal disturbances may be present, characterized by vomiting, anorexia, diarrhea, or abdominal distention. Many infants deteriorate rapidly, appear pallid and develop a shock-like state, and have a large empyema or pyopneumothorax. Prompt surgical drainage as well as antibiotic therapy is necessary to sustain life.

Diagnosis. The clinical presentation of a toxic infant or child with rapidly increasing respiratory distress should always suggest the possibility of staphylococcal pneumonia. Chest radiographs will show patchy bronchopneumonia early, rapidly progressing to dense homogeneous consolidation involving an entire lobe or hemithorax. Most children will develop empyema, and in about 25 per cent of cases pyopneumothorax will occur. Pneumatoceles of varying size are common in the consolidated lung. The findings change rapidly, and frequently radiological re-examination is indicated. The leukocyte count is usually elevated above 20,000, with a marked shift to the left. A white blood count below 5000 suggests overwhelming infection and is a poor prognostic sign. A needle aspiration of the pleural fluid will provide material for diagnostic culture and sensitivity testing.

Course. The course is usually prolonged in spite of successful therapy. Intensive antibiotic therapy and surgical drainage result in survival of 60 to 90 per cent of patients. In survivors the outlook for eventual return to normal lung function is good.

STREPTOCOCCAL PNEUMONIA

Pneumonia due to group A beta-hemolytic streptococci is less frequent than pneumococcal or staphylococcal pneumonia. Streptococcal pneumonia, more often than other bacterial pneumonia, seems to complicate such viral infections as influenza, measles, chickenpox, and rubella, and bacterial infections such as pertussis and pneumococcal pneumonia. It may occasionally occur as primary pneumonia, or secondary to other streptococcal illnesses such as pharyngitis and scarlet fever.

Clinical Pattern. The symptoms are extremely variable and commonly arise late in the course of the predisposing illness. High fever, tachypnea accompanied by chills, and pleuritic pain may be seen early, but often the onset occurs as an insidious exacerbation of the original illness with return of fever and intensification of cough.

Diagnosis. The radiographical findings are often similar to those of staphylococcal pneumonia. Pneumatoceles may be seen on chest roentgenogram in both conditions. Group A beta-hemolytic streptococci can be recovered from the nose and throat cultures, but this finding does not prove the cause of the pneumonia. A rise in the serum antistreptolysin O titer is supportive diagnostic evidence. If pleural fluid is present, the organism can frequently be recovered on culture. Blood cultures are positive in only 10 per cent of patients.

Complications. Empyema occurs in about 20 per cent of children with streptococcal pneumonia. Septic foci in other areas, such as bones and joints, occur occasionally.

HEMOPHILUS INFLUENZAE PNEUMONIA

The incidence of childhood pneumonia due to infection with *Hemophilus influenzae* type B is unknown. This organism is well-established as a cause of serious bacterial infection of infants and children (acute epiglottitis, acute meningitis), but acute pneumonia seems less common.

Clinically, *H. influenzae* pneumonia is difficult to differentiate with certainty from pneumococcal pneumonia. Some observers believe *H. influenzae* pneumonia tends to be more insidious in onset, and the clinical course is usually subacute, lasting several weeks.

Any childhood pneumonia that fails to respond satisfactorily to penicillin or erythromycin therapy should be re-evaluated for the possibility of *H. influenzae* infection. The diagnosis is difficult to establish. Isolation of *H. influenzae* from the blood, pleural effusion, or lung aspirate is confirmatory. A nearly pure culture of *H. influenzae* from the nasopharynx is suggestive evidence. Lung puncture of the consolidated area may be the diagnostic procedure of choice (Klein, 1969).

Management includes appropriate antibiotic therapy and surgical drainage of empyema if it occurs.

OTHER GRAM-NEGATIVE PNEUMONIAS

Other gram-negative pneumonias include those caused by the Klebsiella group, Pseudomonas aeruginosa, Proteus, and *Escherichia coli.* Pneumonia due to these organisms tends to be seen mainly in hospitalized patients in the first few weeks of life and in debilitated infants who have been in the hospital for long periods of time and have received prolonged treatment with humidified oxygen (Williams and Phelan, 1975).

LEGIONELLOSIS

Legionellosis was first recognized as a distinct entity in 1976. The cause is a small, fastidious gram-negative bacillus, *Legionella pneumophila.*

The presenting clinical picture resembles a severe "flu-like syndrome," with dry, nonproductive cough that may gradually become productive. Other symptoms may include pleuritic chest pain, diarrhea, abdominal pain, and central nervous system involvement with confusion or delirium. On physical examination, the patient is acutely ill and febrile, with pulmonary rales or rhonchi. Chest x-rays show patchy infiltrates that tend to progress to nodular consolidation.

The incidence of the disease in the pediatric population is unknown. Preliminary investigations suggest that although severe acute disease is rare, subclinical or mild infections may be fairly common (Muldoon et al., 1981). Diagnosis is currently based on specific seroconversion. Therapy is not well-established, but erythromycin combined with rifampin shows some promise.

TUBERCULOUS PNEUMONIA

Although not technically an acute suppurative pneumonia, pulmonary tuberculosis is included here to stress its continuing importance. The incidence of infection due to *Mycobacterium tuberculosis* in children has decreased dramatically since effective chemotherapy has reduced the number of contagious adults in the general population. The huge influx of Southeast Asian refugees into the United States in the past eight years has introduced a new reservoir of tuberculous patients into many cities in the United States. Our experience with children of this new immigrant population shows an increased incidence of tuberculosis, with the reappearance on our wards of military and meningitic forms of tuberculosis. With early tuberculosis infection, symptoms may be absent, mild, or unimpressive. Low-grade fever, poor feeding, and irritability may be the only symptoms. Sometimes an incidental and unrelated viral respiratory infection will lead to a chest roentgenogram that reveals a parenchymal infiltrate and hilar lymph gland enlargement. This may be misinterpreted as possible pneumococcal consolidation, so that the diagnosis of tuberculosis is initially missed.

More often, the initial tuberculous infection leads to interference with the normal bronchial tree clearance mechanisms and the child suffers a superimposed bacterial pneumonitis (usually pneumococcal). A chest roentgenogram is initially interpreted as lobar consolidation and the diagnosis of tuberculosis considered only after it fails to clear as anticipated. Any lobar pneumonia that is slow to resolve must be considered as possibly tuberculous. Every child with hilar adenopathy or serous pleural effusion must be suspected of having tuberculosis until the tuberculin test has been proven to be negative. All infants and children who develop pneumonia should be tested routinely for tuberculin sensitivity. Tuberculin testing in this group of patients should be done intradermally using tuberculin, purified protein derivative (PPD) and including a positive control. For a positive control, use an intradermal test with common antigens such as candida, tetanus, or streptokinase-streptodornase (SK-SD) to demonstrate skin reactivity (absence of anergy). Today the yield of positive tests for tuberculosis will be small in middle class American society, but the incidence will be higher in socioeconomically deprived areas and among immigrant populations.

PNEUMONIA IN THE IMMUNOCOMPROMISED HOST

Lower respiratory tract infections in the immunosuppressed or immunodeficient child must be evaluated and followed with the greatest care. These children are, of course, subject to all of the usual infections outlined in this chapter; in addition, they have a high incidence of acute and chronic pulmonary infections with many organisms that normally are considered to have low virulence and little propensity for widespread pulmonary invasion. Many of these infections are not sensitive to the antibiotics commonly used in the treatment of childhood respiratory infection, and concomitant infection with two pathogens is common.

After organ transplantation, children on cortisone and immunosuppressant therapy are very susceptible to infection with *Pneumocystis carinii* and cytomegalovirus. Therapy for malignancy with irradiation and antimetabolites results in susceptibility to *Pneumocystis carinii*, Aspergillus, and a variety of other bacteria and fungi. Children with combined immunodeficiency disease are the nost susceptible of all and will develop one infection after another. Physicians must be aware of this problem and must realize that for the child with compromised immunity, there is no such thing as a minor or insignificant respiratory infection.

ANTIBIOTIC THERAPY FOR BACTERIAL PNEUMONIA

Infants under 12 Months of Age. In infants less than one year of age (excluding the neonatal period) who appear seriously ill with pneumonia, staphylococcal pneumonia must be suspected and covered in the treatment program, as well as *H. influenzae.* This would require intravenous nafcillin or methicillin (100–200 mg/kg/day divided into four doses), combined with either ampicillin, chloramphenicol, cephalmandol, or moxalactam in appropriate doses. When the results of culture and sensitivity studies of the blood, pleural fluid, and lung aspirate are available, the treatment program can be revised as indicated.

Children One or Two Years of Age. In this age group, pneumococci are the most common cause of bacterial pneumonia, but staphylococci are still important. Therapy is based on the clinician's evaluation of the severity of the infection. Children who are only mildly or moderately ill, and who could just as likely have Mycoplasma or even Chlamydia as the infecting agent, may be started on erythromycin orally (50 mg/kg/day divided into four doses). If the child fails to improve after 24 to 48 hours, then reorienting the therapy to a broader spectrum with nafcillin or methacillin, plus either ampicillin or chloramphenicol, would seem indicated.

Children over Two Years of Age. Pneumococci are, by far, the most common cause of bacterial pneumonia and, unless the child's condition suggests an overwhelming infection, daily intramuscular injection of procaine penicillin (50,000 units/kg/day up to 1 million units per injection) will usually result in rapid improvement in 24 to 48 hours. When improvement occurs, the child can be switched to oral penicillin V (50,000 units/kg/day divided into four doses) and the dose continued for 7 to 10 days. If the child fails to improve over the first 24 to 48 hours, hospitalization, diagnostic work-up, and broadening the therapy as outlined above is indicated. In the case of some mildly ill children, when the differential diagnosis includes Mycoplasma versus pneumococcal pneumonia, choosing to treat initially with oral erythromycin is reasonable.

Fungal Pneumonias

There are only two fungal organisms that commonly cause symptomatic acute pulmonary infections in children. They are *Coccidioides immitis* and *Histoplasma capsulatum.* The natural occurrence of *Coccidioides immitis* is limited to the arid areas of California's San Joaquin valley, scattered areas of southern California, central and southern Arizona, southern New Mexico, and western and southern Texas. The major endemic areas in the United States for *Histoplasma capsulatum* extend from the western Appalachian slope to the midwestern states that border the tributaries of the Ohio, Missouri, and Mississippi Rivers.

Fortunately, both fungi usually result in pulmonary infections that are so mild that they are either missed or diagnosed as a flu-like syndrome. In the child who develops symptomatic disease, the infection is almost always self-limiting, with the gradual production of a lifelong immunity that prevents recurrence of the pulmonary infection on subsequent exposure to the fungus.

The presenting clinical picture is apt to be the same with either fungus. The child, usually of school age, develops a fever between 101 and 103°F, malaise, nonproductive cough, poor appetite, and a desire to rest rather than play after school. Prominent nonpruritic rashes of the erythema multiforme and erythema nodosum types are commonly seen with coccidioidomycosis but not with histoplasmosis.

Examination of the chest may reveal a few rales but is frequently normal. Chest x-ray usually shows a striking infiltration in one lung with ipsilateral hilar adenopathy. Diagnostic skin tests usually turn positive three to six weeks after infection.

In most children infected with these fungi the infection resolves rapidly, although a few remain febrile and toxic for a much longer period of time and complete convalescence may take two to three months. For reasons that are not understood, an occasional child's immune mechanisms are unable to contain the infection within the lungs and a disseminated fungal infection develops, with serious consequences for the child.

For disseminated coccidiodomycosis and disseminated histoplasmosis, the only proven effective drug currently available is intravenous amphotericin B. Ketoconazole, an orally administered imidazole antifungal agent, appears to hold promise as a safer and more easily administered agent, but experience to date is limited (Committee on Infectious Disease, 1982a).

Acknowledgment

The author would like to acknowledge his indebtedness to Dr. Ann Petru and Dr. Parvin Azimi for their helpful critical review of this chapter.

REFERENCES

Barker, G. A.: Current management of croup and epiglottitis. Pediatr. Clin. North Am., *26*:565, 1979.

Bonham, G. S., and Wilson, R. W.: Children's health in families with cigarette smokers. Am. J. Publ. Health, *71*:290, 1981.

Brook, I., Anthony, B. F., and Finegold, S. M.: Aerobic and anaerobic bacteriology of acute otitis media in children. J. Pediatr., *92*:13, 1978.

Committee on Infectious Disease, American Academy of Pediatrics, 1982a.

Committee on Infectious Disease, American Academy of Pediatrics. Aspirin and Reyes syndrome (special report). Pediatrics, *69*:810, 1982b.

Cramblett, H. G.: Infections of the respiratory tract due to Mycoplasma pneumonia. *In* Kendig, E. L. (ed.): Disorders of the Respiratory Tract in Children. Philadelphia, W. B. Saunders Co., 1972, pp. 260–265.

Davis, H. W., Gartner, J. C., Galvis, A. G., Michaels, R. M., and Mestad, P. H.: Acute upper airway obstruction: Croup and epiglottitis. Pediatr. Clin North Am., *28*:859, 1981.

Davis, S. D., and Wedgwood, R. J.: Antibiotic prophylaxis in acute respiratory distress. Am. J. Dis. Child., *109*:544, 1965.

Denny, F. W.: Infections of the respiratory tract due to mycoplasma pneumoniae. *In* Kendig, E. L. (ed.): Disorders of the Respiratory Tract in Children. Philadelphia, W. B. Saunders Co., 1977, p. 433.

Dingle, J. H., Badger, G. F., and Hordan, W. S.: Illness in the Home. Cleveland, Western Reserve University, 1964.

Downes, J. J., Wood, D. W., Straker, T. W., and Haddad, C.: Acute respiratory failure in infants with bronchiolitis. Anesthesiology, *29*:426, 1968.

Eichenwald, H. F.: Respiratory infections in children. Hosp. Practice, *11*:81, 1976.

Gellady, A. M., Shulman, S. T., and Ayoub, E. M.: Periorbital and orbital cellulitis in children. Pediatrics, *61*:272, 1978.

Gharib, R., Allen, R. P., Juos, H. A., and Bravo, L. R.: Paranasal sinuses in cystic fibrosis. Am. J. Dis. Child., *108*:499, 1964.

Goldberg, F., Berne, A. S., and Oski, F. A.: Differentiation of orbital cellulitis from preseptal cellulitis by computed tomography. Pediatrics, *62*:1000, 1978.

Green, M., and Fousek, M. G.: Hemophilus influenzae type b cellulitis. Pediatrics, *19*:80, 1957.

Guilleminault, C., Eldridge, F. L., Simmons, F. B., and Dement, W. C.: Sleep apnea in eight children. Pediatrics, *58*:23, 1976.

Henderson, F. W., Collier, A. M., Sanyal, M. A., Watkin, J. M., et al.: A longitudinal study of respiratory viruses and bacteria in the etiology of acute otitis media with effusion. N. Engl. J. Med., *306*:1377, 1982.

Hilman, B. C.: Interstitial and hypersensitivity pneumonitis and their variants. Pediatr. Rev., *1*:229, 1980.

Hughes, W. T.: Treatment of Pneumocystis carinii pneumonitis. N. Engl. J. Med., *295*:726, 1976.

Kattan, M.: Long term sequelae of respiratory illness in infancy and childhood. Pediatr. Clin. North Am., *26*:525, 1979.

Klein, J. O.: Diagnostic lung puncture in the pneumonias of infants and children. Pediatrics, *44*:486, 1969.

Klein, J. O.: Microbiology of otitis media. Ann. Otol. Rhinol. Otolaryngol., *89*:98, 1980.

Lang, W. R., Howden, C. W., Laws, J., and Burton, J. F.: Bronchopneumonia with serious sequelae in children with evidence of adenovirus type 21 infection. Br. Med. J., *1*:73, 1969.

Levine, D. P., and Lerner, A. M.: The clinical spectrum of mycoplasma pneumoniae infections. Med. Clin. North Am., *62*:961, 1978.

Maresh, M. M., and Washburn, A. H.: Paranasal sinuses from birth to late adolescence. Am. J. Dis. Child., *60*:841, 1940.

Moffet, H. L.: Clinical Microbiology. Philadelphia, J. P. Lippincott Co., 1975, p. 124.

Montos, A. S., and Ullman, B. M.: Acute respiratory illness in an American community. J.A.M.A., *227*:164, 1974.

Morbidity and Mortality Weekly Report: Pertussis surveillance, 1979–1981. M.M.W.R., *31*:334, July 2, 1982.

Muldoon, R. L., Jaeker, D. L., and Kiejer, H. K.: Legionnaires disease in children. Pediatrics, *67*:329, 1981.

Olson, A. L., Klein, S. W., Charney, E., et al.: Prevention and therapy of serous otitis media by oral decongestant: A double-blind study in pediatric practice. Pediatrics, *61*:679, 1978.

Pantell, R. H.: Pharyngitis: Diagnosis and management. Pediatr. Rev., 3:35, 1981.

Paradise, J. L.: Otitis media in infants and children. Pediatrics, *65*:917, 1980.
Paradise, J. L.: Tonsillectomy and adenoidectomy. Pediatr. Clin. North Am., *28*:881, 1981.
Rachelefsky, G. S., Katz, R. M., and Siegel, S. C.: Diseases of the paranasal sinuses in children. Current Problems in Pediatrics, Vol. 12, No. 5, March, 1982.
Roddey, O. F., Earle, P., and Haggerty, R. J.: Myringotomy in acute otitis media, a controlled study. J.A.M.A., *197*:849, 1966.
Rowe, D. S.: Acute suppurative otitis media. Pediatrics, *56*:285, 1975.
Schachter, J.: Chlamydial infections. N. Engl. J. Med., *298*:426, 490, and 540, 1978.
Shann, F. A., Phelan, P. D., Stocks, J. G., and Bennett, N. M.: Prolonged nasotracheal intubation or tracheostomy in acute laryngotracheobronchitis and epiglottitis. Austral. Paediatr., *11*:212, 1975.
Shuttleworth, D. B., and Charney, E.: Leukocyte count in childhood pneumonia. Am. J. Dis. Child., *122*:393, 1971.
Tetzloff, T. R., Ashworth, C., and Nelson, J. D.: Otitis media in children less than 12 weeks of age. Pediatrics, *59*:827, 1977.
Tooley, W. H.: Lung function in infancy and childhood. *In* Rudolph, A. (ed.): Pediatrics, 17th ed. New York, Appleton-Century-Crofts, 1982, p. 1379.
Williams, H. E., and Phelan, P. D.: Respiratory Illness in Children. Oxford, Blackwell Publications, 1975.
Wohl, M. E. B.: Bronchiolitis. *In* Kendig, E. L. (ed.): Disorders of the Respiratory Tract in Children. Philadelphia, W. B. Saunders Co., 1977, p. 371.

11
VOMITING

Joseph H. Clark, M.D., and Joseph F. Fitzgerald, M.D.

Vomiting, one of the more common pediatric problems, should be differentiated from regurgitation. *True* vomiting is the forceful evacuation of gastric contents, frequently accompanied by nausea, whereas regurgitation is the postprandial loss of part of a feeding, frequently associated with eructation and usually unassociated with nausea.

ETIOLOGY

Most episodes of vomiting in infants and children result from an acute infectious process, most commonly affecting the gastrointestinal or respiratory system, but occasionally the urinary tract or central nervous system. Rare causes of vomiting include congestive heart failure, lead intoxication, uremia, and metabolic disorders such as congenital adrenal hyperplasia, renal tubular acidosis, urea cycle disorders, and diabetes mellitus.

Vomiting related to increased intracranial pressure is usually projectile and unassociated with nausea or colicky abdominal pain. These patients frequently complain of early morning headache that is relieved by vomiting. Vomiting associated with gastrointestinal tract obstruction, e.g., pyloric stenosis, is usually projectile and unassociated with nausea. It may accompany the initial symptoms of acute appendicitis, and it is a prominent symptom in young patients (< 6 years) with peptic ulcer disease (Deckelbaum et al., 1974).

"Cyclic vomiting" is a syndrome characterized by recurrent attacks of severe vomiting without apparent cause, occasionally accompanied by headache, abdominal pain, and fever. The onset is usually prior to age six, and the episodes frequently terminate at puberty. There is often a positive family history for migraine, and many patients develop migraine as adults (Hoyt and Stickler, 1960). The vomiting typically resolves abruptly with the initiation of parenteral fluid therapy. An occasional patient receives benefit from phenytoin sodium.

Emotional disturbance, including anorexia nervosa and bulimia (megaphagia), may result in chronic and recurrent vomiting in older pediatric patients, especially in girls. The vomiting, often brought on by inserting the finger in the back of the throat, typically occurs after the meal has begun or just after it has been completed. Since it can be suppressed, vomiting only rarely occurs in public or in the dining room. The symptom is of little concern to these patients, who are usually thin but rarely emaciated.

Regurgitation or "spitting up" in infancy is benign if the baby continues to gain weight and is otherwise healthy. Usually the complaint disappears by eight months of age. If regurgitation persists and is associated with failure to thrive, recurrent pneumonia, or apnea, an evaluation for gastroesophageal reflux must be initiated (Herbst, 1981).

Rumination, a serious psychiatric disorder of infancy, is thought to be the result of an abnormal maternal-child relationship. These patients suck and mouth their fingers until gastric contents are regurgitated, rechewed, and reswallowed. Persistent rumination may occur in children who are severely retarded or psychotic. A basic treatment principle is to provide the baby with appropriate nurturing care within the hospital setting.

EVALUATION

The duration of vomiting, presence or absence of weight loss, visible peristalsis, an abdominal mass, distention, hernia, history of prior abdominal surgery, and findings suggestive of a systemic disease contribute to the initial diagnostic impression. Particular attention is paid to the character of the vomitus and the relationship of vomiting to meals. Bile-stained vomitus indicates an obstruction distal to the ampulla of Vater. A fecal odor suggests intestinal obstruction, peritonitis with ileus, ischemic injury to the gut, or long-standing gastric outlet obstruction with stasis and bacterial overgrowth. One should determine the pH of the vomitus and test it for occult blood. Careful physical examination, including rectal, should be performed. The initial diagnostic impression dictates further evaluation. Laboratory investigation may be unnecessary.

The initial evaluation for suspected gastroesophageal reflux in a patient older than eight months of age should be a barium study of the upper gastrointestinal tract. This examination evaluates the lower esophageal sphincter and rules out a high obstruction that might cause gastroesophageal reflux. A gastroesophageal scintiscan, utilized as a complementary study, increases the sensitivity of radiographical studies from 50 to 70 per cent (Arasu et al., 1980). Esophageal manometry, the acid reflux test of Tuttle, and extended esophageal pH monitoring are frequently necessary to determine the relative roles of medical and surgical management in complicated cases.

MANAGEMENT

Antiemetics and sedatives are potentially toxic and should not be used in the management of acute vomiting episodes. Diet therapy is most important. Following a brief period of deprivation (three hours for infants and up to six hours for older children), the patient is offered clear liquids in amounts sufficient to maintain adequate hydration. It may be necessary to offer an infant as little as 1 to 2 teaspoons every 20 minutes in order to prevent dehydration. Infants are provided a glucose-electrolyte solution (Pedialyte,* Lytren,† etc.), whereas older children can receive other beverages such as "spent" ginger ale or 7-Up. Both cola and tea have been recommended in the past in spite of the fact that both are considered gastric irritants. An inflamed stomach is sensitive to hot and cold beverages; fluids at room temperature are tolerated best. The diet is gradually increased over 48 hours as tolerated. Highly seasoned foods and known gastric irritants (e.g., aspirin and chocolate) should be avoided during recovery.

Persistent regurgitation is managed by offering thickened feedings (one tablespoon of rice cereal per two ounces of formula), by maintaining an upright or semi-upright position for 45 to 60 minutes after meals, and by elevation of the bed 30 degrees so that the pharynx is slightly higher than the gastric fundus when the infant is prone (Meyers and Herbst, 1982). Further medical management consists of bethanechol (9 mg/M^2/day in three divided doses) or metoclopramide (0.3–0.5 mg/kg/day in three divided doses). The former has been more effective in our experience but has the theoretical disadvantage of inducing bronchospasm in patients with hyper-reactive airways. The major side effects of metoclopramide are tardive dyskinesias and irritability. Surgical intervention is necessary if symptoms continue despite appropriate medical management.

SUMMARY

Although vomiting can accompany serious illness, it is usually associated with a self-limited infectious process of little significance. The correct diagnosis should be made quickly and the patient not subjected to unnecessary and expensive diagnostic procedures. Diet therapy is usually effective, and antiemetics are rarely indicated. Regurgitation may be managed conservatively in infants less than eight months of age as long as the patient is gaining weight and is free of pulmonary symptoms. Projectile vom-

*Ross Laboratories, Columbus, Ohio.

†Mead Johnson, Evansville, Indiana.

iting, however, is usually associated with serious underlying disease dictating careful evaluation in any age group.

REFERENCES

Anderson, O. W.: Antinauseant drugs in the treatment of epidemic or virus gastritis. Pediatrics, *46*:319, 1970.

Arasu, T. S., Wyllie, R., Fitzgerald, J. F., et al.: Gastroesophageal reflux in infants and children—comparative accuracy of diagnostic methods. J. Pediatr., *96*:798, 1980.

Bordfeld, P. A.: A controlled double-blind study of trimethobenzamide, prochlorperazine and placebo. J.A.M.A., *196*:116, 1966.

Deckelbaum, R. J., Roy, C. C., Lussier-Lazoroft, J., and Morin, C. L.: Peptic ulcer disease: A clinical study in 73 children. Can. Med. Assoc. J., *111*:225, 1974.

Euler, A. R.: Use of bethanechol for the treatment of gastroesophageal reflux. J. Pediatr., *96*:31, 1980.

Fleisher, D. R.: Infant rumination syndrome. Am. J. Dis. Child., *133*:266, 1979.

Herbst, J. J.: Gastroesophageal reflux. J. Pediatr., *98*:859, 1981.

Hoyt, C. S., and Stickler, G. B.: A study of 44 children with the syndrome of recurrent (cyclic) vomiting. Pediatrics, *25*:775, 1960.

Meyers, W. F., and Herbst, J. J.: Effectiveness of positioning therapy for gastroesophageal reflux. Pediatrics, *69*:768, 1982.

Rosman, N. P.: Increased intracranial pressure in childhood. Pediatr. Clin. North Am., *21*:483, 1974.

12

DIARRHEA

Joseph H. Clark, M.D., and Joseph F. Fitzgerald, M.D.

Diarrhea is an increase in the frequency, fluidity, or volume of bowel movements relative to the usual habit of each individual (Phillips, 1975). Most episodes of diarrhea develop abruptly and are accompanied by other symptoms and signs suggestive of an infectious process. Less often, the physician is consulted because of chronic diarrhea.

ETIOLOGY

Acute nonspecific gastroenteritis is the predominant cause of diarrhea in a pediatric ambulatory setting. Recent advances in microbiological techniques have led to the successful isolation of a pathogen from approximately 60 per cent of patients with diarrhea (Gall and Hamilton, 1977; Edelman and Levine, 1980). Viral gastroenteritis has two epidemiologically distinct clinical presentations (Blacklow and Cukor, 1981). The Norwalk virus has been causally associated with one third of the cases of epidemic viral gastroenteritis in the United States among school age children, family contacts, and adults. Signs and symptoms, which include nausea, vomiting, diarrhea, abdominal cramps, headache, fever, anorexia, malaise, and myalgia, last 24 to 48 hours.

An intestinal rotavirus has been identified as the cause of a sporadic diarrheal illness that afflicts infants and young children, lasts from five to eight days, and is often accompanied by fever and vomiting. A significant number of affected infants require hospitalization for fluid and electrolyte replacement. This illness, which accounts for 50 per cent of cases of infantile diarrhea requiring hospitalization, is particularly common in temperate climates during winter months.

Escherichia coli, Salmonella, Shigella, *Campylobacter jejuni*, and *Yersinia enterocolitica* are the bacterial pathogens that cause acute gastroenteritis-enterocolitis in North America. Gall and Hamilton (1977) reported that 10.7 per cent of 1215 patients with diarrhea hospitalized at the Hospital for Sick Children in Toronto during 1975 had a bacterial pathogen in their stool. The two most commonly identified were Salmonella and *E. coli*.

Clinical manifestations of *E. coli* infection depend on whether invasive or toxigenic strains have colonized the gastrointestinal tract. The enterotoxigenic infection predominates in infants. These babies pass green, mucoid, foul-smelling stools. Older children can also be infected with enterotoxigenic organisms. Infection with an invasive strain of *E. coli* produces a dysentery comparable to shigellosis. Recent investigations have failed to find a relationship between *in vitro* enterotoxin production and specific *E. coli* serotypes; hence, the serotypic designation of an "enteropathogenic" strain is not clinically useful.

Fever accompanies the watery diarrhea of salmonellosis, and vomiting may occur early. The temperature ranges between 37 and 38°C, and the leukocyte count is 12,000 to 15,000/cu mm. The stools occasionally contain mucus and blood, but rarely gross pus. The illness is usually self-limited and abates after two to five days. Blood cultures are positive in 8 per cent of patients (Saphra and Winter, 1957).

Shigella gastroenteritis begins abruptly with fever and diarrhea. Gross blood is present in the stools of less than half of patients, although polymorphonuclear leukocytes and red blood cells are commonly seen on microscopic examination of a fecal smear. Low-income families living under extremely poor environmental conditions are most commonly afflicted. Infants and children less than five years old are particularly susceptible. Febrile convulsions may be seen early in the course of the illness in 5 to 10 per cent of patients. Occasionally, a seizure precedes the diarrhea and occurs without fever.

Campylobacter enteritis is characterized by fever and voluminous, foul-smelling diarrhea that may contain blood and/or mucus. Diffuse periumbilical or right lower quadrant abdominal pain may be present. Vomiting accompanies the diarrhea early in 30 per cent of patients (Rettig, 1979). The illness is self-limited but relapses may occur for up to one year. Bacteremia is infrequent but may result in meningitis, especially in neonates.

Yersinia enteritis has several clinical presentations. Infants and young children experience a relatively mild, self-limited illness consisting of fever, vomiting, and diarrhea. Their stools may contian blood and/or mucus. Older children and adolescents may have an acute terminal ileitis with right lower quadrant abdominal pain that mimics acute appendicitis or Crohn's disease. Radiological studies reveal a thickened, nodular terminal ileum suggestive of Crohn's disease. Microbiological isolation is difficult, since cold enrichment may be required for greater than one week.

Sporadic cases of acute gastroenteritis can result from colonization of the gastrointestinal tract by *Klebsiella pneumoniae*, pneumococci, staphylococci, *Pseudomonas aeruginosa*, and Candida (Gryboski, 1979). Diarrhea occasionally accompanies antibiotic therapy, especially ampicillin. The mechanism in many cases is unknown, although the emergence of resistant organisms is common. The diarrhea is generally self-limited and clears within several days following discontinuation of the antibiotic. Antibiotic-associated diarrhea is clinically distinguishable from pseudomembranous colitis. Patients with the latter appear toxic and have bloody diarrhea.

Giardia lamblia, the most common parasite identified in the United States, is associated with intermittent watery diarrhea, abdominal distention, flatulence, and, at times, vomiting. Aspiration of duodenal fluid is frequently necessary to establish the diagnosis, since stool examinations are positive in less than half of affected children.

Many causes of chronic diarrhea in infants and children have now been described (Fitzgerald and Clark, 1982; Gryboski, 1979). Many patients with chronic diarrhea require hospitalization for complete evaluation, but the diagnosis of hypercaloric diarrhea, well-water diarrhea, "short-gut" syndrome, altered gastrointestinal microflora, food intolerance, disaccharidase deficiency, parasitic infection, cystic fibrosis, or inflammatory bowel disease may be suggested by the history. Physical examination may point to partial obstruction or "overflow diarrhea" consequent to a chronic fecal impaction.

EVALUATION

A careful history is the most important tool in the evaluation of a patient with diarrhea. Painstaking attention must be paid to the dietary history. It is important to know whether the onset was abrupt or insidious and whether concomitant extraintestinal symptoms consistent with respiratory or urinary tract infections were present. Did other family members experience similar symptoms? A travel history occasionally yields significant information. A complete stool history includes frequency, appearance, consistency, and the presence of blood or mucus. Specific questions about odor and "floating" yield information of only limited value.

Thorough physical examination may point to a likely diagnosis. Careful recording of height (length) and weight on a standard anthropometric chart is valuable. A thorough examination of a patient with diarrhea is never complete without anorectal examination. Digital examination of the rectum rules out an impaction and allows instant stool examination. Stool pH, Clinitest, and Hemoccult reactions are recorded. A low pH (5.5 or less) or positive Clinitest (0.5 per cent or greater) suggests impaired carbohydrate utilization. Microscopic examination of the stool for fat and neutrophils may suggest steatorrhea or an inflammatory process.

Stool cultures are an important diagnostic adjunct when a bacterial etiology is suspected. Hence, they must be plated immediately in order to obtain reliable information regarding the gastrointestinal aerobic flora. It is insufficient to know simply that no pathogens are present. Gram stain of fresh stool provides additional information. This simple test allows one to diagnose an overgrowth of staphylococci, pneumococci, streptococci, or candida, as well as to obtain information about the anaerobic microflora. A *fresh* stool should be examined for ova and parasites. Initial laboratory studies, when deemed necessary, should include CBC, electrolytes, BUN, and serum creatinine. When the history, physical examination, and stool studies suggest malabsorption, a sweat chloride determination for cystic fibrosis, serum carotene, and total serum proteins with fractionation should be obtained. A carotene level greater than 100 μg/dl rules out malabsorption, while a carotene level less than 50 μg/dl suggests malabsorption in the patient consuming adequate dietary carotene. As indicated above, the patient with chronic diarrhea may need admission for complete evaluation (Fig. 12–1).

Gastrointestinal radiographical studies are virtually never indicated in the evaluation of a patient with acute diarrhea; however, studies of the intestinal tract are invaluable in inflammatory bowel disease, and they may be supportive in the evaluation of malabsorptive states.

TREATMENT

Most episodes of diarrhea occurring in infants and children are acute and self-limited. The most effective therapy is dietary. The bowel is put at rest by cutting back on the dietary load and offering clear liquids, e.g., Jello-water or "spent" ginger ale, or a glucose-electrolyte solution such as Lytren* or Pedialyte.† This allows mucosal healing and eliminates compounding factors secondary to the presence of unabsorbed, osmotically active substances in the bowel lumen. The diet is increased as the stool volume decreases. Dairy products and foods with a substantial fat content are added last. A regular diet is frequently tolerated in 48 to 72 hours.

*Mead Johnson Company, Evansville, Indiana.

†Ross Laboratories, Columbus, Ohio.

We do not employ antidiarrhea preparations such as kaolin, pectin, paregoric, or diphenoxylate (Lomotil).‡ None of these preparations has a positive effect on the basic pathophysiology, and they are potentially hazardous. Drugs that slow intestinal motility may prolong the course of infectious enteritides. Empirical antibiotic therapy without a culture is generally not warranted in the outpatient management of acute diarrhea. Antibiotic therapy may alter the flora and lead to a chronic diarrheal state. The toxic patient deserves admission to the hospital and antibiotic therapy as indicated.§

Controversy surrounds the use of antibiotics in mild cases when a stool culture yields a bacterial pathogen such as enteropathogenic *E. coli,* Salmonella, or Shigella. Oftentimes the patient is asymptomatic when the pathogen is identified. Organisms resistant to multiple antibiotics have evolved in the last few years, dictating that we re-evaluate current practice in this regard. Antibiotic resistance is readily transmissible by bacterial conjugation between members of Enterobacteriaceae. Consequently, intraluminal antibiotics place selective pressure on sensitive strains of enteropathogenic *E. coli* and Shigella, leading to the emergence of resistant forms by the acquisition of the appropriate "R" factor (Watanabe, 1971).

In spite of the above, several authors (Drachman, 1974; Gryboski, 1979; Roy et al., 1975) recommend antibiotic therapy for young infants (less than three months of age) and debilitated children with enteropathogenic *E. coli* and Salmonella infections, and for patients of all ages with shigellosis. Ampicillin-resistant strains of Shigella are a frequent occurrence and trimethoprim-sulfamethoxazole is now the drug of choice (Nelson et al., 1976).‖ *Campylobacter jejuni* is sensitive to erythromycin (50 mg/kg/24 hr). Antibiotic treatment of Yersinia is rarely indicated, but trimethoprim-sulfamethoxazole is effective. Giardiasis may be treated with either metronidazole (15–30 mg/kg/24 hr) or furazolidone (5–7 mg/kg/24 hr). The latter is available in a liquid preparation. The patient with giardiasis receives a 10-day course of therapy, while unaffected family members are treated for 7 days.

‡Searle and Company, San Juan, Puerto Rico.

§Early treatment of young adults experiencing traveler's diarrhea with trimethoprim-sulfamethoxazole or with trimethoprim alone is an alternative to prophylactic medication (DuPont et al., 1982).

‖10 mg trimethoprim and 50 mg sulfamethoxazole/kg/day orally in two divided doses.

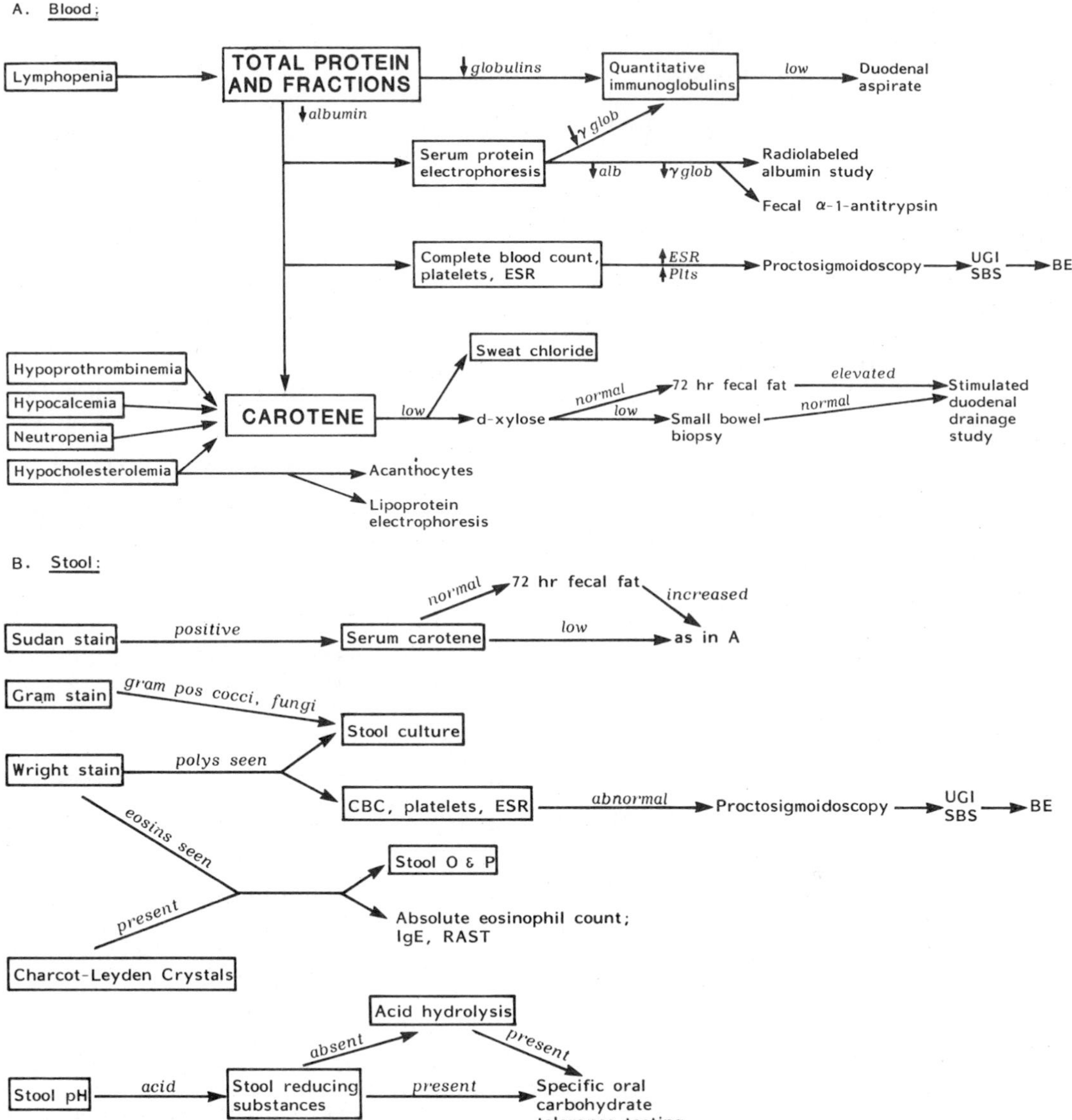

Figure 12–1. Algorithm for laboratory diagnosis of chronic diarrhea. *A*, Blood; *B*, stool. (From Fitzgerald, J. F., and Clark, J. H.: Chronic diarrhea. Pediatr. Clin. North Am., 29:221, 1982.)

The necessity for, and method of, re-establishing a normal intestinal microflora after it has been altered by antibiotic therapy is a matter of some controversy. After determining the antibiotic sensitivities of the predominant organism(s), we administer an appropriate antibiotic (nonabsorbable, if possible) for five days. We then provide viable *Lactobacillus acidophilus* on the fifth day and continue it for eight days. The effect of therapy is evaluated when the eight-day course is completed. It has been our impression that this program is successful, but we have not done a controlled study. Indeed, Pearce and Hamilton (1974) found orally administered lactobacilli to be of no value in a controlled study of 94 children under three years of age hospitalized with acute diarrhea.

Cholestyramine has been advocated in the treatment of intractable diarrhea (Tamer et al., 1974). It is suggested that this nonabsorbable anion-exchange resin binds endotoxin and/or diarrheagenic bile acids in the intestinal lumen. Roy et al. (1975) reported that the drug was ineffective in seven of their patients with persistent diarrhea. While sporadic testimonials regarding the efficacy of this drug are made, more studies are necessary before it is recommended for routine use in the treatment of nonspecific diarrhea. In this same vein, a recent commentary in *Pediatrics* described a "bowel cocktail" of gentamicin, metronidazole, and cholestyramine for the management of infants with persistent diarrhea (Bowie et al., 1981). It must be pointed out that the authors of this statement are responsible for the management of hundreds of infants with persistent diarrhea of mixed infectious origin each year in a setting in which hospital facilities are inadequate to handle the load. Such "shotgun" therapy is not recommended in the management of nonepidemic gastroenteritis-enterocolitis.

SUMMARY

Diarrhea occurring in the pediatric patient is most often acute in onset and self-limited. Dietary management is effective. Antidiarrheal preparations are potentially hazardous and may complicate a relatively mild problem. There is growing concern regarding the use of antibiotics in the treatment of the nonhospitalized patient with diarrhea, even when a stool culture yields a pathogen. Toxic or dehydrated patients deserve admission to the hospital for parenteral fluid therapy.

The initial evaluation of a patient with chronic diarrhea can be effectively accomplished in an ambulatory setting, although admission is often required for special studies.

REFERENCES

Blacklow, N. R., and Cukor, G.: Viral gastroenteritis. N. Engl. J. Med., *304*:397, 1981.

Blaser, M. J., and Peller, L. B.: Campylobacter enteritis. N. Engl. J. Med., *305*:1444, 1981.

Bowie, M. D., Mann, M. D., and Hill, I. D.: The bowel cocktail. Pediatrics, *67*:920, 1981.

Drachman, R. H.: Acute infectious gastroenteritis. Pediatr. Clin. North Am., *21*:711, 1974.

DuPont, H. L., Reves, R. R., Galindo, E. et al.: Treatment of travelers' diarrhea with trimethoprim-sulfamethoxazole and with trimethoprim alone. N. Engl. J. Med., *307*:841, 1982.

Edelman, R., and Levine, M. M.: Acute diarrheal infections in infants. II. Bacterial and viral causes. Hosp. Pract., *15*:97, 1980.

Finberg, L., Harper, P. A., Harrison, H. E., and Sack, R. B.: Oral rehydration for diarrhea. J. Pediatr., *101*:497, 1982.

Fitzgerald, J. F., and Clark, J. H.: Chronic diarrhea. Pediatr. Clin. North Am., *29*:221, 1982.

Gall, D. G., and Hamilton, J. R.: Infectious diarrhea in infants and children. Clin. Gastroenterol., *6*:431, 1977.

Gryboski, J. D.: Chronic diarrhea. Current Prob. Pediatr., *9*:5, 1979.

Harris, J. C., DuPont, H. L., and Hornick, R. B.: Fecal leukocytes in diarrheal illness. Ann. Intern. Med., *76*:697, 1972.

Kohl, S.: Yersinia enterocolitica: A significant "new" pathogen. Hosp. Pract., *13*:81, 1978.

Lerman, S. J., and Walker, R. A.: Treatment of giardiasis. Literature review and recommendations. Clin. Pediatr., *21*:409, 1982.

Nelson, J. D., Kusmiesz, H., Jackson, L. H., and Woodman, E.: Trimethoprim-sulfamethoxazole therapy for shigellosis. J.A.M.A., *235*:1239, 1976.

Pearce, J. L., and Hamilton, J. R.: Controlled trial of orally administered lactobacilli in acute infantile diarrhea. J. Pediatr., *84*:261, 1974.

Phillips, S. F.: Diarrhea: Pathogenesis and diagnostic techniques. Postgrad. Med., *57*:65, 1975.

Rettig, P. J.: Campylobacter infections in human beings. J. Pediatr., *94*:855, 1979.

Roy, C. C., Silverman, A., and Cozzetto, F. J.: Pediatric Clinical Gastroenterology, 2nd Ed. St. Louis, The C. V. Mosby Co., 1975, p. 183.

Santosham, M., Daum, R. S., Dillman, L., et al.: Oral rehydration therapy of infantile diarrhea. A controlled study of well-nourished children hospitalized in the United States and Panama. N. Engl. J. Med., *306*:1070, 1982.

Saphra, I., and Winter, J. W.: Clinical manifestations of salmonellosis in man: An evaluation of 7779 human infections identified at the New York salmonella center. N. Engl. J. Med., *256*:1128, 1957.

Tamer, M. A., Santora, T. R., and Sandberg, D. H.: Cholestyramine therapy for intractable diarrhea. Pediatrics, *53*:217, 1974.

Watanabe, T.: The origin of R factors. Ann. N.Y. Acad. Sci., *182*:126, 1971.

13

HEPATITIS

Joseph F. Fitzgerald, M.D.

Hepatitis can result from non-A, non-B hepatitis viruses, cytomegalovirus, Ebstein-Barr, and other viruses, as well as from the classic infectious entities of hepatitis A and hepatitis B. Certain hypersensitivity and toxic reactions can also closely resemble infectious hepatitis.

Although the vast majority of patients with acute infectious hepatitis recover completely, the physician must be continually alert for that rare patient whose hepatic dysfunction is progressive (Fig. 13–1). The classic patient with infectious hepatitis abruptly develops anorexia,

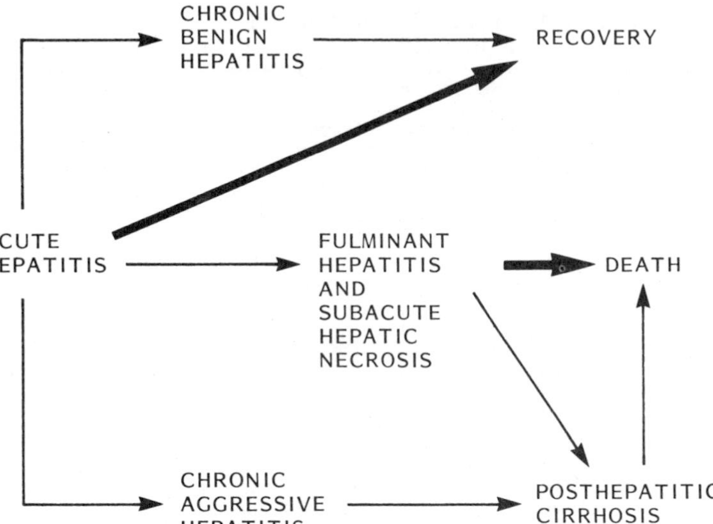

Figure 13–1. The hepatitis spectrum. (From Fitzgerald, J. F., Angelides, A., and Wyllie, R.: The hepatitis spectrum. Curr. Prob. Pediatr., *11*:1, 1981.)

fatigue, malaise, and lassitude 2 to 14 days before jaundice appears. Nausea, vomiting, diarrhea, and, rarely, arthralgia may also occur. Right upper quadrant or epigastric discomfort is common. Fever and "flu-like" symptoms—e.g., cough, coryza, pharyngitis, and photophobia—are frequently observed with hepatitis A virus (HAV) infection. Urticaria, rashes, angioneurotic edema, synovitis, and polyarthritis may be observed during the pre-icteric phase of hepatitis B virus (HBV) infection. An enlarged, tender liver is present in most patients, and the spleen is palpable in 20 to 25 per cent by the time icterus is observed.

The typical patient has modest hyperbilirubinemia (4 to 10 mg/dl), chiefly direct. The aminotransferases (ALT/SGPT; AST/SGOT) are at least tenfold elevated, but usually less than fiftyfold increased (<2000 IU/L). Alkaline phosphatase activity is usually normal or minimally increased, and the prothrombin time, total serum proteins, and albumin are normal. The white blood cell count is usually normal, but a low value may be obtained, as with other viral illnesses. Lymphocytes predominate and atypical forms (virucytes) are commonly seen. Serological tests for identifying HAV and HBV infections should be obtained when the initial laboratory studies support the diagnosis of hepatitis.

Nonspecific supportive care is the cornerstone of therapy. The need for hospitalization is determined not only by the severity of the illness but also by the adequacy of care that can be provided in the home. Sufficient rest is of prime importance. Restriction of quiet activity is unnecessary, as bed rest per se does not result in more rapid recovery than physical activity held within the limit of fatigue. A well-balanced diet with familiar, appetizing foods is recommended. High-protein and low-fat diets are unnecessary. Drugs that are metabolized primarily by the liver should be avoided or used with caution. Antiemetics are ineffective in the management of the nausea and food aversion, and corticosteroids are not indicated in the typical case of acute infectious hepatitis.

Special concern should accompany the first suspicion that a patient's course is atypical. For example, a large firm spleen with a firm, sharp hepatic border in the epigastrium suggests chronic rather than acute liver disease. The presence of ascites and/or muscle wasting also supports chronicity. Persistent fever after the appearance of icterus, especially when associated with a leukocytosis and immature neutrophils, warns of a fulminant course. Fulminant hepatitis is further characterized by a rapidly increasing bilirubin, progressive prolongation of the prothrombin time, and marked elevations of the aminotransferases. A sudden, precipitous decline in the aminotransferases in conjunction with a marked increase in the bilirubin level indicates a poor prognosis. Fulminant hepatitis rarely occurs with HAV infection. While subacute hepatic necrosis is an uncommon sequela of acute hepatitis in children, it does occur; therefore, one must follow patients with hepatitis closely until all laboratory parameters are normal.

Table 13–1. IMMUNOPROPHYLAXIS OF HEPATITIS

	Hepatitis A	
	Treatment	*Guidelines*
Post-exposure	HISG 0.02 ml/kg	Indicated for close personal and household contacts. HISG should be given within 2 weeks of exposure; not indicated after symptoms have appeared.
Pre-exposure	HISG 0.02 ml/kg	Indicated for travelers to endemic areas by unusual routes. Not indicated for travelers on usual tourist routes.
	HISG 0.05 ml/kg	Indicated for prolonged travel (> 3 months) or residence in endemic areas. May be repeated every 4 to 6 months.
	Hepatitis B	
	Treatment	*Guidelines*
Post-exposure	HBIG 0.05–0.07 ml/kg or HISG 0.05–0.07 ml/kg	Indicated following parenteral or mucosal exposure to HBV. First dose within 7 days of exposure followed by a repeat dose in 25–30 days.
	HBIG 0.13 ml/kg or HISG 0.50 ml/kg	Indicated for infants of mothers with acute HBV infection during last trimester of pregnancy.

Approximately one third of patients with chronic aggressive hepatitis (CAH) have a disease onset indistinguishable from that of acute hepatitis. Most of these patients are adolescent females. Extrahepatic features of CAH include acne, amenorrhea, arthritis, dermatitis, pleurisy, colitis, thyroiditis, parotitis, thrombophlebitis, and diabetes mellitus. Hyperproteinemia secondary to hypergammaglobulinemia should suggest the diagnosis. Over 60 per cent of these girls have autoimmune markers, i.e., a positive lupus erythematosus preparation or the presence of antinuclear, antimitochondrial, or anti–smooth muscle antibodies.

While statistics would support the impression that hepatitis is a relatively benign illness in the pediatric age group, an unfortunate few suffer an illness that threatens their lives. Immunoprophylaxis for hepatitis A and hepatitis B are given in Table 13–1. A vaccine for hepatitis B is now available for individuals at risk.

REFERENCES

Fitzgerald, J. F.: Chronic hepatitis. Semin. Liver Dis., 2:282, 1982.

Fitzgerald, J. F., Angelides, A., and Wyllie, R.: The hepatitis spectrum. Curr. Prob. Pediatr., *11*:1, 1981.

Krugman, S., and Gocke, D. J.: Viral Hepatitis. Philadelphia, W. B. Saunders Co., 1978.

Psacharopoulos, H. T., Mowat, A. P., Davies, M., et al.: Fulminant hepatic failure in childhood. Arch. Dis. Child., *55*:252, 1980.

Zieve, L., and Nicoloff, D. M.: Pathogenesis of hepatic coma. Ann. Rev. Med., *26*:143, 1975.

14

URINARY TRACT INFECTIONS

Jerry M. Bergstein, M.D.

Treatment of symptomatic urinary infections is indicated because of the morbidity of the acute infection. Perhaps even more importantly, radiological studies performed subsequent to the detection of infection may lead to the discovery of anatomical lesions (e.g., obstruction, reflux) whose management may prevent on-going kidney damage.

CLINICAL MANIFESTATIONS

After the first few months of life, urinary tract infections are much more common in girls than boys. Beyond the newborn period, urinary tract infections result from fecal organisms ascending the urethra. Although the precise pathogenesis of these infections is unknown, factors that may play a role in the increased susceptibility of females to urinary tract infections include the relatively shorter length of the female urethra and heavy colonization of the perineum by pathogenic organisms. The latter may be related to abnormally high vaginal pH, diminished cervicovaginal antibody, and increased adhesiveness of vaginal and uroepithelial cells to bacteria.

It is important to recognize that the symptoms

of urinary tract infections in children are different from those in adults and that the clinical picture may not suggest the urinary tract as the source of the patient's problems. In newborns, urinary tract infections may be associated with a clinical picture of sepsis, jaundice, vomiting, diarrhea, or failure to thrive. In infants and toddlers, the most common presenting problems are unexplained fever, abdominal pain, failure to thrive, diaper rash, diarrhea, and irritability. It is only in the older child that the presenting complaints resemble those in adults, the most common of which are urgency, abdominal pain, and enuresis.

Physical examination is rarely helpful in the diagnosis of urinary tract infections. Abdominal pain and suprapubic tenderness are occasional findings. Costovertebral angle tenderness may suggest pyelonephritis, and a flank mass may indicate a hydronephrotic kidney. An atonic anal sphincter suggests neurovesical dysfunction. In view of the lack of specific signs and symptoms of urinary tract infections, it is important that this diagnosis be considered in children with unexplained febrile illness.

DIAGNOSIS

The best laboratory technique to confirm the presence of urinary tract infection is the urine culture. Thus, *all children suspected of infection must have a urine culture.* However, other tests can be utilized that suggest the presence of urinary tract infection, and therapy may be started on the basis of these results. But the culture should always be sent!

The most frequently utilized screening test for infection is microscopic evaluation of the urine sediment for leukocytes (pyuria) and bacteria. Several factors limit the reliability of the urinalysis in confirming urinary tract infection. Methods of obtaining the urine, transporting it to the laboratory, centrifuging, resuspending, and analyzing the sediment are extremely variable. Interpretation of the results is clouded by the fact that, although there is a rough correlation between the numbers of leukocytes and bacteria seen in the urine sediment and a positive culture, this correlation is not sufficiently high to confirm the diagnosis of infection. Several studies have demonstrated that urinary tract infection may be present in the absence of pyuria and that pyuria may be the result of processes other than bacterial infection. However, a urine sediment that contains large numbers of white cells and bacteria correlates sufficiently with a positive urine culture that therapy may be initiated on the basis of the sediment findings. But the culture should always be sent!

The quantitative bacterial colony count technique suggests that a colony count exceeding 100,000 per ml of a single organism (more than one organism usually indicates contamination) yields a 95 per cent chance of true infection. This remains the best clinical criterion for the diagnosis of infection in urines obtained by the clean-catch, midstream technique. Counts less than 10,000 per ml generally indicate a contaminated specimen. The significance of counts between 10,000 and 100,000 colonies per ml is unclear, and such cultures should be repeated if possible. If the patient is already on therapy (based on the urine sediment) when a borderline count is obtained, the patient should be considered infected and the course of therapy completed.

Prior to toilet training, urine specimens for culture are commonly obtained using bag devices. Because these devices are easily contaminated, such cultures are significant only if sterile, indicating that infection is absent. Growth of any number of organisms, including greater than 100,000 colonies per ml, must be confirmed by catheterization or suprapubic aspiration cultures. Cultures of urine obtained by the latter techniques indicate infection if the colony counts exceed 1000 per ml. The significance of lower counts is unclear. Even in normal individuals, organisms may ascend the urethra to the bladder, only to be eliminated during voiding. Either technique could obtain some of these organisms, yielding the low colony counts. Since catheterization may introduce organisms into the bladder, the subsequent culture could yield colony counts less than 1000 per ml. Optimally, cultures having counts in this range should be repeated. If the patient is already on therapy when a colony count less than 1000 per ml is obtained, the results of the initial urinalysis should be considered in deciding whether to continue therapy.

No matter which method is used to obtain urine for culture (see Kunin, 1972, for techniques of obtaining urine for culture), it should be sent to the microbiology laboratory on ice and stored at 4°C until cultured. This will avoid proliferation of organisms in the urine after it is voided and a falsely elevated colony count.

TREATMENT

Lower tract infections, the majority of urinary tract infections in children, will be the focus of this discussion. Should upper tract infection (pyelonephritis) be suspected clinically (fever, chills, flank pain, toxic appearance), the child should be hospitalized, a culture obtained, and a parenteral aminoglycoside antibiotic started. An immediate anatomical evaluation (renal scan, intravenous pyelogram, or ultrasound) of the upper tracts should be obtained because pyelonephritis associated with obstruction (e.g., ureteropelvic junction obstruction) cannot be cured until the obstruction is relieved.

The choice of a therapeutic agent in the treatment of lower tract infection depends upon the fact that *Escherichia coli* is the most frequent pathogenic organism (the next most common organisms are Klebsiella, Enterobacter, Proteus, Enterococcus, and *Staphylococcus epidermidis*). Commonly utilized agents to which *E. coli* is susceptible include nitrofurantoin, sulfonamides, ampicillin, and cephalothin derivatives. Nitrofurantoin is preferred as first choice because a greater percentage of coliforms remain susceptible in comparison to the other agents.

Several studies confirm that *10 to 14 days of therapy is adequate for an apparently uncomplicated lower tract infection.* Recent reports suggest that shorter courses of therapy, ranging from one injection of gentamicin or one oral dose of amoxicillin to three days of oral antibiotics, may be equally effective. Until sufficient clinical studies are available to confirm the efficacy of short-term therapies, a full 10-day course is recommended.

It has been common to recommend re-evaluation of the urine (urinalysis and/or culture) during the course of therapy. This is unnecessary if sensitivity studies indicate that the offending organism is susceptible to the antibacterial agent being used. It is important to repeat the urine culture approximately one week after completion of therapy to be certain that the infection has been cured. If the follow-up culture is sterile and subsequent radiographic studies are normal, then surveillance cultures for asymptomatic infections are unnecessary (see below). Further cultures should be obtained only if symptomatic infection is suspected.

X-RAYS

The need for radiographic studies after the first urinary tract infection in a male at any age is clear because of the high frequency of underlying anatomical abnormality. This evaluation should consist of both an intravenous pyelogram and a voiding cystourethrogram.

The need for x-rays after the first infection in females remains controversial. The argument that x-rays should not be performed until after the second infection because urinary tract infections are so common in females is no longer tenable, as 80 per cent of girls who have one infection will have another, usually within a year. The question remains open as to whether the yield ever justifies the performance of x-rays after the first infection in girls. The data available suggest that the chance of detecting a significant anatomical abnormality in girls correlates inversely with age. Thus, radiographic studies are recommended in girls presenting with their first infection under the age of 10 years. In older girls and adults, radiographic studies need be performed only if the patient suffers frequent symptomatic infections.

The radiographic evaluation of a girl younger than three years should consist of an intravenous pyelogram and voiding cystourethrogram. Between ages three and ten years, the initial evaluation should consist of an intravenous pyelogram only. If this study is normal, a voiding study is unnecessary. Low-grade reflux will be missed by this approach but mild reflux in this age group is almost always the result of infection and will disappear if the patient is maintained free of infection. Performance of the cystogram is required if the patient has upper tract abnormalities on the pyelogram or a clinical course of recurrent symptomatic infection despite a normal pyelogram.

A brief word about the role of cystoscopy in the evaluation of the initial urinary tract infection is indicated. *If the radiographic studies are normal, cystoscopy is not indicated.* If reflux is detected in males, cystoscopy is indicated to rule out urethral valves. If reflux is detected in females, cystoscopy is indicated only if the reflux is associated with dilatation of the upper tract. Again, most reflux in females is caused by infection and will disappear if further infection is prevented. The possibility of urethral stenosis in females should not be invoked as a reason for cystoscopy, because that lesion is rare.

PROPHYLAXIS

Despite normal radiographic studies, some girls will have recurrent urinary tract infections, defined as three symptomatic culture-proven infections in a 12-month period. Recurrent infections can be a relapse or reinfection. Relapse refers to recurrence of infection with the same organism that caused the preceding infection.

The organism persists in the upper tract, usually in association with radiographic abnormality of the upper tract. The large majority of recurrent infections in children are reinfections; i.e., each infection is a new one, with the current organism being different from the previous one.

The purpose of long-term (one year) prophylaxis is to prevent these recurrent reinfections. Prophylaxis is accomplished with an agent to which fecal organisms will remain susceptible over the course of therapy. Thus, sulfonamides would not be a good choice because of the rapid development of resistance in the fecal reservoir. The mechanisms whereby successful prophylaxis reduces or eliminates recurrent infections are unknown but may be related to recovery of normal bladder function, alterations in perineal and rectal flora, and impairing adherence of bacteria to uroepithelial cells.

Prior to initiating prophylaxis, existing infection must be eradicated and follow-up culture sterile. An agent of choice for initiating prophylaxis is nitrofurantoin. For the first three months, the same dosage as that used to treat infection (5 to 7 mg/kg/day divided into four doses) is recommended. After three months of prophylaxis, a culture is obtained. If this is sterile, the dose of nitrofurantoin is cut in half and given only twice a day at breakfast and at bed-time. This reduced dosage is continued for the remainder of the year of prophylaxis. Cultures are repeated at three-month intervals during the period of prophylaxis and, of course, promptly should the patient develop symptoms of urinary tract infection. If the urine has remained sterile after completion of one year of prophylaxis, further cultures are unnecessary unless symptoms arise. For the rare patient who will once again suffer recurrent symptomatic infections after completion of one year of prophylaxis, a second year is recommended.

Some patients will suffer recurrent infections while taking nitrofurantoin, while others will not tolerate the drug because of gastrointestinal irritation. These patients should be switched to the combination product containing trimethoprim and sulfamethoxazole. Although studies suggest that this combination is the most effective prophylactic agent, the author prefers to save it for problem patients in the hope of avoiding the development of bacterial resistance. As with nitrofurantoin, a therapeutic dosage is used for the first three months. After a sterile urine culture is obtained, the dose is reduced by half and continued for the remainder of one year of therapy.

MANAGEMENT OF URINARY TRACT INFECTIONS

Clinical Manifestations

History and physical examination may not point to the urinary tract as the source of the illness.

The most common symptoms are unexplained fever, abdominal pain, diarrhea, and enuresis.

Diagnosis

The diagnosis of infection may be suspected by detecting white blood cells and bacteria in the urine sediment.

The diagnosis is confirmed by urine culture.

A colony count of greater than 100,000 colonies per ml of a single organism is the best criterion for infection.

Urine for culture should be sent to the laboratory on ice and maintained at 4°C until cultured.

Treatment

E. coli is the most common organism.

Ten days of nitrofurantoin is recommended.

Be certain to check sensitivity results.

X-rays

After the first infection in a male at any age, perform an intravenous pyelogram and voiding cystourethrogram.

After the first infection in a girl younger than age three, perform both an intravenous pyelogram and a voiding cystourethrogram.

After the first infection in a girl between the ages of three and ten, perform an intravenous pyelogram.

Routine cystoscopy is not indicated.

Prophylaxis

Recurrent infections are defined as three symptomatic culture-proven infections in a 12-month period.

Treat with one year of continuous low-dose therapy.

Screening for Asymptomatic Bacteriuria

Not indicated.

SCREENING FOR ASYMPTOMATIC BACTERIURIA

Several studies indicate that the prevalence of asymptomatic urinary tract infections in girls is between 1 and 3 per cent and that 5 per cent of girls will acquire an asymptomatic infection at some time during the school years (the prevalence of asymptomatic infection in males is so low as not to be considered). With these data in hand, screening for asymptomatic urinary tract infections in girls has been attempted in the hope that (1) early detection and treatment of asymptomatic infection will prevent the morbidity of symptomatic infection, and (2) the subsequent detection of anatomical abnormalities might prevent progressive upper tract damage.

However, *the results of recent studies militate against routine screening for asymptomatic infection.* Asymptomatic infections frequently resolve spontaneously and rarely result in symptomatic infections. Asymptomatic infections may occasionally be associated with upper tract scarring. Yet this scarring, which usually begins before age five, is rarely progressive and does not lead to renal failure. Finally, the treatment of asymptomatic urinary tract infections seems to have no effect on the clearing of reflux, the progression of renal scars, or the later development of hypertension. Thus, the screening of girls for asymptomatic infection cannot be recommended.

REFERENCES

American Academy of Pediatrics Section on Urology. Screening school children for urologic disease. Pediatrics, *60*:239–242, 1977.

Ginsburg, C. M., and McCracken, G. H.: Urinary tract infections in young infants. Pediatrics, *69*:409–413, 1982.

Kunin, C. M.: Detection, Prevention and Management of Urinary Tract Infections. Philadelphia, Lea and Febiger, 1972.

Kunin, C. M.: Duration of treatment of urinary tract infections. Am. J. Med., *71*:849–854, 1981.

Lohr, J. A., et al.: Three-day therapy of lower urinary tract infections with nitrofurantoin macrocrystals: A randomized clinical trial. J. Pediatr., *99*:980–983, 1982.

15

FAINTING

Morris Green, M.D.

Fainting or syncope refers to brief, usually sudden, periods of unconsciousness, loss of postural tone, and falling, due to cerebral ischemia. The history generally provides the most helpful diagnostic information. Careful attention should be given to the circumstances in which the syncope occurred; possible precipitating factors; prodromal symptoms and signs; the suddenness of onset; the duration of the episode; and the occurrence of convulsive movements. A thorough history will often obviate the need for such examinations as an electroencephalogram or fasting blood sugar.

ETIOLOGICAL CLASSIFICATION OF FAINTING

Vasodepressor Syncope (Simple Faint)

Vasodepressor syncope, caused by a sudden and marked fall in blood pressure, is the most common cause of fainting and is usually first noted in adolescence. It may occur when the patient becomes suddenly frightened or threatened by some realistic or fantasized danger. Fainting may also represent a reaction to severe pain or other unpleasant stimulus such as the sight of blood or a needle puncture. Syncope is especially likely to occur in hot, humid, confined quarters; after prolonged motionless standing; when the patient is fatigued; and after fasting. In patients whose syncopal attacks are emotionally induced, anxiety may be overt or evident in frightening dreams. Although psychological factors may cause recurrent fainting spells, especially those not precipitated by apparent cause, they generally do not need to be considered in the single episode.

The simple faint almost always begins with the child standing, although in rare instances it may occur with the patient recumbent. Prodromal symptoms include a feeling of great weakness, generalized numbness, pallor, nausea, excessive salivation, warmth, sweating, lightheadedness, yawning, sighing, blurring of vision, and epigastric discomfort. These antecedent complaints may suddenly terminate in the faint, or they may stop short of that either spontaneously or in response to a head-low position. The interruption of consciousness usually lasts only a few seconds but may persist for several minutes. Clonic movements may ensue if the patient remains unconscious longer than 15 to 20 seconds or if he is held semierect. Symptoms may recur if the patient sits up or stands too quickly. No specific treatment is indicated except to leave the patient recumbent until recovery. With a history of recurrent syncope the child may be instructed to abort the attack by the head-low or recumbent position, walking out of the room when prodromal symptoms are first noted, or attempting to avoid known precipitating situations. The physician will also need to explore the cause for the child's anxiety and proclivity to syncope.

Conversion Reaction

Syncope may also be a symbolic expression of unconscious, repressed instinctual impulses, usually of a sexual or hostile nature and often directed toward a member of the family or other significant person. Such episodes, which are most common in adolescent girls, may also be precipitated by real or fantasized heterosexual experiences. The patient may have a history of repeated episodes of syncope as well as other conversion symptoms. Conversion of the consciously unacceptable impulse to physical expression in the form of syncope permits a partial discharge of these feelings and helps avoid the anxiety that would be engendered by conscious expression or direct gratification of the impulse.

Whereas overt anxiety is frequently noted with vasodepressor syncope, the patient with hysterical syncope often but not always shows little concern. These episodes characteristically occur in the presence of others and are not preceded or accompanied by prodromal symptoms such as nausea, weakness, pallor, and sweating. Hysterical patients may slump or fall in a dramatic fashion, but they avoid injury. They may also faint while sitting or recumbent, unusual positions for vasodepressor syncope. During the episode the patient's eyes may flutter, be held open, or be tightly closed. Moaning, groaning, or other sounds may be noted. Unusual positions and movements may be assumed. The patient may slip in and out of unconsciousness or not be completely unconscious. Interruption of consciousness may persist for seconds or hours. Psychotherapy is indicated to determine the nature of and deal appropriately with the unconscious conflict.

Epilepsy

It is occasionally difficult to differentiate in the history between vasodepressor syncope, breath-holding spells, and epilepsy, since the first two disorders may be accompanied by clonic movements. Syncope due to epilepsy usually lasts longer (generally over 30 seconds) and is more likely to occur with the patient recumbent than is the case with simple syncope.

Cardiac Causes

Occasionally, syncope occurs with exertion in patients with cardiac and flow obstructions such as isolated, marked pulmonic stenosis, and in those with a prolapsed mitral valve, severe aortic stenosis, and hypertrophic obstructive cardiomyopathy, especially after physical exertion, and obstruction of the mitral orifice by a left atrial myxoma. Primary pulmonary hypertension may be characterized by episodes of syncope, especially on effort. Congenital or acquired heart block or cardiac arrhythmias such as paroxysmal tachycardia may decrease cardiac output sufficiently to produce unconsciousness. Attacks of paroxysmal dyspnea in infants with congenital heart disease, e.g., tetralogy of Fallot, may terminate in syncope. Syncope during exercise may be due to an aberrant left coronary artery.

Tussive (Cough) Syncope

Loss of consciousness, usually of short duration, due to cerebral hypoxia may occur after severe paroxysms of coughing, as in children with asthma.

Anemia

Severe anemia may be accompanied by lightheadedness, giddiness, and, rarely, syncope.

Hypoglycemia

Although hypoglycemia does not lead to true syncope, the patient may complain of faintness and exhibit pallor and sweating.

Hyperventilation Syndrome

Hyperventilation may cause lightheadedness, generalized weakness, tingling and numbness of the hands, tetany, or syncope. The physician needs to be alert to the hyperventilation syndrome as a possible cause of syncope in adolescents because patients are more likely to report "blacking-out" spells, seizures, or sensations of smothering, choking, or shortness of breath than overbreathing or tingling and numbness of the hands. Direct questioning or an attempt to reproduce the symptoms by having the patient hyperventilate for a couple of minutes may be necessary. Hyperventilation and syncope may occur after an extreme athletic effort. See also p. 266.

Breath-holding

The breath-holding episode is triggered by some injury, often trivial, or by the child's suddenly becoming angry or frustrated. Vigorous crying is the first manifestation. After a variable period he suddenly gasps or holds his breath until he becomes blue or pale, unconscious, and limp. Convulsive movements or opisthotonus may occur if unconsciousness is prolonged. The history and sequence of events are so characteristic that differential diagnosis generally presents no problem; however, when the precipitating event seems extremely trivial, when there appears to be no triggering circumstance, when the child is said to cry or hold his breath for only a short time, or when the convulsive movements are a prominent clinical feature, differentiation from epilepsy may require an electroencephalogram and further observation.

Some babies seem especially prone to have these spells, and there may be a familial incidence. Although in some cases there appears to be no contributory disturbance in the home or in the mother-infant relation, these need to be explored carefully. Immature parents, maternal depression, inability to set limits on the child, and other difficulties in the maternal-infant interaction need to be dealt with if the spells are to be prevented. Many of these children have an associated iron-deficiency anemia.

Miscellaneous

A. Attacks of syncope lasting from a brief episode to a period of 5 to 10 minutes are rarely associated with the surdocardiac syndrome of congenital deafness, prolonged Q-T interval, and large T waves on the electrocardiogram.
B. Unexplained episodes of unconsciousness have been reported in patients with fused cervical vertebrae.
C. Sudden unconsciousness may be precipitated by needle puncture of the pleural space and after drainage of fluid from the pleural or peritoneal cavities.
D. Postural or orthostatic hypotension is an unusual cause of syncope in children and may occur, as may vasodepressor syncope, when the child has stood motionless for a long time, as in a military or parade formation.
E. Syncopal attacks occur in patients with autoerythrocyte sensitization (psychogenic purpura).

REFERENCES

Engel, G. L.: Fainting, 2nd ed. Springfield, IL, Charles C Thomas, 1962.

Enzer, N. B., and Walker, P. A.: Hyperventilation syndrome in childhood. J. Pediatr., *70*:521, 1967.

Fatnoff, O. D.: The psychogenic purpuras: A review of autoerythrocyte sensitization, autosensitization to DNA, "hysterical" and factitial bleeding, and the religious stigmata. Semin. Hematol., *17*:192, 1980.

Frank, J. P., and Friedberg, D. A.: Syncope with prolonged QT interval. Am. J. Dis. Child., *130*:320, 1976.

Friedberg, C. K.: Syncope: Pathological physiology: Differential diagnosis and treatment. Mod. Conc. Cardiovasc. Dis., *40*:55, 1971.

16

DELIRIUM

Morris Green, M.D.

Delirium, a reversible metabolic encephalopathy, is characterized by a clouding of consciousness that ranges from extreme hyperactivity to coma. Symptoms characteristically fluctuate widely but are generally worse at night. The ability of the delirious patient to sustain his attention is limited, and his conversation may skip abruptly from one topic to another. At one moment he may seem to be in complete contact with his environment, while a few seconds later he does not clearly perceive or understand what is going on. At other times, the impairment in consciousness is steady. Since the sleep-wakefulness cycle is commonly disturbed, the child may be excessively alert and unable to fall asleep at night or may be unusually drowsy during the daytime.

The delirious child may demonstrate great excitement and hyperactivity—running about the room, trying to open the door, struggling with those around him, and thrashing about his bed. The child may pull at his fingertips, reach for imaginary objects, and pick at his clothes. Motor incoordination, incoherent speech, ataxia, tremulousness, and impaired ability to write may be noted. Auditory and visual hallucinations and illusions lead the child to misinterpret shadows; e.g. he may see large bugs on his bed or climbing the walls. Affective states may include fear, anxiety, anger, depression, euphoria, and apathy. Cognitive functions, short-term memory, and comprehension are impaired. The confused older child is unable to answer orientation questions, attend to a task such as sequentially subtracting 7 or 3 from 100, repeat a series of digits backwards, or respond correctly to other components of a mental status examination, e.g., date, time, place.

The etiological classification of delirium is given in Table 16-1. Infectious diseases are an important consideration. In some instances, delirium and fever may be the only presenting symptoms in pneumococcal pneumonia or in encephalitis. Reye's syndrome may be characterized in the prodromal phase by protracted vomiting, lethargy, and disorientation.

A careful history for possible poisoning is indicated in all children with acute delirium, including a review of the contents of medicine cabinets and night tables and all medications taken currently or in the past by the parents or other adults in the household. If no history of a drug ingestion can be obtained, a blood and urine screen for toxic substances should be pursued. Initial symptoms of Jimson weed poisoning include visual illusions, dryness of the mouth, extreme thirst, incoherent speech, confusion, disorientation, stupor, coma, incoordination, and hyperactivity. The pupils are dilated and fixed, and the skin is flushed and dry.

GENERAL MANAGEMENT

The specific cause of delirium, its severity, and the physician's assessment of the parents' ability to care for the child at home will determine the need for hospitalization. Whenever possible, the underlying cause of the delirium should obviously be treated. An ambience of calm should be provided either at home or in

Table 16–1. CAUSES OF DELIRIUM

I. Infectious disorders
   A. Any acute, febrile disease
   B. Pneumococcal or other bacterial pneumonia
   C. Meningitis or encephalitis
   D. Reye's syndrome
   E. Typhoid fever
   F. Rabies
II. Drugs and poisoning
   A. Barbiturates and anticonvulsants
   B. Antihistaminic preparations
   C. Aminophylline toxicity
   D. Corticosteroids
   E. Isoniazid
   F. Jimson weed poisoning
   G. Atropine poisoning
   H. Imipramine poisoning
   I. Amphetamine intoxication
   J. LSD, phencyclidine ("angel dust"), or other psychedelic agent
   K. Gasoline sniffing
   L. Alcohol ingestion
III. Hypoxia, carbon monoxide poisoning
IV. Metabolic, e.g., uremia, hypoglycemia
V. Trauma, e.g., head injury

the hospital. The child needs to be told repeatedly where he is and what is causing his symptoms. He should be assured that he will recover completely in a short time. Delirious patients do best in a quiet room with soft lighting, background music, and absence of shadows and mirrors, and with the mother or other familiar and reassuring, calm person constantly present. A clock, a calendar, and familiar objects in the room may help promote the orientation of older children. Warm packs may occasionally be indicated. In general, sedation should be used with caution. Barbiturates are especially to be avoided. Chloral hydrate, paraldehyde, diazepam, or intramuscular phenothiazine may be used if needed.

17

PRINCIPLES OF EMERGENCY MEDICAL CARE

Paul H. Wise, M.D., M.P.H.

The most dramatic and frightening aspect of clinical practice is providing emergency care to the critically ill child. Fortunately, frank emergencies are rare in most general pediatric practices. Yet, in many ways, emergent conditions are very much an integral part of general pediatric care. A variety of illnesses will be viewed as true emergencies by parents or other caretakers, and the clinician is often confronted with determining whether or not a child is in fact suffering from serious illness. This responsibility requires a basic understanding of the clinical presentations and risks associated with emergent conditions. Pediatricians also provide consultation to the growing number of emergency physicians staffing local emergency facilities. Even when hospital-based physicians direct the child's care, the primary practitioner can often provide the informed support required by all families of critically ill children.

Recommendations regarding emergency equipment should reflect the nature and location of a particular practice. Isolated and some larger practices play an important role in stabilizing critically ill children in the office prior to transfer for definitive care. Other practices may appropriately rely on nearby emergency rooms and require no emergency equipment. The conditions most frequently requiring emergency intervention in a practice setting are those causing respiratory compromise and anaphylaxis. Therefore, basic respiratory equipment, including oral airways, ventilation bag and mask, and oxygen, as well as medications such as epinephrine and anticonvulsants, are useful.

The most helpful way to prepare for potential emergencies is to obtain a working familiarity with local emergency medical systems and backup emergency facilities. Often, important assistance can be provided by emergency medical personnel and transport services based in the community or an affiliated tertiary care center. Great strides have been made in organizing sophisticated regional emergency medical systems. Local practices that have remained in close touch with these services have helped assure that the medical needs and sensitivities of children be fully represented in the development of these new programs.

CARDIORESPIRATORY ARREST

Improvements in prehospital emergency systems, the growing knowledge of cardiopulmonary resuscitation in the general community, and advances in pediatric intensive care have all helped to create an aggressive approach to the resuscitation of children in cardiorespiratory arrest. Although resuscitation is complex and anxiety-provoking, organization of the various aspects of care into a coherent approach improves the quality of the resuscitative effort. One helpful scheme is to view the resuscitation in three interrelated stages (Table 17–1). The first stage is a preparatory phase. Artificial respiration and cardiac massage are begun and other procedures performed to prepare the child for definitive pharmacological intervention. The use of drugs to stimulate cardiac function is considered the second, or interven-

Table 17–1. STAGES IN PEDIATRIC RESUSCITATION

Stage I: Preparation Phase	Stage II: Intervention Phase	Stage III: Stabilization Phase
1. Immediate assessment 2. Initiation of CPR 3. Oxygen and stable airway 4. Role definition 5. History and physical exam 6. EKG 7. Call support services: Anesthesia Respiratory therapy Surgeon Social worker 8. Placement of intravenous line 9. Dextrostix and initial labs: CBC, electrolytes, BUN, creatinine, glucose, calcium, PT, PTT, toxic screen, blood cultures if sepsis suspected, urinalysis, arterial blood gas	1. Medications: Cardiac stimulants Specific antidotes 2. Surgical procedures 3. Supportive measures: Temperature control Intravascular volume control 4. Assessment of cardiorespiratory status: Check pulses with cardiac massage Air movement and chest excursion Arterial blood gases	1. Blood pressure support: Volume control Pressor agents 2. Prepare for transport

tional, stage. The third stage, which begins once a sinus rhythm is obtained, involves efforts to improve perfusion and support the blood pressure.

Cardiorespiratory arrest in children is most commonly respiratory in origin; therefore, the prompt institution of adequate oxygenation and ventilation is of paramount importance. Mouth-to-mouth ventilation should begin as soon as respiration ceases or becomes inadequate. Cardiac massage should be initiated if a pulse cannot be palpated regardless of the presence of heart sounds or complexes on an electrocardiogram. Once artificial respiration and cardiac massage have been instituted, the other components outlined for stage one can be implemented. Substituting bag and mask or endotracheal intubation with 100 per cent oxygen for mouth-to-mouth ventilation, placement of an intravenous line, electrocardiographic monitoring, history, physical examination, and clear definition of professional roles will provide the access and information necessary for the rational use of medications and other definitive interventions.

The first drug that should be administered is oxygen. The institution of adequate oxygenation alone can often stimulate cardiac activity and preclude the need for other cardiotonic medications. Once oxygenation is ensured, sodium bicarbonate, epinephrine, calcium, and dextrose can be administered (Table 17–2). Atropine is useful for bradycardia, whereas lidocaine is indicated when ventricular arrhythmias are present. When difficulty in placing an intravenous line is encountered, epinephrine, atropine, and lidocaine can be given through an endotracheal tube. This route is preferable to intracardiac injection, which may cause significant complications.

The use of the above medications is designed to stimulate a normal cardiac rhythm on electrocardiogram. Cardiac massage should not be terminated, however, until an adequate blood pressure is obtained. Blood pressure support is based upon volume expansion, the use of pressor agents such as dopamine, epinephrine, and isoproterenol, and chronotropic medications designed to increase the heart rate to 150 to 180 per minute in infants and 100 to 120 in young children (Table 17–2).

Throughout the resuscitation process, a concerted effort to maintain communication with the parents must be made. A physician, nurse, or social worker should be designated as the primary person to inform and support the family of the critically ill child during this stressful time.

FOREIGN BODY ASPIRATION

The aspiration of a foreign body is a frequent cause of respiratory distress in young children and the leading cause of injury-related death in infants. The infant and young child are active explorers of their environment and often place objects in their mouth, particularly peanuts, hard candy, gum products, hot dogs, safety pins, and parts of disassembled or poorly designed toys.

The clinical presentation of a child who has

Table 17–2. DRUGS USED IN A RESUSCITATION

Drug	Dose (adult dose)	Preparation	Route*	Indication
Atropine	0.03 mg/kg (0.4 mg)	0.4 mg/cc	IV/IC/IM/ETT	To treat bradycardia and to block vagally mediated bradycardia
Bicarbonate	1–2 mEq/kg/5–10 min (same for adults)	1 mEq/cc	IV/IC	Metabolic acidosis
Elemental calcium	10 mg/kg (300 mg)	CaCl = 27 mg/cc Ca gluconate = 9 mg/cc	IV/IC	Electromechanical dissociation: for positive inotropy and to increase vasomotor tone
Dextrose	0.5 gm/kg (same)	D25 and D50	IV/IC	Presumed hypoglycemia
Epinephrine	0.1 cc/kg (10 cc)	Epi 1:10,000 (10 cc = 1 mg)	IV/IC/ETT	Asystole, bradycardia, hypotension, to coarsen ventricular fibrillation before countershock
Lidocaine	1 mg/kg (50–100 mg)	100 mg/10 cc	IV/IC/ETT	Ventricular ectopy
Narcan	0.01 mg/kg (0.4 mg)	0.4 mg/cc	IV/IC	Opiate intoxication
Pressor Infusions				
Epinephrine	0.01–0.5 μg/kg/min (1–4 μg/min)	1 mg epinephrine in 100 cc D5W; run at body weight (kg) in cc/hr = 0.17 μg/kg/min	IV constant infusion	Hypotension, bradycardia, decreased cardiac contractility
Dopamine	1–30 μg/kg/min (same)	30 mg dopamine in 100 cc D5W; run at body weight in cc/hr = 5 μg/kg/min	IV constant infusion	Low-dose (1–5 μg/kg/min): poor renal perfusion; medium dose (5–15 μg/kg/min): decreased cardiac contractility, bradycardia; high dose (15–30 μg/kg/min): decreased cardiac contractility, hypotension
Isoproterenol	0.01–0.5 μg/kg/min (1–4 μg/min)	Same as epinephrine	IV constant infusion	Bradycardia, hypotension if not caused by hypovolemia

*IV = intravenous; IM = intramuscular; IC = intracardiac; ETT = via the endotracheal tube.

aspirated a foreign body depends upon the relative severity of the obstruction and the adequacy of the subsequent air exchange. Large, elastic, or oddly shaped objects may cause severe obstruction, usually at the laryngeal level, with the child exhibiting the abrupt onset of choking, gagging, high-pitched wheezing, dysphonia, or complete aphonia. The child will initially appear anxious and quite agitated. If the obstruction is not alleviated, progressive signs of deterioration, including cyanosis, lethargy, and ultimately loss of consciousness, will occur.

Although the acute symptoms of severe obstruction can be dramatic, the more common presentation of foreign body aspiration is usually subtle. The actual aspiration may have gone unnoticed or forgotten, whereas the presenting symptoms may reflect the effects either of prolonged obstruction or of secondary infectious or inflammatory processes. The possibility of a foreign body aspiration should be considered in both acute and chronic pulmonary conditions in young children despite the absence of a specific history of aspiration.

The subacute clinical manifestations of a foreign body in the airway are generally related to the anatomical level of obstruction. Laryngeal foreign bodies usually present with hoarseness, discomfort, a persistent, high-pitched, "croupy" cough, and, at times, dyspnea with or without stridor. Tracheal foreign bodies are classically associated with a palpable "thump" and audible "slap" upon expiration as the object strikes the subglottic region; however, persistent wheezing or coughing may be the only symptoms. The bronchus, the right more commonly than the left, is the most common site for a foreign object to lodge. Localized or unilateral wheezing, air trapping, or atelectasis suggests a bronchial foreign body. Bacterial infection may develop distal to the obstruction and clinically mimic pneumonia.

The treatment of the young child who has aspirated a foreign body depends upon the severity of the obstruction. When air exchange is inadequate, as evidenced by the aphonia, cyanosis, or obvious distress, immediate intervention is mandatory. Various mechanical maneuvers have been recommended to expel the foreign body; however, intense controversy persists as to their respective safety and utility. The American Heart Association and the American Academy of Pediatrics recommend four back blows followed by four chest thrusts, both administered with the child's head placed lower than his trunk. The abdominal thrust (Heimlich maneuver) is not recommended because of the danger of injury to the abdominal organs. Blind finger sweeps in search of the foreign body are also discouraged, as they may push the offending object further down the airway. If the back blows and chest thrusts prove ineffective, the jaw should be lifted and mouth opened in an effort to visualize and then remove the foreign body.

Others, pointing out that back blows have been shown to be counterproductive in experimental models, discourage their use. Still others argue that the abdominal thrust has been effective in adults and the dangers to children are minimal. Resolution of these conflicting views must await further study. Until that time it seems reasonable to utilize the back blows and chest thrusts as recommended by the AHA and AAP, but if this intervention proves ineffective, a cautiously administered abdominal thrust is warranted.

If a child with an upper airway obstruction becomes unconscious, mouth-to-mouth or bag and mask ventilation with 100 per cent oxygen is indicated. As few foreign body obstructions are complete, these measures are usually effective if high pressures are used. Chest wall excursion should be monitored to assess the adequacy of air exchange. If ventilation remains inadequate despite repositioning the head and rechecking equipment, an emergency cricothyrotomy is indicated. A large bore needle or catheter (14- or 16-gauge) can be inserted into the trachea through the cricothyroid membrane. Emergency placement of a tracheostomy tube may be attempted if personnel skilled in this procedure are readily available. These invasive emergency procedures are rarely required, however, and should be utilized only when the child's status is deteriorating and the steps outlined above are ineffective.

No attempt to mobilize an aspirated foreign body should be made unless the air exchange is inadequate. If the child is pink, can vocalize normally and produce a vigorous cough, and is not in imminent danger of decompensation, no mechanical maneuvers should be attempted. An effort should be made to localize the nature and location of the object through roentgenographic examination (AP and lateral neck, PA, lateral, lateral decubitus, and fluoroscopic chest), with removal through bronchoscopy under optimal conditions.

SUPRAGLOTTITIS (EPIGLOTTITIS)

Supraglottitis, a local inflammatory process of the entire supraglottic area (not just the epiglottis), primarily caused by *Hemophilus influenzae* type B, usually affects children less than five years of age but can occur in adolescents and adults as well. A rapid, potentially fatal infection that causes progressive airway obstruction at the laryngeal level, supraglottitis generally appears abruptly with fever and dysphagia. The latter usually begins as refusal to eat or drink, followed by pooling saliva in the mouth and drooling. The child usually prefers sitting up with his head and jaw protruding forward in an effort to maximize the caliber of the airway (Fig. 17–1). Laryngeal pain or a cough may also occur, but a gutteral inspiratory stridor is a hallmark of respiratory embarrassment. The triad of fever, dysphagia, and respiratory compromise makes diagnostic consideration of supraglottitis imperative.

The diagnosis of supraglottitis is based primarily upon the history and clinical appearance of the child. Whenever the diagnosis is suspected, an effort should be made to avoid disturbing the child, as struggling or crying increases the likelihood of acute obstruction or exhaustion. Allowing the child to remain in the arms of a parent and deferring all physical and laboratory examination (except perhaps the pulse and auscultation of the chest—both helpful in assessing the adequacy of air exchange) until the airway has been stabilized is essential. Direct visualization of the epiglottis is not recommended in a setting where successful emergency intubation or tracheostomy cannot be ensured. An enlarged "raspberry" colored epi-

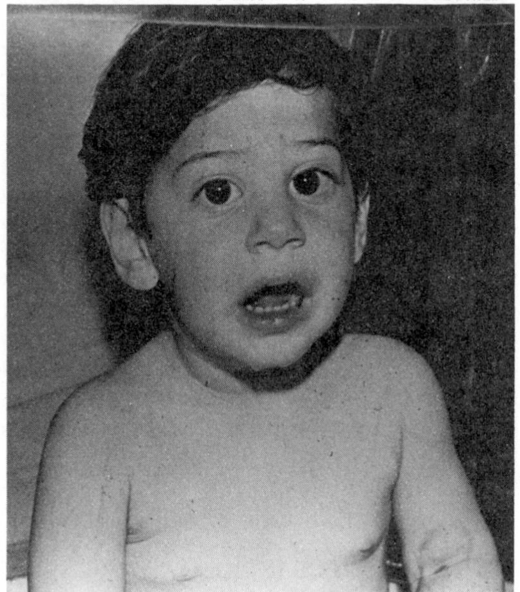

Figure 17–1. Supraglottitis with characteristic posture, protruding jaw, and drooling. (Photograph by permission of Blair Fearon, M.D., Hospital for Sick Children, Toronto, Canada.)

glottis is characteristic; however, the inflammatory process may be confined to the area of the aryepiglottis. A normal-appearing epiglottic tip may therefore be misleading. In addition, irritation of the tongue or pharynx may induce laryngeal spasm, critically obstructing an already compromised airway. If the diagnosis is unclear and air exchange is adequate, a lateral neck soft tissue roentgenogram is indicated. A swollen "thumb-shaped" epiglottis, obscured vallecula, enlarged hypopharynx, and straightening of the cervical spine are the cardinal roentgenographic features of supraglottitis (Fig. 17–2). When the child appears to be in significant or impending respiratory distress, roentgenographic studies should be omitted and all efforts concentrated upon control of the airway.

The primary goal of management of the child with supraglottitis is the stabilization of the airway. All other concerns are of secondary importance. No blood samples should be taken nor intravenous line inserted until a stable airway has been placed. All children with supraglottitis must be admitted to the hospital and receive an artificial airway (either a tracheostomy or tracheal intubation). Admission for observation and antibiotic therapy alone is not recommended. For many years tracheostomy was customary; however, the relative safety and efficacy of tracheal intubation has made this technique preferable in most settings. The choice between tracheostomy and tracheal intubation depends on the competencies of available medical and nursing staff for initial tube placement as well as continued resources for intensive supportive care. In facilities whose staff has little experience in caring for the intubated child, tracheostomy may, in fact, be a wiser choice of airway management. Regardless of which procedure is planned, it should

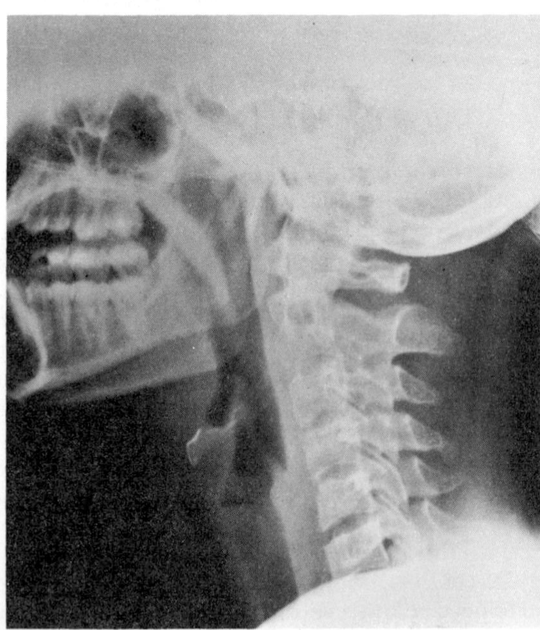

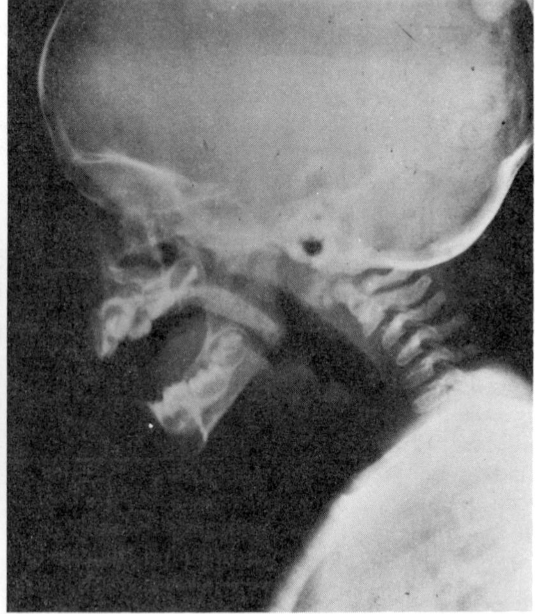

Figure 17–2. Lateral neck soft tissue roentgenograms. *A*, Normal child. *B*, Supraglottitis, with enlarged "thumb-like" epiglottis, obscured vallecula, and enlarged hypopharynx.

be performed in a controlled setting, usually an operating room. Until the operating room is reached, the child should be accompanied by personnel and equipment capable of emergency intubation or tracheostomy, and humidified oxygen administered by mask, if tolerated, or by a funnel held by a parent. Once the airway has been placed, a complete blood count and blood and epiglottic swab cultures should be obtained and a stable intravenous line placed. Chloramphenicol, 25 mg/kg every 6 hours, should be given intravenously. Ampicillin, 50 mg/kg every 6 hours, is adequate if ampicillin-resistant *H. influenzae* is not a local concern. With the airway ensured and antibiotic therapy instituted, improvement is rapid. Extubation is usually possible after 24 to 48 hours, but antibiotic therapy should be continued for at least seven days.

STATUS EPILEPTICUS

Almost 5 per cent of all children experience at least one seizure before they reach the age of 15. Most seizures last only seconds or minutes; however, some seizures may be prolonged. When seizures persist longer than 20 minutes or recur before the patient's full recovery to a normal mental status, the condition is termed *status epilepticus.* Whereas the evidence that a prolonged convulsive state will directly damage neuronal cells is growing, the primary dangers lie in the metabolic disturbances it may induce and the complications of injudicious medical intervention. Hypoxia, hypoglycemia, respiratory and metabolic acidosis, hyperpyrexia, increased intracranial pressure, and hyperkalemia are all recognized complications of status epilepticus; respiratory depression, hypotension, and cardiac arrhythmias are complications of anticonvulsant therapy.

The history should be directed at identifying precipitating events and underlying disease processes. Special attention should be paid to the nature and duration of seizure activity; the presence of fever or other symptoms including stiff neck, headache, and poor appetite; and the possibility of recent trauma or toxic ingestion. A history of previous seizures, medications, and compliance, as well as a careful family history of seizure disorders, should also be reviewed. The physical examination should be directed toward assessing the adequacy of respiratory status and elucidating the underlying etiology of the seizure. Vital signs, the skin (cyanosis, hypopigmented areas, perfusion, signs of trauma), chest wall excursion, and air movement should be carefully examined. Evidence of sepsis or bleeding disorders (petechiae, purpura) should also be carefully considered. A full neurological examination, including pupil size and reactivity, disc margins, muscle tone, and reflexes may provide important diagnostic information.

The treatment of the child in status epilepticus must begin with the assurance of adequate cardiorespiratory function. Continuous monitoring of vital signs, chest excursion, and breath sounds will provide critical data regarding the adequacy of respiratory efforts. At times, arterial blood gas determinations will be necessary to gauge more fully the degree of hypoxemia, hypercapnia, and acidosis that may be present. If significant respiratory embarrassment is suspected, artificial bag and mask ventilation with 100 per cent oxygen should be initiated and, if required, endotracheal intubation performed. Once the airway has been successfully managed, blood for immediate bedside glucose determination (Dextrostix), electrolytes, urea nitrogen, creatinine, calcium, magnesium, toxic screen, and, when appropriate, anticonvulsant levels should be drawn. A stable intravenous line should be started using a dextrose-containing solution (5 or 10 per cent with 0.25 or 0.50 normal saline). A child in status epilepticus may require large amounts of dextrose to maintain blood glucose levels of 100 to 150 mg/dl.

The use of anticonvulsant agents is aimed at terminating seizure activity without significant suppression of cardiorespiratory status. Diazepam (Valium) is effective in quickly terminating seizures; however, it is short-acting and can be relied upon for only a transient effect of 10 to 20 minutes. The initial dose should be 0.1 to 0.25 mg/kg given as a slow intravenous push (no faster than 1 mg/minute). The maximum initial dose is 10 mg. If no response is obtained after 15 minutes, a second dose of 0.25 to 0.4 mg/kg (maximum of 15 mg) can be administered. Diazepam is a well-known cause of respiratory depression and should be given only when staff and equipment required for assisted ventilation are available. Phenytoin (Dilantin) is the most important anticonvulsant in the treatment of status epilepticus. With an onset of action between 20 to 40 minutes, it is quite effective when used in conjunction with diazepam. After diazepam is administered, phenytoin should be given at a dose of 10 to 15 mg/kg infused intravenously over a 20-minute period. As cardiac arrhythmias are the major adverse effect of phenytoin, careful cardiac monitoring is warranted. If the seizure has not been terminated after diazepam and phenytoin administration, paraldehyde and/or phenobarbital can be given. Paraldehyde can be administered rectally in a dose of 0.3 to 0.4 ml/kg (maximum 8 ml) diluted in peanut or corn oil (10 parts oil to 1 part paraldehyde). Phenobarbital is given intravenously over 10 to 15 minutes at a dose of 10 mg/kg. Once phenobarbital is given, great care should be taken in using diazepam, as respiratory depression is far more common when these two drugs are used together than when either is used alone. Intramuscular injection of phenobarbital should be discouraged, as it has an extremely variable uptake and makes more difficult the subsequent use of diazepam. If an intravenous line placement proves difficult, paraldehyde per rectum can supplement careful airway control. If seizure activity persists beyond 60 minutes despite the therapy discussed above, general anesthesia may be indicated; however, in prolonged, unresponsive seizures, a purposeful effort to rule out underlying etiologic conditions is imperative. Neurological infection, trauma, increased intracranial pressure, bleeding from congenital vascular anomalies, toxic ingestions, and hypertension should always be carefully considered.

NEAR-MISS SUDDEN INFANT DEATH

Sudden infant death syndrome (SIDS) is the general term used to describe the unexpected death without identifiable cause of previously well infants. It appears to be the leading cause of death in the United States among infants one week to one year of age. Usually these infants die in their sleep without apparent agonal motion or distress. Occasionally, however, parents will note the child to be cyanotic, limp, and without respirations, and, either through stimulation or the initiation of cardiopulmonary resuscitation, will successfully abort what many feel to be a SIDS episode. A growing body of evidence suggests that these infants are at great risk of subsequent SIDS episodes.

The history should review the events surrounding the episode to gauge its severity and explore the possibility of an underlying disorder. Seizures, sepsis, meningitis, gastroesophageal reflux with secondary choking or aspiration, trauma, or ingestion of toxic substances can all present as a near-miss episode. The physical examination should be directed toward ensuring that the child is in no immediate danger and identifying or excluding an underlying disorder. A careful examination, particularly of the respiratory and neurological systems, is mandatory. An abnormal general appearance, temperature, respiratory rate or rhythm, pulse, or blood pressure suggests an ongoing disease process. Laboratory tests are indicated with any significant near-miss episode. A CBC with white cell differential, electrolytes, bedside and laboratory glucose, calcium, BUN, creatinine, and urinalysis are standard screening tests. Lumbar puncture and blood and urine cultures are required if an infectious process is suspected. A chest roentgenogram will help rule out aspiration, congenital heart disease, and pneumonia.

Infants experiencing a near-miss SIDS episode usually require hospital admission for a short period of observation and monitoring. This allows an opportunity to evaluate the infant more thoroughly and to provide the education and support these families require. If the evaluation suggests sepsis, antibiotic therapy should be instituted until cultures prove negative. Continuous cardiac monitoring for at least 24 to 48 hours is usually warranted, and pneumography and electroencephalography are usually required. Abnormalities in these examinations or observed repeat episodes require that a sophisticated and detailed outpatient management plan be adopted. This is best accomplished at or guided by a medical center skilled in evaluating and managing infants with apnea. Their expertise and commitment to follow-up care offer an invaluable resource for the practicing clinician.

MENINGITIS

The clinical presentation of a child with meningitis depends upon the age of the child. Infants may show only nonspecific signs such as poor feeding, lethargy, irritability, vomiting, and fever; however, a bulging fontanelle, seizure activity, or nuchal rigidity may more specifically indicate the presence of meningitis. In older children, signs of meningeal irritation are usually more prominent, including nuchal rigidity and Brudzinski's or Kernig's signs.

When meningitis is suspected, an examination of the cerebrospinal fluid is required. In bacterial meningitis, the cell count is typically greater than 100 white cells per cubic millimeter, with a predominance of polymorphonuclear leukocytes. At times, the presence of high numbers of white cells will turn the CSF cloudy and in severe cases, grossly purulent. The protein level is elevated (normal range 12 to 23 mg/dl), and the CSF glucose level is usually depressed to less than half the serum glucose level. Gram stain of the CSF is imperative. Important etiologic clues can be obtained, and if *Neisseria meningitidis* or *Hemophilus influenzae* is seen, prophylaxis of exposed family and hospital personnel should be carried out. Rarely pathogenic bacteria (particularly in cases of severe *N. meningitidis*) may be present on Gram stain despite a largely normal cell count. Latex fixation and countercurrent immune electrophoresis techniques have proved useful in rapidly confirming the presence of bacterial products in the CSF.

Viruses, fungi, neoplasms, and *Mycobacterium tuberculosis* may all cause meningitis. Viral or "aseptic" meningitis, which commonly occurs in summer outbreaks, usually presents in a more benign fashion. The CSF cell count is usually below 200 per cubic millimeter with a preponderance of mononuclear cells. Early in their course, some cases of viral meningitis may be characterized by a high number of polymorphonuclear cells. A repeat lumbar puncture six to eight hours after the first will usually reveal a significant shift to mononuclear cells if the infection is indeed viral. Glucose and protein determinations are usually normal.

The treatment of bacterial meningitis must be immediate. Antibiotic therapy should be administered without delay. Intravenous chloramphenicol and ampicillin should be employed until the definitive sensitivities of cultured organisms are known. Careful vital sign measurement is critical, since hypotension and respiratory failure are well-known complications. If the blood pressure is normal, fluid therapy should be held to approximately two thirds of maintenance requirements in the hope of minimizing the danger of increased intracranial pressure. In infants, a baseline measurement of head circumference on admission is useful to help gauge the later possibility of ventricular enlargement or subdural collections.

At times a child with bacterial disease will present in extremis with respiratory insufficiency, obtundation, or hypotension. In these cases, diagnostic tests including CSF examination should be deferred until antibiotics are given and vital signs stabilized.

When the clinical presentation and CSF examination suggest viral meningitis, hospital admission is not usually required. If the child acts and feeds normally and close outpatient follow-up care can be ensured, most of these children can be safely managed at home.

REFERENCES

Bates, J.: Epiglottitis: Diagnosis and treatment. Pediatr. Rev., *1*:173, 1979.

Bell, W., and McCormick, W.: Neurologic Infections in Children. Philadelphia, W. B. Saunders Co., 1975.

Crone, R. K.: Acute circulatory failure in children. Pediatr. Clin. North Am., *27*:525, 1980.

Feigin, R., and Dodge, P.: Bacterial meningitis: Newer concepts of pathophysiology and neurologic sequelae. Pediatr. Clin. North Am., *23*:541, 1976.

Gould, J. B., and James, O.: Management of the near-miss infant: A personal perspective. Pediatr. Clin. North Am., *26*:857, 1979.

Greensher, J., and Mofenson, H. C.: Emergency treatment of the choking child. Pediatrics, *70*:110, 1982.

Heimlich, H. J.: First aid for choking children. Pediatrics, *70*:120, 1982.

Orlowski, J. P.: Cardiopulmonary resuscitation in children. Pediatr. Clin. North Am., *27*:495, 1980.

Rothner, A. D., and Erenberg, G.: Status epilepticus. Pediatr. Clin. North Am., *27*:592, 1980.

18

POISONING IN CHILDREN AND ADOLESCENTS

Frederick H. Lovejoy, Jr., M.D., and Claire Chafee-Bahamon, M.S.

Accidental ingestion or inhalation of potentially poisonous products is one of the most common medical emergencies pediatricians face. Every year 850,000 incidents of poison exposure involving children under five years of age are reported to poison centers. Five to seven per cent in this age group experience such an incident in any given year.

Definition

Poisoning is the result of an ingestion, inhalation, or rectal, dermal, or subcutaneous exposure to a foreign substance, such as a medication, chemical, or biological product of plant or animal origin, in excessive dose.

CLINICAL ASSESSMENT

History

Effective management of the overdosed victim depends on rapid identification of the ingested substance and a clear assessment of clinical severity. Identification and management have been facilitated by (a) improved labeling and identification of dangerous toxins as carried out by the Consumer Products Safety Commission, (b) improved technical staffs and informational sources (computer-generated microfiche systems) as offered by regional poison control centers (Temple and Mancini, 1980), (c) formal training of medical toxicologists with certification by the American Board of Medical Toxicology, as well as advanced training of pharmacists and nurses in the area of clinical toxicology, and finally (d) current data, compiled by the National Clearinghouse for Poison Control Centers as well as by large regional centers, enumerating drugs, household products, and biological toxins to which children and adolescents are most frequently exposed, or from which morbidity, hospitalization, or death may ensue.

When the poisoned patient is presented either by telephone or brought directly to a treatment facility, initial information should include (a) confirmation that a toxic exposure has occurred, (b) identification of the toxic agent(s), (c) determination of the time of ingestion, route, and magnitude (dose of exposure), (d) assessment of the severity of the exposure by ascertainment of the condition of the victim, and (e) determination of the safety of home therapy. With children, the ingested product is generally known. In the case of adolescents, identification is often difficult. For all ages, knowledge of medicines used in the home setting as well as drugs abused locally is helpful. While the precise quantity of ingested product is often difficult to ascertain, estimates are often useful. In the case of liquids, a swallow in a young child is equivalent to 2 to 5 ml. In the case of ingestion of tablets or capsules, it is often helpful to know how many were present in the bottle or container before the incident. When recommending therapy, it is important to use the largest estimated amount to which the victim may have been exposed. When more than one child may have been exposed, it should be assumed that each child consumed the total amount of ingested agent, with each child then treated accordingly. Knowing that the product is not a caustic or a petroleum distillate hydrocarbon and that the child is not convulsing, obtunded, or comatose allows one to proceed in the uncertain situation to removal of the ingested product.

Physical Examination

Pertinent aspects of the physical condition of the child may be determined rapidly over the telephone or by direct clinical examination. The state of consciousness and the rate of progress of clinical illness are of considerable importance. Heart rate, blood pressure, reflexes, response to verbal and painful stimuli, and pupillary signs and response to light are important in the physical examination. Repeated careful physical examinations utilizing known grading systems are helpful in defining the severity of the ingestion and its subsequent rate of improvement or worsening. These systems are also useful in assessing response to antidotal therapy. Grading systems for hyperactivity and coma are presented in Table 18–1.

Signs and symptoms, although often nonspecific, may point to a diagnosis and in certain instances may permit identification of the poi-

Table 18–1. CLASSIFICATION OF HYPERACTIVITY AND COMA

CLASSIFICATION OF HYPERACTIVITY
Grade 1—Restlessness, tremor, hyper-reflexia, sweating, mydriasis, flushing
Grade 2—Confusion, hyperactivity, hypertension, hyperpyrexia, tachypnea
Grade 3—Delirium, mania, tachycardia, arrhythmias, severe hypertension
Grade 4—All of the above plus convulsions, coma, hypotension
CLASSIFICATION OF COMA
Grade 1—Drowsy, but can be aroused and can answer questions
Grade 2—Coma, withdraws to minimal painful stimuli, reflexes intact
Grade 3—Coma, withdraws to maximal painful stimuli, reflexes depressed
Grade 4—Coma, fails to respond to maximal painful stimuli, respiratory and/or cardiovascular depression

son, particularly when a constellation of signs and symptoms (toxidromes) (Table 18–2) is considered together (Mofenson and Greensher, 1975). Specific signs and symptoms often generate a useful list of potential toxic agents. For example, miosis is generally seen with narcotics, cholinergic agents, hallucinogens such as phencyclidine, and a limited number of sedative drugs, including phenothiazines, barbiturates, alcohol, and benzodiazepines (Mitchell et al., 1976). Mydriasis is seen with sympathomimetic agents such as amphetamines, cocaine, and hallucinogens; anticholinergic toxins such as tricyclic antidepressants, antihistamines, atropine and scopolamine type drugs, and certain plants; and withdrawal from narcotics, alcohol, and barbiturates. Lists of clinical manifestations with their most frequently associated drugs or household products are given in a number of reviews (Lovejoy, 1980). The physical examination should also include careful assessment of body or breath odors, which help to identify a limited number of toxins (for example, bitter almonds for cyanide, wintergreen for methyl salicylates) as well as abnormal colors in the urine (orange for pyridium or red for fava beans).

Screening Tests

A limited number of rapid screening tests exist. The roentgenogram of the abdomen will often demonstrate the presence of radiopaque drugs or chemicals, most commonly heavy metals (lead, arsenic, mercury, thallium, etc.), iron-containing products, and less consistently phenothiazines, chloral hydrate, and tricyclic antidepressants. Further, an x-ray taken following gastrointestinal decontamination will demonstrate the adequacy of the various removal procedures. The ferric chloride examination performed on urine or serum is a useful means of identifying salicylates and phenothiazines. Ten ml of urine is boiled to remove ketone bodies, and 5 to 10 drops of 10 per cent ferric chloride solution is then added. A burgundy red color will identify salicylates; a green-purple color, phenothiazines. Methemoglobinemia is identified by exposure of venous blood to room air. A chocolate color in the blood that does not change on exposure to air indicates the presence of oxidized hemoglobin and identifies the need to search for agents (nitrites, nitrates, analine, sulfonamides, phenacetin, nitroglycerin, benzocaine, etc.) capable of producing methemoglobinemia. Measurement of the anion gap is useful to identify toxins, such as methanol and ethylene glycol, whose metabolites (formic and glycolic acid, respectively) are capable of producing this change. The serum sodium plus potassium should equal the bicarbonate plus chloride plus twelve. A gap exceeding twelve indicates the presence of an active anion, suggesting exposure to methanol, ethylene glycol, salicylates, paraldehyde, etc. (Emmett and Marins, 1977). An elevated serum osmolarity above calculated (calculated $= 2 \times$ serum sodium $+$ BUN/3 $+$ blood glucose/18) will identify ingested toxins (ethanol, isopropyl alcohol, methanol) capable of producing an elevated serum osmolarity.

Diagnostic Trials

Ingested toxins may also be identified through the use of pharmacological trials. Examples include (a) naloxone hydrochloride for the identification of narcotics, (b) physostigmine hydrochloride for anticholinergic poisons, (c) deferoxamine for iron poisoning, with subsequent production of a red-colored urine identifying iron complexed to deferoxamine, (d) atropine for reversal of cholinergic effects of organophosphate insecticides, and finally (e) diphenhydramine for reversal of extrapyramidal tract signs induced by phenothiazines (Lovejoy,

Table 18–2. TOXIDROMES

Anticholinergic Agents—Agitation, hallucinations, dilated pupils, dry skin, tachycardia, flushing, fever, arrhythmias
Narcotic Agents—Miosis, coma, respiratory depression
Cholinergic Agents—Salivation, lacrimation, vomiting, diarrhea, miosis, pulmonary congestion
Phenytoin—Slurred speech, nystagmus, confusion, staggering gait
Salicylates—Vomiting, fever, hyperpnea
Extrapyramidal Tract Signs of Phenothiazines—Torsion of the head and neck, ataxia, opisthotonus, oculogyric crisis

1980). Naloxone hydrochloride is used frequently, both as a diagnostic trial and for purposes of therapy, in patients who are comatose and who demonstrate constricted pupils, respiratory depression, hypotension, or central nervous system depression. Doses for each of the five diagnostic trials are given in Table 18–3.

The Toxic Screen

A specific diagnosis is established by laboratory analysis carried out on biological fluids; the qualitative screen is performed on blood or urine, while the quantitative screen is performed on blood. Analysis of gastric contents is no longer carried out. Blood and urine should optimally be obtained two to four hours following ingestion. Qualitative analysis will determine what has been taken. Quantification will determine how much has been taken and will give data relative to the severity of the ingestion.

Small volume distribution drugs (for example, aspirin, acetaminophen, and theophylline) have distributions less than 1 L/kg, are most easily identified from blood (with quantitative data that are useful in assessing severity), and are amenable to enhanced removal through the kidneys or by dialysis. Large volume distribution drugs (for example, tricyclic antidepressants and narcotics) have volumes of distribution of greater than 1 L/kg, and therefore offer data that are less meaningful in interpreting severity.

Table 18–3. DIAGNOSTIC TRIALS—AGENTS AND DOSES

Poisons	Agents	Doses
Narcotic drugs	Naloxone hydrochloride	0.03 mg/kg/dose, I.V., given twice, divided by 2 to 3 minutes
Anticholinergic drugs	Physostigmine salicylate	0.5–2 mg/dose, I.V., given slowly over 2 to 3 minutes
Cholinergic drugs	Atropine	0.05 mg/kg/dose, I.V. (0.4 mg/ml) every 2 to 5 minutes
Iron	Deferoxamine	50 mg/kg/dose, I.M., not to exceed 2 gm
Extrapyramidal tract signs of phenothiazines	Diphenhydramine	2 mg/kg/dose, I.V.

They generally are not amenable to enhanced diuresis or dialysis. Qualitative identification of an ingested product, coupled with clinical assessment and pharmacological data, allows for a logical approach to management. Quantification is useful if a body of literature exists to interpret the meaning of that level and if a therapeutic action (such as the use of an antidote, hemodialysis, or hemoperfusion) is possible. Acetaminophen, aspirin, iron, methanol, theophylline, phenobarbital, carbon monoxide, lithium, heavy metals, and tricyclic antidepressants are examples of toxins for which a serum level is helpful in clinical management.

The ability of the toxic screen to identify accurately and reliably an ingested agent is unclear. In one study, a false negative rate of 30 to 50 per cent and a false positive rate of less than 1 per cent were determined; that is, the toxic screen was able to identify an ingested product with 93 per cent accuracy, while missing an ingested product 30 to 50 per cent of the time (Inglefinger et al., 1980). Failure to identify qualitatively a toxin in a suspected overdose should suggest the need to resubmit a biological sample for repeat laboratory analysis.

TREATMENT

Toxicological Principles

In the case of the child less than five, the overdose is usually accidental, while in the adolescent it is purposeful (suicidal or abuse). The etiology for exposures of children between six and twelve years is unclear. Most clinicians believe, however, that the poisoning in this age group is not accidental, and the physician should approach the victim with an intent to ascertain the existence of potential underlying psychopathology.

Exposure is generally by ingestion, although poisoning may occur by inhalation (carbon monoxide poisoning), by the rectal route (poisoning from aminophylline suppositories), and by the cutaneous route (insecticide poisoning). Ingestions are generally acute but chronic ingestions are recognized with difficulty. Target organs of involvement include the central nervous system (benzodiazepines and barbiturates), the lungs (paraquat, petroleum distillate hydrocarbons), the cardiovascular system (tricyclic antidepressants, digitalis preparations), the liver (acetaminophen, amanita phalloides), the kidneys (ethylene glycol, aminoglycoside antibiotics), the vasculature (iron-containing products), the skin (petroleum distillate hydrocarbons, hydrofluoric acid), the gastrointestinal tract (caustic products), and the hair, eyebrows, and nails (arsenic and other metals).

Awareness of pharmacokinetic principles will improve management of the acute overdose. Absorption in the case of the acute overdose is generally rapid, with onset of symptoms between one and four hours following ingestion. Liquids are absorbed more rapidly than solids, with peak serum levels occurring between one and two hours following ingestion. Delayed absorption occurs in situations where gastric motility is depressed (narcotics and anticholinergic poisons), and with massive ingestions where concretions are formed (meprobamate and aspirin overdoses). Further, in certain instances, onset of symptoms may be delayed, e.g., acetaminophen, paraquat, and amanita phalloides mushroom poisoning. The LD_{50} is less useful for treating the acute overdose because this concept disregards factors such as accuracy of history, rate and extent of absorption of the ingested agent, metabolism or disposition of the ingested agent, and the clinical response of the patient. Once an agent is absorbed, it is distributed in the central (vascular) and peripheral compartments (soft tissues, liver, spleen, and bone). Small volume distribution drugs are distributed primarily in the vascular compartment with their distribution approximating body water. Large volume distribution drugs are distributed in sites predominantly outside of the vascular compartment. With certain drugs this distribution may be extensive (as for example, digoxin, digitoxin, and tricyclic antidepressants). The half-life in overdose is most generally prolonged (an exception being digitalis preparations, for which the half-life is shortened). Prolongation of half-life occurs when mechanisms of removal are saturated. Specific half-lives for most overdoses are not possible to give owing to varying rates of saturation of elimination (saturation kinetics). Elimination of an ingested product occurs through the liver or kidneys. The liver may toxify the parent compound to more active metabolites. Common examples include the conversion of methanol to its toxic product formic acid, glutethamide to its active hydroxylated intermediate, imipramine to its metabolically active product desipramine, ethylene glycol to glycolic acid and other intermediates, and acetaminophen to its toxic intermediates. In these instances, the clinician must prevent the generation of toxic intermediates or augment their removal by dialysis or enhanced urinary excretion. Renal excretion is important for the elimination of certain drugs (examples include many antibiotics, salicylates, bromides, and lithium). Decreased glomerular filtration, as well as an acid urine for salicylates, or an alkaline urine for amphetamines and phencyclidine, may be responsible for delaying normal excretion of these toxins.

Therapeutic intervention is best considered in light of the pharmacological model (Fig. 18–1) whose therapeutic interventions include (a) gastrointestinal decontamination (ipecac-induced emesis, gastric lavage, activated charcoal, cathartics, constant nasogastric suction, and repetitive activated charcoal), (b) alteration in the central and peripheral distribution of drugs (by alteration of protein binding sites or adjustment of pH), (c) enhanced excretion through the gastrointestinal tract (repetitive activated charcoal, binding of endogenously generated metabolites) and alteration of renally excreted drugs (fluid, osmotic, ionized diuresis), (d) the use of dialysis (peritoneal dialysis, hemodialysis, he-

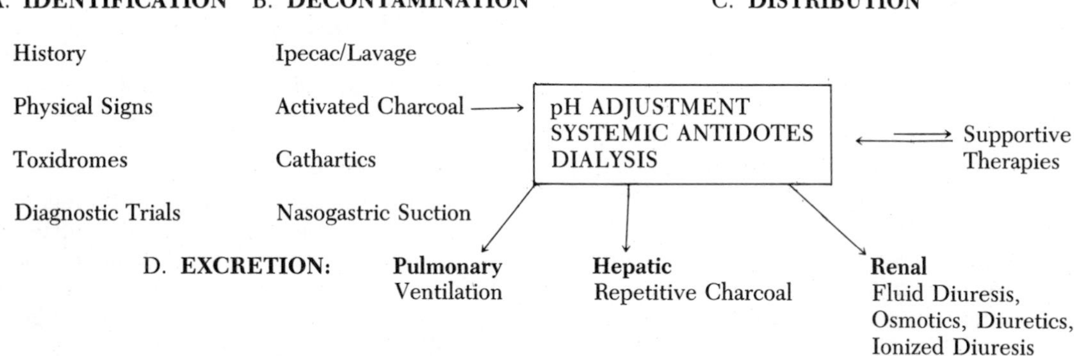

Figure 18–1. Approaches to diagnosis and clinical management for the poisoned patient

moperfusion, exchange transfusion), (e) the use of systemic antidotes, and finally (f) supportive care (for central nervous system depression or stimulation, shock, pulmonary edema, and acidosis).

Decontamination Principles

Decisions concerning the removal of ingested products are among the most common and critical in the initial management of the acute overdose (Easom and Lovejoy, 1979). The patient's level of consciousness is most important in this decision because of the risk of aspiration. Emesis should not be induced if the patient is already obtunded or comatose or if the onset of action of the ingested product is sufficiently rapid that obtundation may occur at the time of emesis. The presence of convulsions is also a contraindication to removal of a toxin by emesis. The risk of leaving the ingested product in the stomach must always be carefully weighed against (a) the risks involved with ipecac syrup–induced emesis and (b) the amount of ingested toxin that can be expected to be removed by the emetic procedure.

Chemical Removal

Chemical removal is the most useful technique for the removal of ingested poisons. Since copper and zinc sulfate cause hepatic and renal toxicity, intravascular hemolysis, and gastrointestinal mucosal damage, they are contraindicated. Salt, a poor and dangerous emetic, is also contraindicated. Apomorphine is a rapidly acting, effective emetic that will induce vomiting in 95 to 100 per cent of patients in two to five minutes; however, being a narcotic, it causes central nervous system depression. This factor limits its routine use for the acute overdose. Naloxone is capable of reversing apomorphine–induced central nervous system depression. Owing to its instability, apomorphine must be freshly prepared. When properly stored in a dark bottle, it has a shelf life of approximately three weeks.

Ipecac syrup is the emetic of choice. It is effective in inducing emesis in 85 per cent of children and adolescents with an initial dose and 95 per cent with a second dose. Emesis occurs within 15 to 20 minutes. Ipecac syrup rarely causes more than two or three episodes of emesis, which generally occur over a 30- to 60-minute time period. In a limited number of human studies, emesis appears to be more effective than gastric lavage. Ipecac syrup is capable of producing emesis with all ingested toxins and is effective following the ingestion of antiemetic drugs such as the phenothiazines.

The dose of ipecac syrup in the child is one tablespoon (15 ml) followed by 100 to 500 ml of clear fluid (depending on age). Milk should not be used as a fluid, as it has been shown to delay the onset of emesis. The time for giving fluids does not appear to be an important factor in producing emesis. While it has long been assumed that motion was important for inducing emesis, one recent clinical study in humans has failed to support the value of this procedure. If emesis has not occurred within 20 minutes, the above dose may be repeated one additional time. If emesis then does not occur, removal of the ingested product by gastric lavage may be indicated. In the adolescent, 30 ml of ipecac syrup should be given and may be repeated once. For the child between 9 and 12 months of age, a single dose of ipecac syrup is given. If emesis does not occur, the child should be seen in a medical facility and careful lavage performed, if removal is still indicated. For children under 9 months of age, lavage rather than ipecac should be used.

Ipecac syrup is safe when given at recommended doses. Total absorption of two doses in the absence of emesis is associated with no toxicity. Central nervous system and cardiac toxicity has been seen only when the above doses have been significantly exceeded. Fluid of extract of ipecac (which is 14 times as concentrated as the syrup) is no longer available and should not be used. Contraindications to the use of ipecac syrup include an altered mental status, convulsions, and ingestion of a petroleum distillate hydrocarbon or caustic agents.

Ipecac is inexpensive (approximately $1.50 per bottle), available without a prescription, and has a shelf life of two to three years, thereby allowing it to be kept in the home for use at the time of the poisoning. It can be administered outside the hospital setting on the advice of a physician or poison center, thereby allowing earlier institution of therapy than if the patient were required to come to the medical setting.

Mechanical Removal

Mechanical removal of the toxin through the use of a blunt object placed in the posterior pharynx to stimulate the gag reflex and promote vomiting is effective in only 10 per cent of cases. It should not be used. Gastric lavage is the method of choice when the patient's state of consciousness is depressed. Lavage requires that the patient be brought to a hospital setting, thereby delaying the removal procedure. It is less effective than emesis for the removal of whole or partially dissolved tablets or capsules. While the procedure is uncomfortable and may entail a risk of vomiting with subsequent aspiration, the clinician does have the ability to discontinue the procedure if medically indicated.

Lavage is indicated for the removal of an ingested toxin at any age when attempts to induce emesis with ipecac syrup have been unsuccessful. In the face of deep coma with loss of the gag reflex, lavage should be undertaken only after the patient has been intubated to protect the airway. The lavage tube has the advantage of providing a route for administration of activated charcoal in the uncooperative or comatose patient. Lavage should be performed with a large orogastic tube (26 to 36 French) with the patient positioned in the head-down posture. Lavage should be carried out with half-normal or normal saline and continued until the return is clear.

Activated Charcoal

Activated charcoal is experiencing increased clinical use in the acute overdose. It is particularly useful in the symptomatic patient to catch up with an ingested product in the small bowel, which is inaccessible to ipecac syrup or lavage. Charcoal is an odorless, tasteless, fine black powder that because of its small particle size and large surface area binds many organic compounds and creates a stable complex that is resistant to dissociation. A partial list of drugs for which activated charcoal has been shown to be effective may be found in a number of reviews (Temple and Mancini, 1980; Lovejoy, 1980). Activated charcoal is effective for most organic compounds and is less effective for alcohols, iron, caustics, cyanide, and heavy metals. The universal antidote (charcoal, magnesium oxide, and tannic acid) is ineffective, and tannic acid is hepatotoxic.

To achieve optimal binding, activated charcoal is best given within one hour of ingestion, following removal of the ingested toxin by emesis or lavage. Charcoal, being black in color, serves as an indicator of gastrointestinal motility and indicates the time at which the ingested product is being eliminated from the body. It should not be used prior to, or concomitant with ipecac syrup, as the charcoal will bind the emetic and prevent its pharmacological action.

Charcoal is administered orally in an amount ten times the weight of the ingested product, or in a dose of a gram per kilogram in the child, or 30 grams in the adolescent. It should be mixed in 60 to 100 ml of water and flavored with cherry syrup to increase its palatability to the small child. Its acceptance is increased if taken by straw with the contents obscured by a cover. If the pediatric patient refuses to swallow activated charcoal, administration of the drug by nasogastric tube may be necessary.

Repeated doses of activated charcoal given every 4 to 6 hours for three or four doses, have found recent use in an effort to interrupt hepatoenteric recirculation of a drug. Evidence exists for the efficacy of this procedure where hepatic metabolism and biliary excretion of active drug into the small bowel exists (tricyclic antidepressants and digitoxin).

Cathartics

Enhanced elimination of a toxin through the gastrointestinal tract, especially with drugs that slow bowel motility, is an important final consideration. Magnesium sulfate or citrate is effective in increasing the rate of transit of a toxic product through the gastrointestinal tract, thus minimizing its absorption. The dose for either cathartic is 250 mg/kg given orally and repeated every three hours until producing a stool. Magnesium sulfate should not be used if renal function is compromised. Salt cathartics are not recommended because they may be toxic if absorbed. Cathartics should follow each dose of activated charcoal when the latter is given repetitively. Cathartics given with activated charcoal do not appear to alter the efficacy of activated charcoal.

Other Methods of Decontamination

Constant nasogastric suction has been shown to be an additional effective approach for preventing absorption of drugs secreted into the stomach (recently demonstrated with phencyclidine).

Many drugs, such as insecticides, are well-absorbed through the skin, and careful washing with soap and water will eliminate this route of absorption. Inhalation as a route of absorption can be prevented by removal of the patient to a noncontaminated environment and by the use of increased concentrations of oxygen. The removal by enema of medications given rectally is a simple and effective method of decontamination.

Alterations in Drug Distribution

The severity and duration of clinical manifestations of an overdose are respectively determined by the toxin's maximal serum concentration and its half-life. Toxicity may be altered in the case of some drugs with low volumes of distribution by alteration of systemic pH. In the case of salicylates and phenobarbital, correction of systemic acidosis will minimize transfer of non-ionized drug into the central nervous system. Decreased protein-binding sites will lead to increased peripheral distribution of toxins, thereby increasing toxicity. If hypoalbuminemia exists, albumin should be given to provide adequate binding for ingested toxins. Care should always be exerted in the therapeutic use of medications in the overdose to be certain that displacement of the toxin from its binding sites does not ensue. Such displacement would result in the redistribution of the toxin to peripheral target organs.

Hepatic Elimination

Hepatic and renal toxins are removed from the body by three major pathways: hepatic, renal, and respiratory. For most agents, one pathway predominates, for example the hepatic route for phenytoin, the renal route for lithium, and the respiratory route for carbon monoxide. For some drugs, such as phenobarbital and salicylates, both renal and hepatic mechanisms operate. Drugs that undergo primarily hepatic inactivation are treated by supportive therapy alone, allowing time for the liver to detoxify the ingested product. Enzyme induction, while theoretically useful, is impractical, as four to five days of induction by drugs such as phenobarbital are necessary to stimulate microsomal activity adequately. For drugs in which hepatic metabolism produces active metabolites (methanol, ethylene glycol, tricyclic antidepressants, glutethimide, parathion, acetaminophen), attention must be given to blocking the production of the metabolites (methanol, ethylene glycol), minimizing the toxicity of produced metabolites by an antidote (acetaminophen), or enhancing gastrointestinal decontamination of the metabolites (tricyclic antidepressants, glutethimide). In these cases, the risk of toxicity will persist until the body has excreted not only the parent compound but the metabolites as well.

Renal Elimination

If the predominant excretory route of the active compound (or metabolite) is the kidneys, forced fluid diuresis may enhance removal by increasing glomerular filtration and minimizing tubular reabsorption of the drug (Rumack and Peterson, 1981; Lovejoy, 1980). Osmotic agents (mannitol or urea) and diuretics (furosemide, ethacrynic acid) increase glomerular filtration and renal tubular flow, thereby enhancing excretion of toxic compounds. Ionized diuresis, the most effective means of enhancing excretion, is based on the principle that a drug in its ionized form in the tubule is unavailable for reabsorption into the body. This principle is applicable for weak acids (aspirin, phenobarbital) with alkalinization of the urine to pH 8. In a similar fashion, alkaline drugs with a high pK (amphetamine, phencyclidine) are effectively removed by acidification of the urine to pH 4 to 4.5. Alkalinization is accomplished through the use of sodium bicarbonate, and acidification is achieved through the use of ammonium chloride alone or ammonium chloride in combination with ascorbic acid.

For drugs that require the respiratory route for removal (carbon monoxide, paraldehyde), an adequate rate and depth of respiration are necessary. In rare instances, assisted ventilation will be necessary to remove drugs eliminated primarily by the respiratory route.

Dialysis

Infrequently, the severity of ingestion will place the patient at sufficient risk to necessitate removal of the toxin more rapidly than can be accomplished by methods of enhanced excretion. Hemodialysis and hemoperfusion and, to a lesser extent, peritoneal dialysis and exchange transfusion can effectively and rapidly remove certain drugs and/or their metabolites. These methods of removal should also be considered when the normal excretory pathway is compromised (renal or hepatic failure), when underlying pathology contraindicates forced diuresis (renal disease, congestive heart failure, congenital heart disease), or when the severity of the ingestion places the patient at excessive risk. Efficacy of dialysis is agreed upon for a limited number of toxins, such as methanol, ethylene glycol, lithium, alcohols, salicylates, and phenobarbital (Rumack and Peterson, 1981; Lovejoy, 1980).

Exchange transfusion is most effective for drugs found primarily in the vascular compartment. Peritoneal dialysis, while a slower method of removing toxins, is capable of simultaneously correcting alterations in electrolytes.

Hemodialysis, limited to patients greater than 10–12 kg, is the most effective of the currently available procedures. Removal of ingested toxins is rapid. Hemoperfusion, the newest method of removal, is generally more effective in clearing a toxin than hemodialysis and is useful for toxins of large molecular size with moderate volumes of distribution.

Antidotes

Desired characteristics of systemic antidotes include high specificity and efficacy with a low incidence of side effects. The amount of antidote required is generally titrated to reduce or eliminate the pharmacological effect of the toxin. Antidotes should never be used prophylactically. A number of detailed descriptions exist in the literature outlining indications, methods of administration, and suggested doses of antidotes (Wason and Lovejoy, 1982; Lovejoy, 1980). The adolescent requires the same dose as the adult for the majority of drugs and antidotes. Naloxone hydrochloride for narcotics, sodium nitrate and sodium thiosulfate for cyanide, methylene blue for methemoglobinemia, atropine sulfate and 2-PAM for organophosphate insecticides, and oxygen for carbon monoxide are antidotes generally needed urgently. The remainder, chlorpromazine for amphetamines, deferoxamine for iron, diphenhydramine for extrapyramidal tract signs of phenothiazines, EDTA, BAL and D-penicillamine for heavy metals, ethanol for methanol and ethylene glycol, N-acetylcysteine for acetaminophen, physostigmine for anticholinergic drugs, and vitamin K for dicumerol and warfarin, all are needed less urgently and should be considered once the patient is well stabilized. The use of the following antidotes, now in an investigational status or of unclear efficacy, should be considered at the time of an overdose: thioctic acid for the Amanita genus of mushrooms, pyridoxine hydrochloride for isoniazid, and diethyldithiocarbamate (Dithiocarb) for thallium. In addition, a number of antisera are available for food poisoning, spider and snake exposures, including antivenoms for black widow spider, scorpion spider, North American pit viper, and coral snakes. Bivalent (A and B) and trivalent (A, B, and E) antitoxins exist for botulin food poisoning.

PREVENTION

Preventive efforts focus on poisoning in children under five years of age.

Epidemiology

Childhood poisoning incidents represent the interaction of an available poison, a temporarily unstable environment, and a susceptible host.

POISON

The most common types of products ingested are shown in Table 18–4. It is particularly important, however, for physicians to recognize and know how to treat poisonings from substances which are both common and known to produce severe symptoms (Table 18–5). Additional products which are rarely lethal but may produce severe symptoms include ferrous sulfate, Lomotil, drain and oven cleaners, and petroleum distillate hydrocarbons. The easy accessibility of hazardous products in the home is a contributory factor in serious childhood poisonings.

Table 18–4. CATEGORICAL FREQUENCY: INGESTIONS BY CHILDREN UNDER FIVE REPORTED TO THE U.S. DIVISION OF POISON CONTROL—1979

Rank	Category	Number of Reports	Percentage of Total (N = 85,262)
1.	Plants (excluding mushrooms)	10,041	11.8
2.	Soaps, detergents, cleaners	5,490	6.4
3.	Antihistamines, cold medications	3,508	4.1
4.	Perfume, cologne	3,507	4.1
5.	Vitamins, minerals	3,454	4.1
6.	Aspirin	3,332	3.9
7.	Miscellaneous analgesics	2,886	3.4
8.	Household disinfectants, deodorizers	2,243	2.6
9.	Fingernail preparations	2,127	2.5
10.	Insecticides	1,988	2.3

Table 18–5. MORTALITY: AGENTS RESPONSIBLE FOR ACCIDENTAL POISON DEATHS IN CHILDREN AND YOUTH, AGES 0–19 YEARS, IN THE UNITED STATES—1978

Category (Most Common Hazardous Product)	Less than 5 years of age	Total for 0–19 years of age
Drugs		
Salicylates (aspirin)	13	14
Antidepressants (tricyclic antidepressants)	10	15
Opiates (heroin, methadone)	4	22
Barbiturates	1	12
Propoxyphene hydrochloride	—	14
Others	20	113
TOTAL DRUGS	48	190
Household Products		
Pesticides, fertilizers (arsenic, cyanide, roach powder)	10	14
Petroleum products and solvents	9	10
Cleaning and polishing agents (furniture polish)	7	8
Corrosives and caustics (battery acid, lye)	3	4
Alcohol	—	9
Others	3	50
TOTAL HOUSEHOLD PRODUCTS	32	95
Gases and Vapors		
Carbon monoxide from motor vehicles	14	186
Carbon monoxide from domestic fuels	6	29
Other carbon monoxide	14	60
Other gases	17	110
TOTAL GASES AND VAPORS	51	385
GRAND TOTAL	**131**	**670**

From Death Certificate Data aggregated by National Center for Health Statistics.

ENVIRONMENT

Stress is frequently associated with poisoning incidents. Common stress factors found in families where poisonings occur include moving in the last three months, one parent away from home, pregnancy, serious family illness in the last month, anxiety or depression in parents, and unemployment (Sibert, 1975). Additional stress factors found in households where a repeat poisoning incident has occurred include a child's power struggle with the mother, parental mental illness, mother's dissatisfaction with her marriage, low ego strength of the mother, and long-term family stress (Sobel, 1970). Twelve to 28 per cent of children who experience a poisoning incident will have another, usually within 12 months. While stress factors are associated with poisonings, family socioeconomic status is not.

HOST

Host factors associated with poisonings are age, personality, and sex. Peak ages for poisonings range from 18 months to three years. Young children who are poisoned tend to be more daring and to strike back when disciplined. In addition, repeaters tend to be boys (Sobel, 1970). The child tends to be most susceptible to poisoning when the use of an agent is immediate in his/her mind. In one study, 81 per cent of medicines had been used within 24 hours and 50 per cent of household substances were in use at the time of the incident (Calnan, 1974).

Preventive Measures

The pediatrician can help prevent accidental poisonings by providing anticipatory guidance concerning child development to parents at well-child visits (Lovejoy and Chafee-Bahamon, 1982). Poison prevention messages are helpful (Table 18–6). In addition, the pediatrician can provide counseling in special circumstances. The physician, aware that a family is going

Table 18–6. POISON PREVENTION MESSAGES FOR STAGES IN CHILD'S DEVELOPMENT

Age and Stage	Poisoning Hazard	Message
4 months—Grabbing	Diaper changing	Keep powders and baby cleaners out of baby's reach in changing area. Don't give containers to infants to occupy them while changing their diapers.
6 months—Crawling	Cleaners in lower cabinets	Reorganize kitchen and bathrooms so cleaners are kept on upper shelves.
12 months—Walking, imitating	Tabletop medications and household products; products in use	Keep tabletops and dressertops free of medicines and nonedible household products. Never leave a child unsupervised while cleaners, paint thinners, or lighter fluids are in use.
24 months—Climbing, taste preferences	Flavored medicines	Store flavored medicines such as children's aspirin, vitamins, and cold medications on very high shelves at all times, and never by a child's bed.

through changes such as pregnancy or moving, can reinforce the importance of adequate supervision for children under five or of obtaining additional help with child care. When prescribing medicines, the pediatrician can remind parents about safe storage. Children are at risk for poisoning during family illness when medicines are left out.

The pediatrician also needs to counsel parents when a poisoning incident has occurred and there is a likelihood that the child will become a repeater. When contacted about an incident, it is important for the pediatrician to obtain a history which will distinguish between the poison exposure resulting from the child's exploration and the exposure that is associated with defiance and stress factors. In the latter case, where it is clear that the parent is having difficulty coping or has not found a successful means for disciplining the child, active counseling by the pediatrician is indicated.

Besides discussing poison prevention, it is important in an early well child visit to discuss appropriate emergency responses to poison exposures. Nearly two thirds of the poisoning incidents seen in the hospital emergency room required no treatment or could have been treated at home (Chafee-Bahamon and Lovejoy, 1983). Therefore, it is important to instruct parents to call their physician or the poison center first rather than going to the hospital. There are over 40 regional poison centers in the United States. Trained information specialists answer the telephone. Based on their experience in handling a high volume of calls and their immediate access to current toxicological information, the specialists can apprise the physician or parent of the appropriate treatment. Such regional centers have been found to provide better telephone information than hospital emergency rooms (Thompson and Trammel, 1983) and to reduce unnecessary visits to the emergency room. Many poison centers provide poison prevention literature that is helpful for parents of young children. In addition to telling the parent what to do in case of a poisoning incident, the physician should make sure parents keep a bottle of ipecac syrup in the home. To ensure that parents do obtain ipecac, physicians may want to distribute bottles in their office or give the parents a "prescription" for the over-the-counter bottle.

In addition to counseling parents, physicians may want to support effective poison prevention efforts. The Poison Prevention Act of 1970 mandated child-resistant packaging for dangerous, frequently ingested toxins. Child-resistant caps have reduced poisoning incidents by 45 to 55 per cent (Walton, 1982). Physicians can support National Poison Prevention Week as well as community poison prevention programs, which, when well-planned, increase the number of households which safely store toxic household products (Fisher et al., 1980).

REFERENCES

Calnan, M. W.: Accidental child poisoning. Com. Health, 6:91–101, 1974.

Chafee-Bahamon, C., and Lovejoy, F. H., Jr.: The effectiveness of a regional poison center in reducing excess emergency room visits for children's poisoning. Pediatrics, in press, 1983.

Easom, J. M., and Lovejoy, F. H., Jr.: Efficacy and safety of gastrointestinal decontamination in the treatment of oral poisoning. Pediatr. Clin. North Am., *26*:827–836, 1979.

Emmett, M., and Marins, R. G.: Clinical use of the anion gap. Medicine, *56*:38–54, 1977.

Fisher, L., VanBuren, J., Nitzkin, J. L., Laurence, R. A., and Swaekhamer, R.: Highlight results of the Monroe County poison prevention demonstration project. Vet. Hum. Toxicol., *22*(Suppl. 2):15–17, 1980.

Goldfrank, L. R.: Toxicologic Emergencies. New York, Appleton-Century-Crofts, 1982.

Ingelfinger, J. A., Isakon, G., Shine, D., and Goldman, P.: Reliability of the toxic screen in drug overdose. Clin. Pharmacol. Ther., *29*:570–575, 1981.

Lovejoy, F. H., Jr.: Acute poisoning. *In* Gelles, S., and Kagan, J. (eds.): Current Pediatric Therapy, 9th Ed. Philadelphia, W. B. Saunders Co., 1980, pp. 654–675.

Lovejoy, F. H., Jr., and Chafee-Bahamon, C.: The physician's role in accident prevention. Pediatr. Rev., *4*:53–60, 1982.

McIntire, M. S., and Angle, C. R.: "Suicide" as seen in poison control centers. Pediatrics, *48*:914–922, 1971.

Mitchell, A. A., Lovejoy, F. H., Jr., and Goldman, P.: Drug ingestions associated with miosis in comatose children. J. Pediatr., *89*:303–306, 1976.

Mofenson, H. C., and Greensher, J.: The unknown poison. Pediatrics for the clinician. Pediatrics, *54*:336–342, 1974.

Rumack, B. H., and Peterson, R. G.: Clinical toxicology. *In* Doull, C., Klaassen, C. D., and Amdur, M. D. (eds.): Casaret and Doull's Toxicology. The Basic Science of Poisons, 2nd Ed. New York, Macmillan Publishing Co., Inc., 1980, pp. 677–698.

Sibert, R.: Stress in families of children who have ingested poisons. Br. Med. J., *3*:87–89, 1975.

Sobel, R.: The psychiatric implications of accidental poisoning in childhood. Pediatr. Clin. North Am., *17*:653–685, 1970.

Temple, A. R., and Mancini, R. E.: Management of poisoning. *In* Yaffee, S. J. (ed.): Pediatric Pharmacology. New York, Grune & Stratton, 1980, pp. 391–406.

Thompson, D. G., and Trammel, H. L.: Telephone evaluation of regional and non-regional poison centers. N. Engl. J. Med., *308*:191–194, 1983.

Walton, W. W.: An evaluation of the Poison Prevention Packaging Act. Pediatrics, *69*:363–370, 1982.

Wason, S., and Lovejoy, F. H., Jr.: Poisoning. *In* Cohen, S. A. (ed.): Pediatric Emergency Management. Bowie, Maryland, R. E. Brady Company, 1982, pp. 37–65.

19

INSECT STINGS AND BITES

Martin D. Broff, M.D.,
and Raif S. Geha, M.D.

STINGING INSECT ALLERGY

Serious allergic reactions to insect stings are not rare. The best estimates suggest that about 0.4 to 0.8 per cent of the population in the United States have anaphylactic reactions to insect stings. Approximately 40 to 50 deaths are reported due to insect stings each year in this country. The frequency of reactions appears to be the same in the atopic and nonatopic populations. Males, especially those under the age of 20 years, are more likely to be affected, probably due to greater exposure. The majority of fatal reactions, however, have occurred in adults, especially those over 40 years.

The major species of stinging insects belong to the order Hymenoptera and include the honey bee, yellow jacket, hornet, and wasp. All but the bee can sting multiple times. The honey bee (*Apis mellifera*) has a barbed stinger that remains in the sting site. As the bee flies off after a sting, it eviscerates itself and dies. Honey bees are found mostly in man-made hives, but wild colonies nest in hollow trees and walls. They are not as aggressive as other Hymenoptera, and will generally sting only if provoked. Stings commonly occur on the soles of individuals walking barefoot in grass that contains a fair amount of clover. Yellow jackets (Vespula spp.) build their nests in the ground, or inside of rotten logs, walls, or crawl spaces. They are very aggressive and account for the largest number of stings. They are scavengers and will be found around garbage cans, picnics, and fruit trees. The yellow hornet (*Dolichovespula arenaria*) and the white-faced hornet (*D. maculata*) build football-shaped paper nests in trees or bushes. They sting when their nest is disturbed by a child running through the bushes or when accidentally or intentionally disturbed during yardwork or home repairs. Wasps (Polistes spp.) build open comb nests in protected places off the ground, especially in the eaves and window sills of buildings. In cold weather they seek warmth indoors.

Types of Reactions

Local Reactions. The most common consequence of an insect sting is mild pain and erythema at the site of the sting, usually accompanied by mild edema. Large local reactions occur in some individuals and can be quite impressive. The edema of a large local reaction can extend over an entire limb but is always contiguous with the site of the sting and never involves distant skin sites or any systemic symptoms. There is an increased risk of a systemic reaction in a small percentage of individuals following increasingly large local reactions. Large local reactions are immunologically mediated, and many individuals may have positive skin tests to insect venom.

Toxic Reactions. This type of reaction, usually the result of multiple stings, may mimic a systemic reaction. The symptoms include faintness, vomiting, diarrhea, fever, headache, edema, and, rarely, convulsions. These reactions are nonimmunologically mediated and are due to pharmacological and enzymatic properties of the components of insect venom in large quantity. Toxic reactions usually clear within 48 hours.

Systemic Reactions. The most dangerous consequence of an insect sting is an anaphylactic reaction. Death due to anaphylaxis may occur within 10 to 15 minutes. Systemic reactions involve multiple systems, including cardiovascular (hypotension, syncope), respiratory (laryngeal edema, bronchospasm), and cutaneous (urticaria, angioedema). Sting victims may also manifest gastrointestinal symptoms, apprehension, or a feeling of impending doom. Anaphylactic reactions are mediated by IgE antibodies to various immunogenic protein components of the Hymenoptera venoms.

Unusual Reactions. There have been rare reports of other types of reactions following insect stings, including serum sickness, vasculitis, encephalitis, neuritis, and nephrosis. The pathogenic mechanism of these reactions is not known.

Diagnosis

Diagnosis is made primarily with the history of the reaction. Considerable effort should be made to extract as many details as possible of the events immediately before and after the sting. What was the patient doing? Where was he at the time of the sting? It is essential to determine the time interval from the sting to the onset of the first symptoms and the temporal progression of symptoms. It is then possible in most cases to determine the type of reaction, i.e., toxic, local, or systemic.

Positive identification of the insect is rarely possible. The insect is very infrequently captured and brought for identification. The history may suggest one insect, but since all of the stinging insects may be found in any location, care must be taken before relying upon the casual observation of the victim. Patients are usually quite adamant that they know the insect, but they have been proven wrong as often as correct.

The physical examination is also important in differentiating sting reactions. A patient presenting in shock will be obvious, with hypotension, tachycardia, and lapse or loss of consciousness. It is important to look for any signs of respiratory distress, such as stridor or wheezing. Note any swelling of the tongue or pharynx. Cutaneous involvement should be determined and may involve urticaria or angioedema at distant sites. The size of a large local reaction should be noted.

Diagnostic Tests

Skin Testing. Hypersensitivity skin testing for immediate type of reaction with purified Hymenoptera venom material is the most sensitive way to detect the presence of IgE antibodies to venom. The indication for venom skin testing is a systemic reaction to a sting. Toxic and local reactions are not indications for testing. Skin testing should be performed by a physician trained in the application and interpretation of immediate hypersensitivity skin tests. A prick test is performed to 1.0 μg/ml venom to screen for exquisite sensitivity. If the prick test is negative, intradermal tests begin at 0.01 μg/ml and increase by tenfold concentrations to a maximum strength of 1.0 μg/ml. A positive reaction is a wheal of 5 to 10 mm or greater with erythema of 11 to 20 mm or greater to a venom concentration of 1.0 μg/ml or less.

A patient should not be skin tested for a period of three to four weeks after a sting, a potential refractory period. During this period the measurable venom specific IgE falls to low levels. Another factor affecting the accuracy of skin testing is the use of antihistamines. Antihistamines interfere with the skin test response and must not be given to patients for a period of 72 hours prior to testing.

RAST Test. Radioallergosorbent (RAST) test to venom is an in vitro assay of serum venom specific IgE. The level of serum IgE to venom may be low or unmeasurable immediately after an anaphylactic sting reaction but will usually peak three to six weeks after such a reaction. RAST results may show elevated levels of specific IgE in individuals with large local reactions, in bee keepers, and in individuals who have previously been treated with whole body insect immunotherapy. The degree of risk of future anaphylactic reaction cannot be assessed by the RAST test. RAST is not as sensitive as skin testing and should not be used to determine if venom immunotherapy is indicated.

Treatment

Treatment of the Acute Reaction. The initial treatment of any systemic allergic reaction should be a subcutaneous injection of aqueous epinephrine hydrochloride 1:1000 at a dosage of 0.01 ml/kg (up to a maximum dose of 0.4 ml) at intervals of 15 minutes. In anaphylactic shock it may be necessary to administer the epinephrine intravenously at a 1:10,000 dilution. Other supportive measures such as the Trendelenberg position, oxygen, and volume expansion must be performed as indicated. It may be necessary to use dopamine by intravenous infusion to support blood pressure in cases of persistent hypotension.

After the treatment of shock, if present, or after the initial epinephrine is given, antihistamine should be administered. Diphenhydramine hydrochloride 25 to 50 mg may be given intramuscularly or orally, and should be continued orally four times daily for a period of 24 to 48 hours.

Bronchospasm, if present, should be treated by intravenous aminophylline if severe, or oral theophylline if mild. Corticosteroids will be of no benefit in the treatment of the immediate reaction but may be used in cases of severe reactions or to prevent late or delayed reactions.

Treatment of Local Reactions. Mild local reactions usually call for little or no treatment. Large local reactions may require the use of cold compresses, elevation of the extremity, and antihistamines to relieve pruritis. Rarely will the use of corticosteroids be justified in local reactions.

Long-term Management. As in all forms of allergy, avoidance is the best possible treatment. A number of simple rules and precautions to follow should be given to the sensitive individual when in a situation of some risk.

When outdoors in areas where insects are prevalent, avoid wearing brightly colored or flowery prints that attract stinging insects. Long sleeves and trousers help to avoid exposing skin. Loose or baggy clothing may trap insects and result in multiple stings. Shoes and socks should be worn, as it is common to see stings where the individual has been barefoot or wearing sandals. Odors, such as scented sprays, perfumes, lotions, and soaps, also attract insects.

Care should be taken in cooking outdoors, at picnics, and near garbage areas. Keep food covered until eating. Keep garbage areas clean and all food waste in closed containers. Spray garbage containers with insecticide.

Other outdoor activities, such as gardening, should be done with caution. Care should be taken not to disturb nests. A sensitive person should not venture out in wooded areas alone. Emergency medication, such as an epinephrine syringe kit, should accompany the sensitive person at all times. The use of the syringe should be demonstrated, to ensure that the patient understands how and when to use it.

Venom Immunotherapy

A new and extremely efficacious treatment for the Hymenoptera venom–sensitive patient is allergy immunotherapy with purified Hymenoptera venom. Compared to placebo and to the previously used Whole Body Extract (WBE), venom injections protected 95 per cent of patients challenged by deliberate stings from having systemic reactions (Hunt et al., 1978). Systemic reactions occurred in 64 per cent of WBE-treated patients and in 58 per cent of placebo-treated patients. The indication for venom immunotherapy is a life-threatening systemic reaction to insect stings (Table 19–1). Mild systemic reactions, such as urticaria alone

Table 19–1. INDICATIONS FOR VENOM IMMUNOTHERAPY

Reaction	Venom Skin Test	Treatment
Local	Not indicated	Avoidance, epinephrine syringe
Urticaria	Negative	Avoidance, epinephrine syringe
Urticaria	Positive	Avoidance, epinephrine syringe
Resp. Distress/Anaphylaxis	Negative	Avoidance, epinephrine syringe
Resp. Distress/Anaphylaxis	Positive	Venom immunotherapy

without any respiratory tract involvement or shock, is not necessarily an indication for venom immunotherapy in children. Because many children will lose hypersensitivity with time and because the duration of treatment is not defined, it is best to avoid treatment in children with mild systemic reactions.

Venon immunotherapy is accomplished by administering the purified venom subcutaneously in a series of weekly injections starting at 0.05 μg and increasing to 100 μg by the fifteenth week. A dose of 100 μg, considered the optimal maintenance dose, is continued at an interval of every four to six weeks. The duration of immunotherapy has not been clearly defined. Systemic reactions have occurred during venom immunotherapy. It is recommended that only physicians skilled in the use of immunotherapy and in the treatment of injection reactions administer venom.

FIRE ANT HYPERSENSITIVITY

The fire ant, present mainly in the Gulf coast area, is of the order Hymenoptera and is reported to cause anaphylactic reactions. *Solenopsis richteri* and *S. invicta* are responsible for most reactions. The insect attaches itself to the victim by biting with its jaws, and then it swings its abdomen around, stinging many times. A sterile pustule develops in 24 hours. In some cases immediate allergic reactions have occurred. The venom of fire ants is different from that of the other stinging Hymenoptera, and therefore sensitivity to fire ants does not imply sensitivity to the other stinging insects. The antigen responsible for fire ant allergy is found in Whole Body Extract as well as in purified venom preparations, so that the more easily obtained WBE may be used for the diagnosis and treatment of fire ant hypersensitivity.

BITING INSECT ALLERGY

Mosquitos, fleas, sand flies, deer flies, and horse flies have all been known to cause local allergic reactions. The hypersensitivity is to the salivary secretions of the insect. Generalized allergic reactions to biting insects have been reported but are exceedingly rare. The mechanism of these reactions has not been well studied. The use of skin testing and immunotherapy has not been established and at this time cannot be recommended. The treatment of insect bites concentrates on avoidance and the use of insect repellants, oral antihistamines, and reassurance that such reactions do not indicate a risk of allergy to stinging insects.

Papular urticaria, a reaction to biting insects that is unique to children, consists of small papules in groups found mainly on the exposed skin of the extremities. It is caused by the bites of fleas, mites, or bedbugs. Treatment is removal of the source of the insects as well as symptomatic treatment with antihistamines and topical corticosteroids.

REFERENCES

Hunt, K. J., Valentine, M. D., Sobotka, A. K., Benton, A. W., Amodio, F. J., and Lichtenstein, L. M.: A controlled trial of immunotherapy in insect immunotherapy. N. Engl. J. Med., *299*:157–161, 1978.

Lichtenstein, L. M., Valentine, M. D., and Sobotka, A. K.: Insect allergy: The state of the art. J. Allergy Clin. Immunol., *64*:5–12, 1979.

Reisman, R. E.: Insect allergy. *In* Middleton, E., Reed, C. E., and Ellis, E. F. (eds.): Allergy, Principles and Practice. St. Louis, C. V. Mosby Co., 1978.

Reisman, R. E.: Stinging insect allergy. J. Allergy Clin. Immunol., *64*:3–4, 1979.

Settipane, G. A., and Chafee, F. H.: Natural history of allergy to Hymenoptera. Clin. Allergy, 9:385–390, 1979.

Yunginger, J. W.: The sting—revisited. J. Allergy Clin. Immunol., *64*:1–2, 1979.

20

THE SKIN: LACERATIONS, ABRASIONS, AND BURNS

Thomas R. Weber, M.D.,
and Jay L. Grosfeld, M.D.

LACERATIONS AND ABRASIONS

Lacerations and abrasions, both minor and major, are extremely common in the pediatric age group. Most physicians should be able to manage minor injuries in their office practice, provided certain basic rules of management are followed. Complicated lacerations involving the eyelids or orbit, nerves or tendons, extensive animal or human bites, or complicated lacerations that might require extensive debridement and/or deep repair should be referred to a surgeon or emergency room facility.

Successful repair of lacerations, both simple and more complex, requires sterile equipment, adequate lighting, the presence of an assistant (other than the parents), proper restraint, and equipment for wound irrigation. It is advisable to keep a sterile "suture set" available (Table 20–1). The procedure and potential risks of scar formation and infection should be carefully explained to the parents, and an informed consent should be signed by a parent and kept in the permanent office records.

Examination of the wound and assessment of the extent of injury should be the first maneuver and ideally is performed using aseptic technique. Sterile gloves and standard surgical mask should be available. Thorough examination of a wound and subsequent repair require a cooperative patient, most easily obtained with sedation in the younger child. Demerol (1 mg/kg), combined with phenergan (0.5 mg/kg) and thorazine (0.5 mg/kg) given intramuscularly is a safe and effective sedative for the one- to four-year-old patient. After waiting 15 to 20 minutes for the medication to take effect, the child should be appropriately restrained. This may be accomplished by wrapping the child in a sheet ("mummification"), or by using a commercially available "papoose board."

In evaluating the wound, the exact details of the mechanism of injury should be kept in mind. Outdoor falls resulting in abrasion or laceration may involve a retained foreign body. Puncture wounds in the extremity may result in nerve or tendon injury; thus, complete neurovascular evaluation of the extremity distal to the injury should be performed. Wounds that are suggestive of child abuse should obviously be managed by a child abuse team in a hospital setting.

The hair should be shaved at least one half inch around scalp lacerations. Eyebrows, however, should never be shaved, because in approximately 15 per cent of cases they will not grow back.

After cleansing the wound with mild soap and water, local anesthesia should be administered. This allows painless inspection of the wound for foreign bodies, permits more vigorous scrubbing, and is obviously necessary before sutures are placed. In general, 0.5 to 1 per cent xylocaine is used by injecting directly through the skin edges with a 25- or 27-gauge needle, after allergy to the drug has been ruled out by questioning the parents. A small amount of the anesthetic dripped directly into the wound provides enough anesthesia for injection of the remaining dose. The total dose should not exceed 3 mg/kg body weight. Epinephrine 1:10,000 may be added to the xylocaine for obtaining hemostasis in highly vascular regions, such as the scalp or face. Local anesthetics with epinephrine should never be used on fingers, toes, ears, or the nose because of the risk of distal necrosis.

The wound should be thoroughly cleansed with an antiseptic solution after the local anesthetic takes effect. Iodine-based antiseptic is most often employed (Betadine). Peroxide 1 per cent is also useful and has the added advantage of being hemostatic. Irrigation with normal saline (0.9 per cent) after cleansing removes loose foreign bodies and dilutes microorganisms. The saline solution can be vigorously flushed into the wound with a syringe and 21-gauge needle. Extremely dirty wounds should be referred to

Table 20–1. SUTURE SET

Syringes—5 or 10 cc
Needles—20 g for drawing up lidocaine, 25 g to administer
Lidocaine—1% is recommended local anesthesia (lidocaine containing epinephrine should never be used on nose, ears, and digits.)
Package of 10 or 20 sponges
Sterile gloves
Sterile towels
Prep equipment, ioprep or betadine
Irrigation equipment
  30 to 60 cc syringe with Luer lock
  Catheter tip adapter
  Sterile bowl
  250 cc normal saline
Suture—4-0, 5-0, 6-0 prolene or nylon
Steri-strips
Sterile instruments (forceps, needle holder, scissors, mosquito clamps)

an emergency room for x-ray evaluation for foreign body and extensive debridement of the contaminated, often necrotic tissue. Most wounds on the bottom of the foot, frequently incurred by running barefoot outdoors, are not sutured at all, but rather left open and allowed to heal by second intention, using frequent soaking and dressing changes at home. Early weight bearing should be avoided.

Hemostasis should be achieved before attempting wound repair, to allow complete visualization of the wound and to prevent post-repair hematoma formation. In most instances, hemostasis can be accomplished by direct pressure. If the wound is bleeding profusely or in a "pulsatile" fashion, exploration should be performed under more controlled circumstances, such as an operating room. Placement of sutures or hemostats deep within an extremity or facial wound to stop bleeding is to be avoided, as injury to nerve or tendon may result. A large abrasion with generalized "oozing" of blood from its surface will frequently respond to topical thrombin gently rubbed directly on the wound with the gloved finger.

Wound debridement should be minimal but should include removal of obviously devitalized tissues. Similarly, foreign bodies (dirt, gravel) imbedded within tissue usually require removal of that tissue for complete debridement. Foreign bodies or necrotic tissue left within a wound after closure will usually cause a wound infection.

The actual wound closure is usually straightforward and uncomplicated, if basic principles are followed. Ideally, the suture line should be without tension and without "dead space" under the skin closure. This may require several layers of suture. Usually the deep layers are closed with plain or chromic catgut (absorbable suture). The skin closure can be accomplished in several ways. Most commonly, fine monofilament nylon suture (4-0 or 5-0 on the trunk and extremities, 6-0 on the face) is utilized. The use of braided suture materials, such as silk, should be avoided because of the increased risk of infection with these materials. In clean, straight wounds, either interrupted or running suture techniques can be used. In irregular superficial lacerations or deep wounds with the deep tissue approximated, interrupted sutures are indicated. In moderately deep wounds or wounds in which the skin is subject to motion (near joints), vertical mattress sutures may prove useful.

Many physicians use subcuticular sutures for clean, straight lacerations. If absorbable suture is used (catgut), the sutures need not be removed, but the wound must be followed carefully to avoid wound infection promoted by the subcuticular foreign body. The placement of cutaneous tapes over the incision is advisable after subcuticular closure, to give a more satisfactory cosmetic result.

Numerous cutaneous tape closure materials are available, and these are highly useful for very superficial wounds with little or no tension. Their use should be avoided over joints. Tincture of benzoin may be used to obtain good adhesion of the tape to the skin, which also must be very dry. The wound must be kept dry for at least seven days to avoid premature separation of the tapes from the skin. No matter which technique is used to close the wound, anatomical apposition of the edges is critical to avoid a "step off" appearance to the scar. Wounds closed too tightly might result in strangulation of the wound edges and tissue necrosis. Thus the sutures should be tied so that the wound edges just touch.

The wound should be covered with a dressing that is functional for the child, provides protection for the wound, and prevents excessive movement. Simple lacerations usually require an occlusive dressing, with tape providing a sterile barrier. Flexible collodion is useful on the face or head, where there is minimal movement. The dressing should be left in place for 48 hours, after which time no further dressing is necessary. Regular skin care can be resumed when the sutures or paper tapes are removed, usually 3 to 10 days, depending on the location of injury. Immobilization of an injured extremity is frequently advisable, and splints, crutches, and slings should be available for this purpose.

Suture removal is an important part of wound care and should be performed under the supervision of a physician. Sutures on the face should be removed three to four days after placement and replaced with paper tapes. Sutures on the trunk or scalp can be left in place for seven days, while those on the extremities should remain for 10 to 14 days, depending on the proximity to joints and the vascularity of the tissues involved.

Tetanus toxoid booster (0.5 cc) should be given if the child has not received a booster in the previous 10 years, or in children with tetanus-prone (dirty) wounds if no booster has been given in the past 5 years. If the child has received no prior injections, he should be given 0.5 cc toxoid for clean (non–tetanus-prone) wounds, with the addition of 250 units tetanus immune globulin in children with dirty wounds. The addition of antibiotics should be considered in extremely dirty wounds, although their efficacy in preventing tetanus remains unproven.

Abrasion injuries, if severe, should be treated in a manner similar to a burn. The wound should be gently cleansed with mild soap and water and all loose foreign bodies removed. An occlusive dressing is then applied, using an antibiotic (Furacin or Silvadene) cream or gauze or a petroleum-impregnated gauze. Daily washings and reapplication of the topical antibiotic are continued until healing is complete, usually in 7 to 10 days. An improperly treated abrasion may become secondarily infected, resulting in deep tissue loss, spreading cellulitis, and ascending lymphangitis. If this should occur, immediate institution of intravenous antibiotics in the hospital is mandatory.

BURNS

Burns are common in the pediatric age group and a serious cause of morbidity and mortality. Most burns are minor and can be treated on an outpatient basis from an office or ambulatory care clinic. First aid for minor burns on an extremity includes immersing the involved area in cool water or running cool water over it. Elsewhere on the body, the parent may cover the involved area with moist, cool, clean cloths or pour cool water over it. The initial evaluation of the child should include a detailed history as to how the burn occurred, what the causative agent was (flame, hot liquid scald, or electrical), associated injuries including possible smoke inhalation, allergies and immunization status, and other medical illness. As with lacerations, any cases suspicious for child abuse should be referred to a child abuse team.

Burns can be conveniently catagorized according to depth and extent in terms of percentage of body surface area. First degree burns involve the epidermis and result in erythema only. They generally do not represent a serious medical problem. Second degree burns are partial thickness injuries (of variable depth, superficial, or deep), usually associated with erythema and blisters. Because pain receptors are retained, second degree burns can be extremely painful. Third degree burns are full thickness thermal injuries that result in a total loss of skin. The most severe third degree burns might involve subcutaneous fat and muscle fascia. Since pain nerve fibers are destroyed, third degree burns are usually painless. Many burns have areas of variable depth; thus, careful inspection and documentation of all areas of burned skin is mandatory.

The extent of a burn can be roughly categorized as minor (less than 10 per cent body surface area second degree burn and less than 1 per cent third degree), moderate (10 to 20 per cent second degree and 1 to 10 per cent third degree), and severe (greater than 20 per cent second degree and 10 per cent third degree). The standard "rule of nines," used to estimate the body surface area in adults, must be modified in children. For example, the head surface area in a one-year-old child comprises 19 per cent of the total and diminishes at 1 per cent per year until, at age 11, it is the same as in the adult, 9 per cent. Each infant leg is 15 per cent of the total surface area, whereas each leg in the adult represents 18 per cent.

The most common burn in the age group under three years is a scald, usually resulting from a curious toddler tipping or pulling hot liquid (soup, coffee, tea, etc.) onto himself, resulting in facial, shoulder, torso, arm, or hand burns. Between ages 3 and 15, flame burns, related to misuse of matches, flammable materials, and fireworks, are most common. These are frequently life-threatening and can result in severe, often deforming injuries.

Evaluation of the burn injury is most appropriate after the burn has been carefully and gently cleansed with warm sterile water and bland soap. Second degree burns covering less than 10 to 15 per cent of the body surface area can be treated on an outpatient basis at home if the family is thought to be reliable. Exceptions would include burns to the face, hands, feet, and genitalia, especially in children under two years of age. These latter cases should be referred to an appropriate center for hospitalization. In addition, particular attention must be directed to circumferential burns with contracture of the eschar; those on the chest may lead to respiratory embarrassment, while those on the extremity may result in vascular compromise distal to the injury. Early referral for escharotomy in these cases may save life or limb.

Ambulatory care for less severe burns should include cleansing as outlined above, followed by application of an antibiotic ointment (Silvadene, Furacin, Neosporin) in a nonadherent, occlusive dressing. Parents are taught to change the dressing twice daily and are encouraged to "force fluids" by mouth over the first 48 to 72 hours following the injury. Blisters should be left intact and allowed to break spontaneously under the dressing. Very small areas of burn in an older child can also be managed in an "open" manner with application of Silvadene cream. The most important aspect in ambulatory burn care is prevention of infection, which can convert a partial thickness to a full thickness injury.

The burn wound should be re-evaluated in the office every two to three days. Superficial second degree wounds should heal in 10 to 14 days by re-epithelization from hair follicles, sweat glands, and other skin appendages, while deep second degree injuries may take three to four weeks to heal completely.

Third degree burns of less than 5 per cent of body surface area can be treated initially on an outpatient basis, with later admission for skin grafting. Full thickness burns that involve more than 5 per cent of the surface area should be referred for immediate hospitalization.

Electrical burns occur most often when toddlers bite an electrical cord, resulting in a burn of the mouth and lip. Initial estimation of the depth of injury may be misleading, because of minimal edema and a white mucosal coagulum. These injuries must be watched closely over the ensuing week, with the parents sufficiently warned of the threat of potential hemorrhagic and cosmetic complications of the burn. Thrombosis and necrosis of deeper tissues, with eventual tissue separation, typically occurs at the seventh to tenth postburn day. This may result in significant hemorrhage from perioral arteries and suggests that hospitalization after the first week may be advisable. A plastic surgeon should be consulted early in the management of the patients. Arm restraints may be necessary to prevent the child from further injuring the involved area.

21 SCREENING EYE EXAMINATION

Eugene M. Helveston, M.D.

The screening examination of a child's eyes is carried out by observation and functional testing. These can be accomplished quickly and effectively without specialized instruments.

ADNEXA

Observation of the child's eye begins with an appraisal of the periorbital area, lids, and lashes. "Lumps and bumps," such as a stye, hemangioma, dermoid, and neurofibroma, are noted. Dacryocystitis causes a swelling in the *inner* canthal area and is associated with tearing and mucopurulent discharge. Flakes from a chronic staphylococcal infection or nits from infestation may be present at the base of the lashes. The upper lid ordinarily covers 2 to 3 mm of the cornea, and the lower lid is usually tangential to or just above the lower limbus. Either bilateral or unilateral drooping of the lid (ptosis) should be noted. When moderate to severe bilateral ptosis is present, frontalis contraction as evidenced by furrowing of the forehead may be employed to elevate the lids. A fold of skin, the epicanthus, in the medial canthal area may give the appearance of strabismus, which may be diagnosed as pseudostrabismus by noting that the light reflex from a small penlight is centered in each pupil.

CONJUNCTIVA

The conjunctiva may have a deep red, flame-shaped collection of blood from a benign subconjunctival hemorrhage. A deep flush in the perilimbal area is associated with an internal ocular inflammation or uveitis, and a diffuse more superficial redness accompanied by a watery or purulent discharge with conjunctivitis. The conjunctiva on the undersurface of the upper lid can be inspected by using a cotton-tipped applicator to evert the upper lid. Conjunctivitis may be due to a variety of bacterial, viral, or intermediate pathogens. Conjunctivitis can initially be treated with sulfacetamide 10 to 15 per cent drops or ointment, bacitracin ointment, or erythromycin ointment. Topical steroids should *never* be used by the primary physician in treatment of conjunctival or corneal disease. If an "eye wash" is needed, an antiseptic and mild astringent solution may be used. Conjuctivitis that does not respond to the above treatment should be investigated for a specific agent and treated accordingly.

CORNEA

The cornea may be abraded by trauma or disrupted by an infectious process, e.g., a chronic bacterial ulcer or a viral ulcer caused by herpes simplex. The latter is especially aggravated by treatment with topical steroids. Such treatment would be analogous to fighting fire with gasoline. Corneal abrasions of mechanical origin may be diagnosed by noting an absence of luster to the cornea and the presence of pooling of fluorescein when checked for fluorescence with an ultraviolet lamp.

PUPIL

The pupil may be observed for movement directly and consensually with a penlight. In the child, the pupil is normally larger than in the adult, averaging approximately 3 to 4 mm in ordinary illumination. Although the pupils should be equal or nearly equal in most instances, minimal pupil inequality is benign provided vision is normal. Marked inequality of pupil size with asymmetrical reaction may indicate neurological disease involving the visual pathways, or Horner's syndrome.

OPHTHALMOSCOPIC EXAMINATION

The ophthalmoscope can be useful for external corneal and conjunctival examination if the examiner uses the +8D lens and holds the instrument approximately 6 to 8 inches from the patient. Two and one-half per cent Neo-synephrine or one per cent Mydriacyl gives adequate pupillary dilation in a few minutes, with only a few hours of suspension of accommodation when the latter is used. A dilated pupil examination is the only practical way to secure adequate study of the optic nerve and macula. The direct ophthalmoscope can also offer the examiner a view of the refracting media from the cornea to the retina. Some estimation of the clarity can be determined and a cataract, corneal opacity, or vitreous opacity may be diagnosed. The retinal examination that can be accomplished with the direct ophthalmoscope is limited to the macula optic nerve and immediate surrounding retina in all but an expert's hands.

MOTILITY

A penlight may be employed to check for straightness of the eyes, that is, the presence or absence of strabismus. A penlight held in front of the patient's eyes approximately one foot away should create a discrete light reflex at the center of each pupil. This is a test for straightness of the eyes. If the pupillary light reflexes do not appear in the center of the pupil, but are deviated toward the temporal limbus in one eye, an esotropia is present. If the light reflex in one eye is deviated toward the nasal limbus, an exotropia is present. Movement of the penlight or other interesting object can determine the presence or absence of free movement of either eye.

VISION TESTING

Functional testing of a child's eyes means primarily determination of visual acuity. In the newborn and infant, awareness of an interesting object and response to a moving series of stripes or pictures may be the only way of testing vision. Occluding one eye in a nonthreatening way will determine whether the nonoccluded eye can see at all. In most instances children will object to occlusion of the only seeing eye. An optokinetic drum is made up of vertical black and white stripes or other alternating, interesting picture objects. On testing, the eyes move in an uncontrolled reflex way, following the movement of such objects. This is a valid, objective means of determining if the child can see. Children under three years old and after the age of walking can recognize small objects, such as a nickel, dime, or quarter when thrown on a carpet. This, as well as observation of a child's behavior, gives some determination of functional aspects of visual acuity. Finding a dime at five feet indicates at least 20/50 vision.

Girls after age three and boys after age three and one-half ordinarily cooperate for the "E" game. In this test, the children must recognize and reproduce the direction of the "fingers" of the "E." It is important to give the child the full line of "E's" in order to rule out the possibility of a functional visual loss, "amblyopia." It is not essential to have a 20-foot room, since a chart may be calibrated for shorter distances and satisfactory visual acuity testing thus obtained. It is more important to determine if the child has equal visual acuity than to ascertain a certain level of acuity as being normal, that is, visual acuity of 20/40 in each eye is probably safer than having visual acuity of 20/50 in one eye and 20/20 in the other. A difference in visual acuity indicates the need for refraction to determine the possible need for glasses or the presence of occult strabismus or organic disease. Difference in visual acuity may not always be corrected immediately by the prescription of glasses. Sometimes patching for functional amblyopia is necessary.

A simple but rewarding test for binocular function may be carried out with an assessment of stereo acuity. A Titmus stereo tester with polaroid glasses can be used to determine the presence or absence of stereopsis. Any child who can see stereoscopically probably has good binocular vision. A simpler test can be carried out by asking the child to place the eraser tip of a pencil he holds directly on the eraser tip of a pencil held by the examiner, as the examiner moves his pencil and holds it still briefly. Accurate pencil placement by the child implies good binocular function.

Color vision testing is relatively unimportant; however, a simple color vision chart may be placed in the waiting room and mothers can administer this test themselves. It should be stressed that 8 per cent of boys and approximately 0.5 per cent of girls have benign red-green "color blindness." Complete color blindness or achromatopsia is incompatible with vision better than 20/200, is invariably associated with nystagmus (dancing eyes), and therefore represents legal blindness.

In the opinion of most pediatric ophthalmologists, adequate preventive eye care in children includes the following indications for eye examinations: (1) Any time the family or the attending physician believes that an eye examination is required—e.g., for strabismus, tearing, or any signs of concern—an eye examination should be done. This can be as early as the first day of life. No child should be considered too young for an eye examination. (2) Each child should have an eye examination before starting school (age four or five). Ideally, this examination would include a dilated fundus examination. In some instances cycloplegic refraction by an ophthalmologist is indicated. If the child is normal, the family can be reassured that routine school visual examinations will be all that is necessary for the child. On the other hand, if some ocular abnormality is detected such as refractive error, strabismus, etc., a plan for routine follow-up examinations or treatment may be established at that time. It is not necessary to have a child seen by an ophthalmologist every year or two merely to confirm that the child's eyes are normal. In cases where a family has a history of severe refractive error or other ocular abnormalities, the eye examination may be done earlier. All children who were born prematurely with or without supplemental oxygen therapy should have a dilated fundus examination as soon as feasible to rule out retinopathy of prematurity.

Of special note is the "white pupil." Among the differential diagnostic aspects of the white pupil are congenital cataract, which requires early treatment; retinoblastoma, which is the most common intraocular tumor in childhood and is invariably fatal if left untreated; retrolental fibroplasia; infestation with *Toxocara canis* or *cati;* persistent hyperplastic primary vitreous; and other rarer causes. A white pupil is an absolute indication for an immediate ophthalmological examination.

Cooperation between the pediatrician and the ophthalmologist who is oriented toward pediatric patients can ensure that children will receive appropriate care.

It should be stressed that no examination of the eyes can uncover learning disability. The eyes see; they do not learn. The eyes should be corrected for refractive error, and should be aligned for both cosmetic and functional reasons, but the use of eye exercises, glasses, and other activities in the hope of enhancing a child's learning abilities is time consuming, costly, and useless.

INJURIES

The eye may be injured by a variety of causes, either mechanical or chemical. The lids, the first line of defense, can be lacerated, abraded, or contused. Superficial horizontal lid lacerations may be simply sutured. Deep horizontal or vertical lacerations, especially those extending through the margin of the lid, and lacerations near the lacrimal drainage apparatus require special attention and should be repaired by a surgeon, usually an ophthalmologist, familiar with the anatomy of this area. In all lid laceration, care should be taken to evaluate the status of the levator palpebrae and to repair it if it is disrupted.

The "black eye," or ecchymosis of the lids, may be the outward manifestation of a much more serious injury such as a contused globe or a blowout fracture of the orbital floor. Diplopia, enophthalmos, or blood in the anterior chamber (between the iris and cornea) mandate referral to an ophthalmologist. While a simple "black eye" in most instances is benign, more serious consequences should always be considered; for instance, a child under two years of age with a black eye and no history of trauma should make the examiner suspicious of a neuroblastoma metastasis or child abuse, denied by the parent.

The conjunctiva may be injured by laceration or abrasion, causing an uncomplicated subconjunctival hemorrhage. These seldom require attention. However, laceration of the cornea presents a serious potential hazard and requires careful repair. Any prolapse of iris or other intraocular material should be left untouched by the initial examiner. A patient with a corneal laceration with or without tissue prolapse should be put at rest, have a patch gently applied over the eye, and then be referred to an ophthalmologist. Less serious corneal abrasions or superficial corneal erosions are relatively frequent. They should be treated as follows: instillation of several drops of topical anesthetic proparacaine hydrochloride 0.5 per cent, dilatation of the pupil with several drops of 2½ per cent Neosynephrine, instillation of several drops of sodium sulfacetamide or Neosporin, placement of a tight patch over the eye, and systemic analgesics as needed. Longer term pupillary dilatation and cycloplegia for comfort may be obtained with 4 per cent homatropine solution. Fluorescein strips to stain corneal defects may be used diagnostically. Some estimation of visual acuity should always be made before treatment, and examination of the fundus and anterior segment of the eye carried out when possible. These children may be treated by the pediatrician or referred to an ophthalmologist. If a corneal problem persists for more than 24 hours, the patient should be seen by an ophthalmologist.

Contusion of the globe can result in a variety of problems including hyphema (blood in the anterior chamber), dislocation or subluxation of the lens, retinal detachment, or globe rupture. Any serious contusion injury to the globe should be managed by an ophthalmologist. As with any severe injury to the eye, the contused eye should be carefully patched and the patient advised not to squeeze the eye.

Chemical injury to the eye is treated with copious irrigation using water, regardless of the cause.

INFECTIONS

The most common cause of conjunctivitis in clinical practice is viral. Viral conjunctivitis requires only symptomatic treatment such as cold compresses and staying in a darkened room, as well as avoiding dissemination of the infection. Certain resistant cases are best treated by an ophthalmologist. The most common cause of bacterial conjunctivitis or "pink eye" in the northern United States is either Pneumococcus or Staphylococcus, while *Hemophilus influenzae* predominates in the South. These infections may be treated with erythromycin, bacitracin, or sulfacetamide ointment or sulfacetamide in the form of 10 to 15 per cent drops. Neosporin in the form of drops or ointment is more effective again *Hemophilus influenzae,* but this drug is also more likely to cause an allergic response. This treatment is used routinely in both eyes, three times a day for 10 days. Symptoms usually disappear in two to three days, but the infection may recur if medication is stopped too early. The same treatment along with the addition of warm compresses should be used in treating styes. In no instance should corticosteroids be used either in combination or alone by the pediatrician. Their use causes a violent increase in severity of herpes simplex corneal infection, leading even to perforation of the globe. Glaucoma and cataracts can also result from prolonged use of corticosteroid drops. Conjunctival cultures may be obtained when severe mucopurulent reactions occur, when the conjunctivitis is of epidemic proportion, or when the host is compromised with systemic disease such as leukemia.

Marginal blepharitis, characterized by dandruff-like flakes at the lid margin, may be treated with topical 10 to 15 per cent sulfacetamide solution, and careful daily removal of the flakes with a cotton-tipped applicator and baby shampoo.

Corneal ulcers may be caused by either viral, bacterial, or mechanical agents. Because of the possibility of scarring or perforation, these infections should be treated by an ophthalmologist.

Iritis or uveitis, the cause of which is usually unknown, is characterized by a deep, perilimbal flush, an inflammatory cell reaction in the anterior chamber, pain, and a small (miotic) pupil. Uveitis is treated by an ophthalmologist. The pain associated with anterior uveitis is usually relieved by dilating the pupil with several drops of homatropine 4 per cent solution.

Lacrimal obstruction in the neonate is treated with warm compresses, sodium sulfacetamide 10 to 15 per cent drops 4 times a day, and gentle massage over the lacrimal sac for 7 to 10 days. If lacrimal obstruction and dacryocystitis persist after two courses of such conservative treatment, the system should be probed by an ophthalmologist. If done before age 6 months, this may be done as an office procedure and offers a complete cure in 90 per cent of patients. After age 6 months, anesthesia is usually required. Lacrimal obstruction that recurs after one or more probings may require temporary silicone tube placement.

Orbital cellulitis is characterized by proptosis and swelling of the lids and conjunctivae. In younger children, orbital cellulitis can have very serious implications. In these cases the possibility of cavernous sinus thrombosis should always be kept in mind. Younger children with orbital cellulitis are ordinarily hospitalized and cared for jointly by the ophthalmologist and pediatrician using intravenous antibiotics.

ALLERGY AND IRRITATION

Many children complain of itching, watering, or vague discomfort of the eyes. There is a strong temptation to treat these nonspecific symptoms with a weak solution of corticosteroid drops. Often, the relief of symptoms is dramatic. However, because of the very real danger of exacerbating a viral corneal infection or causing glaucoma, topical corticosteroids should never be used indiscriminantly. The use of such medicines by ophthalmologists has actually declined greatly in the last decade. Instead of corticosteroids, antiseptic and astringent topical preparations can be very useful in treating nonspecific "allergic" type conjunctivitis. Zinc sulfate 0.25 per cent or one of a variety of premixed commercial preparations may be very helpful for allergic conjunctivitis.

22

HEAD INJURIES

John Shillito, Jr., M.D.

THE PROBLEM

Although injuries to the head may necessitate hospitalization to repair the scalp, skull, or meninges, the principal concern lies not with these overlying tissues but with the brain itself.

Trauma may produce an *immediate* neurological change or "concussion" of unpredictable duration. If unconscious for more than a few minutes with no signs of recovery of consciousness, a child should be hospitalized so that vital functions can be monitored closely and assisted as necessary during the period of reduced consciousness.

Of equal concern is the *delayed* effect of intracranial bleeding or the edema of contused brain. Either can be lethal. Since both increase the intracranial pressure, their differentiation may demand suitable diagnostic studies before appropriate therapy can be chosen.

The possibility of delayed effects presents the commonest dilemma. Is it safe to observe the child at home, or should he be hospitalized for more specialized observation or to be near the

Table 22–1. CONDITIONS NECESSITATING IMMEDIATE HOSPITALIZATION

Continued unconsciousness

Signs of increasing intracranial pressure
1. Progressive loss of consciousness
2. Changes in vital signs: persistent bradycardia; systolic hypertension and widening of the pulse pressure; irregular respiration; fever
3. Persistent vomiting
4. Severe or worsening headache
5. Inappropriate behavior

Other signs of intracranial bleeding
1. Hemorrhages in the optic fundi
2. Meningismus, in absence of neck injury
3. Extreme pallor, especially in infancy, or a rapidly developing, unexplained anemia

Signs of focal brain damage; possible local clot formation
1. Focal neurological deficits: hemiparesis; aphasia; facial asymmetry; unilateral Babinsky sign
2. Dilation of one pupil
3. Convulsions, especially focal

Other considerations
1. Compound skull fracture
   a. Scalp laceration over any skull fracture
   b. Linear fracture into an air sinus
   c. Rhinorrhea or otorrhea, whether or not fracture is demonstrable by x-ray
   d. Blood behind the ear drum or bleeding from the external canal
2. Depressed skull fracture
3. Certain linear fractures
   a. Extensive fracture or fractures from which considerable bleeding may occur both intracranially and in the subperiosteal or subgaleal space
   b. Fracture over the middle meningeal artery which may produce tear of that vessel and produce epidural arterial hemorrhage
   c. Fracture over a major venous sinus (sagittal, lateral) which may permit epidural venous hemorrhage of considerable magnitude and rapidity
   d. Fracture of the occipital bone extending into the foramen magnum. Rupture of a venous lake at the rim of the foramen may cause rapid epidural venous bleeding with compression of brainstem and sudden respiratory abnormalities without the usual localizing neurological signs.
4. Large subgaleal hematoma, especially in infancy
5. Extensive bleeding from scalp laceration
6. Associated cervical spine injury

proper facilities should danger signs dictate immediate intervention? Should he be sent to the hospital for appropriate tests before making the decision about admission? In some cases the correct decision can be made only after review of skull x-rays and even a CT scan (Table 22–1).

Factors such as the nature of the impact may enter into this consideration. Any massive force, such as that caused by a moving automobile or a fall from a considerable height, implies the possibility of serious brain damage and late sequelae and should sway the physician in favor of hospitalization.

The distance between the patient's home and the hospital and the methods of transportation available are important considerations. The ability of the parents to follow instructions, to make reasonable observations, and to remain relatively objective facilitates home observation if otherwise indicated.

Only in infants is it possible to see a state of marked anemia and possibly even hypotension from intracranial bleeding alone. Because a small amount of intracranial bleeding may involve the loss of a large percentage of the infant's circulating blood volume, and because an infant's skull is so distensible, the signs of hypovolemia and even clinical shock may occur before the effects of intracranial pressure are seen. The loss of blood beneath the scalp of an infant may be massive enough to require transfusion. Serial hematocrit values are advisable when any such collection is noted, and hospitalization is wise until the rate of subgaleal bleeding has been established. Concurrent vomiting may dehydrate a child and give a falsely high hematocrit initially.

The possibility of concurrent injuries to other bones and organs should be carefully considered before electing home observation.

WHEN TO TAKE X-RAYS; WHEN TO REQUEST A CT SCAN

The introduction of computer-assisted tomography in the mid 1970s has radically changed the neurosurgeon's approach to cranial trauma and has rendered unnecessary, in most cases, the use of invasive, time-consuming, and less informative studies such as angiography. It can immediately demonstrate an intracranial hemorrhage, even before symptoms appear, and it can show swelling of the brain and hydrocephalus. It may demonstrate the presence of intracranial air even when no skull fracture can be seen by x-ray, thus establishing the presence of a technically compound fracture.

Since the main concern is the state of the intracranial contents, it has been an increasingly common practice to obtain a CT scan first and perhaps bypass skull films entirely. There are certain conditions that skull x-rays can document far better than the CT scan, and their use should not be abandoned lightly.

When to Take Skull X-Rays

From the foregoing, it is apparent that certain types of fractures will require surgical therapy and others medical therapy or very close observation. Although it is inadvisable to make too many rules about when to take x-ray films, the following may be used as a guide:

1. When a depressed fracture is suspected from clinical examination, anteroposterior, lateral, and tangential views of the skull at the area of concern are especially valuable; subgaleal hemorrhage may create a saucer-like area that feels like a depressed fracture which can promptly be ruled out by x-ray.
2. When a large subgaleal hematoma is present it signifies considerable injury; bleeding probably is coming from a fracture, and its presence and size and position can be established by x-rays.
3. When the percussion note of the skull is definitely abnormal, it signifies that either a large linear fracture or a diastatic fracture of one or more sutures exists.
4. When the injury involves the region over a meningeal artery or a large dural venous sinus.
5. When the injury involves an area of the skull containing an air sinus, such as the frontal or mastoid sinuses.
6. When a penetrating injury *may* have occurred, not only to the cranium but also to the orbit, nose, or pharynx, from which a penetrating object may have reached the intracranial contents.
7. When severe head trauma has occurred and neck pain is present, to rule out cervical spine fracture.
8. When the magnitude of forces involved suggests that a fracture may well have occurred even though the child appears clinically less severely damaged.

The mere presence of a linear fracture that does not lie in any of the above-mentioned sensitive areas is not in itself a contraindication to home observation.

When to Get a CT Scan

If the physician is concerned enough to request a CT scan, he should at the same time contact a neurosurgeon about the child, for prompt action may be necessary. In general the scan is looking for the cause of existing or progressive neurological deficit, or for as yet unannounced hemorrhages, suspected because of the location of a fracture. Its purpose is therefore to find an intracranial hemorrhage that may exist and to look for remediable causes of neurological deficits. It is also useful in documenting the presence of cerebral edema or localized contusion with petechial hemorrhage so that appropriate medical therapy can be instituted. It is also useful in its ability to detect minute amounts of intracranial air and the path of unsuspected penetrating foreign bodies. Its use should precede the taking of skull x-rays when the brain is already in trouble. The scan may obviate a period of observation when skull x-rays have demonstrated a potentially dangerous situation.

OTHER TESTS

Electroencephalography has not been useful in the immediate post-traumatic period unless there is some confusion as to whether one is witnessing a postictal or a post-traumatic state.

Ultrafrequency sonar scanning can indicate the position of the midline structures of the brain. This test has been supplanted by the CT scan where it is available.

Lumbar puncture should not be done after recent cranial trauma. The presence of blood in the spinal fluid does not document the presence or absence of intracranial clot, and removal of fluid from the lumbar space may permit an expansion of existing intracranial clot, shifting of the brain, and possible compression of the medulla. If a differential diagnosis is being entertained between trauma, spontaneous intracranial hemorrhage, and meningitis, a screening CT scan to rule out intracranial mass lesions is wise before performing a necessary diagnostic lumbar puncture.

If the child is seen immediately after a head injury, there may be a bradycardia that should be transient. A pulse below 60 is a danger sign until time proves otherwise. The child will usually be pale, listless, and somewhat drowsy and will almost certainly vomit one or more times soon after the injury. If vomiting occurs more than two or three times or is especially violent, it may be advisable to admit the child for observation and possible intravenous rehydration. It is unwise to administer antiemetics unless absolutely necessary for the concomitant drowsiness that many produce will confuse neurological observation.

Instead of drowsiness, a child may manifest irritability and irrational behavior. This should clear within a few hours. Amnesia for the accident itself and retrograde amnesia for several hours prior to the accident are not unusual but are alarming. The cortical blindness produced presumably by contusion or ischemia of the occipital poles is alarming as well but not necessarily indicative of an intracranial clot. If clearing, this sign alone does not contraindicate home observation.

The presence of any localizing neurological signs, such as weakness of an extremity or of the face, difficulty of speech, or upgoing toes on plantar stimulation, contraindicates home observation unless these signs rapidly disappear. Minor headache is not unusual but should be related to the point of injury. The pupils should be equal and reactive. If both are constricted, subarachnoid hemorrhage is usually present. If one or both are dilated and poorly reactive, increasing intracranial pressure should be suspected.

Herniation of the temporal lobe through the incisura of the tentorium will compress and partially paralyze the third cranial nerve, allowing the opposing sympathetic system, which reaches the pupil along the carotid artery and its branches, to dilate the pupil. With complete paralysis of the third nerve, the pupil will be maximally dilated and unreactive to light. Although this can occur from a contusion of the third nerve at the time of injury, this sign should be considered indicative of an intracranial expanding lesion until proven otherwise.

HOME CARE

If it appears to the physician that the child's existing state and the likelihood of sequelae are such that he could be observed at home, there are other aspects of the problem to be considered (Table 22–2).

Although it is well to err on the side of safety, the physician must also consider that the usual admitting procedure at any hospital may unnecessarily agitate an injured youngster who would do better in the quiet of his own home with attentive and capable parents at hand. Also to be considered is the location of the nearest hospital, the availability of transportation to it, and, in some areas, the time of year and the existing or anticipated weather. The identity

Table 22–2. CONDITIONS FOR HOME OBSERVATIONS

1. History of brief loss of consciousness, or none at all
2. Stability or improvement of condition of alertness
3. Normal vital signs
4. Vomiting no more than two or three times immediately after the injury
5. Normal or progressively improving neurological examination
6. Equality of pupils and appropriate size for existing illumination
7. No evidence of penetrating skull injury
8. No evidence of spinal fluid otorrhea or rhinorrhea
9. No blood behind the ear drums or bleeding from external canals

It must be remembered that dangerous sequelae can appear even in the absence of an initial concussion.

and availability of a neurosurgeon should be considered and his help in making this decision about home observation may be sought before there are signs of trouble.

Once home observation is decided upon, the physician should outline for the parents the danger signs and how often these should be looked for. Most parents appreciate this concern and are very willing to carry out instructions.

On occasion, however, their reaction to the discussion disqualifies them as competent or objective observers. In that event, plans can be changed and the child admitted. A list of danger signs is either provided at the hospital emergency ward or can be enumerated for the parents by the physician at their home. The physician should read over the instructions to be sure the parents understand what is expected of them and when to call for assistance. Table 22–3 is a suggested list of instructions.

WHEN TO CALL A NEUROSURGEON

Until enough personal experience has been gained in dealing with children with head injuries, it would be wise to establish communication with a neurosurgeon who is willing to discuss cases even before they become emergencies and to help in the decision as to the necessity of hospitalization. Few neurosurgeons will pass up the opportunity to evaluate a child with questionable symptoms early in the day, before obvious danger signs develop, thus obviating a frantic emergency trip to the hospital.

In general, when any one or more of the above-mentioned danger signs appear, it is wise to make arrangements for hospitalization and contact a neurosurgeon. The availability of the neurosurgeon, the distance to the hospital, the weather, the time of day, and the age of the patient are important factors in such a decision. We should realize that there will be delays varying from 30 minutes to several hours after the child has reached the hospital before he may actually be in the operating room and try to allow for such delays in planning.

SEQUELAE

The majority of children who have sustained the usual head injury with no, or transient, neurological deficit will recover remarkably well

Table 22–3. INSTRUCTIONS FOR CARE OF CHILD WITH HEAD INJURY

Signs of Trouble

Please notify Dr. ______________________ at ______________________ (Tel. No.) if any of the following develop:

1. **Excessive Drowsiness:** Your child may well be exhausted by the ordeal surrounding the injury but should be easily aroused by methods that you would ordinarily use to awaken him from a deep sleep.
2. **Persistent Vomiting:** Children will, in most cases, vomit one or more times after a severe head injury. It should not ordinarily occur more than once or twice, nor should it recur once it has ceased.
3. **Weakness of One Side:** If the child does not use one arm or leg as well as the other or is unsteady in walking, particularly with a limp.
4. **Unequal Pupils:** If one pupil appears to be larger than the other when both eyes are in equal light.
5. **"Seeing Double":** A child may complain of this spontaneously or may squint one eye to prevent seeing double. You may be able to notice that the eyes are not trained on the same object.
6. **Difficulty in Speaking:** The speech should not be slurred, and the child should be able to express himself as well as usual.
7. **Severe Headache:** A headache should ordinarily be relieved by aspirin in appropriate dosage and should not increase in severity.
8. **Convulsions:** If a twitching of the face or arm or leg begins, or if the child forces himself into an odd position without trembling, place him on his side so that he cannot fall. Be sure that there is ample room for him to breathe, placing a firm object, such as a wooden pencil, between the back teeth on one side to keep the mouth open. Stay with the child until the convulsion begins to subside, and call for help as soon as possible.

On the night following the head injury or during the nap period it is advisable to awaken your child (usually every three hours at least) and look for any of these danger signs.

and have no residual problems. During their recovery there may be post-traumatic headache, dizziness, and nausea, particularly when mobilization has begun. These ordinarily subside within a few days, and after recovery has been completed there should be no recurrence of these symptoms.

There certainly is, in childhood, something resembling compensation neurosis of the adult. This usually is a mechanism for gaining attention, which is initially successful. A child may simply hold his head or cry or complain of a headache, and the anxieties of the parents are rightfully aroused until the problem has been settled by the physician.

Should symptoms of headache, stiff neck, personality change, or a neurological deficit occur after the initial period of recovery, one must consider the possibility of a subdural hematoma and take appropriate steps to rule it out. A normal neurological and funduscopic examination, supported by normal CT scan, should be adequate.

After severe head injuries there may have been enough bleeding in the subarachnoid space to produce a temporary communicating hydrocephalus. The increase of intracranial pressure is real and somewhat prolonged even though no intracranial mass exists. It may be necessary to confirm this diagnosis by a CT scan. This type of hydrocephalus is usually transient and can be controlled, if necessary, by serial lumbar punctures, after adequately ruling out an intracranial mass lesion.

Occasionally, fractures into the air sinuses of the skull have allowed an occult spinal fluid leak to occur into the middle ear or the nasopharynx. This leak can produce low intracranial pressure with headache, provide a route of entry for bacteria with resulting meningitis, or allow the entry of air with spontaneous pneumocephalus and accompanying headache.

The most common late sequela of any head injury that involves actual contusion or laceration of the brain is a convulsive disorder. The first seizure may occur even one or two years after the accident. If a severe neurological deficit occurred at the time of injury or if it is known by direct inspection at the time of surgery that the brain was scarred, it is wise to continue the child on anticonvulsants indefinitely. The advisability of discontinuing these drugs can most safely be determined by electroencephalographic evidence of absence of seizure discharges from the area so scarred. A period of tapering the dosage is more advisable than suddenly discontinuing the drug.

Occasionally symptoms can be produced by a leptomeningeal cyst, which should be apparent by plain x-ray film and by CT scan. This is discussed further under follow-up.

Rarely, persistent symptoms following an otherwise insignificant head injury may be attributable to pre-existing intracranial pathology. Some brain tumors have been detected by persistence of symptoms after a head injury which may have been coincidental and relatively insignificant.

RESUMPTION OF ACTIVITY

Usually a child will wish to get out of bed and can do so comfortably only when danger is past. If he is mobilized too soon, recurrence of headache or vomiting signifies that trouble may still lie ahead or that recovery from the contusion is not yet complete. It is wise not to push a child out of bed into normal activity until he is ready.

Once he is up and around the house, it is wise to restrict his activities and visitors to those that will not promote rough play and risk another fall. In the absence of fractures or other complicating features of the head injury, one or two days of symptom-free limited activity should be adequate.

Any recurrence of symptoms should prompt careful reevaluation. Chronic subdural hematomas have been detected in children months after a head injury. Only in the more chronic case is papilledema a reliable sign; other symptoms or signs usually antedate its development in more acute situations.

If a child active in contact sports suffers a series of concussions, the problem of restricting these activities is raised. This must always be handled on an individual basis. If a child, by his repeated head injuries, demonstrates a propensity for accidents, it may be well to remove him from such activities before he seriously damages himself. A concussion is a transient neurological deficit and implies no physical change. If symptoms oulast this initial deficit, there are probably changes present, such as edema of the brain or actual scarring from contusion, and it is certainly unwise to allow the child to resume sports until all symptoms have cleared completely and do not recur with resumption of moderate activity.

FOLLOW-UP

A follow-up visit one or two weeks after a severe head injury, and again after about three months, is a reasonable precaution. Follow-up x-ray examinations are ordinarily made when there has been a considerable diastasis of the fracture line or of the sutures, to ensure that there is no further diastasis that might indicate an expanding intracranial clot. If there has been a fracture with laceration of the meninges, they may be pinched in the fracture, which will cause the separation to persist. This will occasionally permit a cyst of spinal fluid to be loculated; by transmitted pulsations from within the cranium, this cyst can erode the skull, producing a larger bony deficit. This so-called leptomeningeal cyst can be corrected surgically by its removal and repair of the underlying meninges.

Ordinarily fine linear fractures heal promptly, and no follow-up x-ray films are necessary unless the symptoms persist or reappear.

CONCLUSION

In electing to observe the child at home after a head injury, one must consider not only how likely the danger signs are to develop in a given patient but also what measures will have to be taken to get him to the hospital and how long it will take to get him there. It is well to remember that a rapidly developing hematoma can produce respiratory arrest within 30 or 40 minutes after its first signs are detected. Such a catastrophe will usually occur within the first 48 hours after injury; after this period more warning is usually given by slowly developing signs of trouble. Until sufficient experience with head-injured children is gained, it is wise to err on the side of caution and observe such children within immediate access to competent neurosurgical attention.

23

ANIMAL BITES

Douglas A. Boenning, M.D.

Animal bites pose a significant public health problem in the United States. Approximately 1 per cent of the population is bitten annually, with the great majority of victims falling into the pediatric age range. Nearly half of all bites occur in children ages 5 to 15 years. One per cent of all pediatric visits to emergency departments in summer months are related to animal bite injuries, which range from simple lacerations to major trauma with fatal outcomes. With an estimated 80 to 100 million dogs and cats in this country, it is no surprise that they are the species most frequently implicated in biting incidents. Other domestic animals commonly involved in biting are small household pets such as gerbils, hamsters, rabbits, rats, and mice.

Since the clinician is frequently faced with the problem of animal bites, a consistent approach will aid in optimal management. This approach addresses the questions surrounding immediate wound care and prevention of infection (bacterial, tetanus, and rabies) and of future injury.

PRINCIPLES OF IMMEDIATE WOUND CARE

Most wounds are superficial lacerations, abrasions, or punctures. These comprise about 80 per cent of wounds and may be comfortably handled by the office practitioner. Deep lacerations, avulsions, crush injuries, and compound fractures require urgent treatment, surgical repair, and often hospital admission.

All wounds should be irrigated copiously with normal saline or a dilute povidone-iodine solution. High-pressure irrigation with normal saline—using a 30- to 50-ml syringe fitted with an 18-gauge needle—mechanically dislodges bacteria and is particularly helpful in cleaning deep wounds. The clinician should then ensure hemostasis followed by wound closure, if necessary, in a manner that produces the best cosmetic result. Dog bite wounds sutured after thorough local cleansing develop infections no more frequently than sutured lacerations in general.

RISKS OF BACTERIAL INFECTION

In general, there is a low rate of bacterial wound infection in children with dog bites. Although many potential pathogens may be isolated from the dog's mouth or the fresh wound, only about 5 per cent of dog bites become infected. In contrast, 20 to 50 per cent of cat bites or scratches are reported to develop infection. This difference in infectivity between dog and cat bites is partly explained by the higher incidence of puncture wounds associated with cat bites. In relatively small, harmless-appearing puncture wounds, virulent organisms may be inoculated deeply into tissues where a microaerophilic environment promotes their rapid growth. Large open wounds are more easily cleaned and thus have a lower rate of infection. Two other risk factors for infection are wound neglect for greater than 24 hours and wound location on the extremities, particularly those involving the hand.

Wounds that have signs of infection should be cultured and antibiotic therapy prescribed. Two frequently encountered pathogens are *Staphylococcus aureus* and *Pasteurella multocida;* however, because of the large variety of organisms found in the mouths of dogs and cats, no single antibiotic will treat all potential pathogens. If a wound rapidly develops signs of infection, *P. multocida* should be suspected. In general, empirical therapy of the infected wound may be started with an oral cephalosporin pending definitive culture results. If *P. multocida* is isolated, penicillin is the drug of choice. In a prospective study of penicillin prophylaxis in dog bites, 55 consecutive children with nonfacial wounds were allocated to either five days of oral penicillin or local wound care alone. The rates of infection were comparable in both groups (one patient in each) and the overall rate of infection was 3.6 per cent. The low overall rate of infection in itself mitigates against prescribing prophylactic antibiotics for all dog bites (Boenning et al., 1983). Similar findings have been described using prophylactic oxacillin (Elenbaas et al., 1982).

TETANUS STATUS OF THE PATIENT

Tetanus prophylaxis should be considered in all patients. In the child with fewer than three primary immunizations, tetanus toxoid should be administered. Additionally, tetanus immune globulin should be given to that same child if the wound has been neglected for more than 24 hours or the patient has fewer than two primary immunizations. For the child with three or more tetanus immunizations, tetanus toxoid should be administered if 10 years have elapsed since the last booster (5 years if a contaminated or neglected wound is present) (Report of the Committee on Infectious Diseases, 1982).

THE RISKS OF RABIES

All warm-blooded animals are capable of harboring the rabies virus, but in fact, domestic dogs and cats have a low carriage rate. Nevertheless, the fear of rabies is often a reason why parents seek medical attention for their child who has been bitten. In the majority of dog and cat bites, the animal will be a family or neighborhood pet. If the animal appears healthy, it should be observed for 10 days and no antirabies prophylaxis given to the exposed human. If during the 10-day holding period the animal exhibits strange behavior, becomes ill, or dies, the animal's head should be shipped under refrigeration to a qualified laboratory for examination. If a domestic dog or cat is rabid or suspected of being rabid at the time of the bite, then postexposure prophylaxis should be initiated with human rabies immune globulin and human diploid cell vaccine (Plotkin and Clark, 1981). If the dog or cat is a stray or escapes capture, the public health recommendations in the geographical region should guide the management of the patient. Certain wild animals including the skunk, bat, fox, raccoon, and coyote should be presumed rabid until proven negative. Treatment of the exposed human should be initiated immediately. Bites from wild rodents, rabbits, and squirrels rarely require antirabies prophylaxis.

PREVENTION OF ANIMAL BITES

Advice to parents, albeit after the fact in many cases, may prevent recurrence of biting episodes. Ideally, anticipatory guidance should be given during routine well child care. Newborns should never be left unsupervised in the presence of an animal even momentarily. Toddlers should always be watched when they are around a family pet. Preschool and elementary school children should be taught to respect the rights of the animal regarding feeding, territory, and protection of its young. Leash laws should be followed by responsible adults, and these laws should be enforced by authorities in the community.

SUMMARY POINTS REGARDING ANIMAL BITES

1. Thorough cleansing of an animal bite is the most important factor in preventing infection.
2. Wound infections due to *Pasteurella multocida* often develop within 24 hours of the bite.
3. All animal bite injuries should be evaluated for the risk of infection with common bacteria, tetanus, and rabies.

REFERENCES

Boenning, D. A., Fleisher G. R., and Campos J. M.: Dog bites in children: Epidemiology, microbiology, and penicillin prophylactic therapy. Am. J. Emerg. Med., *1*:5–9, 1983.

Callahan, M.: Dog bite wounds. J.A.M.A., *244*:2327–2328, 1980.

Elenbaas, R. M., McNabney, W. K., and Robinson, W. A.: Prophylactic oxacillin in dog bite wounds. Ann. Emerg. Med., *11*:248–251, 1982.

Fleisher, G. R., and Boenning, D. A.: The treatment of animal bites in humans. Compend. Contin. Educ. Pract. Vet., *3*:366–370, 1981.

Marcy, S. M.: Infections due to dog and cat bites. Pediatr. Infect. Dis., *1*:351–356, 1982.

Plotkin, S. A., and Clark, H. F.: Rabies. *In* Feigin, R. D., and Cherry, J. D. (eds.): Textbook of Pediatric Infectious Diseases. Philadelphia, W. B. Saunders Co., 1981, pp. 1267–1275.

Report of the Committee on Infectious Diseases, 19th ed. Evanston, Ill., American Academy of Pediatrics, 1982.

24

MUSCULOSKELETAL TRAUMA IN CHILDREN

Lyle J. Micheli, M.D.

Childhood injuries, and, in particular, injuries to the extremities and back, are now the leading cause of hospital admissions for children and adolescents, and a reason for frequent visits to the office or clinic (Accident Facts, 1978). Pediatric musculoskeletal injuries can be conveniently divided into three etiological categories: (1) high impact, such as falls from a height or motor vehicle trauma; (2) free play activity; and (3) organized sports activities. In relation to the last category, there is growing concern that too many injuries are occurring in children's sports. Much more must be done to prevent these injuries (see Chapter 25).

There is a whole new group of injuries in children engaged in organized sports which rarely occur in the free play situation. These "overuse" injuries, which result from the microtrauma of repetitive training activities, are specific to organized sports training and competition (Micheli, 1983). These "overuse" injuries were more often seen in the past in the adult recreational athlete. They rarely occurred in children engaged in free play activities. When encountered in the adult recreational athlete, these injuries were hypothesized to be a result of the aging process and associated degeneration of body tissues. Clearly, with the present epidemic of overuse injuries resulting from recurrent microtrauma now seen in children involved in organized sports, this simplistic etiological explanation of this type of injury has to be reassessed.

Improper training, usually too much over too short a period of time, appears to be a common contributor to most overuse injuries in sports, including children's sports. Other factors include anatomical malalignment, such as femoral anteversion, genu valgum, pes planus, and muscle-tendon imbalance, particularly excessive tightness resulting from a rapid growth spurt. In running sports, shoewear and playing surface

Table 24–1. RISK FACTORS IN MUSCULOSKELETAL TRAUMA

1. Training errors, including abrupt changes in intensity, duration, or frequency of training.
2. Musculotendinous imbalance—of strength, flexibility, or bulk.
3. Anatomical malalignment of the lower extremities, including differences in leg lengths, abnormalities of rotation of the hips, position of the knee cap, and bow legs, knock knees, or flat feet.
4. Footwear: improper fit, inadequate impact-absorbing material, excessive stiffness of the sole, and/or insufficient support of the hindfoot.
5. Running surface: concrete pavement versus asphalt, versus running track, versus dirt or grass.
6. Associated disease state of the lower extremity, including arthritis, poor circulation, old fracture, or other injury.

can be factors. An excessively hard surface is often implicated in dance injuries. Finally, sports equipment or its failure, defective protective equipment, or inadequate playing equipment can be factors in injury (Table 24–1).

The overuse injuries increase the need for very careful assessment and diagnosis of complaints of pain or limp in the child. Infectious processes and musculoskeletal neoplasms may be overlooked in their early stages if the complaints of an active child are too readily ascribed to the sports or recreational activity in which they are participating (Micheli and Jupiter, 1978).

TYPES OF INJURY

Fractures

The two mechanisms of injury in childhood injuries are single impact macrotrauma and repetitive microtrauma. While single impact fractures, including those involving the growth plate, remain the major concern following many types of injury, stress fractures resulting from multiple microtrauma, including stress fractures of the growth plate, are being seen with increasing frequency in children. In stress fractures, a tiny crack develops in the bone and propagates at a faster rate than the body's normal reparative processes can produce healing (Fig. 24–1*A*). These are often missed initially, since plain radiographs may be unremarkable for two or three weeks following the onset of symptoms.

A high index of suspicion is prudent if there is a history of repetitive activity such as sports training, but any repetitive activity may result in a stress fracture, e.g., a child repetitively jumping from a porch. On physical examination, pain may be elicited by indirect force as in applying a bending force to the lower leg at points above and below the site of a suspected tibial stress fracture. Bone scanning using technetium-99 can be a useful diagnostic aid that is usually positive well before plain radiographs (Fig. 24–1*B*). It must be remembered, of

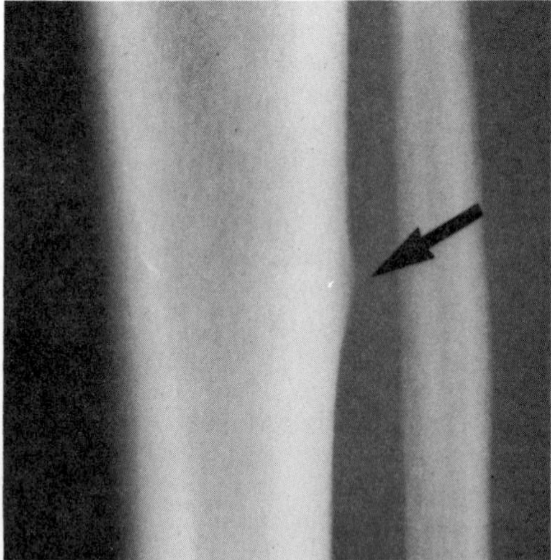

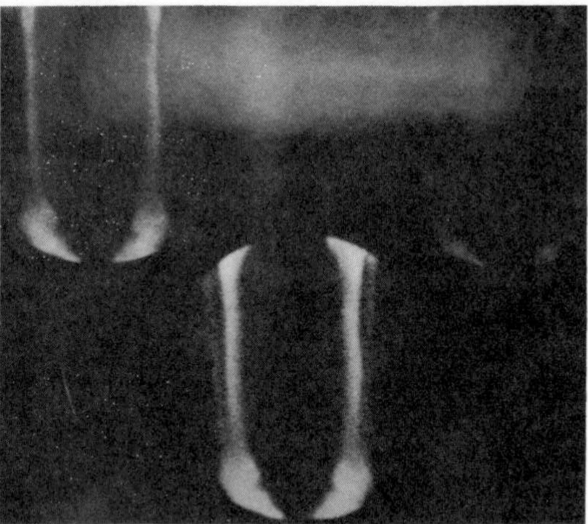

Figure 24–1. *A*, Stress fracture of the tibial shaft. Plain radiographs may only show evidence of healing two to three weeks after the onset of symptoms. *B*, Radionuclear bone scan of the tibia may show increased uptake 24 to 48 hours after a stress fracture.

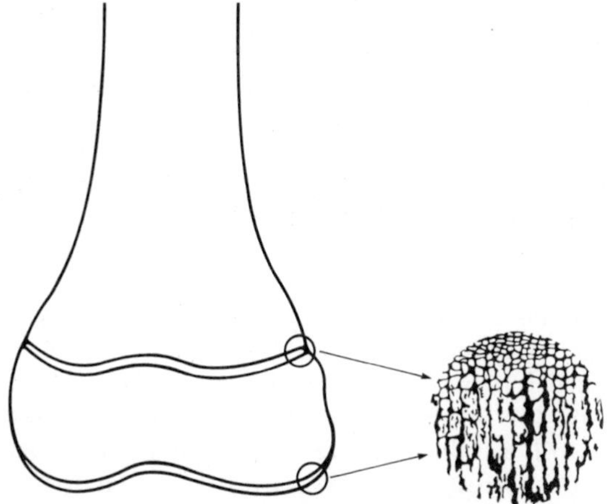

Figure 24–2. In the child, both the growth plate and joint surface consist of growing cartilage, with an increased susceptibility to injury.

course, that osteomyelitis and bone tumors, which must be included in the differential diagnosis of any stress fracture, will also have an increased uptake of radionucleotides (Rosen et al., 1982).

Growth or epiphyseal plate fractures are peculiar to the child. The growth plate, which consists of a somewhat irregular cartilaginous disc located near either end of the long bone between the epiphysis and metaphysis, is responsible for the longitudinal growth of the bone. The histoanatomy consists of multiple columns of cartilage cells in various stages of transformation from immature cells on the one end to degenerated remnants of cells on the other end of the column. The latter form the lattice work for the new bone formation taking place in the shaft (Fig. 24–2). Since this rather intricate structure is less resistant to deforming force applied to the extremities than either the ligaments of the joints or the bony cortex in the shafts of the long bones, mechanical disruption of the child's bones frequently occurs through the substance of the growth plate itself (Bright and Elmore, 1968). If portions of the generative cell layer of the plate are destroyed by the injury, or the subsequent alignment of the fractured growth plate fragments is such that columns of healing bone form across portions of the plate, future growth of the bone may be affected. Loss of limb length, angular deformity, and joint incongruity are frequent sequelae of growth plate injuries (Ogden, 1963). It is this concern for the potential complications of a growth plate fracture in the child that causes many physicians to question the advisability of participation in heavy contact sports before growth has been completed.

The potential for problems following epiphyseal fracture depends on both the extent of growth plate damage and the specific growth plate involved. Fractures involving the growth plate of the proximal humerus rarely result in subsequent growth or joint complication, whereas fractures of the distal femoral growth plate have a high incidence of subsequent problems. In 1963, Salter and Harris classified epiphyseal injuries into five types, with the relative potential for growth plate damage and future growth problems rated as increasing from Type I to Type V (Fig. 24–3). This classification is the one used most frequently today to describe and categorize growth plate injuries.

While the potential danger of these macrofractures of the growth plate is fairly well established, little is currently known about the potential for growth plate injury from repetitive microtrauma such as prolonged running. Proponents of distance running for children, up to and including the marathon distance of 26 miles, 385 yards, seem unaware of the potential for imperceptible but possibly long-term damage to the growth plate and growing articular cartilage of the child.

Joint Injuries

Injuries about joints in the child can include sprains of the joint ligaments, injuries to the major muscle-tendon units that insert near the joint, growth plate fractures, and derangements

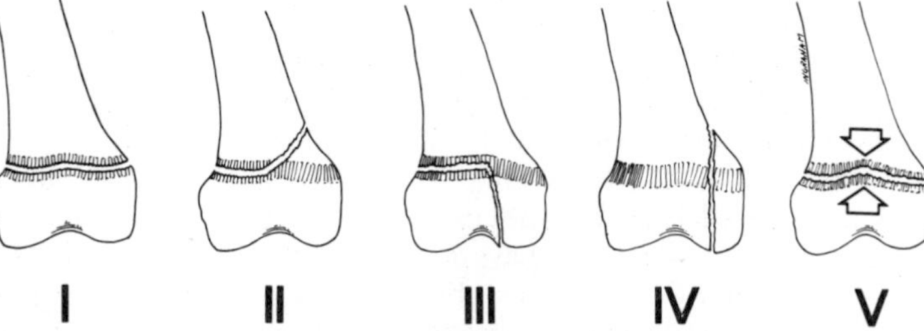

Figure 24–3. The Salter-Harris classification of epiphyseal fractures.

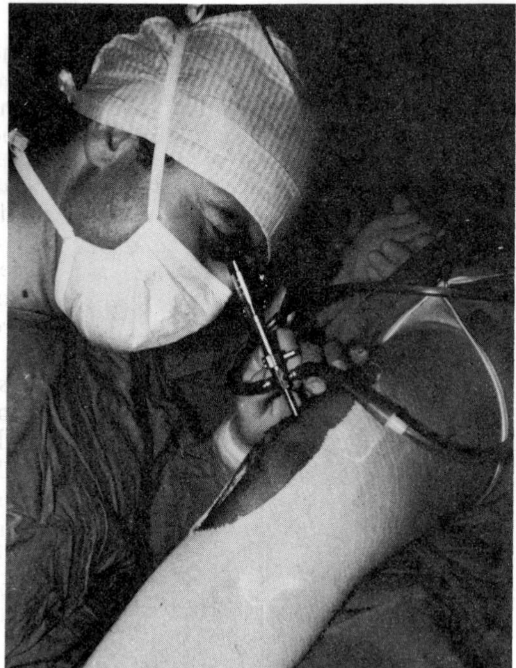

Figure 24–4. The fiberoptic arthroscope is particularly useful in assessing joint disorder in children.

of the internal structures of the joints themselves. When a child complains of pain about a joint, it is very useful to determine whether the pain resulted from a single discrete injury or had a gradual onset, perhaps as a result of repetitive microtrauma or training activities.

With macrotrauma injuries of the joints, the diagnosis of a sprain must be made cautiously in the child. Since during a growth spurt, the ligaments may be stronger than the growth plate, excessive bending or twisting forces may result in fractures through the growth plate rather than in a ligamentous sprain. We have, however, encountered severe ligamentous disruptions of the knee and the ankle in children following injury, and these are being reported with increasing frequency (Mayer and Micheli, 1979). The best way to differentiate between these injuries is early careful examination, localizing the exact site of tenderness and pain.

The development of the arthroscope, including fiberoptic telescopes and video cameras, improved optics, and better operative instruments, has revolutionized the assessment of joint disorders of the knee, ankle, and shoulder in children (Fig. 24–4). A child suspected of having a discoid lateral meniscus as the cause of recurrent limp can now have a comprehensive examination and even resection and shaping of the deranged meniscus through two puncture wounds. In addition to greatly reduced hospitalization and morbidity, this technique may result in fewer residual problems with the knee.

Muscle-Tendon Unit Injuries

The child appears to be at particular risk for muscle-tendon unit problems. In addition to the contusions or strains that may result from direct blows or twists, the process of growth and the insertion of major muscle-tendon units into bone through the epiphyseal growth cartilage places these structures at special risk of injury.

Growth, and in particular the adolescent growth spurt, results in a relative tightening of the muscle-tendon units that span the rapidly growing bones but do not themselves have growth potential (Micheli, 1983). This anatomical fault increases the risk of frank apophyseal avulsion or, more frequently, apophysitis such as Osgood-Schlatter disease, especially in the athletically active adolescent. Stretching exercises done in a systematic fashion appear to be particularly important to prevent injuries to the muscle-tendon unit and the apophysis (Fig. 24–5).

Tendinitis can certainly occur in the young athlete, but much less frequently than in the adult. Usually the site of tendon insertion—the apophysis—becomes symptomatic before the tendon itself, although both may become painful and inflamed. This diagnosis should be made relatively cautiously in the young athlete and only after other possible etiologies, including stress fractures, osteochondritis, and nerve impingement, have been ruled out.

It is important to remember that the inflammatory phase of tendinitis is the body's normal initial healing response to microtears of the tendon fibers. We must respect this response; therefore, rest is an important part of management, particularly in this age group. It is rarely necessary, however, to completely rest or immobilize the injured extremity, and complete rest may actually delay healing. A period of relative "rest" is useful, during which the extremity is used, but with a different stress pattern. A runner with an acute Achilles tendinitis who swims for an hour a day may not be running, but he or she is certainly not resting. Ice packs and gentle compression are useful in the acute stages of tendinitis, and nonsteroidal anti-inflammatory drugs such as buffered aspirin are frequently helpful. We do not use corticosteroid injections in the young athlete.

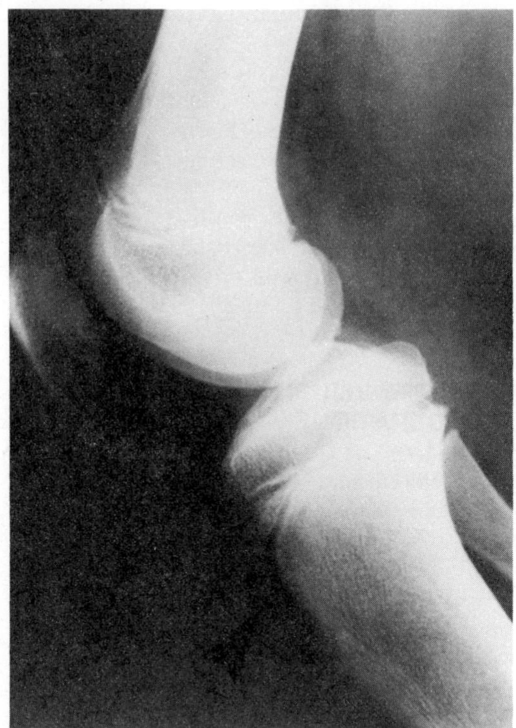

Figure 24–5. Osgood-Schlatter disease, with tenderness and prominence of the tibial tubercle, is an avulsion fracture of the tibial tubercle resulting from repetitive microtrauma.

In addition to these conservative techniques, restoration of the strength and flexibility of the muscle-tendon unit during healing may also aid this process and certainly help prevent recurrence of injury. Stanish (1982) has shown that dynamic eccentric strengthening exercises not only can safely be done during the early healing phase of a tendinitis, but may actually promote healing. Dynamic eccentric exercise is resistive exercise in which the muscle-tendon unit that is being loaded is also lengthening at the same time (Buxbaum and Micheli, 1979).

SITES OF INJURY

The Spine

Neck injuries and complaints of neck pain in the child should always be treated seriously. A careful history, including localization of pain and associated dysesthesia at the time of injury, as well as the direction of injury, whether flexion, extension, or rotation, duration of symptoms, and any previous episode should be determined.

With an acute injury, the neck should be in the neutral position immediately, followed by a careful neurological examination. The soft cervical collar may be used if it truly immobilizes the neck, but a rolled-up towel or even a pair of sweatpants can do a very adequate job, sometimes much better than a commercial apparatus. Plain anteroposterior and lateral radiographs of the spine, including odontoid views, should precede a range-of-motion examination of the neck if serious injury is suspected. If flexion or extension elicits pain, lateral views in flexion and extension should be obtained under careful control to assess ligamentous stability.

These radiographs should be assessed carefully, since increase in excursion of C2 on C3 can be a normal finding in children (Henrys et al., 1977). Particular attention on plain radiographs to possible congenital anomalies, including failure of ossification of the odontoid, as well as spinal dysraphism, should be noted. Recurrent episodes of neck pain following minor trauma, with associated dysymmetry of rotation of the neck, should be referred for further assessment of possible rotatory subluxation of the neck.

If the cervical spine is found to be stable and no major injury has occurred, an initial period of relative rest with application of local heat and mild analgesics to control muscle spasm and pain should then be followed by a progressive program of exercises. We initially use an isometric exercise program done in the six directions of motion with the child providing his own resistance for a count of ten. Dynamic range-of-motion and muscle-strengthening exercises may then be instituted through the painless arc of motion of the neck in all directions.

Thoracic Spine

Injuries to the back and thoracic region are relatively rare. Strains of the muscles of the back, particularly those between the scapula and spinous processes, can generally be diagnosed by careful physical examination. Injuries to the spine itself can occur from falls, including those from a bicycle or porch. Usually the result of flexion or of flexion and rotation, these are diagnosed on plain radiographs, which will show loss of vertebral height anteriorly. These minor vertebral compression fractures of the dorsal spine can generally be handled conservatively with initial rest followed by progressive resumption of activity.

Recurrent microtrauma may also be involved in certain cases of painful adolescent roundbacking or Scheurmann's disease. The characteristic findings of irregularity of vertebral end plates and loss of anterior vertebral height may be a result of a repetitive end plate fracture and secondary spondylodystrophy.

In mild cases of either type of injury, symptomatic treatment, consisting of rest, local heat, and mild analgesics, followed by dorsal extension and lumbar flexion exercises, is usually sufficient. If deformity exists or is anticipated, with kyphosis by Cobb measurement on the lateral radiographs of greater than 50 degrees, extension bracing for a period of 6 to 12 months will often give permanent improvement, with reconstitution of anterior vertebral height and relief of symptoms (Bradford et al., 1974).

Low Back Injuries

Low back injuries in the child and adolescent are being encountered with increasing frequency. These can be divided into mechanical low back pain, associated with increased lumbar lordosis, tight lumbodorsal fascia, and tight hamstrings; intervertebral disc pain; and pain from the bony elements of the spine, including spondylolysis and apophyseal fractures (Micheli, 1979a).

Back pain in the child or adolescent must never be simply dismissed as mechanical in origin. Infectious and neoplastic processes must always be included in a differential diagnosis. Herniation of an intervertebral disc in this age group is frequently associated with trauma, although a constitutional predisposition may also be a factor. Localizing neurological signs and sciatica are often present, but unilateral or bilateral severe hamstring tightness without pain may be the only finding.

Conservative treatment with bed rest, mild analgesics, or anti-inflammatory drugs and even bracing may be effective, but a relatively high percentage come to discectomy.

Bone injury, including spondylolysis, is encountered with increasing frequency in this age group, particularly in the athletically active child. In children involved in recurrent flexion and extension activities of the spine, such as gymnastics, spondylolysis—fracture of the pars interarticularis in the anterior and posterior elements—is most probably a stress fracture (Jackson et al., 1968). Early recognition and relative rest, including bracing, can result in healing of the bony lesion. ^{99}Tc bone scanning is often essential in making an early diagnosis. In addition, pain with hyperextension of the spine, unilateral or bilateral, elicited when the child is standing on each leg, can be diagnostically very helpful.

Tight lumbodorsal fascia and hamstrings, and weakness of the anterior abdominal muscles, can result in tight lumbar lordosis or swayback. Often occurring in association with a growth spurt, this may be a precursor to any of these low back disorders. Preventive measures include low back and hamstring stretching and abdominal strengthening exercises, particularly in the lordotic but athletically active child.

EXTREMITY INJURIES: GENERAL CONSIDERATIONS

Extremity trauma in children can run the full gamut from simple contusion of soft tissue and bone, strain of the musculotendinous units, sprain of the ligamentous supports of the joints, dislocation of the articulating bones of the joints, to fracture of the long bones, with possible associated major neurological or vascular damage. The type of injuries sustained by a child from a given trauma depends upon the relative age and stage of development at the time of injury. As an example, extremity injuries in the neonatal infant often result in a separation of the largely cartilaginous end of the long bone from the shaft of the bone rather than joint injury or fracture of the shaft, because an infant's ligaments are stronger than adjacent bone or epiphyseal plate. These injuries can present problems in the initial diagnosis because of the absence of radiographic abnormalities despite extensive swelling, deformity, or lack of use of the extremity. On occasion, an arthrogram can be helpful in assessing the alignment of the joint. Usually, however, simple traction to align the extremity without deformity is satisfactory treatment. Follow-up reveals the early and rapid appearance of extensive bony callous with early clinical stabilization of the injury (Micheli, 1979b).

In the older child, extremity trauma will frequently result in a fracture of the shaft of the long bone, with joint injury and dislocation relatively rare. In the preadolescent or adolescent child, particularly the child who has toughened his bones and ligamentous structures by athletic training, extremity injuries frequently result in fractures through the epiphyseal growth plate near the end of the long bones rather than in joint surfaces or shaft fractures. A high index of suspicion must be maintained in order to detect these injuries.

Although initial management of extremity

injuries in the child is straightforward, errors frequently occur at this stage of management. The neurovascular status of the extremity and the presence of open injuries of the bones or joints must be determined immediately. A tiny cut from within the skin outward caused by the end of a fracture fragment can have serious results if it is unrecognized and the fracture site becomes infected. On at least two occasions, we have seen gas gangrene with subsequent loss of an extremity result from an unappreciated open fracture.

Absence of extremity pulses is cause for great concern. Dislocations of the shoulder, elbow, hip, or knee may cause serious vascular injury but are inapparent radiographically if they have undergone spontaneous reduction or reduction occurred in the course of manipulation while the patient is being transported.

After the initial assessment is completed, proper splinting of each potentially injured extremity is carried out before sending the child for a radiograph and during further evaluation of the neurological, cardiothoracic, or abdominal status. The newer pneumatic splints provide excellent immobilization of most arm, leg, and knee injuries (Fig. 24–6). In addition, swelling is reduced while the low-pressure splint is in place. In injuries about the elbow and in severely displaced forearm fractures, pneumatic splints should be used only if relative straightening of the extremity will not cause excessive pain or increase the potential for neurovascular injury. When in doubt, it is better to splint the extremity in the position of deformity until consultation is obtained. Rapid splinting of a deformed arm can be carried out with a longitudinal splint of six to eight layers of 3- or 4-inch plaster of Paris padded with web roll or sheet wadding and held in place by loosely applied elastic bandages. Simple sling immobilization generally is sufficient for injuries of the shoulder or upper arm.

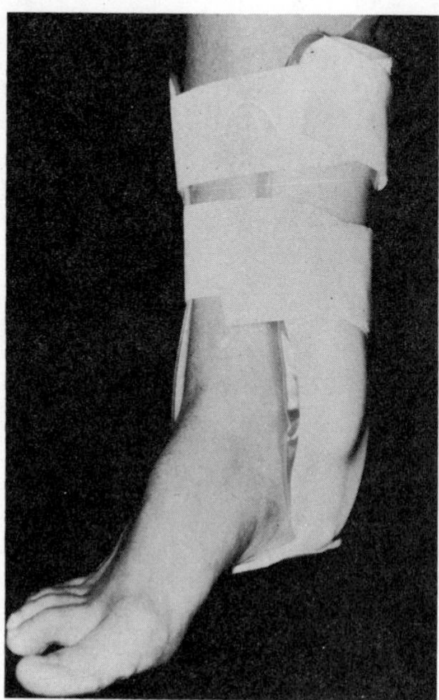

Figure 24–6. This pneumatic ankle splint provides excellent early immobilization, and can aid in rehabilitation later in the course of management.

Upper Extremity Injuries

Injuries about the shoulder in the child can involve the glenohumeral joint, the clavicle and its two joints, or the bony elements of the proximal humerus and scapula.

Fractures of the clavicle lead the list of fractures in this region. These can result from direct trauma, such as a blow or a fall directed on the clavicle, or indirect trauma, such as a fall on an outstretched hand. Clavicle fractures, even badly displaced fractures, can usually be managed by gentle manipulative reduction and splinting in a figure-of-eight splint or brace, without anesthesia. Open reduction is rarely required, and nonunions are extremely rare.

Fractures of the proximal humerus occur relatively more frequently in a child than in the adult, while glenohumeral dislocations are extremely rare. In the younger child, epiphyseal displacements may occur, with propagation through the growth plate. In the older child or adolescent, metaphyseal fractures are more common. In both, rather dramatic remodeling of displaced fractures is observed. Once again, open reduction is rarely indicated.

Acromioclavicular separation or dislocation also occurs relatively frequently in children. Grading of these injuries is useful as a guide to management. A first degree sprain is a mild sprain of the acromioclavicular ligament, without displacement of the joint. Second degree sprains are injuries with partial displacement of the clavicle upward, but with a portion of the ligament complex still intact, while the third degree injury reflects a complete disruption of the ligament complex of the joint (Fig. 24–7).

Recent experience suggests that open reduction of this injury is rarely required (Park et al., 1980). Immediate icing, sling support for comfort, and early range-of-motion and muscle-strengthening exercises should be begun when tolerated.

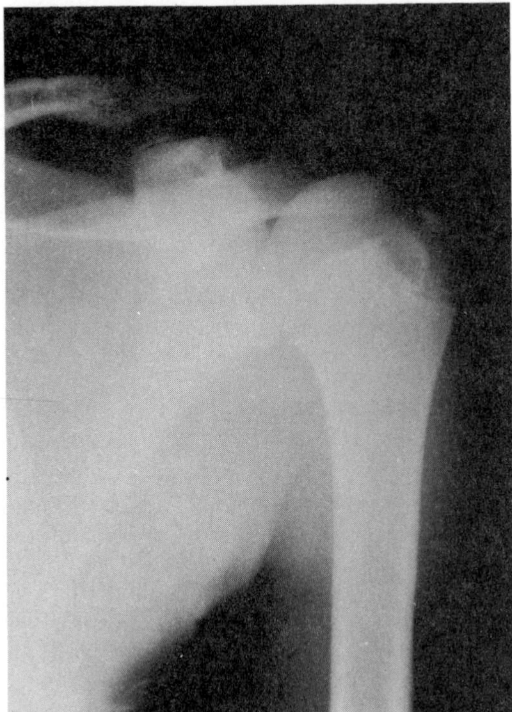

Figure 24–7. Shoulder injuries, including clavicular, humeral, and impingement injuries, are increasing in frequency in children. This roentgenograph demonstrates partial acromioclavicular separation.

Overuse injuries of the shoulder, particularly in the young athlete, are becoming relatively common. The term "Little League" shoulder refers to a microfracture of the proximal humeral growth plate from repetitive throwing (Cahill et al., 1974). Recently, an increased number of impingement syndromes have been noted in young athletes involved in throwing or swimming. It is hypothesized that this impingement occurs between the rotator cuff muscles on the humeral head and the coricoacromial ligament or acromian itself above.

Our own observations on the painful shoulder in the young thrower or swimmer suggest that this injury results from a progressive contracture about the shoulder joint, one which is very amenable to preventive exercises. These young athletes develop a characteristic contracture about the shoulder, with loss of internal rotation at the 90-degree abducted position, and increased external rotation. We believe this reflects a tightened posterior shoulder capsule and loose anterior capsule, and is, in itself, a reflection of an anterior subluxation tendency in these shoulders. A directed exercise program aimed at restoring a full range of motion, as well as good strength, to the involved shoulder is useful. The patient is placed on active resisted internal rotation with the shoulder abducted to 90 degrees.

ELBOW INJURIES

A painful, swollen elbow in a child must be considered an emergency, for injuries about the elbow can result in permanent disability or even loss of the extremity. These injuries can result in a sprain or a completely displaced supracondylar fracture of the distal humerus with progressive neurovascular compromise of the forearm and hand (Fig. 24–8) (Micheli et al., 1979).

Initial management includes determination of the distal neuromuscular status, including radial pulse, capillary refill, and sensory and motor activity of the ulnar, radial, and median nerves. Immobilization in a position of relative comfort should be the next step. This position is often *not* that of flexion to a 90-degree angle in a sling. In fact, 90-degree flexion may increase the potential for swelling and further neurovascular compromise. If possible, ice should be applied immediately, as well as a gentle compression dressing. A splint made of a folded newspaper, Ace bandages, and bags of crushed ice may be ideal.

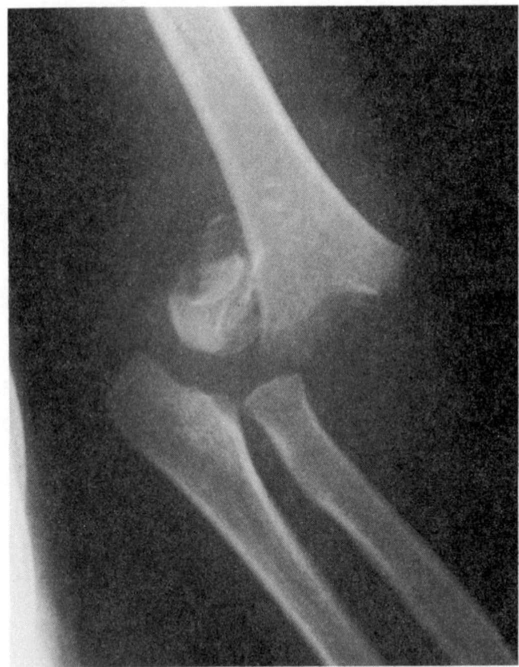

Figure 24–8. A displaced supracondylar fracture of the humerus must be considered a medical emergency.

High-quality radiographs, often with multiple views, are essential for diagnosis and subsequent management. It is important to include the joints at both ends of an injured extremity; e.g., with elbow injuries, this means shoulder and wrist. The incidence of ipsilateral fractures of the forearm with elbow injuries is higher than often realized (Micheli et al., 1980).

In these injuries, the absence of a radial pulse alone does not indicate ischemia, but the loss of a pre-existent pulse along with pain in the hand, pallor of the fingers, and pain with extension of the fingers indicates impending ischemia.

In the event of impending ischemia, removal of possible constricting bandages or splints and careful extension of the elbow should be undertaken. If, despite these measures, signs of vascular compromise persist beyond one hour, emergency surgical decompression of the muscles and fascia of the forearm must be considered.

A variety of different fractures may occur about the elbow, in addition to supracondylar fractures, which are less emergent in nature but which often require careful assessment and reduction. In any elbow injury associated with swelling, circumferential bandages or cast should be avoided, as splints or a sling is much safer and equally effective.

"Little League" elbow, a general label applied to the overuse injuries sustained by some young pitchers, can include osteochondritis of the capitellum, with or without associated loose bodies in the joint, injury and premature closure of the proximal radial epiphysis, overgrowth of the radial head, and irritation or frank avulsion of the medial epicondyle. The mechanism of injury appears to be the repetitive valgus strain applied to the elbow by throwing, with compression medially and traction laterally (Tullos and King, 1972).

If detected early, relative rest and exercises to improve the strength of the entire arm, as well as attention to throwing technique which minimizes the valgus strain at the elbow, can stop the process. A child with a history of repetitive throwing who presents with pain about the elbow with associated swelling and complete loss of motion must be examined very closely using AP, lateral, and both oblique x-rays of the elbow, as well as possible elbow arthrogram, to determine injury.

FOREARM, WRIST, AND HAND

Injuries to the forearm, wrist, and hand in children, although potentially serious, rarely carry the risk of loss of limb. As with any extremity injury, initial neurovascular assessment is essential. Displaced wrist fractures, in particular, may result in median nerve injury. Pain with rotation of the forearm, particularly with supination, is an important sign. Radiographs of the elbow and wrist are essential in forearm injuries. An innocuous-appearing fracture of the ulna may be accompanied by a dislocation of the proximal radius—the Monteggia fracture—and must never be overlooked.

Fractures about the wrist follow a certain age-related pattern. In the infant or toddler, the minimally displaced buckle or torus fracture is common, and simple splinting of the wrist is usually adequate. In a child, metaphyseal fractures of the ulna and radius, often completely displaced, usually require reduction under anesthesia. In the younger adolescent, fractures through the distal growth plate are more common and usually require complete anesthesia for reduction in order to minimize injury to the growth plate.

In the older adolescent, fractures of the carpal navicular are more common, and persistent pain, with associated snuff box tenderness, is reason for thumb spica cast immobilization and repeat radiographs, including navicular views, in two weeks.

In the child, the diagnosis of dislocated fingers should be made with caution, as a fracture through the growth plate may mimic a dislocation, and an attempt at reduction of the "dislocated" joint may cause further injury. The diagnosis of "chip" fracture, by radiograph, should be approached with similar caution, as the chip may be the avulsed site of insertion of a major tendon or ligament.

LOWER EXTREMITY INJURIES

Injuries about the hip and pelvis are less common than other lower extremity childhood injuries, particularly in the ambulatory patient. Avulsions of major muscle-tendon units, including the hamstrings at the ischium, the sartorius, the rectus femoris at the front of the hip, and the abdominals at the pelvic rim, can be a cause of acute pain and disability in free play activities or sports (Clancy and Foltz, 1976).

These avulsions can usually be managed by a period of rest, including bed rest and use of crutches, followed by progressive restoration of motion and strength to the involved extremity.

Although sprains of the ligaments about the hips can occur, they are relatively rare. Of greater concern is displacement of the proximal femoral epiphysis, which appears to be more common in active children. Recurrent limp with complaints of hip, thigh, or even knee pain and loss of internal rotation of the flexed hip are diagnostic findings.

Activity-related limp and hip pain may also be the first sign of Legg-Calve-Perthes disease or aseptic necrosis of the femoral head. A number of cases of Legg-Calve-Perthes disease, initially thought to be sports injuries, are seen in sports clinics because symptoms began in association with sports activities.

Thigh injuries include muscle-tendon unit injuries as well as proximal and distal stress fractures of the femur. Thigh contusions should always be treated with immediate immobilization, icing, and relative rest, as well as gentle compression. Disability from a thigh contusion may last for a year or more, and recovery may be additionally delayed by the development of myositis ossificans in the contused muscle (Wilkes, 1976).

In minor contusions, swelling is usually minimal, and active and passive flexion of the knee, although painful, is full. In moderate contusions, the knee can be flexed beyond 90 degrees, but flexion is limited when compared to the opposite extremity, and there is usually a drop of the knee into flexion, or "quad lag," when the leg is held extended above the examining table. In the severe contusion, active or passive, knee flexion is less than 90 degrees, and pain may be severe.

Severe contusions should be treated with bed rest, immobilization, and intermittent icing for up to five to seven days. We do not use heat or warm water whirlpools in any stage of the rehabilitation of thigh contusions.

When strength and range of motion have been restored to the injured extremity, sports may be resumed, but a protective thigh pad applied directly to the extremity should be used for at least a year following injury, as reinjuries can be more severe than the initial injury.

Knee Injuries

Injuries about the knee in the child and adolescent, particularly when they result from single-impact macrotrauma, are frequently misdiagnosed and undertreated. Injury to the knee may cause a fracture of the growth plate, with the ligamentous structures of the knee remaining intact. Careful clinical assessment and attention to radiographic detail of the growth plate are generally sufficient to make a diagnosis of epiphyseal injury. In a significant number of cases, however, severe ligamentous injuries can occur without associated fracture. By the time the child is examined, swelling about the knee and joint effusion make clinical assessment difficult, and effusion and swelling may actually impart a false clinical stability to the knee. Initial radiographs certainly are unremarkable, and the injured child is all too often splinted and given crutches, with subsequent evaluation one to two weeks following injury when satisfactory ligamentous repair may no longer be possible.

Careful clinical history is often vital in making the proper diagnosis of these injuries. A severe twisting injury induced by a high level of extrinsic force, accompanied by a "pop" in the knee and a sensation of the knee tearing or coming apart, is highly suspicious. Frequently there is a sensation of instability of the knee immediately after injury, and the patient describes his knee as wobbly and tending to give way when he or she attempts to put weight on the extremity.

Recent studies have suggested that the presence of blood in the knee is a reflection of serious derangement in at least 90 per cent of observed cases (DeHaven, 1980). When a high index of suspicion is present for a serious knee disruption, either of ligaments or of internal structures, consideration should be given to acute arthroscopy. This can be done very effectively, even under local anesthesia. We generally use xylocaine with epinephrine in the skin and subcutaneous tissues and fill the joint itself with 0.5 per cent marcaine solution.

In addition to being the most common site of macrotrauma injury in the young North American athlete, the knee is also the most frequent site of overuse injury. The vast majority of these overuse injuries involve the extensor mechanism, however, whereas the macrotrauma injuries about the knee usually involve the ligaments or internal structures.

With growth, and particularly with the growth spurt, the muscles spanning the knee joint must adjust to the most rapidly growing bones in the body. The presence of the heavy fascia lata laterally and relatively lighter tissues medially results not only in longitudinal traction, but also lateral deviation of the knee, particularly of the quadriceps mechanism and its sesamoid bone, the patella (DeHaven et al., 1979) (Fig. 24–9).

If this tendency to proximal and lateral deviation of the quadriceps mechanism is excessive, recurrent lateral subluxation or even dislocation of the patella may occur. Lesser

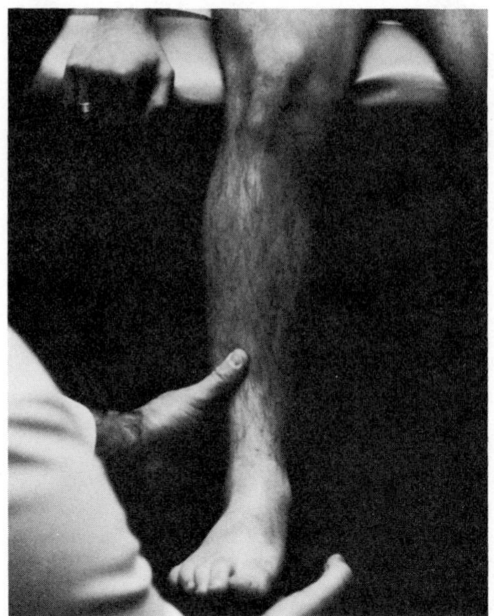

Figure 24–9. This young athlete with parapatellar knee pain has a more lateral insertion of his patellar tendon (increased "O" angle) and a resultant increased increased tendency to lateral deviation of the patella in its groove.

degrees of this growth-related deformation may be expressed as low-grade knee ache, made worse by stair climbing or prolonged sitting in one place ("theatre sign").

This knee pain may often begin after a particular episode of overuse, such as double basketball practices on an upsprung wooden floor or suddenly beginning hill running. For clinical purposes, this entity has been labeled patellofemoral stress syndrome. We find this a useful classification and preferable to the frequently used diagnosis of chondromalacia. Chondromalacia properly refers to a pathological condition of articular cartilage, including the patella, in which there is softening, fibrillation, or frank erosion of cartilage. While a patellofemoral stress syndrome may result in chondromalacia of the patella or underlying femoral articular cartilage, this is by no means a direct or a necessary relationship.

There is also more recent evidence that deformations of shape of the patella itself frequently occur secondary to the soft tissue contractures resulting from this growth process; therefore, this frank bony deformation might in itself be preventable if these soft tissue imbalances about the knee and extensor mechanism were corrected (Reider and Marshall, 1977).

Based on this hypothesized pathogenesis of the patellofemoral stress syndrome, a logical approach would be to attempt to strengthen the medial structures of the quadriceps and upper leg and stretch the lateral structures. We have found this a very successful treatment, with progressive resistive adductor and quadriceps muscle strengthening, done with the knee extended, and stretching exercises of the fascia lata and hamstrings (Fig. 24–10). The ability to lift 12 lbs in a straight leg raise fashion, done in 3 sets of 10 repetitions, is generally associated with disappearance of symptoms. This level is approached in a slow and progressive fashion, of course, and without pain, since at times, the quadriceps and particularly the vastus medialis, which is specific to terminal extension, may be so weak that only the weight of the leg itself can be lifted initially.

If, after six months of exercise, the knee

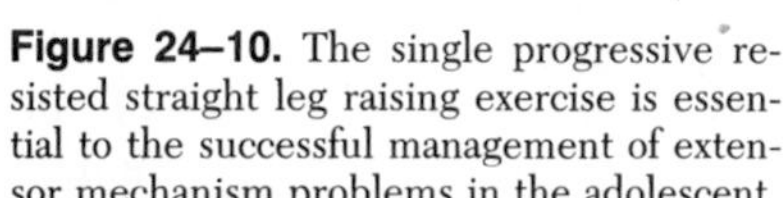

Figure 24–10. The single progressive resisted straight leg raising exercise is essential to the successful management of extensor mechanism problems in the adolescent.

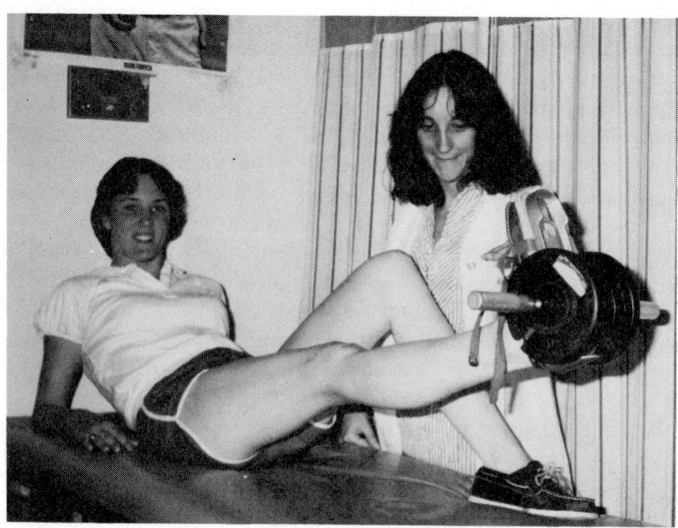

remains painful and the goal of 12 lbs is not reached, a lateral release is performed and exercise then resumed. With this approach, 92 per cent of our children were satisfactorily treated with exercise alone and of the remaining 8 per cent who came to lateral release, 82 per cent were able to restore strength and resume painless activities (Micheli and Stanitski, 1981).

Onset of Osgood-Schlatter disease appears to follow a similar pattern, although appearing more frequently in boys with the onset of growth spurt. Recently, however, we have noted a new population presenting with Osgood-Schlatter disease—younger girls, age 10 to 12, who are involved in vigorous jumping training, as in figure skating or gymnastics. A similar static straight leg raising strengthening program for treatment and rehabilitation, as well as a stretching program for tight, weak quadriceps muscles, is used. We now rarely use a preliminary stage of casting, not wishing to make a tight, weak muscle tighter and weaker, and we believe we can attain the same relative immobilization with "relative rest"—substituting swimming or biking for running activities.

In both patellofemoral stress syndrome and Osgood-Schlatter disease, an envelopment brace that leaves the patella open, such as the Marshall or Palumbo brace, has a role in the early stages of management or as a safety device when play is resumed (Fig. 24–11).

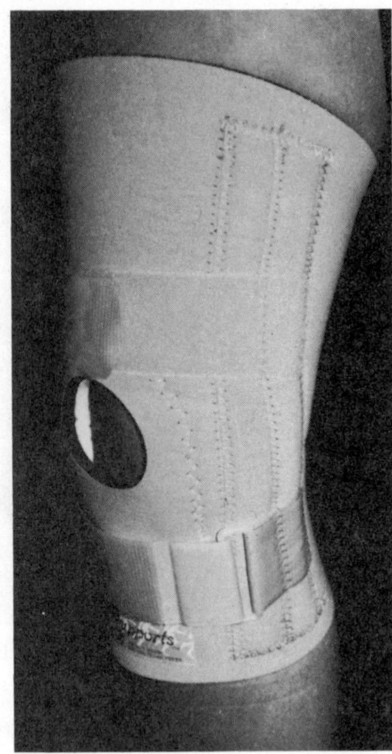

Figure 24–11. The Marshall knee brace can be helpful in managing patellar disorders in adolescents.

Osteochondritis dissecans of the knee, which is often traumatic in origin, can present as low-grade aching in the knee with a history of intermittent swelling. Rarely, frank locking of the knee occurs. The diagnosis may initially be confused with patellofemoral stress syndrome. Radiographs are usually diagnostic (Matteir and Frymoyer, 1973) (Fig. 24–12).

While the more traditional management of this lesion includes a period of immobilization if it is nondisplaced, more recent techniques, which have been facilitated by the development of the arthroscopy, include resection under arthroscopic control if the lesion is loose, or transarticular drilling or pinning again, under arthroscopic control, if the lesion is intact. More experience with this approach is needed before it can be recommended as a program that increases the rate or incidence of union.

Ankle and Foot

Caution must be used in making the diagnosis of a sprained ankle in a child. Certainly, an injury that results in inversion of the foot and pain and swelling about the lateral aspect of the ankle may tear the ligamentous structures on the lateral aspect of the ankle, but it may also cause a minimal displaced fracture through the distal fibular growth plate. Usually, careful examination can determine whether the maximal site of tenderness is over the distal growth plate or the ligaments immediately inferior to the bone. If excessive swelling has developed before the patient is examined, it is best, if the possibility of growth plate fracture exists, to err on the side of caution and immobilize the ankle in a non–weight bearing cast from toes to midcalf for a period of three weeks. One of our studies of ankle sprains showed that the most common etiological factor in these injuries was tightness of the calf muscles.

Overuse injuries of the foot and ankle in the child are not uncommon. The most common complaint is heel pain, often in a child involved in field sports such as soccer or lacrosse. Tenderness over the os calcis apophysis, at the tendo-achilles insertion, along with a tight gastrocnemius-soleus mechanism, is usually sufficient to make the diagnosis of os calcis apophysitis (Matteir and Frymoyer, 1973). This condition can frequently be bilateral.

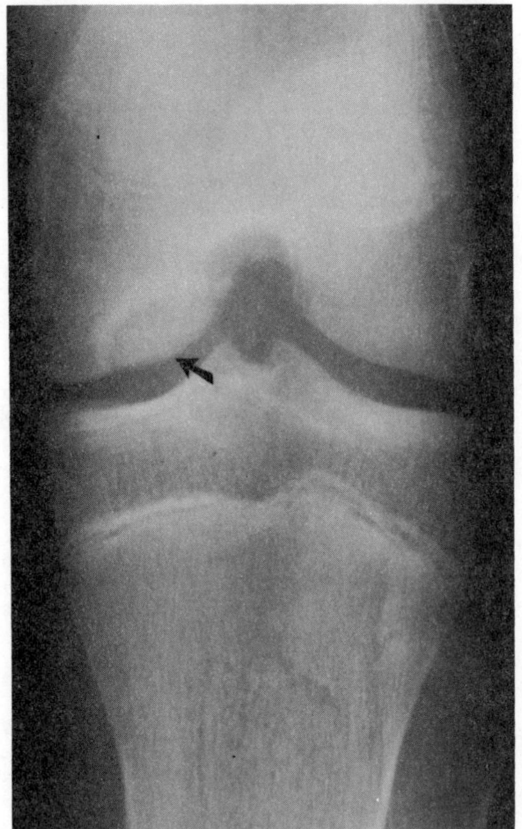

Figure 24–12. Osteochondritis dissecans of the medial femoral articular surface in the adolescent.

A stress fracture of the os calcis can present with similar complaints but can usually be ruled out by presence of tenderness on the sides of the os calcis. If any doubt exists after the diagnosis, radiographs, including the axial Harris view of the os calcis, should be obtained. Occasionally, bone scan may be necessary in children with foot pain. Such rare conditions as a stress fracture of the navicular may be diagnosed best in this way.

While the primary etiological factor in os calcis apophysitis appears to be a tight tendoachilles, usually associated with a growth spurt, maltraining is also a factor. In addition, inspection of the playing shoes will often reveal a shoe with a "negative cant," with the heel actually lower than the toe box, due to cleat wear or shoe design. This condition usually responds very rapidly to a program of directed heel-cord stretching and dorsiflexion strengthening exercises, as well as a temporary heel lift. A short program of intermittent icing and mild anti-inflammatory medication may also be indicated.

Occasionally, the child athlete will develop tendinitis—most commonly of the tibialis posterior or peroneal muscles. This usually responds readily to conservative management, particularly if treatment is initiated early. In addition, we have seen a number of children involved in distance running present with what appears to be an avulsion injury to the medial malleolus. Once again, this raises the possibility of new types of avulsion overuse injury in the child engaged in heavy running training.

PREVENTION OF INJURIES IN THE CHILD

It is important to attempt to determine which risk factors are specifically involved in a given musculoskeletal injury in a given child, including the overgrowth injuries. We have learned to be suspicious of certain patterns of sport-specific injuries. The complaint of low back pain in the young gymnast must be assessed very carefully, and a high index of suspicion of spondylolysis must be entertained. Painful lower extremities in the young runner must be carefully assessed for the possibility of stress fracture. Pain about the shoulder or elbow in the throwing athlete must be assessed for the possibility of "Little League" shoulder or elbow. Painful shoulder in the young swimmer or painful knees in a young swimmer or ballet dancer similarly deserve early assessment, as simple directed exercises and relative rest can often completely eradicate the tendency toward ongoing pain and tissue injury.

In addition, the observation that a child athlete is entering a relative growth spurt, made possible only by regular assessment and recording of these assessments, can be extremely important in anticipating problems while in this growth spurt. The child is particularly in need of supplementary flexibility exercises or a decrease in intensity of training.

As noted above, there is often a multiplicity of risk factors responsible for the occurrence of a given injury in an individual child. One must be careful not simply to ascribe the occurrence of injury to the growth spurt or muscle-tendon imbalance when other etiological factors such as anatomical malalignment or coexistent disease state might be present. It must always be remembered that the child is at particular risk of skeletal infectious processes and neoplasms, particularly bony tumors. It would be a tragedy, indeed, if a child with a low-grade aching knee pain due to osteogenic sarcoma of the proximal tibia were to be treated with straight leg raising exercises and shoe orthotics, simply because this pain presented in the course of athletic activities.

Careful longitudinal studies are needed if we are able to determine both the maximum and minimum levels of athletic training and physical activity that should be done during childhood. Experienced horse trainers do not jump horses with open growth plates, because of the overuse injuries that can occur and eliminate the horses from a successful competition in the future. We should be as concerned about safe levels of physical activity for our children.

REFERENCES

1. Accident Facts. Chicago, National Safety Council, 1978.
2. Bradford, D. S., Moe, J. H., Montalvo, F. J., et al.: Scheurmann's kyphosis and roundback deformity—results of Milwaukee brace treatment. J. Bone Joint Surg., *56A*:740–758, 1974.
3. Bright, R. W., and Elmore, S. M.: Physical properties of epiphyseal plate cartilage. Surg. Forum, *19*:463–464, 1968.
4. Buxbaum, R., and Micheli, L. J.: Sports For Life. Boston, Beacon Press, 1979.
5. Cahill, B. R., Tullos, H. S., and Fain, R. H.: Little League shoulder. Am. J. Sports Med., *2*:150–153, 1974.
6. Clancy, W. E., and Foltz, A. S.: Iliac apophysitis and stress fractures in adolescent runners. Am. J. Sports Med., *4*(5):214–218, 1976.
7. DeHaven, K. E.: Diagnosis of acute knee injuries with hemarthrosis. Am. J. Sports Med., *8*:9–14, 1980.
8. DeHaven, K. E., Dolan, W. A., and Mayer, P. J.: Chondromalacia patella in athletes—clinical presentation and conservative management. Am. J. Sports Med., *7*:1–12, 1979.
9. Henrys, P., Lyne, E. D., Lifton, C., and Salciccioli, G.: Clinical review of cervical spine injuries in children. Clin. Orthop., *129*:172–184, 1977.
10. Jackson, D. W., Wilkes, L. L., and Cirincione, R. J.: Spondylolisthesis in the female athlete. Clin. Orthop. Rel. Res., *117*:68–73, 1968.
11. Matteir, R., and Frymoyer, J.: Fracture of the calcaneus in young children. J. Bone Joint Surg., *55A*:1091, 1973.
12. Mayer, P. J., and Micheli, L. J.: Avulsion of the femoral attachment of the posterior cruciate ligament in an eleven-year-old boy. J. Bone Joint Surg., *61A*:431–432, 1979.
13. Micheli, L. J.: Overuse injuries in children's sports: The growth factor. Orthop. Clin. North Am., 1983 (in press).
14. Micheli, L. J., and Jupiter, J.: Osteoid osteoma as a cause of knee pain in the young athlete. Am. J. Sports Med., *6*:199–203, 1978.
15. Micheli, L. J.: Low back pain in the adolescent: Differential diagnosis. Am. J. Sports Med., *7*:362–364, 1979a.
16. Micheli, L. J.: Musculoskeletal injuries. *In* Randolph, J. G. (ed.): The Injured Child. Chicago, Year Book Medical Publishers, 1979b.
17. Micheli, L. J., Skolnick, M. D., and Hall, J. E.: Supracondylar fractures of the humerus in children. Am. Fam. Phys., *19*:100–114, 1979.
18. Micheli, L. J., Stanitski, C. L., and Santore, R.: Epiphyseal fractures of the elbow in children. Am. Fam. Phys., *22*:107–116, 1980.
19. Micheli, L. J., and Stanitski, C. L.: Lateral retinacular release for parapatellar pain. Am. J. Sports Med., *9*:330–336, 1981.
20. Ogden, J. A.: Skeletal injury in the child. Philadelphia, Lea and Febiger, 1963.
21. Park, J. P., Arnold, J. A., Coker, T. A., Harris, W. D., and Becker, D. A.: Treatment of acromioclavicular separations: A retrospective study. Am. J. Sports Med., *8*:251–256, 1980.
22. Reider, B., and Marshall, J. L.: Patella tracking. Surg. Forum, *28*:502, 1977.
23. Rosen, P. R., Micheli, L. J., and Treves, S.: Early scintographic diagnosis of bone stress and fractures in athletic adolescents. Pediatrics, *70*:11–15, 1982.
24. Salter, R. B., and Harris, W. R.: Injuries involving the epiphyseal plate. J. Bone Joint Surg., *45A*:587–595, 1963.
25. Stanish, W. D.: Treatment of tendinitis with dynamic eccentric resistive exercise. Presented at the American Orthopedic Society for Sports Medicine Annual Meeting, Lake of the Woods, Arkansas, 1982.
26. Tullos, H. S., and King, J. W.: Lesions of the pitching arm in adolescents. J.A.M.A., *220*:264–271, 1972.
27. Wilkes, L. L.: Myositis ossificans trauma in a young child. Clin. Orthop., *118*:151, 1976.

25

SPORTS MEDICINE

Nathan J. Smith, M.D.

Few things have changed as drastically in the past 50 years as the way children play and the meaning that modern play has in their lives. The restricted urban environments in which most children live allows little opportunity for self-directed, spontaneous play. Many of today's play opportunities are highly organized, adult-dominated sport programs patterned after the familiar models of varsity and professional sports. Such programs can provide fun, opportunities for familiarity with many sports, and the energy-expending exercise essential for good health and fitness. However, the very nature of the professional-varsity sport model presents a significant risk of adult domination with vicarious imposition of adult goals and aspirations as well as generating performance expectations contrary to the physiological and emotional maturity of the young participants.

Participation in competitive sports has very significant meaning for adolescents as they participate in rapidly expanded athletic programs in middle schools and junior and senior high schools. Scholastic sports participation is more than just an opportunity for energy-expending exercise. For the early adolescent this may be the only available opportunity in a mechanized, automated environment to test their new and developing physique. Sport provides ready access to parental and peer acceptance. Coddington (1972) in his study of adolescents' perception of life-stress situations, found that failing in a competitive activity with one's peers was perceived as more stressful than moving to a new community and new school, failing a grade, or death of a close friend. Failure to make the team was ranked nearly as high as loss of a parent through divorce or being involved in a pregnancy. Success and failure in sport must be recognized as a matter of considerable concern to the adolescent and a potential source of considerable anxiety.

WHEN IS THE CHILD "READY" FOR SPORT?

The informed physician is able to provide parents, children, and leaders of community sport programs with sound recommendations regarding sport programs and sport participation based on the investigations of exercise scientists and research into various aspects of growth and development.

Prior to the age that girls begin their adolescent growth spurt there is no significant difference in the size and strength of boys and girls of similar ages. From a purely physical basis in relation to proficiency and risk of injury, there is no reason why boys and girls prior to the age of 12 should not compete on the same teams and against each other. Inasmuch as girls will not participate in collision sports after the onset of adolescence there is little reason for their participation in these sports in the elementary school age, nor do these sports have particular merit for boys at this age. It is prudent to be sensitive to attitudes still present in some areas that little boys should not be defeated in games by little girls. Boys competing with girls in these situations may suffer some painful ridicule from parents and other adults important in their lives.

Boys do not have the potential to develop significant increases in strength in either upper or lower extremities until the initiation of pubertal endocrine changes with increased production of androgens, although some increased strength in abdominal muscles and back muscles has been found developed in response to training in 10- and 11-year-olds. In the preadolescent the potential for responding to training with increased endurance is limited by the underdeveloped muscle mass and the limited potential for energy metabolism. This is due in part to the low activity of phosphofructokinase in the prepubescent muscle. In addition, neuromuscular limitations exist at this age, limiting information processing and the efficiency of acquiring motor skills by the young sport participant. Because of these physiological limitations prior to mid and late adolescence the desirable goals of sport are limited to fun, enjoyment, socialization, and a low-key introduction to a variety of sport skills. Involvement in prolonged training and practice schedules directed to championships and elite performances is inappropriate at this age for well-documented structural and physiological reasons.

During early adolescence opportunities for intense athletic involvement increase. Almost 80 per cent of all junior high schools have interschool competitive athletics even though there have been at least nine official bodies that have issued policy statements to the effect that such interschool sport programs are not appropriate for this age. Parents of the early adolescent will begin to wonder how good an athlete their son or daughter is going to be and may urge them into highly competitive programs before they are physically capable of responding to the demands of training. Parents and their concerned children should know that the adolescent will first grow in height and, on the average, this rapid gain in height will be followed in 14 to 15 months by a rapid gain in weight. The weight gain will be primarily an increase in fat in girls with relatively little muscle gain, and in boys the rapid weight gain is associated with decreasing fatness and a marked increase in muscle mass. After these growth changes of adolescence, it becomes inappropriate for boys and girls to compete on the same teams and against each other in the large numbers of sports in which proficiency and risk of injury are dependent on body size and strength. In response to the argument that girls who are good enough should be allowed to play on the boys' team, it could be said that boys who are good enough should be allowed positions on the girls' teams. If this were accepted, boys with the greater size and strength would occupy most of the positions on both teams and most girls would not get to play on either team.

The new muscles developed by boys as they experience their rapid increase in body weight only gradually develop their potential for strength, endurance, and efficient energy metabolism. These muscles are poorly supplied with capillaries and increased capillarization of muscle will develop only in response to training and muscle work. Twelve to 14 months after the peak rate of weight gain in boys there will be the potential for the newly acquired muscles to respond to a training program with increases in strength and endurance. The neuromuscular maturity will have been acquired that will allow the prompt acquisition of new sport skills. For the average male this stage of maturity compatible with a rewarding and satisfying experience in an intensely competitive athletic program will occur no sooner than the age of 16 years. Athletic potential will continue to increase for several years beyond this age. This emphasizes the tragedy of too early intense involvement in sport with psychological "burn out" by age 14 or 15 before even the earliest physical potential for athletic performance has been reached.

THE PRE-ADOLESCENT ATHLETE

The vast majority of children will become participants in organized sport before they are graduated from the elementary school. Although the goals of play for this age should be limited to "fun," enjoyment, and the early familiarity with some sport skills, the very nature of organized sport provides a setting vulnerable to a variety of abuses. Excessively long seasons and practice sessions, inappropriate matching of competitors, physical and performance expectations that are unrealistic, parental excesses, and lack of trained coaching and administrative personnel in the programs are common problems in the community-based youth sport programs for young children. In light of how extensive these programs are in this country, involving as they do essentially every community and the majority of children, it is regrettable that there has been little research done as to the emotional or physical consequences of youth sport participation. Clinical experience and the few studies that have been made indicate that the risk of injury is not significant even in the collision sports such as football when played by pre-adolescents. These "athletes" have neither the size, the strength, nor the motivation to cause many injuries. Excessive emotional stress coming from competitive play has not been documented. One investigation found that batting in a Little League baseball game was not nearly as stressful as playing a solo on a musical instrument. The most threatening emotional consequences of participation in a highly structured sport program for the young child will be found in the home in the matter of parental and sibling reactions to a child's athletic performances. The parent and family reaction to sport will determine whether being a young athlete is to be a healthful, maturing challenge or an overly stressful and destructive experience. Much of this critical behavior will center on reactions to losing and poor performances. Children will not gain from a sport experience until they are completely confident that their worth in the eyes of the parents and family is not dependent on the outcome of some athletic performance or contest. Once this level of psychological maturity has been reached, they can then have the confidence to cope with the losing that inevitably comes to all athletes and can confidently enjoy the benefits of being involved in sports.

Anticipatory counseling regarding youth sport participation for the elementary school age child has become an essential component in child health care. The physician, it is hoped, is somewhat familiar with the youth sport programs in the community and is knowledgeable about the physical and emotional maturation characteristics of the pre-adolescent child as they will relate to sport participation. Parents will profit from learning the proper goals for sport participation at this age as the subject is introduced into health counseling of the five- to eight-year-old patient. Parents can be advised to address questions such as the following before their children become involved in youth sport programs. What are the goals and qualifications of the staff that run the program? Who wants the child in the program—the parent, the child, the coaches, the program directors? Do the parents and child appreciate the commitments of time and perhaps money that are involved? What will this do to family life? Is this child ready to be "coached"? Are the parents prepared to be parents of a "bench warmer" or a "loser" and accept the decisions of the coach about their child? What will the parents do if their child wants to quit? How do they get out of a sport program without being a "quitter"?

Organized sport participation is not an essential for a healthy, fulfilling childhood. Yet there are many youth sport programs organized on a very low-key, recreational basis with fun as their primary goal and so designed that all children get to play and participate. Physicians have the responsibility of alerting parents to the pitfalls as well as the advantages of sport participation for their young children. They may often be in a position to provide expertise to the community that will minimize the negative aspects of sport programs active there.

THE PREPARTICIPATION HEALTH EVALUATION

Most scholastic sport programs demand some type of health evaluation prior to participation. These examinations are intended to protect the health of the athletes and deal with liability concerns of the school. There are more than seven million young people involved each year in high school sport programs, and they are the healthiest segment of their age group. In order to meet the needs of the athlete, the school, and the physician and to deal with the large numbers of participants involved, the examination must be specifically sport directed and be designed only to determine the candidate's suitability for sport participation. The compulsory preparticipation health evaluation cannot be the answer to providing comprehensive health services to this large population of adolescents. There is neither the time nor the economic resources available to make this a realistic goal. For those privileged adolescents who will have care by a personal physician available during adolescence, the preparticipation sport evaluation can well be part of that care plan, but it must include those elements particularly related to assessing suitability for athletic participation.

Group examinations are recommended as being an efficient and effective method of meeting the health evaluation needs of many teams or a school's population of athletes. Garrick (1977) has described in detail how such a group examination can be carried out with efficient use of physician time while satisfying the desired goals of the examination. A screening history limited to five questions identifies the athlete who needs further evaluation (Table 25–1). The physical examination gives particular attention to the cardiovascular system and the orthopedic examination. After the first year of sport participation in high school, the most frequently encountered abnormality in the physical examination will be evidences of an inadequately rehabilitated previous sport injury; muscle atrophy and weakness or instability and altered range of motion of an injured joint. Assessment of maturity status by Tanner staging is an essential for male athletes.

It is recommended that the sport-directed preparticipation health evaluation be required of each athlete entering a school's sport program. At the beginning of each subsequent school year only a history review of sport injuries, other accidents, and illnesses is required, with the complete physical evaluation required only every three years.

There are few, if any, health conditions that will completely exclude a junior or senior high school student from some type of sport participation. None will gain more from a good sport experience than the adolescent with a chronic health problem. The young person with diabetes mellitus can participate in any of the school's sport programs. Many asthmatic patients participate in competitive swimming. The patient with a well-controlled seizure disorder can par-

Table 25–1. SCREENING QUESTIONS FOR ATHLETIC PHYSICAL EXAMINATION

1. Have any members of your family had a "heart attack" or "heart condition" prior to the age of 50?
2. Do you have to stop while running around a quarter-mile track twice?
3. Are you taking any medications?
4. Have you ever "passed out" or have you ever been "knocked out"?
5. Have you ever had any illness, condition, or injury that:
   a. Required you to go to a hospital as a patient overnight or to the emergency room for x-rays?
   b. Required an operation?
   c. Caused you to miss a game or more than one practice?

These five questions are completed by the athlete in the group examination or can be completed in the waiting room or asked by an office assistant. Any of the above questions answered in the affirmative are pursued in detail by the examining physician.

ticipate in any sport of his or her preference. If seizures are not well controlled, water sports such as swimming, rowing, and water polo are to be avoided, as are those in which falls could occur, i.e., gymnastics and equestrian sports. Individuals missing one of the paired organs, those with hepatosplenomegaly, and these with hemorrhagic disorders should be disqualified from the collision sports.

MATURITY STATUS AND SPORT PARTICIPATION

Assessing maturation status is an essential part of the preparticipation evaluation for male candidates in junior and senior high school sport programs and community-based programs involving individuals in these age groups. Those who are slow, late maturers should be identified and counseled regarding participation in collision sports. They should be advised of their performance handicap and the increased risk of injury in relation to more mature individuals of similar chronological age.

Small, late-maturing boys will often be attracted to wrestling programs. Competitors in this popular sport are matched on a weight basis and, thus, the small, late-maturer's size is not an apparent handicap. However, competing in the lower weight classes with a more mature athlete of the same weight puts the late maturer at a distinct disadvantage, since he is destined to have few winning experiences and is at increased risk of injury in a collision sport with a high injury risk. In all collision sports (wrestling, football, lacrosse, ice hockey), males should be well into Tanner stage four or five before they are suitable candidates for competition at the high school level.

Each year, there is a candidate for almost every high school football team that is very large, very obese, and a slow, late maturer. With little strength, little endurance potential, and immature skeletal development, he makes a very poor football player, will have an unrewarding experience as a noncompetitive athlete, and is at high risk for injury, particularly early-season heat disorders. The most frequent victim of fatal heat stroke in early season football practices has been the obese middle lineman in his first year of football. This late-maturing, grossly obese and large individual should be medically disqualified and directed to an appropriate conditioning program.

The very tall, late-maturing boy who is to reach an eventual height of over six feet, seven or eight inches is the obvious candidate for the high school basketball team. As Caucasians, essentially all of these very tall boys will be late maturers. As a late-maturing individual he will not experience his peak velocity of growth until he is in high school. He can be faced with an overwhelming challenge in attempting to perform up to the expectations of his size. Entering high school, this young man is at least two to three years away from having the strength and endurance potential to perform well in high school competition. These young men, their coaches, and their parents should be informed of the status of maturation associated with strength and endurance and when this very tall, late maturer may be expected to achieve a degree of physical development compatible with being competitive in sport. Limiting competition demands and practicing skills under the guidance of an understanding coach, while living with informed parents, can maintain a positive interest in sport for this individual with the physical potential to gain much from an athletic experience.

The physician should recognize the very early maturing boy among his patients. As a boy, the early maturing individual can be expected to be the grade school all-star athlete. Sport performance is very directly related to maturation status, with the early maturing individual having a great advantage as he competes against individuals of the same chronological age, but smaller, less strong, and with less endurance. With limitless opportunities to participate in highly organized youth sport programs the early maturing individual can become a true sport "star" by age 10 or 12 and, along with his parents, has a completely distorted projection of his future athletic potential. As others "catch up" in maturity during the early years of high school, the bright young star will fade. Losing the limelight of sports, he can be a serious disappointment to himself and his parents and vulnerable to serious depression during adolescence. These individuals should be encouraged to compete against individuals of similar maturation status early in their sport experience. They can be directed to compete against older, but similarly mature individuals at tennis and to work out with the high school junior varsity team while they are still in junior high school. In this way, they can keep their sport aspirations and expectations in proper and realistic perspective.

NUTRITION CONCERNS OF THE ATHLETE

Athletes recognize that their diet influences their athletic performance by providing the energy needed for competition and training as well as affecting their body size and composition. Becoming involved in an athletic endeavor can be a very positive motivating force in upgrading the often questionable nutritional practices of the adolescent.

Parents of the pre-adolescent "Little League athlete" may make inquiries as to how diet can be managed to maximize the performance of their very young competitor. A well-planned diet and family meal should be part of the lifestyle of every pre-adolescent. Diet planning should not be directed at making a young child a better shortstop or quarterback.

The older, high school aged athlete, physically capable of intense competitive efforts, will profit from nutrition counseling. It is important for these individuals to know that intense training and competition doesn't increase the need for any essential nutrient. There will only be an increased need for food energy intakes to meet the needs of high energy–expending workouts and increased fluid intakes for water replacement. Thus, the many vitamin, mineral, and protein supplements promoted to athletes are needlessly expensive, potentially dangerous, and completely useless for the healthy young athlete. Common nutrition concerns among athletes include gaining weight to increase performance potential, replacing fluid and electrolyte sweat losses, maximizing glycogen content of muscles as an energy substrate in endurance competitions (glycogen loading), and proper food intake prior to competition. Specific guidelines to be followed in regard to these questions are available both in the lay (Smith, 1977) and medical literature (Smith, 1981).

Widespread nutrition abuse is encountered in weight-matched competitions such as in scholastic wrestling programs. Young wrestlers attempt to minimize their body weight to increase their competitiveness by being matched against smaller opponents. Starvation and dehydration with a variety of excesses using diuretics and cathartics are not uncommon practices. The athlete will be most competitive in a weight-matched sport when he takes into competition the maximum of strength, endurance, and quickness for every pound of body weight. This merely means having the minimal level of body fat compatible with the highest degree of fitness. The level of body fat that satisfies this goal is an estimated level of fatness of 5 to 7 per cent of body weight as body fat. This estimate is most conveniently and accurately made during the high school years using a skinfold caliper. Reducing body fatness to this level for the young aspiring wrestler is best done at a rate no faster than two pounds per week while having a caloric intake of no less than 2000 kilocalories each day. Increasing energy expenditure by appropriate preseason conditioning exercise and controlling dietary intake will create the needed negative energy balance to reduce body fatness to the fit level for competition. During the high energy–expending competing season the young athlete will maintain his competing weight while taking in a generous diet that will support his athletic activities, as well as his normal adolescent growth. Allowing sufficient time to reach a desired level of fatness and competing weight before the season starts is essential. Body composition cannot be safely or effectively altered in a brief period of time.

THE PHYSICIAN TO THE TEAM

Physicians are often asked to provide medical services to a team or a sport program. Injury management is only one small part of the physician's overall responsibilities and not the most frequent medical concern of athletes. Management of minor infections, skin care and control of contagious skin infections, nutrition and hydration needs, maturation assessments, rehabilitation programs for previous injuries, and appropriate conditioning activities for athletes of different ages and sexes are all questions that will be dealt with. Information needed to approach these issues knowledgeably is readily available and requires a minimal effort for the physician to deal with these issues appropriately for the athlete and coaches.

The physician's relationship with the school administration and the coaching staff should be clearly defined. It is important to recognize the role of the coaches in the health and safety of the school's sport programs. The coach is the only responsible adult who is present at every practice session and every contest. The coach establishes all policies for the program, including those that will deal with the health, safety, and medically related aspects of performance of the athletes. The physician's efforts will be most effective when there is good communication and an effective working relationship established with the coaches. It will be highly desirable if steps are taken to ensure that the coach is well-informed regarding safe conduct of practices and other health-related matters. The coaches want to be informed. There is no more important function for the team's physician than to make sound medical information available to the coach and to train the coaching staff in on-field recognition and management of injuries. The coach is the one adult who is always there.

The school's athletes soon come to know that their performance is dependent on having a completely healthy body. Any and all health problems interfere with the performance of the athlete. Thus, the most important principle involved in the care of the intensely committed high school athlete is to recognize that *there is no such thing as a minor health problem* when it involves an athlete. A medical complaint that would justify a visit to the office can be a very major concern in the athlete. A minimally infected hangnail on the throwing hand of the high school's quarterback on a Friday morning is a very major health problem for the athlete, the parents, the coach, the school, and the community. Learning to accept the health complaints of the athlete in the perspective of athletic performance and competition will involve seeing medical problems in a new perspective for most physicians. Acquiring this skill will gain them the respect and sincere appreciation of an exciting new population of grateful patients. An athlete never has a minor health problem. Dropping out of a sport for even a short time is never an acceptable treatment for any health problem!

REFERENCES

Coddington, R. D.: The significance of life events as etiologic factors in the disease of children. J. Psychosom. Med., *16*:205, 1972.

Garrick, J. G.: Sports medicine. Pediatr. Clin. North Am., *24*:737, 1977.

Magill, R. A., Ash, M. J., and Smoll, F. L. (eds.): Children in Sport: A Contemporary Anthology. Champaign, Ill., Human Kinetics, Publishers.

Michener, J.: Sports in America. Greenwich, Conn., Fawcett Publications, 1976.

O'Donoghue, D. H.: Treatment of Injuries to Athletes. Philadelphia, W. B. Saunders Co., 1976.

Smith, N. J.: Some health care needs of young athletes. Adv. Pediatr. *187*:228, 1981.

Smith, N. J.: Food for Sport. Palo Alto, Cal., Bull Publishing Co., 1977.

Strauss, R. H. (ed.): Sports Medicine and Physiology. Philadelphia, W. B. Saunders, 1979.

26

SEXUALLY TRANSMITTED DISEASES IN ADOLESCENTS

Mary-Ann B. Shafer, M.D., and Charles E. Irwin, Jr., M.D.

The increase in sexual activity over the past decade, with 70 per cent of females and 80 per cent of males (Zelnick and Kantner, 1980) initiating sexual intercourse in adolescence, has resulted in a number of health problems, including the marked increase in prevalence of sexually transmitted diseases (STDs). Between 1965 and 1979, the incidence of reported *Neisseria gonorrhoeae* tripled; in adolescent males 15 to 19 years old the rate doubled; in adolescent females 15 to 19 years old the rate increased fivefold (Shafer et al., 1982). Gonorrhea represents only one of a large group of STDs. Recent reports indicate that *Chlamydia trachomatis* may be the most common STD (Schachter, 1978). In one clinical study, *C. trachomatis* was isolated from 22 per cent of endocervical cultures, whereas *N. gonorrhoeae* was isolated from 3 per cent (Saltz et al., 1981).

Complications of sexually transmitted diseases, especially acute salpingitis, may result in permanent damage to the reproductive system in the adolescent female, including increased risk for infertility and ectopic pregnancy (Shafer et al., 1982). Physicians caring for adolescent patients in an office can be highly effective in preventing both sexually transmitted disease and their sequelae by incorporating appropriate sexual history, physical examination, laboratory evaluation, and patient education, which includes common health problems associated with STDs.

SEXUALLY TRANSMITTED DISEASE–RELATED HISTORY

The task of obtaining a sexual history from the sexually active adolescent can be a difficult one for both the physician and the patient. The physician must establish a trusting relationship with the adolescent. This can be best accomplished by assuring the adolescent of the confidential nature of all sexually related information obtained during the history. Since STDs include a myriad of agents and syndromes, presenting signs and symptoms may be absent, unobserved, or denied by the adolescent because of limited knowledge of normality and STDs. In addition, fear, embarrassment, or perceived inaccessibility of health care for the adolescent's problem may affect utilization of available health services. The pediatrician has a unique opportunity to begin discussions of sexuality with the prepubertal youth and the sexually inexperienced adolescent. These questions may include normal pubertal development and the changing nature of relationships with parents and peers. As the youth enters puberty, questions related to sexuality, reproductive health, sexual activity, contraception, and STDs need to be reviewed routinely as part of any health assessment.

Assessment of the sexually active adolescent begins with a complete general medical history emphasizing areas associated with sexually transmitted diseases. The physician's history should include an inventory of sexual habits, with emphasis on frequency of sexual activity, number and sex of partners, sexual orientation, and types of intercourse. Information regarding previous STDs and treatment, contraception, date of last menstrual period, and pregnancy history will be helpful in determining appropriate components of the physical examination and laboratory tests. A history of symptoms which includes the triad of frequency, burning, and dysuria accompanied by a genital discharge forms the hallmark of STDs in males and females. Specific signs and symptoms of STD syndromes are outlined in Table 26–1. However, many individuals with sexually transmitted infections have few or no symptoms. Studies have estimated that approximately 80 per cent of females and 50 per cent of males with *N. gonorrhoeae* have no signs or symptoms. Therefore, the young person with a history of multiple sexual partners, a new partner, past history of STDs, or homosexual male orientation is at high risk for an STD and should be screened with appropriate physical examination and laboratory tests.

Table 26–1. SIGNS AND SYMPTOMS OF STD SYNDROMES

STD-Related Signs and Symptoms in Past 30 Days for Males and Females	
Generalized malaise, fever	Anorexia or nausea ± vomiting
Purulent discharge from eye(s)	Abdominal pain ± RUQ pain
Pain, erythema of joint(s) ± swelling	Dyspareunia
Pruritis, rash: generalized or perineal	Constipation/diarrhea ± pruritis, rash, pain per rectum
Males	*Females*
Serous/mucopurulent urethral discharge	Vulvar pruritis, rash, erythema, swelling, pain
Testicular/epididymal pain ± swelling	Lower abdominal pain ± RUQ pain, pain with walking
Perianal pruritis, rash, trauma, tenderness	Unusual cramping, prolonged bleeding with last menstrual period
Jaundice	Vaginal discharge: malodorous, increased amount, ± mucopurulent

EXAMINATION OF THE SEXUALLY ACTIVE ADOLESCENT

The examination of all sexually active adolescents should include a complete physical assessment with careful attention to the skin, lymphatic, gastrointestinal, and genitourinary systems. STD infections span the spectrum from no apparent disease to genitourinary symptoms and signs requiring immediate hospitalization. Examinations of the sexually active adolescent male and female are outlined in Tables 26–2 and 26–3. A pelvic examination should be performed as a part of the annual assessment of any sexually active adolescent female and whenever signs and symptoms of a lower genital tract infection occur. In the adolescent male, routine rectal examinations are not indicated unless the patient has signs and symptoms indicative of perianal infection or engages in anal intercourse. Indications for laboratory evaluation are outlined in Table 26–4. Additional laboratory evaluation for specific problems is included under "Vulvovaginitis and Cervicitis," "Acute Salpingitis," and "Non-gonococcal Urethritis."

Table 26–2. EXAMINATION AND STD PATTERNS IN THE SEXUALLY ACTIVE ADOLESCENT FEMALE

Vital Signs	
Temperature:	Fever, especially ≥38.5°C
Skin	
General:	Maculopapular lesion on trunk, face, palms, soles, mucous membranes (syphilis, scabies)*
Extremities:	Erythematous, vesiculopustular, or hemorrhagic papules on distal extensor surfaces with mono- or polyarticular arthritis (disseminated gonococcal disease)
Lymph Glands:	Enlarged ± tender generalized or inguinal nodes
Eyes:	Conjunctivitis with purulent discharge (gonorrhea, chlamydial infection)
Pharynx:	Painful/painless vesicles/ulcers on soft palate; erythema, exudate on tonsils (herpes, syphilis)
Abdomen:	Enlarged, tender liver; lower abdominal mass(es) ± peritoneal signs (hepatitis, Fitz-Hugh–Curtis syndrome, PID)
Gentourinary System	
Perineal skin/hair	Scabies; lice; warts; painful/painless vesicle(s) or ulcer(s) (herpes, syphilis)
Periurethral glands	Abscess with purulent discharge from duct ± urethra (gonorrhea)
SPECULUM EXAMINATION	
Vaginal	Discharge with abnormal color, odor, amount, pH, and wet mount examination (vaginitis—see specific STDs); mucosa with erythema, edema, punctate hemorrhages (trichomonas); warts (condyloma acuminatum); ulcer(s) (syphilis, herpes)
Cervix	Punctate hemorrhages, vesicles(s), ulcer(s), chancre, friability of cervix, with mucopurulent discharge, i.e., swab to discharge from os is yellow/green (cervicitis—see specific STDs)
BIMANUAL EXAMINATION	
	Tenderness of vagina, cervical motion tenderness, enlargement and tenderness of uterus or adnexa, with rectal examination to confirm vaginal findings (see vaginitis, PID)

*Most common STD(s) associated with these clinical signs are listed in parentheses.

Table 26–3. EXAMINATION AND STD PATTERNS IN THE SEXUALLY ACTIVE MALE ADOLESCENT

Vital signs, skin, lymph glands, eyes, pharynx, abdomen	See Examination of Female, Table 26–2
Genitourinary system	
Penis: Glans and shaft	Meatal erythema; rash: small painful/painless vesicle(s), ulcer(s), chancre, warts; discharge: color, odor, amount
Scrotum/testes	Erythema, swelling, tenderness, especially of epididymis; rash (see Penis)
Rectal examination	Perianal rash (see Penis) Fissure, tears, decreased tone, tenderness ± discharge or bleeding; prostatic enlargement, tenderness ± discharge elicited after prostatic manipulation

COMMON STD PROBLEMS

General

Gonorrhea, chlamydia, syphilis, and genital herpes are outlined in Tables 26–5 to 26–8, including etiology, epidemiology, syndromes, common symptoms/signs, and treatment (Saltz et al., 1981; Centers for Disease Control, 1982; Noble, 1982). Other STDs, including trichomoniasis, nonspecific vaginitis, candidiasis, venereal warts, scabies, pubic lice, and molluscum contagiosum, are outlined in Table 26–9, including etiology, syndromes, and treatment (Centers for Disease Control, 1982; Noble 1982). In addition, the most common STD genitourinary problems of vulvovaginitis, cervicitis, acute salpingitis, and non-gonococcal urethritis are discussed in more detail in the following sections.

Vulvovaginitis and Cervicitis

Vulvovaginitis, a common gynecological problem in adolescence, is frequently sexually

Table 26–4. INDICATIONS FOR LABORATORY EVALUATION IN SEXUALLY ACTIVE ADOLESCENTS*

	Male	Female
Urinalysis	Where indicated; sterile pyuria is sign of chlamydia	Same as male
VDRL or RPR (if positive, confirm with FTA-ABS)	Past history of STD, homosexual, at diagnosis and 30 days postdiagnosis of STD (not positive in early primary syphilis)	Same as male, prostitute
Gram stain	Urethral discharge or first-part voided urine sediment: WBCs, intracellular gram-negative diplococci indicate gonorrhea; WBCs, no bacteria indicate chlamydia	Cervical/vaginal discharge not usually definitive because of presence of normal flora on stain
Gonorrhea culture	Contact history, any GU symptoms, homosexual Culture urethra and other sites	Routine pelvic exams, contact history, any GU symptoms, acute salpingitis Culture endocervix and other contact sites
Chlamydia culture	Same as gonorrhea, especially in non-gonococcal urethritis	Same as gonorrhea Culture urethra in "nonbacterial" urethral syndrome
CBC, ESR, other	When indicated for evaluation of systemic STDs	Same as male, especially when considering acute salpingitis
Pregnancy test	Not applicable	When indicated, before use of tetracycline and metronidazole
Papanicolaou smear	Not applicable	Annually in all, especially in known genital herpes Cervicitis: herpes, gonorrhea, chlamydia, condyloma
Wet mounts of discharge (saline and KOH)	Not indicated	With lower genital tract signs/ symptoms or STD contact history
Phenaphthazine paper to discharge (pH paper)	Not indicated	With lower genital tract signs and symptoms

*Frequency of "routine" testing is dependent on sexual behavior. Homosexual males, prostitute youth, youth in detention, and youth with multiple sexual partners may require frequent evaluation.

transmitted in the adolescent female. In the adult population, the distribution of causal agents include *Candida albicans* (35 to 40 per cent), *Gardnerella vaginalis* (30 to 35 per cent), and *Trichomonas vaginalis* (10 to 20 per cent) (Hurd, 1979). Vulvar lesions are associated with syphilis, condyloma accuminatum, pediculosis pubis, scabies, molluscum contagiosum, herpes, and less commonly chancroid, granuloma inguinale, and lymphogranuloma venereum. "Vaginal" discharge may originate from the cervix infected with chlamydia, trichomonas, or gonorrhea. The discharge may also represent normal endocervical eversion tissue or increased cervical mucus production associated with oral contraceptive use. Vaginitis may be suspected with a history of recent onset of a vaginal discharge, with or without an offensive odor. It is frequently associated with vulvar pruritis and erythema, frequency, burning, and dysuria. On speculum examination, the mucosa may be edematous and erythematous, with the discharge characterized by a foul or "fishy" odor, depending on the etiological agent. Except in moniliasis, vaginal pH (which is measured with pH paper) is usually greater than 4.5. With wet mount microscopic examination, hyphae, clue cells, or flagellated trichomonads indicate specific disease. Cervicitis is present if the cervix is easily friable (bleeds easily when touched gently with a swab) or has a mucopurulent discharge from the endocervix (green/yellow color on white swab). Changes in cervical exfoliative cytology as demonstrated on the Papanicolaou smear have been associated with specific STD agents, especially herpes. The

Table 26–5. GONORRHEA

Etiology	*Neisseria gonorrhoeae*, a gram-negative diplococcus
Epidemiology	1,500 cases in females and 1,000 cases in males per 100,000 population, 15–19 years old. (These figures underestimate prevalences, as they represent "reported cases" only and do not control for sexual activity.)
Syndromes	*Uncomplicated:* asymptomatic carrier state, urethritis, pharyngitis, proctitis in males and females, and cervicitis in females *Complicated:* acute salpingitis and Bartholin's/Skene's gland abscesses in females; perihepatitis (Fitz-Hugh-Curtis), ophthalmitis, arthritis-dermatitis, meningitis, and endocarditis in both males and females
Common Symptoms/Signs	*Males:* frequency, burning, purulent discharge *Females:* cystitis, vaginal discharge, cervicitis *Asymptomatic:* estimate of 80% of females and 50% in males

Treatment—Selected CDC Regimens

A. Uncomplicated Infection
   1. Ampicillin 3.5 gm P.O. and Probenecid 1.0 gm P.O.
      followed by
      Tetracycline 500 mg P.O. q.i.d. × 7 days or Doxycycline 100 mg P.O. b.i.d. × 7 days
      OR
   2. Aqueous procaine penicillin G (APPG) 4.8 million U I.M. at two sites and Probenecid 1.0 gm P.O. (treatment of choice for anorectal gonorrhea in homosexual men)

B. Complicated Infections: These infections require hospitalization and high-dose intravenous therapy.

C. Special Considerations:
   1. Allergy to penicillins: Treat with alternative nonpenicillin regimens.
   2. Coexistent STD infection: Current recommended regimens for treatment of gonorrhea include drug effective against chlamydia because of the high rate of coexistent infection with gonorrhea and chlamydia. If syphilis is suspected with gonorrhea, it is important to note that benzathine penicillin is not an effective gonorrhea regimen.
   3. Pharyngeal gonorrhea: This is not effectively treated with ampicillin.
   4. Penicillinase-producing *Neisseria gonorrhoeae* (PPNG): PPNG strains show high treatment failure rates with ampicillin alone.
   5. Treatment of sexual partners: Males and females exposed to gonorrhea should be examined, cultured, and promptly treated with one of the above regimens.
   6. Follow-up of positive cultures: All males and females should be recultured from infected site(s) 3–7 days after completion of treatment. Cultures should be obtained from the anal canal of all women who have been treated for gonorrhea.
   7. Treatment failures: The patient with persistent gonorrhea after treatment with a non-spectinomycin regimen should be treated with spectinomycin 2.0 gm I.M. PPNG should also be considered and post-treatment isolates should be tested for penicillinase production. However, in most cases, recurrent gonococcal infection is due to reinfection from an untreated sexual partner. Improved contact tracing and patient education must be emphasized.
   8. Treatment in pregnancy: Use penicillins, not tetracyclines; spectinomycin may be used with penicillin allergy or PPNG; erythromycin may be added for coexistent chlamydial infection.

Table 26–6. CHLAMYDIA

Etiology	*Chlamydia trachomatis*, an obligate intracellular bacteria
Epidemiology	Estimate that 15% of sexually active adolescent females have cervical infections. Major cause of non-gonococcal urethritis (NGU) in males
Syndromes	*Uncomplicated:* asymptomatic carrier states in males and females. Cervicitis in females, non-gonococcal (NGU) or post-gonococcal (PGU) urethritis, ophthalmitis in males and females *Complicated:* acute salpingitis, perihepatitis, acute epididymitis, proctitis
Common Symptoms/Signs	*Males:* frequency, burning, dysuria with mucoid or purulent urethral discharge (NGU); but may be asymptomatic *Females:* Nonbacterial cystitis, cervicitis, but frequently asymptomatic

Treatment

A. Uncomplicated Infection
   1. Tetracycline 500 mg P.O. q.i.d. for 7 days
      OR
   2. Doxycycline 100 mg P.O. b.i.d. for 7 days
B. Complicated Infections: These infections frequently require prolonged ambulatory care or hospitalization for intravenous therapy.
C. Special Considerations
   1. Pregnancy: Erythromycin, 500 mg P.O. q.i.d. × 7 days, should be substituted for tetracycline.
   2. Treatment for sexual partners: Partners should be examined, cultured, and promptly treated with one of the regimens above.
   3. Follow-up: All infected persons should be recultured 3 to 7 days after completion of treatment. Treatment failures most likely represent noncompliance or an untreated partner.

Table 26–7. SYPHILIS

Etiology	*Treponema pallidum*, mobile spirochete.
Epidemiology	The ratio of gonorrhea to syphilis in the 15- to 19-year-old age group is 100:1. Prostitutes, bisexual and homosexual males, and their sexual contacts are at risk for infection.
Syndromes	Primary, secondary, latent, late (neurosyphilis, cardiovascular syphilis)
Common Symptoms/Signs	*Primary:* chancre is the classic lesion, a painless ulcer with indurated border in genital or nongenital areas; appears 10–90 days after exposure; atypical lesions are common, may be multiple; chancre is infectious. *Secondary:* follows primary within 6 months with a myriad of clinical signs lasting 2–6 weeks; infectious; diffuse maculopapular, follicular, or pustular rash; condyloma in anogenital area; generalized lymphadenopathy. *Latent:* from disappearance of secondary signs to development of late (neuro- or cardiovascular) syphilis.

Treatment

A. Primary, Secondary or Latent, less than 1 year
   1. Benzathine penicillin G 2.4 million units I.M. at one visit
      OR
   2. Tetracycline 500 mg P.O. q.i.d. × 15 days
B. Follow-Up
   1. Treatment for sexual partners: Treat all partners with one of the above regimens.
   2. Follow-up: Physical assessment (include pelvic examination where indicated); obtain VDRL or RPR.

Table 26–8. GENITAL HERPES

Etiology	*Herpes virus hominis,* a DNA human virus; type 1 virus is isolated most frequently from lesions above the umbilicus, while type 2 is generally isolated from genital lesions.
Epidemiology	Primary herpes may be acquired during adolescence; frequently asymptomatic; once infected, recurrences are likely.
Syndromes	Asymptomatic carriers and urethritis in males and females; balanitis and other penile/scrotal lesions in males; vulvovaginitis, cervicitis in females. Clinical presentation is divided into primary and recurrent herpes.
Common Symptoms/Signs	Vesiculoulcerative lesions on perineum, vagina, and cervix in females and prepuce, glans, penis, penile shaft, and scrotum in males; paresthesias, pruritis, genital pain, dysuria, tender adenopathy, fever, urethral or vaginal discharge; constitutional signs more common and intense in primary; episodic recurrences with varying frequency.

Treatment

A. Primary Infection
5% acyclovar ointment to lesions 6 × day for 7 days to begin as early in disease course as possible. (This treatment *may* only shorten course of symptoms, does not decrease rate of recurrence.)
B. Recurrent Infection: Symptomatic relief only (acyclovar not proven efficacious).
C. Special Considerations
1. Treatment of sexual partners: Condoms recommended if either partner has active disease but efficacy of use not proven.
2. Follow-up: Females with genital herpes need to inform their clinician of infection history during pregnancy; may be associated with cervical dysplasia and infected women should have annual Papanicolaou smears.

STDs most commonly associated with vulvovaginitis and cervicitis are gonorrhea, chlamydia, herpes, trichomonas, gardnerella, and candida.

Acute Salpingitis

Acute salpingitis, or the more nonspecific term, acute "pelvic inflammatory disease" or PID, is a sexually transmitted inflammatory process involving the endocervix, endometrium, and endosalpinx, with subsequent spill of tubal exudate into the peritoneal cavity. It is estimated that 30 to 40 per cent of all acute salpingitis occurs in females less than 20 years old and is a major cause of involuntary infertility.

In addition to infertility, the chronic sequelae that may result from acute salpingitis include chronic pelvic pain, dyspareunia, pelvic adhesions, pyosalpinx, tubo-ovarian abscess, chronic salpingitis, and ectopic pregnancy. Current research confirms the importance of the polymicrobial etiology of acute salpingitis, including *Chlamydia trachomatis, Neisseria gonorrhoeae, Mycoplasma hominis,* anaerobic bacteria (Bacteroides, gram-positive cocci) and facultative gram-negative rods *(Escherichia coli, Hemophilus influenzae).* Differential diagnosis of acute salpingitis includes acute appendicitis, acute cholecystitis, acute pyelonephritis, ectopic pregnancy, mesenteric lymphadenitis, ovarian cyst, ovarian tumor, septic abortion, and pelvic thrombophlebitis (Sweet et al., 1979).

In order to standardize the diagnosis of acute salpingitis, the following criteria should be met: (1) history of lower abdominal pain, (2) lower abdominal tenderness (rebound preferentially), (3) cervical motion tenderness, and (4) adnexal tenderness. In addition, one or more of the following should be present: (1) fever, (2) leukocytosis, (3) elevated erythrocyte sedimentation rate, (4) inflammatory mass on sonogram, and (5) culdocentesis revealing bacteria and white blood cells in the peritoneal fluid (Shafer et al., 1982). Treatment is based on the polymicrobial etiology of acute salpingitis and not the specific organism isolated from the cervix. *We currently recommend hospitalization for all adolescents with salpingitis to assist in compliance with medication and rest and to decrease the incidence of infertility.* Hospitalized treatment regimens are outlined in Table 26–10. If hospitalization is not feasible, the current ambulatory regimens recommended by the Centers for Disease Control for treatment of acute salpingitis are outlined in Table 26–11.

Non-gonococcal Urethritis (NGU)

Urethritis not associated with *Neisseria gonorrhoeae* is usually associated with *Chlamydia trachomatis, Ureaplasma urealyticum,* or, less

Table 26–9. OTHER SEXUALLY TRANSMITTED DISEASES

Etiology	Syndromes	Treatment	Comments
Trichomonas vaginalis	Asymptomatic, urethritis/cystitis, and proctitis in males and females; vaginitis, cervicitis in females	Metronidazole 2.0 gm P.O. × 1	Partners: examine and treat Pregnancy: do not use metronidazole Antabuse-like effect of metronidazole
Gardnerella vaginalis	Nonspecific vaginitis (NSV) in females	Ampicillin 500 mg P.O. b.i.d. × 7 days (50% failure rate) OR Metronidazole 500 mg P.O. b.i.d. × 7 days	Clue cells on wet mount Vaginal pH > 4.5 and "fishy" odor when KOH added to discharge
Candida albicans	Urethritis in males and females; balanitis in males; vulvovaginitis in females	Males: clotrimazole cream to skin b.i.d. until asymptomatic (3–7 days) Females: 1 clotrimazole vaginal tablet per vagina h.s. × 7 days OR Clotrimazole cream 1 applicator per vagina h.s. × 7 days	May need to treat GI candidiasis or partners if recurrences; more common in oral contraceptive users
Human wart virus	Condylomata accuminata (genital warts) in males and females	10–25% podophyllin in tincture of benzoin q week for 2–4 weeks; wash area after 4 hours	Do not use in pregnancy; in urethral meatus, intraurethral, vaginal, cervical, oral, or anorectal, refer for removal
Sarcoptes scabiei	Scabies in males and females	Lindane 1% lotion/cream applied thinly from neck down; wash after 8 hours.	Treat all sexual partners and household members. Do not use lindane in pregnant or lactating females.
Phthirus pubis (Pediculus pubis)	"Crabs" in males and females in pubic hair, eyelashes, and moustache	Lindane shampoo and comb pubic hair, wash bedding and clothes, repeat treatment in 1 week	Treat all sexual partners and household members. Do not use in pregnant or lactating females.
DNA-positive virus	Molluscum contagiosum in males and females	Curettage lesions	May be found on nongenital skin; not always STD.

Table 26–10. ACUTE SALPINGITIS: EXAMPLES OF COMBINATION REGIMENS FOR IN-HOSPITAL TREATMENT*

In-Hospital Regimen	Followed by Ambulatory Regimen	Comments
1. Doxycycline: 100 mg I.V. b.i.d. plus Cefoxitin: 2.0 gm I.V. q.i.d.	Doxycycline: 100 mg P.O. b.i.d. to complete 10–14 days of therapy	Optimal coverage for *N. gonorrhoeae* and *C. trachomatis;* may not be optimal for anaerobes, pelvic mass, or acute salpingitis associated with intrauterine device (IUD)
2. Clindamycin: 600 mg I.V. q.i.d. plus Gentamycin/tobramycin: 2.0 mg/kg, followed by 1.5 mg/kg I.V. t.i.d.	Clindamycin: 450 mg P.O. q.i.d. to complete 10–14 days of therapy	Optimal coverage against anaerobes, facultative gram-negative rods; may not be optimal for *C. trachomatis* and *N. gonorrhoeae*
3. Doxycycline: 100 mg I.V. b.i.d. plus Metronidazole: 1.0 gm I.V. b.i.d.	Continue both drugs at same dosage orally, to complete 10–14 days of therapy	Optimal coverage for anaerobes and *C. trachomatis;* not optimal for some strains of *N. gonorrhoeae*, including PPNG and some facultative gram-negative rods

Continue I.V. drugs for minimum of 4 days and at least 48 hours after fever defervesces; then begin oral regimens to continue as ambulatory patient. All patients must be reassessed within 48–72 hours with a complete physical assessment, including a pelvic examination to ensure correct diagnosis and favorable response.
Management of sexual partners: All partners should be examined, cultured for *N. gonorrhoeae* and *C. trachomatis*, and treated accordingly with a gonorrhea and chlamydia regimen.
Follow-up: A pelvic examination including a test of cure culture(s) from positive sites should be performed 3–7 days after treatment completion.

*Centers for Disease Control, 1982.

commonly, *Herpes virus hominis* or *Trichomonas vaginalis* (Govan and Kessler, 1980). NGU may present as a milder disease than gonorrhea in men, with a mucoid discharge with or without symptoms. Men frequently complain of frequency, burning, and dysuria. However, symptoms and signs used to differentiate NGU and gonorrhea are unreliable. An examination of the discharge by Gram strain and culture is required to make the specific diagnosis (Table 26–4). If the Gram stain of the urethral discharge or first-part voided urine sediment contains WBCs and no bacteria, trichomonads, or gram-negative intracellular diplococci, the diagnosis of NGU is most likely. Confirmation is made with negative gonorrhea cultures and positive cultures for chlamydia when possible. Treatment is discussed in Tables 26–5 to 26–9.

MANAGEMENT OF THE SEXUAL PARTNER

Sexual partners of adolescents with sexually transmitted disease should be identified, examined, cultured, and treated by the appropriate regimen. Partners should be evaluated in

Table 26–11. ACUTE SALPINGITIS: EXAMPLES OF COMBINATION REGIMENS FOR AMBULATORY TREATMENT*

Ambulatory	Followed By	Comments
1. Cefoxitin: 2.0 gm I.M. OR 2. Ampicillin: 3.5 gm P.O. (Amoxacillin: 3.0 gm P.O.) OR 3. Aq. procaine penicillin G 4.8 million units I.M. at 2 sites PLUS Add probenecid, 1.0 gm P.O. to each regimen above	1. Doxycycline: 100 mg P.O. b.i.d. OR 2. Tetracycline: 500 mg P.O. q.i.d. to complete 10–14 days of therapy	Cefoxitin (or equivalent) plus doxycycline/tetracycline, active for *N. gonorrhoeae* (including PPNG); Ampicillin, amoxacillin, or aq. procaine penicillin plus doxycycline not optimal for PPNG

Management of sexual partners: See Table 26–10.
Follow-up: All patients treated on an ambulatory basis should be re-evaluated in 48–72 hours. Those not responding should be hospitalized. A pelvic examination including test of cure culture(s) from positive sites should be performed 3–7 days after treatment completion.

*Centers for Disease Control, 1982.

the same setting as the adolescent patient when possible or referred to an appropriate site such as a public health clinic. Sexual abstinence or the use of condoms by the male partner during the treatment course is important. Follow-up and preventive health counseling are essential for both partners. In discussing STDs with the partner, a nonjudgmental approach will accomplish the best treatment and follow-up results.

MANAGEMENT OF THE HOMOSEXUAL PATIENT

The homosexual male has unique STD problems, and therefore identification of sexual preference is an important component of a complete health assessment. Homosexual males are at greater risk of acquiring pharyngeal gonorrhea, syphilis, hepatitis B, and gastrointestinal parasites (Owen, 1980). A vaccine is now available for hepatitis B and should be given to all HBsAg-negative homosexual or bisexual adolescent males. In addition, recent reports of immunosuppression and Kaposi's sarcoma in homosexual males should alert the physician to examine the skin carefully for unusual lesions and generalized, nontender lymphadenopathy (Friedman-Kien et al., 1982).

THE PEDIATRICIAN AND SEXUALLY TRANSMITTED DISEASE IN ADOLESCENTS

Sexually transmitted disease is a major morbidity and public health issue of epidemic proportions in youth today. The pediatrician can play an important role with adolescents in his or her office practice. Utilizing anticipatory guidance prior to sexual activity, the pediatrician can discuss with the adolescent the common sexually transmitted diseases, prevention methods, early signs and symptoms, and possible sequelae to specific infections.

Recognition of youth at risk for STD is essential. Recent data suggest that youth who engage in risk-taking behaviors, including substance abuse, school nonattendance, and reckless automobile driving, and youth in detention are likely also to engage in premature sexual intercourse with the resultant increased risk of developing STDs. In addition, the homosexual male youth or the young male experimenting sexually with a male sex partner is at higher risk for STDs (Govan and Kessler, 1980). Emphasis must be directed toward prevention, early detection, and appropriate treatment in an effort to avoid permanent sequelae, especially infertility and possibly neoplasia.

RESOURCES FOR THE PEDIATRICIAN

Management of sexually transmitted disease, including agents, diagnosis, treatment, and prevention, changes rapidly. Textbooks oriented toward clinical practice are available (Noble, 1982). Up-to-date treatment regimens are periodically published in the Centers for Disease Control publication *Morbidity and Mortality Weekly Report.* In addition, staff members of local public health clinics for sexually transmitted disease are frequently excellent resources for assistance with patient education literature, diagnosis, management, and contact tracing.

REFERENCES

Centers for Disease Control: Sexually transmitted disease: Treatment guidelines, 1982. Morbidity Mortality Weekly Report (Suppl.), *31*:355, 1982.

Friedman-Kien, A. E., Laubenstin, L. J., Rubenstein, P., et al.: Disseminated Kaposi's sarcoma in homosexual men. Ann. Intern. Med., *96*:693, 1982.

Govan, D. E., and Kessler, R.: Urologic problems in the adolescent male. Pediatr. Clin. North Am., *27*:109, 1980.

Hurd, J. K.: Vaginitis. Med. Clin. North Am., *63*:423, 1979.

McCormack, W. M.: Penicillinase-producing *Neisseria gonorrhoeae*—a retrospective. N. Engl. J. Med., *307*:438, 1982.

Noble, R. C.: Sexually Transmitted Diseases (2nd ed.). New York, Medical Examination Publishing Co., Inc., 1982.

Owen, W. F.: Sexually transmitted diseases and traumatic problems in homosexual men. Ann. Intern. Med., 92:805, 1980.

Report of the Centers for Disease Control Task Force on Kaposi's Sarcoma and Opportunistic Infections. Special Report. N. Engl. J. Med., *306*:248, 1982.

Saltz, R., Linneman, C. C., Brookman, R. R., and Rauh, J.: *Chlamydia trachomatis* cervical infections in female adolescents. J. Pediatr., *98*:981, 1981.

Schachter, J.: Chlamydial infections. N. Engl. J. Med., *298*:428, 490, 540, 1978.

Shafer, M. A. B., Irwin, C. E., and Sweet, R. L.: Acute salpingitis in the adolescent female. J. Pediatr., *100*:339, 1982.

Sweet, R. L., Mills, J., Hadley, K. W., Blumenstock, E., Schachter, J., Robbie, M. O., and Draper, D. L.: Use of laparoscopy to determine etiology of acute salpingitis. Am. J. Obstet. Gynecol., *134*:68, 1979.

Zelnick, M., and Kantner, J. F.: Sexual activity, contraceptive use and pregnancy among metropolitan-area teenagers, 1971–1979. Fam. Plan. Perspect., *12*:230, 1980.

27
THE ACUTE SCROTUM

Michael E. Mitchell, M.D.

The sudden onset of swelling in the scrotum of a child with or without pain should alert the physician to the possibility of a surgical emergency. The differential diagnosis (torsion of the testis, torsion of the appendix testis, epididymitis, orchitis, scrotal edema, vasculitis, trauma, or tumor) must be appreciated to facilitate rapid evaluation and ensure proper therapy.

Torsion of the testis commonly occurs by two distinct mechanisms at two different ages. The first, the extravaginal torsion, in which the testis with its membrane twists on its vascular pedicle, occurs in the perinatal period. Although surgery is the usual treatment, it is not commonly effective, as the torsion usually occurs well before birth. The second, the intravaginal torsion, is associated with a "bell clapper" testis, in which the testis twists *inside* its membrane. This complication occurs with peak incidence between the ages of 12 and 17 years. The clinical course is acute, with rapid unilateral scrotal swelling and pain, which initially may mimic an abdominal crisis. The testis will be tender, observed to be high in the scrotum, and sometimes lie transversely. The condition need not be associated with a history of trauma and should not be associated with fever or elevated white count, and urinalysis should be normal. Immediate surgical intervention to untwist the spermatic cord and pex both testes is indicated (Johnston, 1982).

Torsion of the appendix testis, a small pedunculated appendage of testicular development (Müllerian derivative) or more uncommonly of epididymal development (appendix epididymis—Wolffian duct) can occur. If evaluated before massive swelling occurs, point tenderness only without testicular tenderness may be observed, as well as a "blue dot sign" caused by the hematoma visualized through the scrotal skin. If conclusively diagnosed, torsion of the appendix testis and epididymis needs no surgical intervention.

Bacterial infection of the epididymis is an important consideration in the differential diagnosis of testicular torsion. Acute tender scrotal swelling with a positive urinalysis, fever, and/or leukocytosis should lead to this diagnosis. Doppler blood flow studies or nuclide scrotal scan may show increased persuion of the involved testis. After treatment with antibiotics, careful evaluation for congenital malformation of the urinary tract must be made. Inflammation of the epididymis without infection (chemical epididymitis) can occur and make differentiation from torsion difficult.

Viral orchitis in the prepubertal male is uncommon. Even with a history of parotid swelling, true torsion must be ruled out.

Unilateral and bilateral testicular pain and swelling have been noted in the patient with Henoch-Schönlein purpura. Differential diagnosis is difficult in these patients (Loh and Jalan, 1974). Scrotal isotope scanning can be very helpful (Naiman et al., 1978).

Tumor of the testis must be considered in all patients with testicular enlargement even in the early age group. Although uncommon, minimal trauma with subsequent bleeding into the testis may point to pathology not previously recognized. Careful follow-up examination may be the only way to differentiate clearly the traumatized normal testis from testicular tumor. Tumor of the testis is *always* to be explored through the groin, *never* the scrotum.

Idiopathic unilateral scrotal swelling can occur, but in the earlier stages the palpation of a nontender testis will obviate the need for a surgical exploration for torsion (Evans and Snyder, 1977).

The prompt evaluation of the patient with a unilateral painful scrotum should include a careful history, physical examination, urinalysis, and complete blood cell count. If torsion of the testis cannot clearly be ruled out, then immediate surgical intervention is indicated. Other diagnostic studies such as Doppler flow evaluation or radionuclide scrotal scanning should be reserved for patients in whom torsion is seriously in doubt. It is the timing that is critical

(Krarup, 1978). If the testis is to be salvaged, torsion must be relieved and blood flow restored immediately.

REFERENCES

Evans, J. P., and Snyder, H. M.: Idiopathic scrotal edema. Urology, 9:549, 1977.

Johnston, J. H.: Acquired lesions of the penis, the scrotum and testis. *In* Williams, D. I., and Johnston, J. H. (eds.): Pediatric Urology. London, Butterworths, 1982, pp. 467–475.

Krarup, T.: The testis after torsion. Br. J. Urol., *50*:43, 1978.

Loh, H. S., and Jalan, O. M.: Testicular torsion in Henoch-Schönlein syndrome. Br. Med. J., *2*:96, 1974.

Naiman, J. L., Harcke, T., Sebastianelli, J., and Stein, B. S.: Scrotal imaging in the Henoch-Schönlein syndrome. J. Pediatr., *92*:1021, 1978.

SECTION IV

BIOPSYCHOSOCIAL-DEVELOPMENTAL DISORDERS

In 1948, Milton Senn, a pioneer in the introduction of psychodynamic concepts into pediatric practice, envisioned that pediatricians would develop a balanced competency in both the psychosocial and the biomedical aspects of child health. Thirty years later, the Task Force on Pediatric Education reported that more than half of general pediatricians regarded their residencies as inadequate in training and experience in the developmental and behavioral aspects of pediatrics. Although Senn's vision has not yet become a reality, the improvement of training in the psychosocial aspects of child health is a prominent item on today's agenda for pediatric education. Although there has been some discussion of developing a subspecialty of "behavioral pediatrics," we favor the inclusion of biopsychosocial pediatrics in the training and practice of all pediatricians.

Beyond the residency, the practitioner who wishes to enlarge his understanding of the psychosocial aspects of pediatrics may choose from a range of continuing medical education activities, including seminars, lectures, grand rounds, courses in pediatric interviewing, mini-residencies, fellowships, and self-study. Study groups of pediatric practitioners, which meet weekly under the direction of a qualified pediatrician, child psychiatrist, or other mental health professional to discuss patients being seen by one of the participants because of a behavioral or developmental problem, are highly effective. The practitioner may also schedule consultation sessions from time to time with a child psychiatrist to discuss selected patients.

Textbooks and journals that emphasize the developmental and behavioral aspects of pediatrics are becoming increasingly available. Some of these are listed below.

Selected Books

Allmond, B. W., Buckman, W., and Gofman, H. F.: The Family is the Patient: An Approach to Behavioral Pediatrics for the Clinician. St. Louis, C. V. Mosby Co., 1979.

Aten, M., and McAnarney, E.: Behavioral Approach to Adolescents. St. Louis, C. V. Mosby Co., 1981.

Diagnostic and Statistical Manual of Mental Disorders, 3rd Ed. (DSM III). Washington, D.C., American Psychiatric Association, 1980.

Friedman, S. B., and Hoekelman, R. A. (eds.): Behavioral Pediatrics. New York, McGraw-Hill Book Co., 1980.

Grossman, H. J., Simmons, J. E., Dyer, A. R., and Work, H. H. (eds.): The Physician and the Mental Health of the Child. I. Assessing Development and Treating Disorders within a Family Context. Chicago, American Medical Association, 1979.

Grossman, H. J., and Stubblefield, R. L. (eds.): The Physician and the Mental Health of the Child. II. The Psychological Concomitants of Illness. Chicago, American Medical Association, 1979.

Hersh, S. P., and Simmons, J. E. (eds.): The Physician and the Mental Health of the Child. III. Issues and Skills in Relating Primary Medical Care to the other Human Services. Chicago, American Medical Association, 1981.

Kenney, T. J., and Clemmens, R. L. (eds.): Behavioral Pediatrics and Child Development, 2nd Ed. Baltimore, Williams and Wilkins, 1980.
Levine, M. D., Carey, W. B., Crocker, A. C., and Gross, R. T. (eds.): Developmental-Behavioral Pediatrics. Philadelphia, W. B. Saunders Co., 1983.
Prugh, D. G.: The Psychosocial Aspects of Pediatrics. Philadelphia, Lea and Febiger, 1983.
Sahler, O., and McAnarney, E.: The Child from 3–18. St. Louis, C. V. Mosby Co., 1981.
Senn, M. J. E., and Solnit, A. J.: Problems in Child Behavior and Development. Philadelphia, Lea and Febiger, 1968.
Simmons, J. E.: Psychiatric Examination of Children, 3rd Ed. Philadelphia, Lea and Febiger, 1981.
Talbot, N., Kagan, J., and Eisenberg, L.: Behavioral Science in Pediatric Medicine. Philadelphia, W. B. Saunders Co., 1971.
The Future of Pediatric Education. A Report by the Task Force on Pediatric Education, 1978.
Thomas, A., Chess, S., and Birch, H. G.: Temperament and Behavior Disorders in Children. New York, New York University Press, 1968.

Books Explaining Behavior for Parents

Becker, W. B.: Parents are Teachers. Champaign, Ill., Research Press, 1971.
Patterson, G. R.: Living with Children (Revised). Champaign, Ill., Research Press, 1976.
Schaefer, C. E., and Millman, H. L.: How to Help Children Cope with Common Problems. New York, Van Nostrand Reinhold, 1981.

Selected Journals

Monographs in Developmental Pediatrics
Journal of the American Academy of Child Psychiatry
Journal of Developmental and Behavioral Pediatrics
American Journal of Orthopsychiatry
Journal of Child Psychology and Psychiatry
Zero to Three. Published by the National Center for Clinical Infant Programs.

Morris Green, M.D.

28

THE PEDIATRIC INTERVIEW

Morris Green, M.D.

For the general clinician, the interview is the most frequently used tool in understanding and managing the problems, vulnerabilities, strengths, and invulnerabilities of children and families, whether these be biomedical or psychosocial. It has been said that 90 per cent of diagnoses are made by interview data. An effective interview requires an extensive data base, thoughtful experience, good judgment, self-assurance, sensitivity, and a deep interest in personal care. Most interviews in pediatric practice at times of health supervision visits or acute illness care are relatively brief. The data and the relationship in such instances can be cumulative based on a continuing care role. At other times, in relation to Level II or III problems or consultations, the interview will be of greater length. As a reflection of the interview's central importance in ambulatory pediatric practice, the list of principles of interviewing included in this chapter is extensive. It is hoped that the reader will find these principles helpful in all levels of pediatric care. In addition to facilitative techniques, these guidelines stress the importance of personal style and individual approaches. No guideline can substitute for experience and only experience can teach interviewing, but experience without guidance may not result in the physician's becoming a skilled interviewer.

Some Generalizations

The interview is a powerful diagnostic and psychotherapeutic tool—an effective method of collecting data needed for diagnosis and establishing a relationship.

An effective interview represents a blending of cognitive and technical skills with the patient's and the physician's feelings and personalities.

Organic and psychosocial possibilities should be considered together.

In clinical medicine, biomedical competence is a prerequisite for psychotherapeutic effectiveness and for diagnostic open-mindness.

The expert physician balances his scientific objectivity with an empathetic, tactful exploration of his patients' feelings.

The interview is a progressive, cumulative process.

The interview aspect of the practice of medicine is intensely personal.

The nature of the interview depends upon the clinician's personality and experience and the personality of the patient.

The skilled interviewer has a cultivated perceptiveness; a scientific curiosity about people; and a highly developed ability to *see*, to *hear*, to *feel*, to *empathize*, and to *read* the patient.

The goal is verbal, nonverbal, and affective *communication*.

The interview is an *active* process, an experience, a relationship. It should be flexible, spontaneous, and intuitive.

The patient will scrutinize the doctor's face for evidence of interest, concern, indifference, censure, agreement, acceptance, anger, disapproval, shock, friendliness, surprise, reassurance, and response.

The physician may use his facial expression to facilitate the interview. An appearance of quiet attention demonstrates an interest in what the patient is saying. On the other hand, an expression of concern may reinforce his reaction to a child's prolonged absence from school.

Interviewing techniques should not show. The process should be seamless.

When there are many problems, focus on one at a time.

Ask open-ended questions that permit meaningful answers in preference to those that can be answered by "yes" or "no."

Determine what the patient wants and his readiness to accept help.

Are the parents psychologically or developmentally minded? If the physician surmises at the beginning that his interest in psychosocial and family interactions would be perceived as both irrelevant and intrusive, those considerations should be reserved until later. The initial concern should, in that event, be limited to biomedical factors and an exploration of feelings not pursued at that time; otherwise, these patients and the parents may feel affronted.

Do not interrogate. Prod or probe sparingly. Medical practice is not a court of law.

Minimal movement by the interviewer is advisable.

The patient's questions and expectations must be answered at some level.

Even though it is not always the real problem (and the real problem may not become apparent to parent or physician until later), the chief complaint should remain the focus of the interview. The physician should return to that topic by the end of the session.

Interviews should be scheduled for a defined period of time and concluded within that limit.

The success of an interview is likely to be compromised if the physician feels pressured by lack of time.

The physician must charge appropriately for his time.

Both parents should be asked to be present.

BEGINNING THE INTERVIEW

The interview begins with introductions and a few transitional social remarks. With the parent, this may be very brief. When seeing a child or adolescent alone, this introductory period may continue for a few minutes.

The experienced clinician has in mind one or more diagnostic hypotheses based on the presenting symptoms and the patient's age. These may change in response to additional information and observation.

"Would you tell me what has been concerning you about Cynthia?"

"What else. . .?"

"Now, you've mentioned two concerns, one, ____________, and two, ____________. What else?"

If the mother does not accompany the father, find out why.

Overly vigorous note taking may suppress significant parts of the history, especially if there is a psychological problem; on the other hand, if parents appear wary of psychological implications, initial meticulous note taking may allay their concerns until the tone of the interview changes.

It is difficult to write and observe the patient simultaneously, and observation may be as important as what is said.

Jot down pertinent dates and names, but save time at the conclusion of the interview for writing or dictating.

LISTENING

If given the chance, patients often spontaneously disclose their problems.

The interviewer needs to *hear* the message, which includes the order in which the problems are mentioned by the patient, recurrent references, and significant omissions.

The skilled interviewer is very attentive to how words and phrases are used to conceal, to reveal, or to suggest the patient's thoughts, feelings, or history: (1) The patient's spontaneous association of statements and events. (2) The first statement of the patient and the last one on leaving. (3) The patient's opinion of and attitude toward previous clinicians. (4) Possible litigation in process, e.g., custody, accident, school phobia, probation. Be circumspect. (5) A significant pause before answering a question. (6) Quick, unsolicited, and defensive protestations: "We have a wonderful marriage." "There couldn't possibly be anything emotionally wrong." "One thing I'm certain about, it's not his nerves!" "That doesn't bother me now." "That's all over now." "Everything is fine." "The other children are doing well." "I'm very happy." (7) When a patient says, "I don't see what that has to do with my problem," it's probably relevant. (8) Unexpected use of medical terminology by someone who is not a health professional. (9) An impersonal, clinical quality to the history. (10) One person speaking for another who is present, e.g., "He thinks . . ." (11) Avoiding answering a question through subtle change of the subject or appearing to misunderstand while feigning eagerness to answer.

If the interviewer believes that the answer to a question is not a candid one, rephrase the question: "How do you *really* feel?" or return to the question later.

Sometimes a question to which a patient initially chooses not to respond may be answered later or in a subsequent interview.

Nonstop talking may be a cover for the patient's anxiety, perhaps acting as a defensive screen so that the interviewer will not have a chance to ask potentially troublesome questions.

The patient may not disclose the primary or real reason for coming until convinced that the interviewer will be empathetic.

Patients who feel understood by the physician will usually share their real concerns and problems.

The patient may be totally unaware of what may seem self-evident to the clinician.

The way patients perceive events may be very different from the way the interviewer sees them.

A different account of the history may be given by each parent and by the child.

Persistent symptoms may be due to secondary, conscious gains.

The primary clinician may initially have an advantage over the psychiatrist if the parents and child believe that the complaint, e.g., recurrent abdominal pain, has an organic etiology.

Some patients simply do not understand or are unable to accept an etiological relationship between psychosocial factors and somatic complaints.

Some families do not have a language of affects. Their attention is captured by somatic complaints rather than a person's feelings.

There is a hidden psychosocial morbidity in many families.

Parents of infants who fail to thrive or who are retarded, psychotic, or handicapped are likely to have feelings of anger, shame, inadequacy, anxiety, despair, and guilt.

When a patient says, "Let me ask you about a hypothetical situation" (or a question about someone else), the question is probably related to the patient's own problem.

ASSUMPTIONS

While most patients come with the wish and the expectation to be helped, they may have reservations about both. They have their own agenda of concerns and ideas of what would be helpful.

These considerations may condition the success of the visit.

Patients often present a facade.

Seek to identify the *primary* patient and the *central* problem.

Regard the initial history as tentative and incomplete. The most important material may not be disclosed until later.

The patient may initially not be able to describe his problem comfortably or adequately. He may not be sure what it is.

THE SETTING

Courtesy and cordiality of the appointment secretary and receptionist are essential.

Punctuality of the physician contributes to a positive relationship.

Greeting of each patient individually by name should be accompanied by eye contact and a friendly gesture such as a firm handshake and a smile. The greeting should not be perfunctory.

A quiet setting and the assurance of privacy are facilitative.

Comfortable chairs of the same height should be arranged to permit eye contact between the physician and the patient without strain.

Soft lighting is helpful.

The patient should not face sunglare.

The hospitable ambience of the room and comfortable furniture facilitate openness.

Depending upon the comfort of the patient and the kind of communication sought, the doctor should not sit too close or too distant.

A distance of 5 or more feet fosters an impersonal atmosphere, whereas sitting next to the patient is more facilitative.

It is generally not a good idea to sit behind a desk when interviewing children or adolescents.

The interview should not be interrupted by phone calls or someone opening the door.

Patients may talk more freely during or after the intimacy and reassurance of the physical examination. Listen carefully at these times or at the conclusion of the examination. Ask if there is anything else they wish to ask or tell you about.

See the parents and the child together and separately.

If the parent is hesitant about talking, excuse the child from the room.

If the parents appear comfortable when relating sensitive matters in the child's presence, he or she has probably heard the material before.

THE FACILITATIVE INTERVIEWER

The ideal physician is perceived as mature, unhurried, accepting, nonjudgmental, courteous, gracious, genuine, responsive, and trustworthy.

The doctor's expertise should be sensed by the patient as reassuring rather than intimidating or patronizing.

The facilitative doctor's interest is shown by the alertness with which he follows what the patient is saying, by his facial expression, and by the tone of his voice.

Different people seem to respond to different approaches. There are some who respond best to an assertive interviewer, others to one who is gregarious, and others to one who is quiet and unpretentious.

The patient's name and that of the parents and siblings should be specifically used at points during the interview as a way of personalizing the process.

The empathetic doctor senses the patient's feelings—anxiety, depression, anger, or fear: "You seem kind of sad today."

He respects the patient's dignity.

He is not too smoothly articulate.

He allows patients to talk, following their leads.

He is not prematurely reassuring.

INTERVIEWING CHILDREN

Children may be initially apprehensive and fearful about the interview: "I'll bet you were a little nervous about coming here."

Introduce yourself. Explain what you do. Be yourself—an adult who likes children.

Give children time to get acquainted.

The doctor's comfortable friendliness will place the child at ease.

While children will usually talk readily, an occasional child, especially if shy or anxious, responds only to direct questions and then circumspectly.

The doctor may play with very young children for a few minutes to get acquainted. Blocks, a ball, crayons, a pad of paper, picture books, or a doll and bottle are useful facilitators.

Since very young children can easily imagine that a stuffed animal or a hand puppet can talk and listen, part of the interview can be conducted through that medium if it seems appropriate.

Topics to talk with children about include (1) the members of his family, (2) school experiences: "How are the teachers (the subjects, the other students)?"; successes; (3) friends; (4) sports and recreation; (5) possible career plans; (6) favorite television programs; (7) admired singers or actors; (8) pets.

Create the opportunity for the child to talk about some of his or her strengths, especially at the beginning of the interview: "Tell me about some of the things that you're best at."

"Many girls your age are concerned about ____________. I imagine that you may be also? Tell me about it."

Role playing: "Let's imagine that you're the doctor . . . Dr. Susan . . . and a girl your age . . . let's call her Marcia . . . tells you she has____________ (patient's symptom). What would you think might be causing her trouble?" Then later, "What do you think would help her?"

"If your teachers asked you to write a story about your life . . . family, what would you write?"

"How are things going?" "What kind of things do you do for fun—your favorite activities?" "What kind of activities do you dislike?" "Tell me how you spend a typical school day, say yesterday. A typical Saturday and Sunday?"

"What do you and your mother (father) do for fun?" "Do you have a special friend?" "To whom do you talk about things?" "How are the other children in your school, neighborhood?" "Tell me about your mother (father, brother)." "Tell me about your relationships—how you get along with your_______ (siblings, parents, peers)."

"What would you like to do when you're finished with school?"

"What kind of discipline do your parents use?" "For what?" "Do you think that's fair?" "Is it effective?" "Do mother and father have the same ideas about this?" "What do you think the rules ought to be?"

"It's natural for everyone to get angry sometimes. What are some of the things that make *you* angry?"

"What do you do when you get mad?" "How could I tell if you were angry?" "What keeps you from letting people know when you're angry?"

"If a fairy godmother were here and granted you three wishes, what would they be?"

"How do you differ from and how are you like your sister (brother)?"

"What makes you sad (worried, happy)?" "Many children worry about their parents—their health, something happening to them—or they may worry about themselves. Whom do you worry about the most?"

"Who has been sick in your family?" "Have there been any deaths in your family?" "Draw me a picture." "Tell me a story about your picture."

INTERVIEWING ADOLESCENTS

The ground rules should be clarified at the start: the patient is free to discuss the interview with his parents if he wishes, but the doctor will not unless the patient concurs or, in the doctor's judgment, the parents need to be told for reasons of the patient's health or safety. The physician would then share with the patient his intention to do so.

After the introductory amenities, which give the patient time to look around, the doctor may simply ask, "John, I wonder if you would tell me why you came to see me (or why your parents brought you to see me)."

If the patient denies knowing why, report what the parents said or ask what he thinks it might be . . . his best guess.

If he still says he does not know, respond with a statement such as, "I understand that you're having a problem at school."

Adolescents will usually discuss their thoughts and feelings readily, especially when their parents are not present and confidentiality is ensured.

If angry or offended about coming, the adolescent may deny that there is a problem.

If the patient has been brought by subterfuge, dissociate yourself from that tactic: "I'm sorry. That wasn't appropriate. Tell me why you think this happened."

If the doctor believes the child may be depressed or angry, the following statement that fronts for a question may be facilitative: "I would guess that things aren't going so well for you." Usually the child will give his answer nonverbally by a quick glance at the physician. This cue can be followed by the statement: "Tell me about it."

The doctor should not feel challenged to make the patient talk, nor press about subjects that he obviously does not want to acknowledge. The traditional review of symptoms is a neutral introduction that may enhance the initial communication.

"Your life is none of my business unless you would want to talk with me about how things are going."

"I can appreciate that you weren't wild about coming here . . . that you don't feel it makes sense . . . but since we have this time, I'd be interested in hearing about how you think things are going."

If the patient does not respond, it is generally fruitless to continue at length. Close the visit graciously, give the child your phone number, and tell him you'd be pleased to see him again if he would like to come back.

Questions about sexualilty, drugs, and alcohol may be expected by the adolescent.

Some questions for adolescents.

"How have you felt lately?"

"How would you describe yourself . . . your usual mood . . . your feelings?"

"Tell me about some of the things that you're really good at."

"Do you have a job?" "What do you do?"

"How do others—your family, your friends—feel toward you?"

"What are your responsibilities or chores at home?"

"What sort of privileges do you have at home?"

"What rules do your parents have for you? What happens if you bend them?"

"I don't know your mother (father, sibling) well. What are they like?"

"How do they feel about this problem?"

"What do they think of your friends?"

"Have you had a recent date?" "What did you do?"

'How would you change your life if you could?" "How about in regard to your mother (father, boyfriend)?"

"What does (name of disease or symptom) mean to you?"

"I know this is the reason why you came to see me, but I'm interested in learning what you've thought might be causing this problem."

"Do you think that it's something serious?"

"What have you been told about it? Explain what that means to you."

"What are some of the changes that have occurred in your life lately?"

"What do you do for physical activity?"

"What are your dietary preferences?"

"Everyone has stress. What makes you feel most under stress? What do you find helps you cope?"

"Typically, adolescents have concerns from time to time about their body, their size, their growth, and their development, and I would suppose that you have too. What thoughts have you had about your health?"

"If that's too personal, we'll not talk about it now." "What do the other teenagers at school think about drugs (drinking, sex)? What's your attitude about that?" "What's your knowledge of sexuality?" "Are you sexually active?" For the female adolescent, these questions may be linked to those about menstruation.

"Do you smoke?"

"What else were you expecting of this visit?"

"I don't know" or "I forgot" are generally evasive statements. If the adolescent remains guarded, be patient. There is a reason, e.g., parental admonition not to talk, uncertainty about confidentiality, lack of trust in the doctor, shame, anxiety, or being forced to come.

OBSERVE ACTIVELY

Visual clues are highly important.

Patient's attitude on meeting the interviewer: Smile? Pleased? Cool? Suspicious? Overly friendly? Unfriendly? Reserved? Indifferent? Depressed?

Be aware of feelings engendered in oneself during the interview—anger, anxiety, dislike, admiration, frustration, impatience.

Much is communicated nonverbally and affectively.

Does what you see and feel match the patient's words?

Appearance and behavior that may be significant:

Perspiration.

Blushing or paling.

Controlled, uneven, or blocked speech.

The plaintive voice; talking in a whisper.

The patient's gait.

Tics.

Frequent swallowing.

Tenseness, fidgetiness.

Preoccupation.

Avoidance of eye contact.

Sudden glance at the interviewer or someone else in the family following a statement or question.

Clenching, rubbing, wringing hands, scratching, nail biting.

Mendicant posture.

The kind of clothing worn. Among adolescents, dark clothes may be a sign of depression.

Sudden request by parent or adolescent for permission to smoke.

Reddening of eyes or crying.

Frowns.

Smiles.

Apparent concern or unconcern about symptom.

Double messages, e.g., mother laughing while telling child to behave, smiling when talking about his bad behavior.

The light that seems to go on in a patient's mind when he has made a significant association or achieved a new insight.

Interaction between parents and child and between child and physician during the visit.

Developmentally inappropriate behavior, e.g., older child on parent's lap; difficulty in separating child from parent; the mother laying a young infant on the examination table and then walking away.

The way in which the infant or young child is held or helped during the interview and physical examination.

Does the mother have "parenting presence"?

Response of child to parent's requests.

The child's play and activity.

ITEMS DIFFICULT FOR PATIENTS AND PARENTS TO VERBALIZE

The possibility of a serious disorder in their child, e.g., mental retardation or malignancy.

Emotional problems, including alcoholism and depression.

Their own health problems.

Sexual problems.

Marital difficulties.

Financial stresses.

Child abuse.

Sexual abuse.

Anger, especially at members of the family.

If the patient's concerns are thought to be conscious and relevant, it may be appropriate for the interviewer to provide an opening: "Many parents (children) in this situation have this sort of question (worry), and it would be only natural if you did also. . . ."

QUESTIONS FOR PARENTS

When reviewing the prenatal period or early infancy, "Was that a convenient time for you to be pregnant?" "How did your pregancy go?" "What was your labor with__________ like?" "Your delivery?" "Did you have anyone to help you during this time?"

Answers to questions about feeding, sleeping, toilet training, and discipline may be informative.

"Often our children remind us of someone in our family or ourselves. Whom does_____ remind you of?"

"How does__________get along with other children?"

"What sort of temper does__________ have?"

"Was__________ever very sick?"

"Why do you think that is?"

"What do you think would be helpful?"

"How do you think all this has affected __________?"

"How do you think__________feels about that?"

"Tell me how__________spends his day."

"Have you and__________been separated for any length of time?"

"Does__________become upset when you leave?"

"What changes would you like to see in your child (spouse, yourself)?"

"This has been going on for some time, and I was just wondering why you came in now?"

"Whose idea was it to come?"

"I know this is why you came to see me, but this has been going on for some time . . . you've been thinking about it a lot, so I'd be interested in what possibilities you've thought of?"

"This has been going on for a time, and it would be helpful to know what you have been doing about this?"

"Does this behavior also occur when others are caring for him? At school?"

"Would you tell me what has *really* been worrying you about __________?"

"What were you expecting of this visit?"

Questions about the relationships parents experienced as children with their own parents and siblings—how they were reared—may be highly relevant. "How were things for you when you were growing up?"

A review of the parent's life history. Ask about the physical and emotional health of each parent at each stage of the child's development.

"Do you have a chance to go out without the children? Why not?"

"How have things been going between the two of you?"

"What are the arrangements for privacy in your home?"

"What have you told__________(the child) about your illness (his illness, the divorce, the stillbirth, the adoption, etc.)?"

How physically and psychologically available are the parents to the child?

CLARIFICATION

The clarifying function of the interview helps patients gain a realistic view of their situation.

One way to encourage elaboration on a topic is to shift one's posture and appear quizzical: "You know, I'm a little puzzled about what you consider your main concern. What would you say is the major difficulty?" or "I guess that I don't understand that. Would you please clarify it for me?"

If the patient disclaims an opinion on what the cause of his problem is ("I don't know." "I have no idea."): "I recognize that you don't know, but since it's been going on for some time, I'm sure you've had some notions about it; it would be helpful to have your ideas."

Understand what the patient means by the words he uses. Verify that he understands the ones the physician uses.

When the patient uses qualifying terms such as "reasonably well," "a little," "somewhat," "really," "fair," "in most respects," "average," "so-so," "OK . . . I guess," "like everybody else," ask for clarification.

Seek specificity about content and feelings rather than vague references.

If clarifying information is not obtained when there is a good physician-patient relationship, it is probably not consciously available to the patient.

Parents and child feel better if they have a diagnosis, some idea as to the cause of a problem and what can be done about it.

When he surmises that the patient has not disclosed the pertinent facts or that a specific diagnosis would seem blunt or premature, the physician may sidestep an answer by a statement such as, "I'm not sure yet" or "This is obviously a complex matter, and it will take time to understand."

Significant differences of opinion in the family can be noted with a comment such as, "Both of you seem to have a little different view of this matter."

To have the patient elaborate, repeat the patient's preceding word or phrase.

Use one or two syllable sounds—uh huh, yes, hum, ah.

Possible responses to encourage patient disclosure:

"Why do you say *that*?"
"Why do you ask?"
"How do *you* feel about it?"
"And so . . ."
"Such as . . ."
"So . . ."
"Well . . ."
"Give me an example."
"Tell me more about that."
"For instance . . ."
"Therefore . . ."
"Why is that?"
"You feel . . ."
"You mentioned____________?"
"As I get it,____________."

If the patient seems angry about something that he has not verbalized: "You seem to be angry about something. Since I don't know why, tell me."

If the patient brings up material that does not forward the purpose of the interview, neither indicate an interest in it nor seek elaboration.

If the patient is tearful or cries, the doctor may wait a moment and then comment: "This is difficult to think about" or "This seems to be upsetting you. Would you tell me about it?"

Offering facial tissues to quickly may prematurely shut off an elaboration of what is upsetting.

HELPING THE PATIENT TO FEEL BETTER

By the end of the interview each patient should feel better about himself or herself and should experience the interview as worthwhile.

Commend the patient in some way. Try to build up his self-esteem, e.g., "What a beautiful child!" or "That's quite an achievement."

To a child: "I thought, when you walked in, that you were probably an athlete."

Patients who feel positively evaluated by their doctor are more likely to comply with his recommendations.

In addition to their problems and failures, patients should be encouraged to report their successes and strengths.

The patient with multiple hypochondriacal symptoms needs to be encouraged to carry on in spite of his symptoms.

The clinician's interest and understanding is especially appreciated by the parents of retarded children.

Such interest may be shown nonverbally by holding or cuddling the baby and by talking to the child.

THE DIFFICULT PATIENT

Understanding the reason for their difficult or inappropriate behavior helps the physician work productively with patients who otherwise would be even more disturbing, frustrating, and anger-provoking.

The physician will at times feel calm and relaxed, whereas at other times and with different patients he may be tense, impatient, and angry.

The patient's anger may be a manifestation of anxiety; cockiness, compensation for insecurity; and "sweetness and light," a cover for hostility.

The patient's difficult behavior usually derives from previous relationships with authority figures other than the physician.

The patient's overevaluation or underevaluation of the physician is usually unrelated to what the doctor says or does.

With patients who are angry, uncooperative, belittling, sarcastic, provocative, suspicious, disrespectful, attacking, irritating, resentful, blustering, or challenging, the doctor should maintain his equanimity and avoid defensiveness, although it may be almost impossible not to flare with anger. At the same time, one does not accept abuse.

When the parent's anger is a cover for anxiety, his demeanor may change dramatically in response to the physician's calm, empathetic remark: "I'm sure that you must be very worried about your child's illness." "Tell me about it." or "You're obviously very angry about something. Tell me what you think is wrong." "What happened?" Then listen without becoming defensive.

If one senses at the beginning of the interview that the patient is angry, try to disarm him by conveying your understanding of how he feels, by being careful not to be perceived as critical, by going slow, by avoiding interpretations that suggest that the parent's emotional problems may be contributory, by initially confining questions to the presenting complaint, and by being serious and concerned.

Compulsive or highly narcissistic patients are difficult to help. They see no merit in changing or in accepting suggestions.

Some patients, regretably, will be unable to form a trusting relationship with the doctor.

Some patients show no obvious emotion and give minimal, almost telegraphic answers that conceal more than they reveal.

Other patients talk incessantly but circumvent efforts to elicit their feelings.

A patient's needs and expectations may be so great or unrealistic that no physician can satisfy them.

EXPRESSIONS OF EMPATHY

"How did you manage?"

"That must have made you angry (sad, happy)."

"That must have been a trying time for you."

"You must have been hurt (upset)."

"It's hard to talk about this."

"People don't seem to understand how you feel."

"You seem to be receiving a lot of unwanted advice."

"You seem to be kind of hard on yourself."

"I'd guess you find it difficult to trust anyone."

"The death of someone so close is hard to take."

"I suppose you were scared that you might lose ____________."

"This has been kind of a secret fear, I take it."

An understanding nod.

CAUTION

A history of failure to follow previous regimens generally implies future noncompliance.

If a patient reports dissatisfaction with or anger at previous doctors, be prepared for a similar reaction.

Rather than agree, disagree, or ignore such pejorative remarks, the physician might quietly observe: "Well, you seem to have been unhappy with that experience."

It may be difficult to establish a constructive, continuing relationship with a nomadic patient who has consulted a succession of doctors. Often such patients seek agreement with their own perceptions rather than an objective opinion.

The patient who is too friendly, overly interested in the doctor's personal life, too courteous, too agreeable, or too flattering may be trying to control or vitiate the relationship. If unsuccessful in this, his or her behavior may change abruptly.

The pace of the interview should not exceed the tolerance of the patient.

Respect the patient's defenses. It is unwise to push him to reveal more than he is prepared to disclose.

Do not point out inconsistencies in a patient's story.

Do not try to hurry the process. A certain amount of time is required. It is better to schedule additional sessions than to do too much at once.

Discuss with the patient only those feelings that he has verbally expressed, even though you sense other feelings of which he is unaware or which he does not wish to disclose. Premature verbalization of the patient's undisclosed feelings may cause resentment and defensiveness.

The chronically depressed patient may have a considerable reservoir of anger. Proceed with caution.

Take care when exploring matters not closely relevant to the patient's present concerns, especially in the initial interview.

Do not be manipulative or devious.

Provide help at the level the patient is prepared to receive it. Do not give advice you believe the patient cannot follow.

Because a very anxious patient has difficulty in concentrating, address only one item at a time. Explanations should be brief.

It is generally wise to avoid judgmental terms such as "good," "bad," "right," "wrong," and "fault." Do not express to the parents or child criticism of anyone.

In situations such as a divorce or a parent-child conflict, there are two sides, often widely divergent, to the story.

Let sleeping dogs lie. Know when not to intrude. Otherwise, one may arouse so much anxiety and resistance that the patient will not return.

Although helpful on occasion, humor should be used sparingly and with discretion. Avoid teasing, facetiousness, jocularity, sarcasm, or comments that make the patient think that you are laughing at him, making light of his complaint, or not acting in a professional manner.

Avoid familiarity. Keep the relationship professional, not social.

Avoid discussion of one's personal life and experiences.

Do not discuss other patients in any way, even if asked about someone specifically. Your ability to keep confidences is being tested.

Try to be aware of your own emotional blind

spots, prejudices, and situations that tend to make you anxious and/or angry.

In general, avoid the use of the personal pronoun "I," e.g., "*I* think" or "If *I* were you."

Set a limit on the length of the interview. Spending an unlimited amount of time is wasteful of the physician's and the patient's time, expensive, and countertherapeutic.

If the parents have little insight into their problems, proceed with caution.

Do not comment on slips of the tongue or inconsistencies in the patient's or parents' story.

Have reasonable goals and expectations for each patient.

Do not exceed the boundaries of one's competency.

The pediatrician is not a marriage counselor.

Do not deny the reality of the patient's complaints, e.g., "pain," "weakness," "dizziness," etc.

Give advice sparingly about psychosocial issues.

Avoid hasty, superficial advice or reassurance. The patient may have knowingly withheld the information necessary for a meaningful response.

Confrontation of parents with a direct interpretation of psychosocial etiologies, even when obvious to the doctor, is usually undesirable.

Patients tend to be defensive about gratuitous interpretations.

Patients may be antagonized if they are not ready to accept the doctor's observations.

Authoritative advice may be given if the patient understands exactly what the doctor is saying, is not seriously emotionally disturbed, has been communicative, and has asked for such counsel.

Do not take at face value all the statements a patient makes.

Unless adequately expressed, a patient's anxieties are not lessened by random reassurance.

Be alert to the manipulative patient who seeks—at times through slanted, inaccurate, or incomplete data—to influence the doctor to do what the patient wants, e.g., delay in hospitalization for the patient with anorexia nervosa, procedures and tests in the Munchausen's syndrome by proxy. When thwarted, even gently, some of these patients may become very angry.

Be cautious about listening to "secrets" from one of the parents transmitted privately in an attempt to control the doctor. Although there are exceptions, it may be appropriate to suggest that they bring up the material with other members of the family during the interview.

The patient who asks your opinion about someone else's behavior or problem is likely talking about himself.

The patient who requests or demands to be told exactly what to do may have no intention of following that advice. "Well, do you think you would follow those suggestions?" "Well, it's not quite that easy. It's going to take time to understand the problem better and to see just what would be helpful."

If a mother indicates that the father will not agree to come in for the next visit, she may be expressing her ambivalence about his presence. Convey your belief that she can get him to come or offer to call him directly. "I'd like to have his ideas about Tom's situation."

Is the patient and his family ready for referral? Do they believe they need psychiatric help? Do they know what is involved—potential benefits, limitations, and time required? Do they have misconceptions?

While premature or too abrupt psychiatric referral should be avoided, any possible ambivalence the physician may feel about the effectiveness of such help or any reluctance to share the child's management should not interfere with recognition of the patient's readiness for such help.

Although psychiatric referral may be declined, the pediatrician has the responsibility, at the appropriate time, to convey his recommendation clearly.

Parents are extraordinarily sensitive to any implication that they have caused their child's emotional problem.

If psychiatric help is either unavailable or declined, the pediatrician may continue to be helpful.

Be cautious about initiating a discussion of institutionalization of a retarded child unless the parents indicate their readiness for such discussion.

FACILITATING DISCUSSION OF POSSIBLE PSYCHOLOGICAL ETIOLOGICAL FACTORS

If a parent states that her child is "nervous": "Who else in the family would you say is nervous?" or "Who's the *nervous* one in your family?" or "Who does the *worrying* in your family?"

If the parent raises the possibility of an emotional cause, do not pounce on that suggestion. Be a little tentative: "Well, I guess that's possible. Would you explain a little more why you suggest that?"

"Sensitive" or "blue" or "down" may be less charged words than "anxious" or "depressed." "Tension" and "stress" usually do not create defensiveness.

"You seem kind of tense (worried)."

If the patient repeatedly denies the presence of problems when the physician believes they exist: "OK—everything may not be as great as you say, but you seem to think that everything is fine."

Before inquiring about a sensitive matter: "Could I ask you kind of a personal question? If it's too personal, you need not answer, but it would be helpful for me to know."

"Well, those are natural feelings."

FAMILY INVENTORY

Ask about symptoms or illnesses, emotional and social adjustments of parents, siblings, grandparents, and other significant persons. "How is your health, Mr. X?" "What kind of symptoms do you have?" "Are you seeing a doctor?" "What medicine are you taking?" "How do *you* feel?" "How are things going with you?"

If a parent seems sad or anxious, verbalize that observation and invite the parent to talk about it.

Family life topics to explore:

- Time and cause of deaths of significant persons.
- Separations and losses that the child has experienced.
- Parents' work, including hours.
- How the parents have been getting along.
- Who lives in the house (including persons not in the family and new additions to the household).
- Family crises.
- Sleeping arrangements.
- Privacy practices.
- The father's participation in the family.
- Thoughts about discipline.
- Does the mother have time for herself away from the children?
- Do the parents have joint or individual social interests?
- Social supports.
- Community ties—church, clubs, and other organizations.

"You've been telling me about what you regard as Tom's troublesome traits. Tell me about his good points—things you really like about him."

"Mr. Smith, you're a crucially important (key) person in Tom's life, and I'd like to hear your thoughts about how he is getting along."

"If you could, what would you change about your family?"

"What do you believe your husband (wife, son, daughter) thinks about that?"

In the interviewer's judgment, does the family's equilibrium depend on the continuing presence of the symptom?

BEING PSYCHOLOGICALLY HELPFUL

The physician's personal warmth, empathy, integrity, and sincerity are important ingredients of a therapeutic physician-patient relationship.

In being identified by the patient as reliable and trustworthy, the physician has developed a helping relationship.

The physician's ability to promote confidence and facilitate communication of facts and feelings enhances his effectiveness.

The physician's understanding of people permits him to avoid being moralistic, judgmental, or authoritarian.

The opportunity in the interview for the patient to sort out thoughts, communicate fears and worries, and discharge feelings with an interested and facilitative physician, a person who has a special status in society, may be a powerful therapeutic experience.

The patient experiences the supportive interest of the physician in being valued as a person.

The physician's acceptance of the patient and his problem is therapeutic.

The physician's ability to get a child to like, trust, and admire him, to be comfortable and friendly, to relate in a strongly positive fashion, and to identify with and assume, at least to some extent, his ideas and attitudes toward health and his view of the child's symptoms and life situation offers a special therapeutic relationship.

Continuity of care and the appropriate investment of time and interest facilitate a constructive relationship.

The doctor's supportive interest in carefully identifying the patient's successes, strengths, and resources in addition to his weaknesses, worries, feelings, puzzlements, and vulnerabilities helps establish a health-promoting bond among physician, parent, and child, contributes to a patient's self-esteem, fosters his ability to assume an active role in the resolution or amelioration of his problem, and promotes the development of new capabilities.

The interview offers an opportunity for self-reflection, discovery, and clarification. It helps the child be more open with his feelings.

It is not necessary for the doctor to understand all the psychodynamics of a problem in order to be therapeutically effective.

The patient's spontaneous insight is more important than the physician's interpretation.

Be aware of the patient's feelings and your own.

The right word or phrase at the right time may be extremely helpful.

The physician may, at times, be directive, giving members of the family assignments to be done before the next session, e.g., greater participation of the father, increased social experiences for the parents, enhanced communication within the family, efforts to alter behavior that is troublesome, and more open discussion of some issues about which there is conflict in the family.

IF THE INTERVIEW IS NOT GOING WELL

Does the patient sense that the doctor is more interested in psychosocial matters than he had anticipated or can understand?

Is the patient comfortable?

Did the interviewer do anything verbally or nonverbally to interfere with rapport?

Did the patient come against his own wishes? Failure to volunteer information or to elaborate may be signs of this. If one suspects coercion, ask the patient to clarify his feelings about coming.

Is the patient angry? Depressed? Psychotic? Retarded? Very shy?

Is the patient reluctant to talk in the presence of another family member?

Is the patient still evaluating the physician?

Are the doctor and patient incompatible?

Is the patient intimidated?

Does the patient doubt the doctor's competence or interest?

Is the patient worried about confidentiality?

Does the patient really want help at this time?

Is the patient psychologically or developmentally minded?

Is the patient hesitant or unable to express feelings?

Some patients erect a barrier of rationalization and intellectualization.

The psychologically disturbed patient may omit significant details, alter others, and resist the efforts of the interviewer to learn additional facts.

When the history is extremely diffuse, it may be because the patient is very anxious.

The patient may be afraid of what the physician may learn; e.g., he or she may fear that such exploration and clarification will lead to a divorce or that the doctor will think less of him or her.

An adolescent patient may be shy, embarrassed, unaccustomed to talking with an adult, depressed, and/or anxious.

There may be cultural or language barriers.

PERIODS OF SILENCE

If there is some hesitancy in getting the interview started, look at one of the parents or the child: "__________, why don't you start off?"

Pauses should not be too quickly interrupted.

If a pause is prolonged, one of the following may facilitate resumption of discussion:

"Now you've been telling me about ______. Could you tell me something about __________?"

"You said__________?"

"You mentioned__________?"

"Won't you go on."

"You were about to say something."

"These things are hard to talk about."

"Well . . ."

"So?"

Use encouraging gestures, such as a nod or a smile.

ENDING THE INTERVIEW

By keeping aware of the time, the doctor can bring the discussion to a natural end within the time set without seeming abrupt or incomplete.

"Well, I see that our time is up." The doctor should stand up and move to open the office door.

It may be helpful to offer a brief summary of the interview to illuminate important points made, to indicate the doctor's satisfaction with it, and to commend the patient:

"You've been very helpful."

"There are some other matters that we ought to discuss, so I believe that further sessions would be helpful."

"Think some more about all this, and we'll

discuss it next time. Some other ideas will probably come to mind."

Both the doctor and the patient—the parents and the child—should have a clear understanding of what they are to do next or between visits.

"You have your assignments, and I'd like for you to work on them between now and next ____________."

If return visits are inconvenient or unnecessary, arrange follow-up by phone: "Call me back Thursday at 4:00 and let me know how things are going."

If the patient raises another problem at the end of the interview—"Oh, by the way. . ."—do not attempt to deal with it then. Rather, suggest that he or she bring it up in the next session or make an appointment for another visit, but recognize that it may be the most pressing issue for the patient.

The usual interval for supportive interviews is weekly.

Less frequent visits make continuity difficult to maintain.

Time is often an important diagnostic and therapeutic ally.

Return visits may permit the interviewer to see each parent alone: "Why don't each of you take turns bringing Tom to see me."

The end of the interview *is* the end of the interview.

The temptation to have a social chat will be there during the let-down period after the intensity of the interview; however, such practice tends to undermine the interviewer's effectiveness.

Prepare a summary, including key words, promptly after session.

REFERENCES

Engel, G. L., and Morgan, W. L., Jr.: Interviewing the Patient. Philadelphia, W. B. Saunders Co., 1973.

Korsch, B. M., and Alvey, E. F.: Pediatric interviewing techniques. Curr. Probl. Pediatr., 3:3, 1973.

Senn, M. J. E.: The contribution of psychiatry to child health services. Am. J. Orthopsychiatry, *21*:138, 1951.

Senn, M. J. E.: Emotions and symptoms in pediatric practice. Adv. Pediatr., 3:69, 1948.

Senn, M. J. E.: The psychotherapeutic role of the pediatrician. Pediatrics, 2:147, 1948.

Simmons, J. E.: Psychiatric Examination of Children, 3rd Ed. Philadelphia, Lea and Febiger, 1981.

29

MOTHERING DISABILITIES

Morris Green, M.D.

Mothering disabilities particularly affect infants in the first year of life, leading to some of the signs and symptoms listed in Table 29–1. Whether manifested as inadequate caloric intake, anorexia, or rumination, mothering disability is the most frequent cause for failure to thrive in infants. Indeed, periodic determination of an infant's weight is a simple screening method for problems in mother-infant interaction. Developmental delay may also occur, especially in vocalization, smiling, and the use of large muscles. The infant may show other evidences of environmental deprivation such as "hot cube" behavior, a hesitancy in grasping one of the one-inch cubes used in infant testing when offered by the examiner.

Mothering disabilities often represent the sequelae of many historically predisposing factors. These past life experiences do not always lead to problems, but they increase the odds against successful mothering. They represent, in a sense, vulnerabilities analogous to maternal diabetes or hypertension.

Predisposing factors reported by women who experience difficulties in their mothering roles frequently include *a history of a poor relationship between the mother and her own mother.* The experiencing of emotional deprivation, rejection, derogation, lack of affection, and constant criticism appears to be a major handicap to successful mothering. The parents of physically abused children seem almost always to have had a highly unsatisfactory rearing experience when they were young. Many young mothers and fathers are *socially isolated* from the support that might come from friends, neighbors, or older relatives experienced in mothercraft. Families who abuse their children have great difficulty in turning to others for help in crisis situations. Other parents are alienated from their own parents and from social organizations.

Table 29–1. INFANT SIGNS AND SYMPTOMS OF MOTHERING DISABILITIES

1. Failure to thrive
2. Feeding problems
3. Developmental delay
4. Rumination
5. Recurrent vomiting or diarrhea
6. Irritability, excessive crying, excessive excitability
7. Apathy, listlessness, lethargy, excessive sleepiness
8. Sleep problems
9. Increased visual alertness ("radar-like") or withdrawal and disinterest in people
10. Decreased cuddling behavior
11. Poor physical care
12. Evidence of physical abuse
13. Passive behavior or rapid shifts in behavior
14. Breath-holding episodes
15. Nutritional anemia
16. Separation problems: clings, insists on being held all the time
17. Excessive maternal worry about illness in infant
18. Temper tantrums
19. Mother a poor historian
20. Mother who holds infant stiffly and facing away from her

A long-term *emotional disturbance* or maladaptation such as alcoholism, drug abuse, intellectual limitation, immaturity, psychosis, or character disorder may also be present. Unresolved *maternal grief*, perhaps over the previous loss of an infant due to sudden infant death syndrome or the recent death of her husband or one of the mother's own parents may impair mothering. More unusually, mothering may be distorted because the new baby comes to represent for the mother an important person in her past, e.g., her own mother, who died prematurely. Such mothers are secretly convinced that their babies will also die prematurely.

Other cogent historical factors include *marital discord or separation; maternal physical illness*, especially illness thought to be possibly injurious to the baby or to the mother; *many pregnancies* at short intervals; a very much *unwanted pregnancy; family illness*, especially when the expectant mother has to provide care for the sick relative; a disruptive *move* late in pregnancy; a *threatened miscarriage*; a serious *complication of pregnancy*, including the raising by the physician of the question of fetal death; and the other stressors common to most social-psychological problems, e.g., *financial worries, unemployment*, and frequent moves.

The current life situation of a pregnant woman or new mother affects greatly her child-rearing behavior. Such women may be vulnerable to a breakdown in their mothering capacities when overwhelmed by unexpected perinatal contingencies. Table 29–2 lists the contemporary situations in which mothering may be vulnerable and in which the pediatrician should be especially diagnostically alert.

The potentially deleterious effect that the birth of a *premature baby* may have on mothering arises from such considerations as the receiving of a guarded prognosis, the anticipatory mourning that may occur, the sense of failure that the woman may endure, and the separation and infrequent contact with the baby that may be experienced. Such babies also appear to be at higher risk of physical abuse than those who are born at full term.

The birth of an *infant with a congenital anomaly* or birth injury may lead to parental feelings of inadequacy, distortion of child-rearing practices, lack of communication within the family, increased physical demands on the mother, and social isolation of the parents. If a baby is severely retarded, the feedback and positive reinforcement that mothering requires are seriously hampered.

An *early critical illness*, a long-term life-threatening illness in the baby, or a *difficult delivery* in which complications threatened the life of the mother or baby are psychologically as well as physically dangerous. Unexpected recovery from an illness in which the mother thought the baby would die may be followed by the "vulnerable child syndrome," in which

Table 29–2. PERINATAL CONTINGENCIES

1. Prematurity
2. Birth defect
3. Critical illness; difficult delivery
4. Maternal depression
5. Multiple births
6. Lack of involvement and support of the father
7. Marital discord
8. Social isolation
9. Infant's temperament
10. Financial worries
11. Motherhood thought unrewarding
12. Illness in mother or family
13. Guilt about returning to work or not working
14. Mother subjected to multiple stressors in the absence of social supports
15. Mother views immediate future as unpredictable and life's contingencies as uncontrollable

the mother believes that her baby is highly vulnerable to illness and likely to die prematurely. This constellation of symptoms includes difficulty in separation of the infant or child from the mother, sleep problems, delay in the child's acquisition of self-help skills, inability of the mother to discipline the child, and maternal overconcern about the child's health. Because such mothers are unable to tell whether the baby is well or ill, they may call the physician frequently about symptoms that appear to the doctor to be trivial or about signs, such as "rapid breathing," which the physician does not confirm.

Maternal depression in the first year of an infant's life is frequently associated with characteristic symptoms in the child. There is a marked lack of discipline, and the child demonstrates severe temper tantrums, negativism, and abusive behavior toward the mother. Hyperactivity, crying, and harrassing irritability, worse on days when the mother is most depressed, are present. Difficulty in separation, overprotection, and delay in acquisition of self-help skills are other prominent symptoms. The mother's depression is usually not disclosed unless the physician makes appropriate inquiry. These women appear to have lost their *mothering presence*, that nonverbal projection of an effective mother somewhat analogous to *command presence* in the military. As a result, they are unable to provide the leadership and sense of security that children require. They are too ill emotionally to function effectively as mothers, and they urgently need psychiatric help.

Failure of the infant to meet parental expectations contributes to mothering disability. An infant's temperament, sex, activity, reactivity, and style of responsiveness obviously have major influences on mothering. Thomas et al. have pointed out that the infants who have the greatest susceptibility to behavioral disturbances are those with extreme irregularity in biological functions, e.g., sleeping and feeding; withdrawal from new stimuli; negative mood; excessive and loud crying; and intense reactions and nonadaptability to change, e.g., new foods, routines, places, activities. Some mothers who abuse their children seem to expect the child, in a kind of role reversal, to reassure and comfort them.

Prevention of developmental problems manifested in the first year necessitates that the pediatrician identify in the prenatal interview those high-risk mothers who are vulnerable to a parenting disability (see Chapter 5). Remedial or supportive measures introduced at that time will, it is hoped, reinforce their strengths and help contain their vulnerabilities. Such data also augment the physician's diagnostic alertness after the birth of the baby.

Since a mother will not likely spontaneously volunteer that she is depressed or that there are other stressors that limit her ability to nurture her infant, signs and symptoms in the baby may provide the only clue. Mothers who are experiencing difficulties need to sense the physician's empathy for how they are feeling and what they are experiencing. Expressions of interest by the physician such as, "How are *you* feeling?" or "You sound kind of tired." or "You seem a little blue." may open a channel for communication and support. Clarification and identification of the problem, coupled with an expression of interest and an accepting relationship, impressively facilitate successful mothering. The right word or phase at the appropriate time may be extremely effective.

Greenspan has published a helpful screening outline of clinical landmarks for adaptive and disordered infant development for the periods from birth to three months (homeostasis); two to seven months (attachment); three to ten months (somatic-psychological differentiation); and nine to 24 months (behavioral organization, initiative, and internalization). Table 29–3, adapted from this screening outline, describes disordered maternal behaviors that suggest maladaptive patterns.

Once symptoms such as failure to thrive, severe sleep difficulties, or discipline problems are present, one may anticipate secondary reactions in the mother such as feelings of inadequacy, extreme frustration, guilt, anxiety, and anger. These nonverbalized feelings, which may masquerade as overt hostility or apparent dis-

Table 29–3. MATERNAL BEHAVIOR ASSOCIATED WITH MOTHERING DISABILITY

1. Inability to comfort infant
2. Inability to provide developmentally appropriate environmental stimuli
3. Overstimulation of baby
4. Maternal responses not contingent upon or reciprocal with infant's needs or states; misreading or missing of infant's signals
5. Care given mechanically and impersonally without positive interaction
6. Failure to look or smile at, talk to, reach out for, hug, or caress infant; withdrawn, aloof demeanor
7. Overly anxious or overprotective maternal behaviors
8. Mother's response limited to one modality (feeding, swinging) regardless of infant's immediate need

interest, need to be understood. Such mothers are extremely sensitive to any implication of blame. They need acceptance, availability, and support, not criticism.

In the presence of a mothering disability, one needs to arrange a nurturing environment that will provide for the infant positive emotional, social, and physical stimulation. Since at this time she may not perceive them independently, this may include explaining to the mother her baby's needs and helping her read behavioral cues. This is especially needed in the case of a handicapped infant. In other situations, one may arrange for a homemaker or mother's aid. A public health nurse may be asked to visit the home periodically. During periods of stress, the mother should have the opportunity to call the physician or nurse. Day care for infants and young children, nurseries for temporary care during a family crisis, and mothers' groups are other important community resources. Families with what Greenspan has called multiple-risk-factors, i.e., major socioeconomic stresses, emotional illness, and limited coping functions, require comprehensive supportive services for the mother, including health, mental health, and social services; educational, vocational, and legal help; guidance in meeting the baby's developmental needs; and direct developmental therapy for the child, including infant stimulation, home start programs, therapeutic preschools, and psychotherapy. In some circumstances, it may be necessary to admit the baby temporarily to a hospital or other caring facility. Social reasons for hospitalization are often as necessary and valuable as those for medical emergencies.

REFERENCES

Coleman, R. W., and Provence, S.: Environmental retardation (hospitalism) in infants living in families. Pediatrics, *19*:285, 1957.

Green, M.: Care of infants and children with long-term handicaps. Bull. N.Y. Acad. Med., *55*:832, 1979.

Green, M., and Solnit, A. J.: Reaction to the threatened loss of a child: A vulnerable child syndrome. Pediatrics, *34*:58, 1964.

Greenspan, S. J.: Psychopathology and Adaptation in Infancy and Early Childhood. Principles of Clinical Diagnosis and Preventive Intervention. New York, International Universities Press, Inc., 1981.

Greenspan, S. J.: Developmental morbidity in infants in multi-risk-factor families: Clinical perspectives. Publ. Health Rep., 97:16, 1982.

Steele, B. F., and Pollock, C. B.: A psychiatric study of parents who abuse infants and small children. *In* Kempe, C. H., and Helfer, R. (eds.): The Battered Child. Chicago, University of Chicago Press, 1968, pp. 103–147.

Thomas, A., Chess, S., and Birch, H.: Temperament and Behavior Disorders in Children. New York, New York University Press, 1968.

Wolkind, S.: Depression in mothers of young children. Arch. Dis. Child., *56*:1, 1981.

30

BREATH-HOLDING SPELLS

Morris Green, M.D.

Breath-holding spells are common in infants, especially during the latter part of the first year and the early months of the second year, and may persist in unusual situations until the age of four years. Episodes may be triggered by some injury, often trivial, a reprimand or sudden fright, anger, or frustration. Vigorous crying is the first manifestation. After a variable period, there is a sudden gasp or breath-holding until the child becomes blue or pale, unconscious, and limp. Rigidity, convulsive movements, or opisthotonus may rarely follow if unconsciousness is prolonged. Some children, especially those who experience large numbers of these episodes, may only gasp or cry briefly before holding their breath.

The presenting complaint is usually convulsions or blacking out rather than breath-holding or syncope. The history and sequence of events are so characteristic that the differential diagnosis generally presents no problem; however, when the precipitating event seems extremely trivial, when there appears to be no triggering circumstance, when the child is said to cry or hold his breath for only a short time, or when the convulsive movements are a prominent clinical feature, differentiation from epilepsy may require an electroencephalogram and further observation.

Some babies seem especially prone to have these spells, and there may be a familial incidence. The parents need to be told authoritatively that the episodes, although frightening, are not life-threatening. Although in some cases there appears to be no contributory disturbance in the home or in the mother-infant relation, these need to be explored. Immature parents, maternal depression, inability to set limits on the child, manipulativeness on the part of the child, and other difficulties in maternal-infant interaction need to be dealt with if the spells are to be prevented. Many of these children have an iron deficiency anemia that appears to be an associated rather than a causative disorder.

The first step in management should be an attempt to improve maternal-infant interactions and to address problems in the family. With such interventions, the episodes will usually stop. After a base line is obtained of the circumstances temporally related to each episode, appropriate environmental changes may be introduced to avoid precipitating situations, activities, and places. The baby should also be given immediate positive reinforcement for appropriate behaviors. Because behavior that is not reinforced will eventually be given up, the parents and other caretakers should be instructed to ignore the spells every time they occur. This may not be easy to do without feeling guilty. Initially, the episodes may increase in frequency, but if this approach is maintained, they will eventually diminish. This approach is inadvisable if the child demonstrates multiple problem behaviors.

REFERENCES

Livingston, S.: Breathholding spells in children. A differentiation from epileptic attacks. J.A.M.A., *212*:2231, 1970.

Lombroso, C. T., and Lerman, P.: Breathholding spells (cyanotic and pallid infantile syncope). Pediatrics, *39*:563, 1967.

31

PICA

Morris Green, M.D.

Pica, the persistent ingestion of non-nutritious substances such as dirt, sand, grass, clay, plaster, paint, salt, or coal, occurs in pregnant women and young children, usually in the toddler and preschool age group. The child with pica is at risk of visceral larva migrans, lead poisoning, or other toxicity. Although the etiology of pica is not clearly established, a non-nurturing environment with insufficient maternal supervision and availability, frequent moves, inadequate play resources, poor nutritional practices, and major emotional problems in the family appear to be contributory factors. These children have a higher-than-normal incidence of such oral behavior as use of a pacifer, thumbsucking, persistent use of the bottle, and sucking on various objects; discipline problems; and temper tantrums. Iron deficiency and pica are often present in the same child, but oral or intramuscular iron is not a specific treatment for pica. Improving the nurturance of the child through attention to psychological and environmental factors in the parents and home are the mainstays of therapy.

REFERENCES

Cooper, M.: Pica. Springfield, Ill., Charles C Thomas, 1957.

Gutelius, M. F., Millican, F. K., Layman, E. M., Cohen, G. J., and Dublin, C. C.: Nutritional studies of children with pica. Pediatrics 29:1012, 1962.

32

PSYCHOGENIC PAIN DISORDERS

Morris Green, M.D.

Children with somatic complaints due to psychosocial factors are initially seen by the pediatrician because of the parent's assumption of an organic cause. Table 32–1 lists the kinds of presentations that suggest a psychogenic etiology. In some instances, psychogenic pain is thought to be penitence for conscious or unconscious guilt due to angry or sexual feelings directed toward a relative or other significant person. In other cases, the process of identification explains why the kind and localization of the pain corresponds to that experienced by a parent or other significant person. Anxiety may increase the child's awareness of normal physiological sensations, such as intestinal peristalsis, decrease his threshold for pain, or increase muscle spasm, leading to a cycle of pain, spasm, and more pain. A conversion mechanism may also be operative. Pain may persist when it affords the child conscious secondary gains or acts as a distractor that permits the family to avoid confrontation and conflict. Some families do not talk about feelings but rather deal only with somatic complaints. The child may have learned that the parent will respond in a caring fashion to somatic complaints but ignore those of an affective character.

Diagnosis

Psychogenic pain disorders are best approached developmentally through an understanding of the challenges and environmental stresses that a child is confronting at a given time. These are best determined in the pediatric interview, a process that allows both the collection of data and the development of a therapeutic relationship between the doctor and the child and family. The physician may open the interview with a statement such as: "In seeing many children with abdominal (or other) pain, I've found that it's sometimes due to physical causes, sometimes to stresses at this age, and sometimes to both. But *pain is pain* no matter what the cause, so it's my practice to examine all possibilities thoroughly . . . physical . . . psychological . . . whatever."

This preface precludes the possible conclusion on the part of the parents or child that the doctor, in a snap decision, has concluded that the pain is "in the child's head" or that the child is "making it up." It conveys the message that psychosocial considerations are a legitimate part of the diagnostic process and recognizes that such possibilities are more easily accepted at the onset than after a negative work-up for organic disease. Ruling out an organic etiology before considering those of a psychological or developmental nature may be antidiagnostic and antitherapeutic.

As his most effective psychotherapeutic tool, the interview helps the physician understand the patient's and the parents' past and current life situations along with their feelings, beliefs, and anxieties while they sense his expertise and interest. Sharing personal facts, feelings, and problems with the physician often results in a dramatic lessening of anxiety and pain. In addition to illuminating links between the child's pain and the environmental or developmental stresses being experienced, the interview provides parents, who may be unaware of their child's problems because of a preoccupation with their own difficulties, the opportunity to concentrate on their child, themselves, and their interactions in a clarifying fashion. The physician's personal warmth, empathy, and capacity to understand how the patient feels helps him foster the child's identification with his knowledge of what is healthy.

The following kinds of personal, developmental, and family stresses and problems are of interest in the interview:

I. Separation experiences that represent for the child a major life change and stress.
   A. The death or the anticipated death of a significant person—a parent, sibling, grandparent, friend, or pet.
   B. Divorce or anticipated divorce or desertion.
   C. Social or vocational commitments that result in unavailability of the parents to the child. Such parents are psychologically little involved with

Table 32–1. PRESENTING COMPLAINTS SUGGESTING A PSYCHOGENIC DISORDER

1. When the description of the somatic complaint does not characterize an established biomedical disease.
2. When the reason for the child's being seen remains unclear to the physician.
3. When the complaint has been associated with frequent absences from school.
4. When the symptom has been present for some time without change.
5. When the complaint, in itself, carries a high probability of a psychogenic etiology: urinary frequency, hyperactivity, chronic abdominal, chest, or musculoskeletal pain, or headaches.
6. When multiple somatic complaints involving multiple body systems are reported.
7. When the description of the symptoms seems exaggerated.
8. When the parent's or child's concern about the complaint is greater or less than ordinarily anticipated.
9. When the child has been previously seen for the same complaint by many physicians.
10. When the complaint is described by the parent in a clinical, impersonal fashion with an excessive use of medical terminology.
11. When the parent expresses dissatisfaction or anger at the physicians previously consulted about the complaint.
12. When the child with a chronic complaint is brought in by the father with the explanation that the mother is "ill."
13. When the complaint has previously led to multiple investigations and hospitalizations, including invasive procedures.
14. When the parent or child expresses the belief that the doctor will not be able to help them.
15. When the parents insist, without being asked, that the symptom is *not* due to the child's "nerves."

their child and frequently absent from the home.

D. The fear of premature death in a child who has recovered from a critical illness or who has a long-term, life-threatening disease—the vulnerable child syndrome.

E. Lack of communication within the family.

F. Recent move of the family or a close friend.

G. Entrance into middle or junior high school.

H. The child placed outside his family.

I. Addition of a step-parent, other adult, or adopted sibling to the family.

J. An older sibling's marriage, entrance into college, or departure for military service.

K. Major change in parental career or life style.

L. Social isolation of the family.

II. Family illness

A. Vulnerable parents or siblings.

1. Medically vulnerable due to a physical illness, e.g., cancer or myocardial infarction in a parent or a long-term handicapping condition such as mental retardation or myelodysplasia in a sibling. Each parent should be asked specifically about his or her own health, the kind of pain experienced in the past or currently, and whether they are seeing a physician or taking medicine. The child should also be asked about complaints and illnesses in each of his parents, grandparents, and siblings.
2. Parents or siblings may unrealistically and secretly be thought by the child to be vulnerable to a premature death due to an accident or a sudden illness.

B. Psychological symptoms and disorders in the family, e.g., anxiety, depression, alcoholism, psychosis. Helpful exploratory questions include: "Who's the nervous one in your family?" or "Who does the worrying around your house?"

C. Parental hypochondriasis or preoccupation with illness.

III. Marital discord is obviously a major stress for children.

IV. Lack of mutuality in parent-child interactions, e.g., over-expectation, over-restriction, unfavorable comparison with a sibling, or the child's awareness that his parents are disappointed in him.

V. The child may be hesitant to show anger in the belief that such feelings are wrong. This is especially difficult for the child whose parent is chronically or seriously ill or who lives in a family in which the direct expression of anger is suppressed.

VI. The child's inability to make and keep friends.

VII. The adolescent's concerns about sexuality.

VIII. School and learning problems.

IX. Economic distress in the family.

X. An "overachieving" child's fear of impending failure in academic or other competitive activity.

The child or adolescent and the parents will often spontaneously disclose these when they are consciously aware of them. Indeed, it is best for the child or parent to suggest the possibility of a psychogenic etiology themselves: "Could it be his nerves?" If they pose such a question, it is usually best not to make an immediate affirmative response but to be somewhat tentative: "Well, that's an interesting idea. You may have something there. I'd like to hear more of your ideas about that." Otherwise, the parents may believe they have been entrapped.

During the interview, it is useful to learn why the parents come now when the pain has been present for some time, what the parents and child think is wrong, how the pain has affected the child in his daily life, and what the parents and child expect the doctor to do. The physician will also need to surmise what the symptom brings in secondary gain and whether the complaint is masking a school phobia. (How much school has this pain caused Susie to miss?)

The motivations for a visit in the presence of a recurrent or persistent complaint include the following:

1. There is a life crisis in the family, e.g., divorce, serious illness, death, or economic calamity.

2. Feelings of anxiety or depression in a parent or child have caused amplification of the symptom and magnification of the worry.

3. School attendance authorities have demanded a medical appraisal because of the child's frequent absences from school.

4. A question of a serious biomedical illness has been recurrently raised by relatives or friends, or the parent has encountered information that causes her to seek reassurance.

5. The parent or child with a need to feel cared for comes to the physician for support and nurture.

6. The family has reached the limit of its tolerance for the child's symptom.

A meticulous physical examination is important, not only for the detection of abnormal findings but also for reassurance. Since parents and adolescents may talk more freely during or after the physical examination, significant historical information may be volunteered at that time. A thorough examination conveys the physician's interest in the patient and his complaint. In conjunction with the history, it may preclude or limit the need for other procedures.

Laboratory or x-ray examinations should be limited to those necessary to clarify the diagnosis and not be ordered simply because the parent "expects" such tests or to "reassure" them. Needless procedures tend to reinforce psychogenic pain. If examinations mentioned by the parents are not to be done, the doctor should explain why.

Once the physician is satisfied on the basis of the history, the physical examination, or other evaluations that the pain is psychogenic, the findings need to be presented to the parents and the child in a way that is understandable and acceptable. One may begin with a statement such as, "I have good news for you. Susie's examination is completely normal, so I am pleased to say that other tests won't be necessary. As is common with children her age, her pain seems to be associated with some of the stresses we've been discussing." One may continue: "I'm impressed that Susie is an alert, sensitive girl. We obviously wouldn't want to change that, even if we could, but being bright and sensitive can be a mixed blessing. As we all know, persons who have a sensitive personality can appreciate art and music and beauty more than others, but they are also sensitive to discomfort and pain. With her sensitivity, it's natural that some of the things that you've been telling me about may be affecting her. We don't want to make Susie less perceptive, but more comfortable, in less pain. What we have to do here is work on these things that are troublesome."

If there is open communication within the family, improvement often ensues without further professional help once the contributing stresses become evident. In other cases, the physician may wish to be more directive, e.g., have the child return to school; refer the parents for medical or psychiatric help; recommend a tutor; suggest that the parents decrease their demands on the patient; or suggest that parents be more involved with their child. Other options are for return weekly appointments to see the pediatrician and, if appropriate, referral of the child for psychiatric help. When adverse circumstances such as inadequate income, death, or divorce are unalterable, the physician considers with the parent or child how they may better cope with a situation that will not change.

Another approach would be to say, "I don't know how all this started. It sounds like with a viral infection, the flu, or something like mono, but with the pain hanging on so long, I have a hunch that some of the stresses we've been talking about must be playing a part in all this." Another approach might be, "I don't know if the things we have been talking about are related to Johnny's pain or not, but as a pediatrician I know that they're important to his development and deserve our further attention."

In some situations, the doctor may expect limited or no success in the management of psychogenic pain, e.g., the patient brought reluctantly at the insistence of the school because of absenteeism, the family not ready to confront their problems, the child living in a chaotic situation, or a parent who for her own reasons seems to need a child with a persistent symptom. The presence of a substantial secondary gain is a strong disincentive to recovery.

INFANTILE COLIC

Infantile colic, a nonspecific disorder occurring during the early months of life, is characterized by episodic fussiness or prolonged, vigorous crying. Presumably due to intermittent abdominal pain, the episodes, which usually begin in the late afternoon or evening, may persist for hours. The infant appears to be in great pain. His face is flushed, abdomen distended, fists clenched, and extremities tightly flexed. Large amounts of flatus may be passed.

While the etiology of infantile colic is usually obscure, possibilities include underfeeding, overfeeding, or poor feeding techniques, e.g., improperly sized nipple holes, bottle propping, inadequate burping. Uncommonly, cow milk allergy may be etiologic. Persistent irritability may be secondary to maternal depression or family tension. Other more unusual causes of recurrent crying include such physical problems as an anal fissure, otitis media, inguinal hernia, and brain damage.

That fussy periods are common in young infants should be mentioned to new mothers, especially if the physician's assessment of the neonate's behavior—e.g., excitement, lability, consolability, and limited self-quieting activity—suggest that the infant is a candidate for paroxysmal fussiness. The physician may then suggest how the mother may promote relaxation and avoid excessive stimulation of her baby.

If colic occurs, the parents should be told that a number of measures may be tried, although in most cases a specific cause is not identifiable. Important among these is the firm prescription of respite periods for the mother, e.g., a nap in the daytime while the baby is sleeping, a free afternoon once a week, or the use of a babysitter in the late afternoon. Support from the physician and others during this trying time, coupled with acceptance of colic as a developmental variant, helps the parents master this temporary affront to family tranquility.

A number of other approaches may be suggested. Some infants are quieted by rhythmic rocking, humming noises, patting, or walking. For others, a pacifier seems to help. Frequent feeding should be avoided. Being held firmly against the parent's chest, either wrapped snugly in a blanket or supported in a pouch, or having their back gently massaged while placed prone on their parent's lap may secure relief. If the infant is breast fed, a trial elimination of foods such as cabbage and onion from the mother's diet may be worthwhile. Substitution of hypoallergenic milk may be tried if cow milk allergy is considered to be a possibility.

In selected instances, the doctor may resort to medication to interrupt the cycle. Elixir of phenobarbital (20 mg/5 cc) in a dosage of ¼ teaspoonful, three times a day, may be given for a specified number of days. Whiskey or gin, from a dropperful to a teaspoonful in an ounce of warm, sweetened water has its advocates. Although antihistamines and anticholinergics/antispasmodics (Bentyl syrup) have also been utilized, their effectiveness has not been demonstrated by controlled studies.

CHEST PAIN

Of the chief etiologies of chest pain in children, muscle strain, fatigue, and spasm are the most common. Although rare in children, when exertional pain with associated tachycardia or syncope suggests a cardiac basis, laboratory examinations to be considered include a PA and lateral chest roentgenogram, an M-mode echocardiogram, a two-dimensional echocardiogram, an exercise tolerance test, 24-hour Holter monitoring, serum cholesterol determination, and, possibly, cardiac catheterization. Children with psychogenic precordial pain may have a parent or other close relative who has a cardiac disorder or is troubled by angina. As a rule, psychogenic pain does not awaken a child at night.

REFERENCES

GENERAL

Balint, M.: The Doctor, His Patient and The Illness, 2nd Ed. New York, International Universities Press, 1964, Chap. 4.

Engel, G. L.: Pain. *In* MacBryde, C. M., and Blacklow, R. S. (Eds.): Signs and Symptoms, 5th Ed. Philadelphia, J. B. Lippincott, 1970, p. 44.

Engel, G. L.: "Psychogenic" pain and the pain-prone patient. Am. J. Med., *26*:899, 1959.

Green, M., and Beall, P.: Paternal deprivation—a disturbance in fathering. Pediatrics, *30*:91, 1962.

COLIC

Schmitt, B. D.: Infants who do not sleep through the night. Deve. Behav. Pediatr., *2*:20, 1981.

CHEST PAIN

Driscoll, D. J., Glicklich, L. B., and Gallen, W. J.: Chest pain in children: A prospective study. Pediatrics, *57*:648, 1976.

Engel, G. L.: Pseudoangina. Am. Heart J., *59*:325, 1960.

33

SLEEP DISORDERS

Morris Green, M.D.

PHYSIOLOGY OF SLEEP

Except in the newborn period and early infancy, when the cycles are less defined, normal sleep consists of regular cycles of REM (rapid eye movement) and NREM (non–rapid eye movement) sleep. After the age of two years, the sleep pattern is similar to that in the adult—approximately five sleep cycles each night with about three fourths of the time occupied in NREM sleep. The ratio of REM to NREM sleep in infants is 1:1, whereas in adults it is 1:4. The REM-NREM sleep cycle in infants is 50 to 60 minutes, whereas in adults it is 90 to 100 minutes. During REM sleep, rapid, synchronous movement of the eyes and marked activity of the brain are noted. Most dreams occur during REM sleep. NREM sleep, during which rapid eye movements do not occur and the brain is in a resting phase, is composed of four EEG stages: stage 1 or transitional; stage 2, during which sleep spindles are noted; and stages 3 and 4, which are characterized by high-amplitude slow waves.

ETIOLOGICAL CLASSIFICATION OF SLEEP DISORDERS

I. Hypersomnias

A. Narcolepsy most frequently has its onset in the second decade of life. The attacks, during which the patient experiences a sudden and irresistible urge to sleep, are brief, perhaps 30 seconds in duration if the child is standing and one to two hours if reclining. Occasionally, the patient can voluntarily delay the onset. Fifteen to 20 episodes may occur per day.

Associated symptoms may also appear. *Catapexy,* which is characterized by sudden weakness or loss in muscle tone that lasts from seconds to minutes, may be precipitated by emotional states such as laughter, anger, or surprise. During these episodes, the patient may experience a jaw drop, feel "weak in the knees," or fall to the floor unable to move. Consciousness is maintained. *Sleep paralysis,* a brief attack of flaccid paralysis that occurs when the patient is falling asleep or awakening, may be accompanied by a feeling of intense fear or by visual and auditory hallucinations.

B. The Kleine-Levin syndrome (periodic hypersomnia and bulimia) is characterized by episodes of excessive sleep and overeating, which occur from two to four times a year and last several days to weeks. During this time, the child usually sleeps continuously, awakening only to go to the bathroom or binge eat. The cause of this syndrome, which is limited to males, is not known. Spontaneous remission usually occurs after two or three years.

C. Depression is the most common cause of hypersomnia in adolescents.

D. Obstructive sleep apnea is characterized by daytime hypersomnolence, headache on arising in the morning, fatigue, and secondarily, poor school performance. Sleep, accompanied by periods of loud snoring, is repeatedly interrupted by apnea and partial awakening. Sleep apnea may be caused by a sleep-induced intermittent hypotonia of the tongue muscles leading to partial or complete upper airway obstruction; enlarged tonsils and adenoids; glossoptosis in the Pierre Robin syndrome; and extreme obesity (the obesity-hypoventilation or Pickwickian syndrome).

E. Post-encephalitic sleep disturbance may be characterized by hypersomnia.

F. Post-traumatic syndrome after head injury may include hypersomnia.

G. Drug-induced sleepiness is an important, and often overlooked, cause of sleeping in the classroom.

II. Disorders of arousal related to emergence from stage 3 or 4 NREM sleep.

A. Somnambulism (persistent sleep walking), more frequent in school age boys than in girls, occurs in 1 to 6 per cent of the population within the first three hours of sleep in the transition from stage 3 or 4 NREM sleep to more superficial levels preceding the first REM sleep cycle. Single episodes of sleep walking are estimated to occur in 15 per cent of school age children. The child suddenly awakens, sits up, climbs out of bed, and walks about with his eyes open but uncomprehending and poorly coordinated. Mumbled and monosyllabic responses may be given to questions. Unless protected, he may hurt himself. Episodes last from seconds to 30 minutes and are not remembered by the child. One to four episodes may occur per week. Although the cause of somnabulism is not clear, a developmental etiology is likely, since sleep walking tends to be outgrown within a few years. In children with persistent somnambulism, diazepam may be therapeutic. Psychomotor epilepsy is also a diagnostic consideration with a history of sleep walking.

B. Night terrors occur during arousal from stage 3 or 4 NREM sleep early in the night, occasionally 90 to 100 minutes after the child goes to sleep. Most frequent in children from 3 to 8 years of age, night terrors also occur in older infants and adolescents. The child suddenly sits up, screams in terror, is clearly highly anxious, and cannot be consoled. Tachycardia, sweating, and agitation are noted. Episodes last from a few seconds to 10 or 30 minutes and are not remembered by the child. Probably a developmental phenomenon, night terrors disappear with further central nervous system maturation. Occasionally, a stressful environmental event can be identified as the precipitating cause.

C. Nightmares are frightening dreams that occur during REM sleep. The child, more easily aroused than with night terrors, usually becomes fully awake and vividly recalls the content of the dream. An occasional nightmare is within normal limits, but persistent or frequent episodes suggest an environmental problem. Although drugs are usually not indicated in the treatment of these episodes, diazepam may be used if nightmares are especially severe.

D. Enuresis occasionally occurs as the child arouses from stage 3 or 4 NREM sleep prior to entering the first REM sleep period 1 to 3 hours after going to sleep (see Chapter 34).

E. Somniloquy or talking while asleep occurs during arousal from REM sleep.

III. Developmental/psychological. The frequency of these problems is high.

A. Colic may interfere with an infant's sleep pattern, usually with going to sleep (see Chapter 32).

B. Resistance to sleep. Infants between the ages of six and nine months may object to going to sleep. Since sleep is a separation experience, it is understandable that the infant may be uncomfortable or anxious about going to sleep. Anticipatory guidance given at health supervision visits should prepare parents for this possibility. A regular bedtime routine should be recommended along with firmly conveying that the baby is expected to go to sleep. Favorite toys and play things (a teddy bear or a special blanket) may help in the transition to sleep. If the mother is unable to set normal developmental limits or fears that the baby's crying will disturb her husband's studying or the neighbors, persistent resistance to sleep may develop. Resistance to sleep is frequent in the infants of depressed mothers.

C. Night waking. Beginning at about nine months, infants awaken in the middle of the night and then refuse to go back to sleep. The problem is compounded when the child is able to crawl out of his crib. The frequency of night waking in infants between 6 and 12 months of age has been reported to range from 25 per cent (Carey, 1974) to 50 per cent (Moore and Ucko, 1957). These infants were found to have low sensory thresholds (Carey, 1974). Episodes often begin during an illness. If the parent is firm about her expectation that the baby go back to sleep, the problem is a transient one. If, however, she is not firm or attempts to remedy the problem by taking the baby into the parent's bed, night wakening may persist. The parent should be advised to check the baby if his crying is persistent and reassure him by her presence, but to try not to pick him up. If necessary, the parent may sit down next to the baby's crib for a moment or two. Playing with the baby at this time will prolong the problem. Since one of the parents may also have a sleep problem, an appropriate question is "Who else in your family has trouble sleeping?" Awakening during the night is a frequent manifestation in infants of depressed mothers. Medication has no role, although it is tempting to parents and physician. No child seems to suffer from this sleep problem. It is the parent who worries and loses sleep.

D. Sleep problems are common in the vulnerable child syndrome (see Chapter 29). The child often sleeps in the parents' bedroom, either with the mother, with both parents, or in his own crib or bed which is kept next to the mother in her direct line of vision. The parents may report that the baby does not sleep well, but a closer inquiry often reveals that it is the parent who awakens several times a night to check on the child, often managing to arouse him to be sure that he is alive. The interview in these cases may reveal that the mother is unable to sleep at night unless she feels the baby is safe and sound. It becomes apparent that many such mothers unwittingly keep the baby awake each night through a series of visual, auditory, and tactile stimuli that convey her insistence that the baby not fall alseep, probably because of her fear that she would feel the baby was dead.

E. Night time rocking and head banging. Some babies may normally rock themselves to sleep. If this habit is exaggerated, excessive environmental stimulation should be suspected.

F. Night time wandering. Some preschool age children, seen because of hyperactivity or destructiveness, are reported to climb out of bed during the night, wander around the house, turn on the electric or gas range and, if they can find matches, start fires. These children usually have major emotional disturbances, and psychiatric help is generally required.

IV. Insomnia. Older children and adolescents with persistent insomnia may be tense, worried, moody, or depressed. From 5 to 12 per cent of adolescents may report trouble sleeping. Sleeping pills should not be prescribed.

V. Sleep reversals occur in some children with hepatic failure or post-encephalitic behavior. Delirious children may be drowsy during the daytime and unable to sleep at night.

VI. Psychomotor seizures are a rare diagnostic possibility in children with night terrors or somnabulism episodes that appear to be more than transient developmental problems.

REFERENCES

Anders, T. F.: Night-waking in infants during the first year of life. Pediatrics, *63*:860, 1979.

Anders, T. F., and Weinstein, P.: Sleep and its disorders in infants and children: A review. Pediatrics, *50*:312, 1972.

Anders, T. F., Carskadon, M. A., and Dement, W. C.: Sleep and sleepiness in children and adolescents. Pediatr. Clin. North Am., *27*:29, 1980.

Carey, W.: Night waking and temperament in infancy. J. Pediatr., *84*:756, 1974.

Frank, Y., Braham, J., and Cohen, B. E.: The Kleine-Levin syndrome. Am. J. Dis. Child., *127*:412, 1974.

Gilleminault, C., Eldridge, F. L., Simmons, F. B., and Dement, W. C.: Sleep apnea in eight children. Pediatrics, *58*:23, 1976.

Kales, A., and Kales, J. D.: Sleep disorders. N. Engl. J. Med., *290*:487, 1974.

Kravath, R. E., Pollak, C. P., and Borowiecki, B.: Hypoventilation during sleep in children who have lymphoid airway obstruction treated by nasopharyngeal tube and T and A. Pediatrics, *59*:865, 1977.

Moore, T., and Ucko, C.: Night waking in early infancy: Part I. Arch. Dis. Child., *32*:333, 1957.

Nagera, H.: Sleep and its disorders approached developmentally. Psychoanal. Study Child., *21*:393, 1966.

Price, V. A., Coates, T. J., Thoresen, C. E., and Grinstead, O. A.: Prevalence and correlates of poor sleep among adolescents. Am. J. Dis. Child., *132*:583, 1978.

Rabe, E. F.: Recurrent paroxysmal nonepileptic disorders. Curr. Probl. Pediatr., *4*:3, 1974.

Sallustro, F., and Atwell, C. W.: Body rocking, head banging, and head rolling in normal children. J. Pediatr., *93*:704, 1978.

Schmitt, B. D.: Infants who do not sleep through the night. Dev. Behav. Pediatr., *2*:20, 1981.

Simpser, M. D., et al.: Sleep apnea in a child with the Pickwickian syndrome. Pediatrics, *60*:290, 1977.

Sleeping Pills, Insomnia, and Medical Practice. National Academy of Sciences. Washington, Office of Publications, 1979.

Spock, B.: Sleep and sleep disturbances in young children. Postgrad. Med., *21*:272, 1957.

Young people who sleep badly. Editorial. Br. Med. J., *2*:1450, 1978.

Zarcone, V.: Narcolepsy. N. Engl. J. Med., *288*:1156, 1973.

34

ENURESIS

Morris Green, M.D.

Enuresis is a common condition whose precise etiology is not known, but a considerable amount of epidemiological evidence suggests that the usual patient with nocturnal enuresis suffers not so much from "disease" as from a variation in normal development. Several population studies have demonstrated that over 5 per cent of children have nocturnal enuresis after the age of five, but that by the end of adolescence this percentage has diminished to less than 1 per cent. Such delay in achieving nighttime bladder control often has a familial predisposition. While relapse, or secondary, enuresis often occurs after psychologically upsetting events and stresses, such as separation, there is little evidence that psychological factors are of major importance in primary enuresis. Obviously, secondary psychological consequences such as shame, fear, and parental coerciveness may occur as enuresis persists.

Organic disorders that may cause involuntary urination include obstructive uropathy, a pelvic mass, diabetes mellitus, diabetes insipidus, and psychogenic water drinking. Children with myelomeningocele and a neurogenic bladder frequently have urinary incontinence, as may those who are mentally retarded.

DIAGNOSIS

As with other developmental symptoms, diagnosis and treatment should proceed simultaneously, with the interview serving as the principal tool to collect data and to establish a constructive relationship between the doctor and the child and family. Through the interview, the physician clarifies for himself and for the patient the multiple etiological possibilities and determines the familial incidence of enuresis, the family's and the child's understanding of the problem, their interest in overcoming this symptom, the methods that have already been tried, and their notions about what might work. Through this process, the doctor sets the stage for the child's active participation in the mastery of his own problem and promotes the child's identification with the physician. Observation of the boy's urinary stream is also indicated if the history suggests difficulty in initiating urination or an interrupted urinary stream.

LABORATORY EVALUATION

The evaluation of children with enuresis should probably include a urinalysis for specific gravity, glycosuria, proteinuria, and pyuria, and urine culture, although this examination is rarely positive. Negative findings are usually of importance in reassuring the physician and the patient. The American Academy of Pediatrics Committee on Radiology has recommended that routine radiologic studies not be obtained in the presence of a normal urinalysis and urine culture, normal physical examination including the external genitalia, and absence of a neurological abnormality. If symptoms such as frequency, urgency, dribbling, dysuria, hesitancy in beginning or straining on urination, a poor urinary stream, a history of previous urinary tract infections or a preponderance of daytime wetting suggest true urinary incontinence or obstructive urologic disease, dynamic urinary tract studies, excretory urography, and voiding cystourethrography are indicated. Such causes of enuresis are very rare.

MANAGEMENT

In the absence of symptoms or signs that suggest organic disease in children five or six years of age or younger, management of bed wetting consists of an explanation that the symptom is most likely occurring on a developmental or familial basis and that spontaneous cure can be anticipated. The frequency of dry nights or periods has some predictive value as to the spontaneous cessation of the symptom. Stresses that the child is confronting should be explored and, if possible, ameliorated. Punitive measures or ridicule, although done out of the parents' frustration, are to be discouraged.

For children above the age of five or six, the physician's principal role is to help the child who is motivated take responsibility for mastering the bed wetting and to convey his confident expectation that he will be able to accomplish this successfully. Encouraging the child to think of ways to control his bed wetting helps elicit his active participation. The child's suggestions might include reducing his fluid intake after dinner, setting an alarm to awaken himself at night, having the parents awaken him, or practicing holding his urine for longer periods of time. Bladder training, advised as a method to increase the child's functional bladder capacity, may give the child a feeling of self-responsibility. It may also be suggested that the child keep a diary in which he records the steps he has taken to control the symptom, with gold stars to indicate successes. This diary should be reviewed periodically by the physician during brief office visits and appropriate positive reinforcement given.

This approach is recommended for most patients seen because of enuresis. Because there is a high spontaneous cure rate and children respond well to a program of positive reinforcement that includes their active participation, conditioning devices and medications are not frequently indicated. Conditioning devices should be advised before prescribing imipramine. This kind of apparatus, which is sensitive to the passage of a few drops of urine, sounds an alarm that awakens the child and leads to contraction of the external bladder sphincter and suppression of the micturition reflex. Examples of such devices include the *Nytone* alarm (Medical Products, Inc., Salt Lake City, UT 84119), which has a buzzer on the wrist and sensors on the child's underwear, and the *Wet-Stop* alarm (Palco Laboratories, 5026 Scotts Valley Dr., Scotts Valley, CA 95066), which has a buzzer on the collar and sensors on a small plastic card that fits into a pocket on the front of the child's underwear. Both of these alarms are relatively inexpensive. They are not indicated in children under the age of eight but may be used in older children if the child and parents are motivated. Conditioning has had a success rate of about 70 per cent achieved slowly, i.e., in the third or fourth months of use, and a relapse rate of 10 to 15 per cent. The conditioning device should continue to be used for three to four weeks after the enuresis stops. There is evidence that its use does not cause or increase psychological symptoms; in fact, by fostering a sense of control, psychological well-being is probably increased.

If a pharmacological agent is to be prescribed, imipramine may be given one hour before bedtime in a dosage of 25 mg for children 6 to 8 years of age, 50 mg for those from 8 to 12, and 50 to 75 mg over the age of 12. The initial prescription should permit a one-week trial. If improvement occurs, the medication may be continued for two months. The response rate ranges between 25 and 40 per cent. The high relapse rate experienced with abrupt cessation of the medication may be lessened if the drug is tapered to every other night and then every third night for several weeks. Its potential toxicity is the main contraindication to the use of this agent. Since imipramine poisoning can be lethal, the parents must be carefully instructed as to the serious toxic possibilities inherent in its use and the absolute need to keep it out of the reach of young children.

Diurnal or daytime enuresis presents a different problem than nocturnal enuresis, although they may coexist. Most children are dry during the day by the age of two and one-half years except for the occasional time when they do not want to interrupt what they are doing to void. In addition to those listed above for nocturnal wetting, organic etiological disorders for diurnal enuresis include an ectopic ureter, urinary tract infection, urethritis in girls due to bubble bath products, and fecal impaction. These are uncommon. Giggle incontinence may rarely occur in girls when they laugh vigorously. In adolescent girls, daytime wetting may occasionally be due to bouts of bladder spasm.

Diurnal enuresis is usually due to anxiety associated with such environmental stressors as marital discord, separation, divorce, parental illness, death of a relative, maternal depression, or inappropriate parenting, e.g., harsh punishment or abuse. Treatment consists of identifying and dealing with the sources of the child's anxiety and discontinuation of whatever punitive measures may have been used.

REFERENCES

Committee on Radiology, American Academy of Pediatrics: Excretory urography for evaluation of enuresis. Pediatrics, *65*:644, 1980.

McLain, L. G.: Childhood enuresis. Curr. Probl. Pediatr., 9:4, 1979.

Schmitt, B. D.: Daytime wetting (diurnal enuresis). Pediatr. Clin. North Am., *29*:9, 1982.

Schmitt, B. D.: Nocturnal enuresis: An update on treatment. Pediatr. Clin. North Am., *29*:21, 1982.

Shelov, S. P., et al.: Enuresis: A contrast of attitudes of parents and physicians. Pediatrics, *67*:707, 1981.

35

SCHOOL REFUSAL (AVOIDANCE)

Morris Green, M.D.

School refusal, at times inappropriately referred to as school phobia, requires prompt pediatric intervention. In this disorder the child refuses to attend school or to go outside during school hours. Although a child or adolescent may be brought to the doctor with refusal to attend school as the chief complaint, a somatic symptom more commonly is given as the reason for the visit.

School avoidance may be accompanied by such symptoms as vomiting, abdominal pain, and pallor, which quickly abate once the child is told he will not have to go to school. When persistent or recurrent symptoms such as fever, sore throat, fatigue, abdominal pain, or dizziness are given as the chief complaint, absence from school is usually not mentioned by the parents as a problem. In such instances of *masked* school refusal, it is diagnostically helpful for the physician to ask how much school the illness has caused the child to miss. When the parent responds to that unanticipated question, usually after a pause, the physician's response—e.g., "Three weeks! That's really serious."—should emphasize his belief that the absence from school is a problem of the highest priority.

Separation anxiety is the most common cause of school refusal. Many five- and six-year-old children show a transient reluctance to separate from their mothers to go to school during the first few months of the first year. This group rarely have physical symptoms and are relatively easy to manage by firmness on the parents' part and the understanding support of the teachers. However, other children seen because of persistent school refusal demonstrate a developmentally inappropriate level of dependency. They worry that something devastating will happen to their mothers or that the parent will leave home while they are at school. The mothers themselves may also find it difficult to tolerate the separation because of their hostile-dependent relationship. It is helpful if these irrational fears can be fully illuminated in the interview. "Tell me what you are afraid will happen? What else? And. . .?" The child may quietly report that he is afraid of a teacher who seems irritable and has scolded other children or of classmates who push other children around, but generally such school-based fears do not account for school refusal. This is not to deny that a frightening experience going to and from or in the school may have been the precipitating cause of the problem.

School avoidance may also be a late manifestation of the vulnerable child syndrome, in which the child and the mother share an unspoken agreement that the child is safe only in the presence of the mother. Reluctance to attend school may also occur in children with chronic illness owing to feelings of anxiety or vulnerability, concern about their appearance (alopecia, cushingoid facies, understature), and inability to keep up because of frequent absences due to recurrent hospitalization or visits to the doctor.

Environmental stressors that may contribute etiologically to school refusal include the birth of a sibling, physical or mental illness of a parent or sibling, death of a significant person, separation or divorce, parental alcoholism, a move that requires transfer to a new school, entrance to a middle or junior high school, harrassment on the way to school, and the lack of privacy when undressing or showering for physical education classes. Depressed mothers, especially if they have thought of suicide, may feel safer when someone is in the house with them.

An occasional older child who has missed school because of an acute illness may find it difficult to resume a previous pattern of overachievement. Depression or an incipient psychosis are other diagnostic considerations in the older child or adolescent with school refusal. Truancy differs from school refusal in a number of ways. With truancy, the parents are usually unaware of or indifferent to the child's absence from school. Although the child ostensibly leaves for school, he never arrives there or he returns home during school hours. Truants have usually been poor students with a history of disciplinary and learning problems at school. Many are involved in antisocial and delinquent behavior symptomatic of a rebellion against authority. Some may be chronically depressed. Others come from multi-problem families. Children with school refusal, in contrast, generally are excellent students who enjoy school but are afraid to leave home.

TREATMENT

Patients, and often their mothers, may resist the return to school. The parent may fear that forcing the child to do so may be physically or emotionally damaging: "You wouldn't let your daughter go to school if *she* had fever, would you, *Doctor!*" Most children with school refusal, however, can be readily managed by the pediatrician or family physician. Recognized as competent in physical disorders, the primary care physician is in an especially advantageous position because the parents usually believe that the child has a somatic illness. Although the physician may quickly recognize that the problem is one of school refusal, the child's somatic complaints should be accepted as real. It is usually not necessary to use terms such as "school refusal" or "school phobia" or to volunteer an explanation of the psychodynamics involved, nor does therapeutic success require that all the underlying problems within the family be uncovered. Since the etiological role of separation anxiety in school avoidance will not be consciously recognized by the patient or his parents, overexplanation may lead to defensiveness and anger.

After a conspicuously meticulous physical examination, the parent and child should be clearly told that the child's physical examination is absolutely normal and that the child is physically healthy and should return to school. If this report elicits a smile from the parent and a sense of relief, the problem is well on the way to a solution; on the other hand, if the parent appears unhappy or disappointed, resolution of the school refusal may be much more difficult.

The physician should strongly emphasize his conviction that school attendance is extremely important and that the child should return to school immediately, i.e., the next day. The parents—both the mother and the father—should be instructed that although the child may be reluctant to go and may complain of being ill, they must be firm. The child is not to have a choice. If the child is reluctant to go to school by himself, the parent should accompany him to the classroom. If the mother cannot do this, the father or someone else should do so. The physician must convey his confident expectation that the child will return to school.

If the child appears ill on awakening, the doctor should be called. If the child complains of symptoms after he is in school, he should be sent to the nurse's or the teacher's lounge until ready to return to the classroom. A mild or moderate tranquilizer may be used for a short period of time if the child's separation anxiety is especially intense; likewise, desensitization may be necessary, with the return to school staged over four or five days. Desensitization is explained to the child and parents as a proven method of helping a person overcome his fears, that the child will return to school by gradual steps, that when he is comfortable with the first step, he will take another and so on until he is no longer scared. The doctor and child may then jointly work out the steps. First, the child may dress but not go to school; second, the child may go to the school with his parent but not go in; third, the child may go into the school but not stay; fourth, the child might visit his teacher at lunch time but not stay; fifth, the child may go to class but stay for only one hour, etc. These recommendations should, of course, be discussed with the school personnel after the office visit. Once the child is back in school, the somatic complaints usually cease and no further school refusal occurs.

In the case of the older child absent from school for an extended period, the following approach is generally effective. After the history and physical examination have been completed, the doctor turns to the child, pauses as if momentarily in thought, and then announces his decision: "Susie, I know that you're not back to normal yet. I'm generally pretty conservative about such matters, but I tell you what I'm going to do. I'm going to *let* you go back to school . . . of course not full time immediately, but gradually . . . two hours a day the first couple of days, then three hours, and so on. School's so important, I can't let you miss any more. I'll write this out as a schedule, and that's what we do. I'll call the school right now to discuss our decision with them."

The patient may be more comfortable if provided with a simple reentry diagnosis that can be shared with peers who ask why the child had missed so much school. The physician may also suggest that the parents hold a *recovery party* to which the child's close friends are invited: "Dr. Smith tells us that Susie is on the road to recovery, so we're having a party to celebrate her getting well and returning to school! Won't you come and help us celebrate!" This public attention precludes the child's continued absence from school and facilitates his return.

Although these approaches are usually successful, an occasional failure may be anticipated. In that event, the matter may have to be referred by the school authorities to the truant officer and legal action invoked. In the presence of severe separation anxiety and dependency, chronic depression, an incipient or frank psychosis, or multiple psychosocial problems within the family, psychiatric referral and psychotherapy of the child and family are indicated.

REFERENCES

Eisenberg, L.: The pediatric management of school phobia. J. Pediatr., *44*:758, 1959.

Green, M., and Solnit, A. J.: Reactions to the threatened loss of a child: A vulnerable child syndrome. Pediatrics, *34*:58, 1964.

Kleiman, M. B.: The complaint of persistent fever: Recognition and management of pseudo-fever of unknown origin. Pediatr. Clin. North Am., *29*:201, 1982.

Nader, P. R., Bullock, D., and Caldwell, B.: School phobia. Pediatr. Clin. North Am., *22*:605, 1975.

Schmitt, B. D.: School phobia—the great imitator: A pediatrician's viewpoint. Pediatrics, *48*:433, 1971.

Simmons, J. E.: School phobia and depression. *In* Green, M., and Haggerty, R. J. (Eds.): Ambulatory Pediatrics II. Philadelphia, W. B. Saunders Co., 1977, p. 208.

Weitzman, M., Klerman, L. V., Lamb, G., Menary, J., and Alpert, J. J.: School absence: A problem for the pediatrician. Pediatrics, *69*:739, 1982.

36

DEPRESSION IN CHILDHOOD AND ADOLESCENCE

Ella Copoulos, M.D., and Karen Hein, M.D.

Depression in children and teen-agers is becoming a more frequently recognized and diagnosed health problem. The myth perpetuated by adults that childhood is the happiest period of an individual's life is being replaced by recognition that seriously depressed children and adolescents exist.

According to classic psychoanalytical theory, the child's limited psychosexual maturation precludes the development of depression. Other theories stated that the child's immature cognitive and emotional development made it difficult for him to express feelings of sadness and depression directly, leading to the clinical presentation of "masked symptoms" of depression, such as conduct disorders, delinquency, drug abuse, promiscuity, truancy, aggressiveness, irritability, temper tantrums, hyperactivity, somatic complaints, enuresis, and school refusal or failure. However, the distinction between children whose abnormal behavior is associated with depression and children whose abnormal behavior exists separately without associated depression was not made clear by this conceptualization.

A consensus is now emerging that (1) the depressive "masks" or "equivalents" may represent merely the presenting symptom or "chief complaint" of a depressed child; (2) careful assessment of the child, taking into consideration developmentally determined differences in emotional expression and cognition, will usually reveal depression if it is present; (3) severe childhood depression (major depressive illness) represents a distinct clinical syndrome that closely resembles major depression in adults; and (4) childhood depression may be associated with, but not defined by, other dysfunctional behavior.

ROLE OF THE PEDIATRICIAN

Since pediatricians are frequently the first health professional to see children referred for appetite or weight changes, sleep disturbances, loss of energy, sudden changes in behavior, school problems, or suicidal behavior, the physician should have the diagnostic skills necessary to assess the youngster for depression and to distinguish between depression that is a transient mood or normal response to a difficult life situation and a persistent mood disorder with corresponding decreased levels of functioning. The pediatrician can perform the initial interview and physical examination and obtain appropriate laboratory evaluations to detect possible underlying organic disease. The child's symptoms should not be attributed to organic mental disorders caused by endocrine disorders, central nervous system disease, or the effects of drugs. The pediatrician should be able to counsel the child and his family about the existence of depression as a real illness and advise them of the necessity of psychiatric consultation and therapy when indicated. The pediatrician can also be instrumental in increasing environmental support for the depressed child through discussions with family members and school personnel. In the event that the child is without suitable environmental support systems, and/or is at risk of attempting suicide, custodial or protective arrangements should be made by the pediatrician until therapy can be arranged.

DEFINITION OF DEPRESSIVE SYNDROME

The primary features of the depressive syndrome among children are sustained mood changes, including a general sense of ill-being, sadness or unhappiness, pervasive anhedonia (a lack of interest or pleasure in usual activities), and self-deprecatory feelings of helplessness, hopelessness, worthlessness, and excessive guilt. Associated symptoms and signs may include changes in vegetative and psychomotor functioning and cognition: appetite or weight changes, sleep disturbances, somatic complaints, fatigue, psychomotor agitation or retardation, loss of ability to concentrate, and thoughts of death or suicide. When there is a significant change from the child's normal behavior or level of functioning that persists for several weeks, these signs and symptoms probably represent depression.

It may occasionally be difficult to distinguish between the depressive syndrome described and the depressed mood that may accompany other childhood psychiatric disorders and medical conditions, including anorexia nervosa, hypothyroidism, viral illness, brain tumor, diabetes, asthma, ulcerative colitis, and neurological disease. These conditions may generate or be associated with depressed mood as well as coexist with the fully developed depressive syndrome. It should, however, be possible to distinguish between these on the basis of severity, number, chronology, and duration of symptoms, as well as other specific diagnostic criteria.

INCIDENCE

Various estimates for the incidence of depression in childhood range from approximately 2 to 17 per cent in the normal child population, 7 per cent of children admitted for a medical illness to a general pediatric inpatient ward, 23 per cent of a delinquent adolescent population, to as high as 40 to 60 per cent of selected pediatric populations of psychiatric clinics, residential treatment centers, and psychiatric hospitals.

Depressed mood and depressive syndrome, common problems among hospitalized and chronically ill children, can frequently be attributed to separation from parents, other family members, friends, and the normal environment, and restriction of usual activities. Compared to nondepressed hospitalized children, depressed hospitalized children have a higher frequency of somatic complaints unrelated to their medical problem. This point has important implications for the avoidance of unnecessary diagnostic procedures and therapies.

DEVELOPMENTAL PERSPECTIVE

The manner in which the depression presents is related to the child's emotional and cognitive development. The older the child, the closer the depression resembles the clinical picture of depression in adults.

Depression in Infancy

Spitz entitled the profound behavioral changes seen in infants deprived of their mother or other nurturing figures anaclitic depression (Spitz, 1946). This syndrome of apathy, withdrawal, decreased responsiveness and motor activity, weight loss, and progressive physical deterioration is uncommonly seen today; however, some infants with "failure to thrive" may be suffering from a form of depression found in situations where poor maternal attachment and neglect or abuse predominate.

Depression in Childhood

The preschool child is also very sensitive to separation from the predominant caretaker (usually the mother), as well as to other situations of perceived loss (e.g., a pet or friend). In contrast to the infant, the young child is more effective in expressing sadness with unhappy facial expressions and tears, or verbal expressions of feeling rejected, unwanted, or unloved. In extreme situations there may be signs of loss of interest in activities, passive withdrawal, or, alternatively, expressions of irritability, with oppositional behavior and temper tantrums. The young child has a fairly low tolerance for stress and frustration, and may respond to unsettling changes in his environment with regressive behavior such as bed-wetting or a desire to return to bottle or breastfeeding.

The school age child has an expanded ability to express depression verbally as well as by facial expression and behavioral changes. In addition, older children whose impulse control is poorly developed may "act out" their depressed feelings in destructive or antisocial ways in an attempt to ward off painful emotions. Depressed school age children are also prone to develop somatic complaints and problems in school.

Depression During Adolescence

The teen-ager may experience frequent changes in mood as a normal response to the changes of adolescent development. The physical changes of puberty often lead to preoccupations with the body and fearful anxieties, especially if development is precocious, delayed, or nonsynchronous with peers. Working toward self-individuation and economic and emotional independence can induce feelings of sadness, loss, insecurity, and guilt, as well as feelings of confidence and strength. The normal ups and downs of peer friendships and intimate relationships may produce swings in emotion. These usually situational and transient mood changes are not harmful unless they seriously compromise the adolescent's ability to cope with the present or plan for the future.

The adolescent's cognitive and emotional maturation influences the way in which more pervasive long-lasting depression is expressed. For example, in order to fully experience "hopelessness," it is necessary to have a conceptualization of the future. But it is not until adolescence that the changeover from concrete to abstract thought processes occurs, enabling children to develop an expanded time sense that includes past, present, and future. Compared to younger children, the adolescent may manifest depression with a wider range of emotional and behavioral features. In addition to somatic complaints and acting-out kinds of behavior, the adolescent may verbally express feelings of excessive guilt, sinfulness, or worthlessness. The clinical picture increasingly resembles adult depressive illness. This may include the use of drugs and alcohol in attempts to relieve uncomfortable feelings, and an increased potential for suicide compared to younger children.

ETIOLOGY

There are numerous theories to explain the etiology of childhood depression, but they have not as yet been able to pinpoint conclusive predisposing factors. In view of the present level of knowledge, it is probably most helpful to consider childhood depression as the final common pathway of multiple genetic, biological, psychological, and environmental influences.

Biological Basis of Depression

Theories supporting a biological or biochemical basis for depression stem from the hypothesis that disturbances of monoamine neurotransmitter metabolism in the brain, producing changes in neuroendocrine homeostasis, result in the expression of major affective illness. Neuroendocrine and other biological markers that have been associated with endogenous depression in adults are currently being studied in children. These include hypersecretion of cortisol (Puig-Antich et al., 1979), blunting of the growth hormone response to insulin-induced hypoglycemia (Puig-Antich et al., 1981), and decreased urinary excretion of MHPG (3-methoxy-4-hydroxyphenylethylene glycol), a major metabolite of the central neurotransmitter norepinephrine (McKnew and Cytryn, 1979). Changes from normal sleep patterns found in endogenously depressed adults (decreased REM sleep latency, increased REM sleep activity, disturbances in sleep continuity) are also being investigated in children with the aid of sleep EEG studies (polysomnography).

The findings from these and other studies are preliminary, and currently there are no clinically useful laboratory tests for the diagnosis of childhood depression. However, current evidence suggests that with continued development, these and related tests have the potential for identifying patients at risk, aiding diagnosis, and ultimately predicting response to specific pharmacological therapies.

DIAGNOSIS OF DEPRESSION—DSM III

Recent advances in the diagnosis of childhood depression include the standardization of diagnostic criteria (Table 36–1). Application of the new criteria aids in distinguishing between depression as a normal temporary human emotion, depression as a clinical symptom, and depression as a specific syndrome or disorder as it occurs in children and adolescents at various stages of development.

The third edition of the Diagnostic and Statistical Manual of Mental Disorders (DSM III) proposes use of the same basic diagnostic criteria and classification system for depressive disorders in children and adults. The DSM III does, however, recognize that the diagnosis of childhood depression may involve some associated features unique to children of different developmental levels (Table 36–2).

To meet the DSM III criteria for major depression, the child's clinical presentation must include the major symptom of persistent dysphoric mood (usually depression) or persistent anhedonia (loss of interest or pleasure in usual activities), plus at least four of the following symptoms present almost daily for a minimum of two weeks:

1. Poor appetite or increased appetite (or unintentional weight loss or gain of large magnitude)
2. Insomnia or excessive sleep
3. Psychomotor agitation or retardation
4. Loss of interest or pleasure in usual activities
5. Loss of energy or increased fatigue
6. Feelings of self-reproach, worthlessness, or excessive guilt
7. Decreased ability to concentrate
8. Recurrent thoughts of death or suicidal behavior

In addition, there are other associated symptoms that may or may not be present, including

Table 36–1. DSM III DIAGNOSTIC CRITERIA FOR MAJOR DEPRESSION

Presence of:	Dysphoric mood (depressive) or Anhedonia (loss of interest or pleasure in usual activities)
Plus four of the following:*	Poor appetite or increased appetite (weight loss or gain) Insomnia or excessive sleep Psychomotor retardation or agitation Loss of interest or pleasure in usual activities (including sexual activity) Loss of energy or increased fatigue Feeling of worthlessness, self-reproach, or excessive guilt Decreased concentration Recurrent thoughts of death or suicide or suicidal behavior

*Three of first four in children under age six.

Table 36–2. ASSOCIATED FEATURES OF DEPRESSION

All Ages:	Depressed appearance Tearfulness Anxiety Irritability Fear Brooding Panic attacks Phobias Hallucinations
Prepuberty:	Conduct problems Separation anxiety School problems Somatic symptoms
Adolescence:	Aggressiveness or antisocial behavior School problems Social withdrawal Substance abuse Somatic complaints

tearfulness, anxiety, irritability, brooding, fear, phobias, panic attacks, and excessive somatic concerns. Rarely, psychotic symptoms such as a markedly distorted sense of reality, hallucinations, or delusions may be present. The underlying depressed mood is usually conveyed by the content of the hallucinations or delusions. The presence of psychotic symptoms classifies the patient as having a major depression of the psychotic subtype.

The DSM III includes several diagnostic distinctions between children and adults. In children under age six, at least three of the first four symptoms listed must be present. A persistently sad facial expression may be used as evidence for dysphoric mood in children who deny feeling sad or in very young children who are unable to express themselves verbally. For children less than six years old, psychomotor retardation and loss of interest may be expressed as hypoactivity and apathy, respectively (Table 36–3).

Table 36–3. EQUIVALENT SIGNS OF DEPRESSION IN CHILDREN UNDER AGE SIX

Child	Adult
Persistent sad face	Dysphoric mood
Failure to gain weight	Anorexia
Apathy	Anhedonia
Hypoactivity	Psychomotor retardation

Other behavioral or psychological disturbances may commonly be found in association with major depression in children. Separation anxiety may appear in depressed prepubertal children, marked by the child's extreme anxiety over being even briefly separated from parents or home, fear that something bad will happen to the parents in the child's absence, and often resulting in refusal to attend school. Depressed adolescent boys may demonstrate overtly antisocial behavior.

Differential Diagnosis

Bipolar disorder (previously labeled manic-depressive illness) is defined as one or more episodes of mania (elated mood with associated extremes of behavior) with or without a history of major depression; it is rare in prepubertal children. The incidence of bipolar disorder increases during adolescence and reaches a peak in early adulthood. The distinction between bipolar disorder and major depression is important because the initial choice of therapy differs. If the severity of symptoms warrants a trial of medication, lithium carbonate is indicated instead of a tricyclic antidepressant.

Cyclothymia and dysthymia, less severe affective syndromes compared to the bipolar and major depressive disorders, may also present in late adolescence. Cyclothymic disorder is characterized by alternating periods of "highs" (hypomania) and "lows" (depression), whereas dysthymic disorder (previously called neurotic depression) is characterized by fairly persistent depressed mood. Both may be associated with substance abuse and with various personality disorders. They may be important to diagnose and treat because they are by definition chronic mood disturbances, with the potential for disrupting normal development and creating long-term emotional and social disability.

The hallucinations and delusions that may accompany the major affective disorders (major depression, bipolar disorder) in youth suggest the possible diagnosis of schizophrenia. However, in most cases the content and timing of the psychotic symptoms allow the correct diagnosis to be made. In schizophrenia, auditory hallucinations more likely contain commenting or conversing voices without depressive content. Although schizophrenia may be associated with episodic depressed mood, the psychotic symptoms clearly occur when the patient is not depressed as well as when he is depressed.

ASSESSMENT

Improved diagnostic techniques for assessing childhood depression are being developed. The clinician should question the child directly concerning subjective symptoms of depression, rather than attempting to infer this information from the traditional play interview technique. Additional history (chronology of symptoms, previous psychological status) and observations of behavior obtained from parents, teachers, and other people important in the child's life are considered helpful and sometimes necessary supplements but should not replace the child's own description of present thoughts, feelings, and mood.

The Schedule for Affective Disorders and Schizophrenia for School-Age Children (K-SADS or Kiddie-SADS, developed by Puig-Antich and Chambers), is an example of an interview instrument for diagnosing depression in children 6 to 16 years old (Table 36–4). A series of alternatively phrased questions covering the major symptoms of depression is administered individually, first to the parent and then to the child, in a semistructured interview format. The responses obtained are rated according to severity, then given a summary rating item by item. The use of this kind of systematic evaluation enables the clinician to apply specific diagnostic criteria, measure the severity of depression and, if repeated over time, monitor for improvement, recovery, or recurrence of major depressive illness.

Table 36–4. DEPRESSION ASSESSMENT: QUESTIONS FOR THE CHILD

Depressed Mood
- Do you feel sad (or moody, blue, down, empty, bad)?
- What makes you feel sad?
- How often do you cry?
- Can you cheer up? Feel happy when something good happens?
- Do you have worries?
- How do you feel about yourself?
- Do you think you will ever feel better?
- Do you feel guilty about things that aren't your fault?

Anhedonia
- Do you feel bored?
- Were you bored before you started feeling sad?
- What do you like to do?
- Do you do things that are fun now?

Suicidal Thoughts and Behavior
- Do you think about dying? Hurting yourself? Killing yourself?
- Do you have a plan to do it?
- Have you tried to kill yourself? How? Did you tell anyone?
- What happens when you die?
- Do you really want to die? Would it be better for you or your family?

Adapted from Puig-Antich, J., and Chambers, W. J.: Schedule for Affective Disorders and Schizophrenia for School-Age Children (K-SADS-P). New York, New York Psychiatric Institute. In press.

TREATMENT

Various psychological and pharmacological therapies have been used in the treatment of childhood depression. Some have focused more on alleviating the child's internal feelings of depression and vegetative symptoms, while others have concentrated on changing associated behaviors and teaching the skills required for normal social functioning.

Pharmacotherapy—Imipramine

There is substantial evidence that pharmacotherapy can play an important role in the treatment of major depression in adults. If a definite diagnosis of major depressive disorder according to DSM III criteria can be made in a child or adolescent and if the severity of symptoms threatens the continued development, health, or life of the youth, then a carefully monitored trial of tricyclic antidepressant medication might be indicated.

Physicians caring for children on imipramine should become familiar with the drug's side effects and toxicities. Most of the minor effects occasionally encountered lessen with time or with slight decreases in dosage. They may, however, be very annoying to the child or cause parental alarm, resulting in noncompliance with the planned regimen. These include the anticholinergic symptoms of dry mouth, constipation, urinary retention, and blurry vision, as well as drowsiness, dizziness, nervousness, orthostatic hypotension, and gastrointestinal discomfort. Imipramine commonly causes certain cardiovascular side effects, including increases in heart rate and blood pressure, and changes in cardiac conduction (widened QRS complex, prolonged PR and QTc intervals) visible on electrocardiographic tracings. Electrocardiographic monitoring is essential during imipramine therapy for childhood depression in order to stay within bounds of provisional EKG safety limits (Puig-Antich, 1980) and to avoid life-threatening cardiac toxicities.

Prior to beginning medication, the child's medical history should be reviewed, and a baseline electrocardiogram and physical examination should be obtained. Besides diagnosing any previously undetected illness contributing to the depression, the physician should look for possible medical or environmental contraindications to the use of imipramine (i.e., untreated hyperthyroidism, hypertension, cardiac arrhythmia or heart block, or lack of adult supervision for an impulsive or suicidal child). The physician should also be aware of common drug interactions (i.e., possible potentiation of CNS depressant effects of alcohol and other sedatives and of sympathomimetic effects of decongestants containing epinephrine) and possible adverse effects of imipramine on the control of other medical problems (i.e., imipramine may lower the seizure threshold in children with seizure disorder or unpredictably alter the control of blood glucose in diabetic children).

The recommended initial dose of imipramine in the treatment of childhood depression is 1.5 mg/kg/day. This dose should be gradually increased by 1 mg/kg/day increments over one to two weeks (to a maximum recommended dose of 5 mg/kg/day) until the maintenance plasma drug concentration reaches the therapeutic level [combined imipramine and desipramine level of 200 ng/ml (Puig-Antich, 1980)]. Therapeutic drug level monitoring (imipramine plus the major active metabolite desipramine) plays an important role in imipramine therapy, since therapeutic response depends on an adequate blood level, but the therapeutic ratio is small. Before each dose increase, the presence of symptomatic side effects should be determined, and the child's blood pressure, pulse rate, and electrocardiogram should be monitored. A positive response to medication (defined as a decrease in depressive symptoms) may not be observed until two to four weeks after a therapeutic blood level is reached. In children who respond, imipramine therapy is generally continued for several months before tapering the medication and observing for relapse or recurrence off medication.

Although imipramine may be safely used to treat depression in children when appropriate indications and guidelines are followed, the physician should be aware of two additional potential complications of drug therapy. The first is imipramine overdose. The second, imipramine withdrawal, may result from rapid discontinuation of the drug. The symptoms of the withdrawal syndrome, which include nausea, emesis, abdominal cramps, headache, agitation, fatigue, and anorexia, can usually be avoided by slowly tapering the medication over several weeks.

Drug treatment can be justified only if it is part of a comprehensive treatment plan that includes some form of psychotherapy or counseling. Medication, even if successful in alleviating the depressed mood and vegetative symptoms, may have little positive effect on the child's residual impaired social functioning.

Imipramine may be useful in the treatment of a prolonged, profound major depressive episode in youngsters older than age six when serum levels can be monitored and signs of toxicity evaluated at frequent intervals.

Psychotherapy

Some form of psychosocial intervention or psychotherapy is generally indicated in the treatment of childhood depression. This is a necessary adjunct to pharmacotherapy in the case of major depressive illness, where therapy should address the residual problem areas of low self-esteem, inadequate social skills, and poor interpersonal relationships unrelieved by antidepressant medication. Psychotherapy is considered the mainstay of treatment for neurotic or characterologic depression and may facilitate the successful resolution of developmental or acute situational depressions. Extensive clinical experience indicates that psychotherapy is beneficial in many cases.

An example of a comprehensive, developmentally focused therapy is the "multimodal" treatment for depressed children (Petti, 1981). Multimodal treatment encompasses supportive psychotherapy, environmental support (family counseling, parent skills training), psychoeducational intervention (modifying the child's school experience to encourage positive feedback from teachers and peers, and academic achievement), behaviorally oriented milieu therapy (to increase adaptive behavior and internal control), social skills training (verbal and nonverbal communication, conflict resolution, assertiveness), and pharmacotherapy if indicated. Here an important goal is to raise the child's self-esteem and sense of competence and to increase his chances of experiencing positive reinforcement and pleasure.

There are several additional benefits of a behavioral approach to childhood depression.

The first is that with proper coordination many, if not all, of the individual components may be adapted to outpatient care in order to minimize disruption of the child's life. The second is that the interventions are primarily active and directive. Therefore, effective therapy does not necessarily depend on the total understanding and cooperation of a depressed child. The third is that several basic elements of the techniques used are already in or may be easily added to the pediatrician's repertoire of therapeutic skills. These include supportive counseling of patients and families, mediating parent-child conflicts, suggesting diagnostic testing and assisting in alternative school placements, and helping arrange supervised peer group activities for socially isolated children.

SUICIDAL BEHAVIOR

Suicide is the most feared potential outcome of severe depression in children and adolescents. In addition to being a sign of major depression, suicidal ideation and behavior may be associated with other psychiatric disturbances, including acute adjustment disorder, conduct disorder, and psychosis unrelated to depression. Children and adolescents with poor impulse control, or those who make desperate attempts to manipulate what is from their perspective an intolerable situation or environment, may also demonstrate suicidal behavior. Nonetheless, depression is one of the major identified risk factors for suicidal behavior.

Incidence and Demographic Factors

Suicide is currently the third leading cause of death among teen-agers in the United States. The U.S. suicide rates for youth 10 to 19 years old more than tripled between 1950 and 1977. Estimates of the frequency of suicide are probably conservative. There are no reliable national data for children under age 10, since suicide is not officially listed as a possible cause of death in this age group. Young children do, however, commit suicide. For every youth who commits suicide, there are an estimated 50 to 200 more who attempt suicide. Those who survive may be affected emotionally and physically and are at increased risk of making additional attempts or succeeding at suicide in the future.

Suicide occurs among youth of all races, ethnic groups, religions, and socioeconomic backgrounds. It is thought that females outnumber males in suicide attempts by a ratio of 3 to 1 but that boys outnumber girls in actually completing suicide. This may be related to the observation that males, especially teen-agers and young adults, tend to use violent methods such as guns, knives, or hanging, whereas females commonly attempt suicide with less violent methods such as pill ingestion, from which spontaneous recovery or resuscitation may be more likely.

Identifying Patients At Risk

There is no available psychiatric or social profile that enables the physician to predict with certainty which youth will actually attempt suicide, nor to predict the outcome. In most cases, however, there are clues that the child is in trouble. If the physician thinks that a youth might be considering suicide, whether on the basis of clinical signs of depression, preoccupation with death, or verbal or behavioral hints of intent, the physician should raise the question directly. This will not "cause" suicide to occur and, in fact, often produces relief on the part of the disturbed youngster.

Factors that have been positively correlated with the risk of suicidal behavior in youth include major psychiatric illness, extreme family disruption or situations of physical abuse, alcohol or drug abuse, prior attempts, and a history of depression or suicidal behavior in parents. Recent changes in mood and behavior, especially those corresponding to the symptoms and signs of depression, may signal increased risk: depressed mood; feelings of profound helplessness, hopelessness, worthlessness; inability to concentrate; recent onset of school failure or refusal; and sudden increasing isolation from friends and family members. Rarely a youth may conceive of death as a temporary and reversible situation, a state similar to life, or a pleasurable experience. Although these ideas are not the primary cause of suicide, they may enable the child to carry out the act.

There may be a triggering event identifiable as the proximate "cause" of the suicide attempt: loss of a significant relationship, actual or anticipated conflict with parents, school failure, unwanted pregnancy, or threat of punishment. Triggering events may, from the adult standpoint, make sense only in the context of the child's long history of problems and current inability to cope. From the youth's point of view, suicide may be considered as one of several alternative solutions to intolerable problems, chosen only after other attempts, such as running away from home, have failed.

Immediate danger of suicide in children at risk is suggested by positive thoughts about suicide or preoccupation with death, actual suicide threats, explanatory notes, arrangements for death such as giving away pets or prized possessions, or specific suicide plans including knowledge of methods and precautions against discovery. Suicide encompasses a broad spectrum of behavior, including ideation, threats, gestures, and attempts, as well as successful suicide. For any individual child there is no reliable way of determining the actual risk except in retrospect; therefore, it is essential that even threats be taken seriously. In children it may be misleading to infer seriousness of intent from the lethality of the method planned or used, since the youth may not have sufficient knowledge to predict realistically the probable outcome of his actions.

The pediatrician may be able to help prevent suicide by identifying youth at high risk, directly questioning them concerning intent and established plans, and being alert to recognize behavioral clues of impending suicidal behavior.

Management of the Suicidal Patient

The care of any suicidal youth involves immediate intervention to demonstrate appropriate concern and to protect the youngster's life, a thorough psychosocial assessment, and the initiation of a treatment plan. The pediatrician may wish to obtain early psychiatric consultation to help accomplish these goals, especially for the youth who requires hospitalization or remains actively suicidal after a failed attempt.

If the pediatrician becomes aware that a suicide attempt is in progress, it may become necessary to involve the police or emergency squad in attempts to persuade the youth not to carry out the plan. Discussion that focuses on the problem situation rather than on the actual plans for suicide may be helpful, stressing, for example, that alternative, "better" solutions can be found. It is advisable to make hopeful statements, while at the same time firmly instructing the youth not to hurt himself. Once the immediate crisis is over, the youth should be examined and treated for possible medical sequelae of the attempt.

If following the suicide attempt the youth is judged to be out of physical danger, a decision has to be made as to whether or not psychiatric hospitalization is necessary. (Hospitalization on a medical/pediatric unit is acceptable if appropriate suicide precautions, such as 24-hour direct observation, can be provided.) Hospitalization can be therapeutic merely by providing a sanctuary from pressures that may have precipitated the suicide attempt. It indicates to the patient that he or she will be cared for and protected and communicates to the family the seriousness of the child's problem. The hospital provides a neutral setting in which to perform a complete psychosocial evaluation, clarify the environmental issues underlying the attempt, and begin to involve the family in planning for therapy. It is extremely difficult to accomplish this in a single emergency session in an outpatient setting.

If, however, following the attempt, the youth is no longer actively suicidal, seriously depressed, or psychotic, has some insight into his behavior, and has concerned parents who will provide adequate supervision, it may be possible to complete the evaluation and initiate therapy without hospitalization. In order for this alternative course to be chosen, the physician should be confident that a strong external support system exists, and that the youth has control over impulsive thoughts and actions. The physician should also make sure that, both for an outpatient evaluation and during the posthospitalization period, a youth without insight is not returned to the exact same environment that may have precipitated the attempt.

REFERENCES

American Psychiatric Association: Diagnostic and Statistical Manual of Mental Disorders, 3rd Ed. Washington, D.C., 1980.

Carlson, G. A., and Cantwell, D. P.: Unmasking depression in children and adolescents. Am. J. Psychiatry, *137*:445, 1980.

Mattson, A., Seese, L. R., and Hawkins, J. W.: Suicidal behavior as a child psychiatric emergency. Arch. Gen. Psychiatry, *20*:100, 1969.

McKnew, D., and Cytryn, L.: Urinary metabolites in chronically depressed children. J. Am. Acad. Child Psychiatry, *18*:608, 1979.

Petti, T. A.: Active treatment of childhood depression. *In* Clarkin, J. F., and Glazer, H. I. (Eds.): Depression, Behavioral and Directive Intervention Strategies. New York, Garland Press, 1981.

Pfeffer, C. R.: Suicidal behavior of children: A review with implications for research and practice. Am. J. Psychiatry, *138*:154, 1981.

Puig-Antich, J., Chambers, W., Halpern, F., Hanlon, C., and Sachar, E. J.: Cortisol hypersecretion in prepubertal major depressive illness: A preliminary report. Psychoneuroendocrinology, *4*:191, 1979.

Puig-Antich, J., Chambers, W., Halpern, F., Hanlon, C., and Sachar, E. J.: Prepubertal endogeneous major depressives hyposecrete growth hormone in response to insulin-induced hypoglycemia. Biol. Psychiatry, *16*:801, 1981.
Puig-Antich, J., and Chambers, W. J.: Schedule for Affective Disorders and Schizophrenia for School-Age Children (K-SADS-P). New York, New York Psychiatric Institute.
Puig-Antich, J.: Affective disorders in childhood: A review and perspective. Psychiatr. Clin. North Am., *3*:403, 1980.
Spitz, R.: Anaclitic depression: An inquiry into the genesis of psychiatric conditions in early childhood, II. Psychoanal. Study Child., *2*:313, 1946.

37

CONVERSION SYMPTOMS

Morris Green, M.D.

Persistent symptoms in children may have either an intrapsychic or a biomedical etiology. Conversion symptoms are considered to be overt manifestations of an unconscious psychic process in which the patient's repressed wishes, fantasies, or conflicts—principally in relation to sexual, aggressive, or dependency issues—are symbolically expressed. What cannot be expressed verbally and directly is conveyed nonverbally and indirectly. When such intrapsychic conflicts are repressed, the discomfort that awareness of anxiety or guilt would engender is lessened. This is the *primary gain*. The increased attention and solicitude afforded the patient and the dispensation that the symptom provides to avoid threatening, anxiety-provoking, or unpleasant interactions is the *secondary gain*.

CASE

Three weeks before being seen, Brenda S., a 14-year-old girl, began to vomit several times a day and complained of epigastric discomfort. She reported that her only intake was carbonated soft drinks. Her mother also reported that Brenda had "passed out" twice and, on occasion, experienced difficulty in breathing.

Although the child had lost five pounds of weight, she was not dehydrated, and the physical examination was normal. In the interview, it was noted that the child avoided any expression of her feelings but tended to intellectualize. She was very idealistic and set very high moral standards for herself and others. A year prior to the onset of the illness, the mother had experienced almost identical symptoms following her divorce from Brenda's father. At that time, the mother sought psychotherapy because of severe depression. Shortly before the onset of the present illness, Brenda learned that the man whom she had considered to be her father was not and that her mother was unmarried when she was conceived.

Brenda and her mother were assured that an organic disorder was not present but that the etiology was stress-related. A schedule of activities was initiated, since the child had been remaining in bed. The family was advised to discontinue the special attention, i.e., cards, gifts (10 stuffed animals), and phone calls, that were perpetuating the sick role. Psychiatric consultation was offered but declined. Although Brenda would not outwardly accept the explanation for her illness, her symptoms abated over the next few days.

SYMPTOMS

Conversion symptoms include paralysis or weakness of an extremity, blindness, blurring of vision, deafness, aphonia, whispering, anesthesia or paresthesia of a region, abnormal gait, tics, pain (abdominal, chest, or musculoskeletal), headache, urinary retention, fatigue, hyperventilation, anorexia, dysphagia, convulsions, syncope, vertigo, nausea, and vomiting. The symptom chosen may be unconsciously modeled after that in a relative or other significant person, current or in the past, or one that the child has previously experienced. There is often a precipitating emotional stress, e.g., sexual abuse, a family crisis, marital discord, critical school examinations, an illness, physical trauma, surgery, or other major life change. The onset may be either acute or insidious, and the symptoms may be persistent, intermittent, or shifting.

DIAGNOSIS

Diagnosis requires the simultaneous exclusion of an organic etiology and confirmation of the presence of those psychological findings consistent with a conversion reaction. In many instances, the symptom(s) is clearly inconsistent with an organic disorder, and the criteria for a conversion reaction are readily evident; in other cases, the differentiation may be very difficult, especially since the symptomatology of either may be almost identical. Organic and psychological disease may, of course, co-exist, and the early manifestations of some serious organic disorders such as dystonia musculorum deformans, central nervous system degenerative disease, a brain tumor, or an osteoid osteoma may be misinterpreted.

Conversion reactions most commonly occur in school age children and adolescents. They are unlikely in children under five years of age. Although emphasized in the past as characteristic, the psychological attitude of *la belle indifference* or a seeming lack of concern is not a reliable diagnostic feature. Likewise, the patient may not demonstrate a "hysterical" personality. For diagnostic or therapeutic purposes, it is unnecessary for the pediatrician to clarify the symbolic meaning of the symptom. Children with conversion symptoms often have few close friends. There may be very close ties with the mother.

TREATMENT

The prognosis is best when the onset is acute; when there is a clearly identified precipitating stressful experience; when the child has been previously emotionally healthy; and when the family is developmentally or psychologically minded. The diagnosis and treatment of conversion symptoms is best done on an ambulatory basis, since hospitalization tends to fix the symptom. In the interview, effort should be made to identify possible precipitating emotional stresses. Unnecessary diagnostic procedures are to be avoided. The child should be firmly expected to be active, and bed rest is proscribed. Exercise activity programs are helpful. Reinforcement of the child's sick role in the family should be avoided, e.g., by a decrease in (1) attention to symptomatic complaints, (2) parental questions about how the child is feeling, and (3) gifts and cards. Instead the child should receive attention and praise for his improvement. When the symptoms are persistent and restrictive, pediatric hospitalization and psychiatric referral may be necessary (see p. 301). Often both the child and the parent, usually the mother, may need psychotherapy. Since the conversion mechanism is an unconscious one, the parents or child will not spontaneously associate the emotional stress with the symptom. Indeed, the occurrence of such a stress may be denied. Recognizing this, direct interpretation of the psychological mechanisms involved in the pathogenesis of the problem should not be pursued. Rather, attention should be authoritatively directed to helping the child cope with life stresses. Psychiatric referral may be introduced by a statement such as follows: "Often, some of the stresses we have been discussing will cause symptoms such as Mary has. At this point, I am convinced that psychiatric help is necessary for her full recovery."

REFERENCES

Friedman, B. S.: Conversion symptoms in adolescents. Pediatr. Clin. North Am., *20*:873, 1973.

Lazare, A.: Conversion symptoms. N. Engl. J. Med., *305*:745, 1981.

38

HYPERVENTILATION SYNDROME

Morris Green, M.D.

Hyperventilation may cause lightheadedness, generalized weakness, tingling and numbness of the hands, tetany, or syncope. The physician needs to be alert to the hyperventilation syndrome as a possible cause of syncope in adolescent boys and girls, because patients are more likely to report "blacking-out" spells, seizures or sensations of smothering and inability to breathe, choking or attacks of shortness of breath than overbreathing or tingling and numbness of the hands. The complaint of rapid breathing is virtually never volunteered. Some children complain of chest pain, fatigue, weakness, and palpitations. Direct questioning or an attempt to reproduce the symptoms by having the patient hyperventilate for a minute or two may be necessary. The numerous episodes of hyperventilation syndrome that occur in some adolescents may be due to anxiety, in some cases about sexuality.

The physician's reassurance and explanation and the patient's subsequent understanding of the mechanism for the pathogenesis of the symptoms usually permit the process to be voluntarily controlled. Rebreathing into a paper bag may also be suggested. Counseling sessions may be indicated to help the child cope with his or her concerns.

REFERENCES

Enzer, N. B., and Walker, P. A.: Hyperventilation syndrome in childhood. A review of 44 cases. J. Pediatr., *70*:521, 1967.

Missri, J. C., and Alexander, S.: Hyperventilation syndrome. J.A.M.A., *240*:2093, 1978.

39

ANOREXIA NERVOSA

Katherine A. Halmi, M.D.

Anorexia nervosa is a medical and psychiatric disorder characterized by a loss of control over dieting behavior which results in a substantial weight loss, peculiar patterns of handling food, intense fear of gaining weight, disturbance of body image, and amenorrhea. Anorexia nervosa is one of the few psychiatric illnesses whose course may be unremitting until death.

CLINICAL FEATURES

The generally accepted diagnostic criteria for anorexia nervosa are presented in Table 39–1. Anorectic adolescents lose weight by drastically reducing their total food intake, with a disproportionate decrease in the intake of foods with a high carbohydrate and fat content. The term "anorexia" is a misnomer, since the loss of appetite in anorexia nervosa is rare before the patient is emaciated. Some patients cannot exert continuous control over their restriction of food intake and will engage in episodes of binge-eating, i.e., eating a large amount of carbohydrate-rich food in a short period of time. Such binge-eating episodes are usually followed by self-induced vomiting, another way in which anorectics attempt to lose weight. Other anorectics do not binge-eat but self-induce vomiting after a normal meal. Other purgative behaviors such as abusing laxatives and diuretics are frequently used by the adolescents to lose weight.

Anorectic patients exhibit peculiar behavior in relation to food; e.g., they hide candies and cookies in their pockets and around the house or they refuse to eat with their families or in public places. When forced to eat with others, they will frequently hide food in their napkins or pockets and spend a great deal of time

Table 39–1. DIAGNOSTIC CRITERIA FOR ANOREXIA NERVOSA

1. Refusal to maintain body weight over a minimal normal weight for age and height. A 50th percentile weight for age and height should be determined from pediatric growth charts. A weight 10 per cent below this is considered a minimal normal weight. If growth retardation is present, base the normal weight on a projected growth curve based on height and weight data obtained prior to anorexia nervosa.
2. A noticeable and substantial weight loss.
3. A disturbance of body image in which the patient feels fat even when she is emaciated.
4. Intense fear of becoming obese which does not diminish as weight loss progresses.
5. Amenorrhea.

rearranging the food on their plate. When confronted about this peculiar behavior, anorectic patients often deny that their behavior is unusual or they flatly refuse to discuss the matter.

Anorectic patients constantly think about food and how fat they are. This preoccupation with slenderness is revealed by their frequent checking on themselves in the mirror and by incessant talking about feeling fat and flabby. Their preoccupation with food leads them to collect recipes and spend much time preparing food and elaborate meals for others.

Anorectic patients have an intense fear of gaining weight and becoming obese, even in the face of increasing cachexia. The overactivity of the anorectic is directed toward losing weight. Because of a disturbance in body image, they fail to recognize that the degree of their emaciation is beyond just "slenderness." Even when emaciated, they describe the sensation of "feeling fat." When confronted, some anorectics will admit that they are too thin, but this intellectual acknowledgment usually coexists with a feeling of being fat; therefore they seldom change their behavior and gain weight. Many anorectics steadfastly deny any symptomatology.

Amenorrhea may be the first symptom of anorexia nervosa, appearing before noticeable weight loss has occurred. Usually, however, anorectic adolescents are referred for amenorrhea after they have sustained a weight loss. In the emaciated state, anorectic patients regress to the pattern of luteinizing hormone (LH) secretion found in prepubertal girls; this pattern reverts to a more mature one with weight gain. Although restoration to a normal body weight is a prerequisite for the resumption of menstruation, factors other than nutritional state, most likely psychological in nature, contribute to the prolonged amenorrhea (Falk and Halmi, 1982).

Often the anorectic adolescent comes to medical attention when the weight loss is finally noticed by a parent. This may not occur for many months. As the weight loss becomes profound, physical signs such as hypothermia, dependent edema, bradycardia, hypotension, lanugo, and a variety of metabolic changes occur. Often the severely emaciated anorectic will have a leukopenia with a relative lymphocytosis and a low fasting serum glucose level, and less often they will have elevated serum cholesterol and carotene levels. A metabolic alkalosis is not uncommon in those patients who self-induce vomiting or abuse laxatives and diuretics. Persistent vomiting may lead to erosion of the enamel of the teeth and eventually more serious problems of tooth decay and loss of teeth (Halmi and Falk, 1981). Many anorectic patients are subjected to unnecessary extensive laboratory and x-ray examinations because the diagnosis of anorexia nervosa is not considered or the clinician wants "to rule out the organic before considering the emotional."

Endocrine changes such as a low to low-normal serum thyroxin level, a low serum triiodothyronine level, an increased mean 24-hour plasma cortisol concentration, an increased cortisol half-life, a reduced metabolic clearance rate of cortisol, and an incomplete suppression of ACTH and cortisol levels by dexamethasone will all revert to normal with weight gain. The lack of response of growth hormone to L-dopa and to insulin does not change with weight restoration and may reflect, along with the amenorrhea, a hypothalamic impairment.

EPIDEMIOLOGY

Anorexia nervosa occurs predominantly in females, with only 4 to 6 per cent of the anorectic population being male.

The onset of anorexia nervosa is usually between the ages of 10 and 30, with a disproportionate increase in onset occurring at ages 14½ and 18 (Halmi et al., 1979). The peak ages of onset occur at a time when the adolescent is attempting to become more independent. At age 14½, most young women are about to enter high school and at age 18 they are preparing for a job or college. Since great emphasis is placed on the association of beauty and thinness in our culture, almost all young women diet in order to improve their appearance and thereby gain more social acceptance. The stress of dieting is certainly a precipitating factor in the development of anorexia nervosa.

From reports of consecutive admissions to student health centers, there is indirect evidence that the incidence of anorexia nervosa has been increasing in the past 10 years. The best estimate of prevalence is that one severe case of anorexia nervosa is present in every 200 girls between the ages of 12 and 18, as shown in a study in English boarding schools (Crisp et al., 1976).

COURSE

The course of anorexia nervosa varies from spontaneous recovery without treatment, recovery after a single episode with a variety of treatments, a fluctuating course of weight gains followed by relapses, to a gradually deteriorating course resulting in death due to starvation.

The most consistent indicator of good outcome is an early age of onset, and the most consistent indicators of poor outcome are late age of onset of the illness and previous hospitalizations for anorexia nervosa. Outcome is less favorable in anorexia nervosa patients who binge and vomit and in those patients whose parents will not respond to parental counseling (Halmi, 1980).

DIAGNOSIS

The diagnosis of anorexia nervosa is frequently difficult because the anorectic patients, unmotivated for treatment, often deny many of the characteristic symptoms of the disorder. It is important, therefore, to interview family members or friends who have observed the adolescent's behavior. Because of the family's common denial, even this source may not provide sufficient information. It is usually necessary then to hospitalize the patient for diagnostic observation.

Depression may lead to some weight loss; however, depressed adolescents are not preoccupied with the calorie content of food, nor do they collect recipes and spend an inordinate amount of time cooking and preparing foods. Some adolescents meet all the criteria for both anorexia nervosa and a major depression. In such cases both conditions should be treated.

Schizophrenic patients usually have delusions about the food they are eating but they are seldom concerned over the calorie content of the food and are rarely preoccupied with the fear of becoming obese. They do not demonstrate the hyperactivity present in the anorectic adolescent. An occasional anorectic patient will also meet the criteria for schizophrenia and should be appropriately treated for both.

Bulimia, the rapid consumption of large amounts of food in a short period of time, is present in about half of anorexia nervosa patients. Bulimia, a diagnostic entity, is differentiated from anorexia nervosa by the fact that bulimic patients maintain their weight within a normal weight range, even though large fluctuations may occur. Bulimic patients have irregular menstrual cycles, but they are not amenorrheic for periods of three months or longer. Anorectic patients with bulimia form a distinct subgroup. Self-induced vomiting, laxative abuse, and diuretic abuse are far more prevalent in bulimic-anorectic patients than in those without bulimia. The bulimic-anorectic patients display more impulsive behavior, such as alcohol and street drug abuse, stealing, suicide attempts, and self-mutilation; are more extroverted and show less denial of their illness and have a hearty appetite; and show greater anxiety, depression, and guilt and have more somatic complaints (Casper et al., 1980). Vomiting is often denied by the patient with anorexia nervosa and is frequently done secretly.

TREATMENT

Since most anorectic patients are disinterested in, and even resistant to, treatment, they are brought to the doctor unwillingly by agonizing relatives or friends. In order to obtain their cooperation in treatment, it is important to emphasize to the anorectic adolescent the benefits of the treatment, such as a decrease in the obsessive thoughts about food and body weight with a subsequent improvement in being able to concentrate on other matters with less effort, a decrease in depressive symptoms and irritability, and a restoration of prior peer relationships. As their illness progresses, anorectic adolescents withdraw from their friends and are much less active socially. If extremely emaciated, the anorectic will be upset that she no longer has the energy to be active. Reassurance that her previous activity level could be restored with treatment will also help persuade her to enter a treatment program. The parents' support for the treatment program is essential, especially since firm recommendations must be carried out.

The treatment of anorexia nervosa must be multifaceted. Medical management and personal, behavioral, and family therapies are all necessary treatment modalities. The immediate aim of treatment should be to restore the patient's nutritional state to normal. Mere emaciation or the state of being mildly underweight (15 to 25 per cent) can cause irritability, depression, preoccupation with food, and sleep disturbance. It is exceedingly difficult to accomplish a behavioral change with psychotherapy in an emaciated patient experiencing the psychological effects of emaciation. Nutritional rehabilitation and rapid medical recovery can occur in a structured environment in an inpatient treatment program.

Initial outpatient therapy may be successful in adolescents (1) who have had the illness for less than four months, (2) who are not binge-eating and vomiting, and (3) whose parents are likely to participate effectively in family therapy. The three criteria listed above are based on clinical experience and should be helpful in deciding whether an outpatient program has a chance of success. There are no controlled treatment studies assessing the effectiveness of an initial outpatient treatment program compared to an initial hospitalized treatment program.

The more severely ill patients present a difficult management problem. Patients who are vomiting require daily monitoring of weight, fluid and calorie intake, and urine output. Initially it is more efficient and medically safer to give the patients total nutrients in the form of a formula such as Sustacal, which contains adequate amounts of vitamins, minerals, proteins, fatty acids, and carbohydrates, all conveniently blended so that the patient cannot selectively discard any item. If the formula is given in six equal feedings throughout the day the patient will not have to ingest a large amount at any time. In order to avoid gastric dilatation the patients should be started on a daily caloric intake to maintain their low present weight with 50 per cent of that calculated amount added. This amount can be increased every five days or weekly. Hyperalimentation is rarely necessary except for the patient with severe medical complications.

Hospitalization of anorectic adolescents is advantageous in that it isolates them from a potentially noxious environment. Each patient should have a behavior analysis during the first few days after admission to the hospital so that appropriate positive and negative reinforcements can be selected and the child placed into an *individualized* behavior therapy program. Behavior therapy is most effective in the medical management and nutritional rehabilitation of the patient, although there are times when other target behaviors can be changed with behavior therapy. Most adolescents need a daily reinforcement for weight gain. A medically safe rate for weight gain would be ¼ pound or 0.1 kilogram per day. Initially, weight gain rather than eating behavior should be reinforced so that the patients will not self-induce vomiting, obtain their rewards, and continue to lose weight. The patient's weight is an objective measure. Making positive reinforcements contingent only on weight gain is helpful in reducing staff-patient stressful interactions. Behavior therapy is also useful in stopping vomiting behavior. After a period of time on Sustacal, the patients can be transferred to eating food from a tray prepared by a dietician. The next step is to have the patient select her own foods to maintain a normal weight. The latter is done after the patient has been maintaining her weight within a normal weight range for at least one week.

Drugs can often be useful adjuncts in the treatment of anorexia nervosa. A preliminary analysis of a controlled treatment study has shown that cyproheptadine, an antihistaminic drug, is effective in inducing weight gain and decreasing depressive symptomatology in doses of 32 mg per day (Halmi, 1982). Since cyproheptadine has so few side effects, it is an especially attractive drug to use for anorectic patients. In the same study, there was an indication that amitriptyline may also be effective in inducing weight gain. It is important to start amitriptyline at a very low dosage, as low as 40 mg per day in a severely emaciated patient, and gradually build the dosage up to a therapeutic range of around 150 mg per day.

The first drug used in treating anorectic patients was chlorpromazine. Although there has been no controlled double-blind study to prove the efficacy of chlorpromazine in inducing weight gain in anorectics, clinical observation has associated weight gain with the use of this medication. Also, chlorpromazine clinically seems to be effective in the severely obsessive-compulsive anorectic patients.

Although there is no convincing evidence that family therapy as a sole form of treatment is effective, most experienced clinicians believe that counseling family members is a necessary component to an effective treatment program. Family therapy is usually used in conjunction with behavior contingencies and individual psychotherapy. It is important that each family be carefully analyzed for characteristics unique to that family and that the therapy correspond to the individual needs of the family. Because considerable variation of maladaptive interactional patterns exist within anorexia nervosa families, a treatment strategy for each individual family should be created.

Classic psychodynamically oriented therapy for treating anorexia nervosa has been regarded as ineffective by experienced psychoanalysts (Bruch, 1970). Individual psychotherapy should focus on making the patient aware of her behavior and the effect it has on maintaining her illness. A therapist must deal with the patient's denial of illness, fear of failure, fear of becoming independent of the family, and fear of accepting the expected responsibilities of a growing adolescent. The patient's need to control her environment by her maladaptive living pattern must be brought to her awareness.

Continuing outpatient individual therapy for varying periods of time, depending on the severity of illness, is needed after the hospitalized treatment phase. The patient's anxiety and preoccupation with her weight do not disappear immediately after she regains her weight. Likewise, continuing outpatient family therapy is needed. An effective outpatient program includes behavioral contingencies for medical management, family therapy and personal psychotherapy.

It is likely that early diagnosis and vigorous early intervention have been effective in reducing the mortality of this disorder. The longer the maladaptive eating patterns and emaciation continue, the more difficult it is to restore the patient to a medically and psychologically healthy state. Patients who do not improve in a treatment program should be referred to a specialized eating disorder treatment program.

ROLE OF THE GENERAL PEDIATRICIAN

It is obvious from the varying course of anorexia nervosa that the role of the pediatrician will differ according to the severity of the anorectic's illness. A pediatrician can be helpful in establishing an early diagnosis by inquiring of the adolescent as to whether she is dieting and noting whether the adolescent has had a recent weight loss. Parents can be questioned as to whether their daughter has shown a greater interest in cooking or collecting recipes or has tried to obtain a new job as a waitress. Parents may have observed that their adolescent girl gazes into the mirror frequently and comments on her slenderness or that she comments incessantly about looking fat and feeling flabby. A recent change in eating behavior, such as the adolescent's refusal to eat with her family or in public places, should bring a high index of suspicion of anorexia nervosa. At this point a nutritionist could obtain a detailed diet history from the patient over the past week. If the patient is unreliable, a diet history may have to be obtained from the parents or the patient's peers. If an adolescent has rapidly increased her exercising or physical activity concomitantly with her dieting, it is very likely that she is developing anorexia nervosa.

The pediatrician should ask the adolescent what weight she would like to be. If this weight is unreasonably low, the pediatrician should show the adolescent on the height and weight charts what the proper weight range should be for that person. If she vigorously protests and refuses to answer further questions about her eating behavior, there should be serious concern about the development of anorexia nervosa. The number of calories necessary to maintain the lowest weight within a normal weight range should be calculated and an additional 50 per cent should be added for activity. A nutritionist can give the patient three or four examples of the amount and kinds of foods that the patient could eat for breakfast, lunch, supper, and a snack to meet the caloric requirements to maintain a normal weight. It is important not to emphasize calorie counting but rather to have the patient visualize the amount of different food types she should be eating in order to maintain a normal weight. The pediatrician should then see the patient weekly to monitor her weight and to obtain further information about her eating behavior. It is wise for the pediatrician to explain to the adolescent the medical complications associated with prolonged dieting in an underweight condition. A pediatrician should also try to obtain information about the child's relationship to her parents and her peers and about any recent stresses that may have occurred. If the adolescent is still losing weight after seeing the pediatrician for a month, the adolescent should be referred to a psychiatrist. The psychiatrist should evaluate the parents as well as the adolescent with the eating disorder. The criteria for hospitalization of a patient with anorexia have already been mentioned.

Dividing the responsibility between the pediatrician and the child psychiatrist for the care of a patient with an eating disorder is possible when the roles of each specialist are clearly defined. Most anorectic patients are very successful at pitting staff against staff. Therefore, it is extremely important that the treatment team be a cohesive unit. When the child is admitted to the hospital, it is advisable for the pediatrician, the child psychiatrist, and the nursing team to meet together and establish a treatment program that is feasible for the setting, for the patient, and for the staff. A treatment program should be presented to the patient and the parents and no changes should be made unless they are done in a team meeting. Sometimes it is better for the pediatrician to be responsible for the ward management in the weight gain program and the child psychiatrist to be responsible for the individual psychotherapy and the family therapy. If the adolescent is to be hospitalized in a pediatric hospital, the hospitalization should be as brief as possible, with emphasis on rapid weight restoration. In this kind of setting many doctors have found that the only way they can handle these patients is to keep them in bed until they have reached their target or normal weight. If the patients are allowed out of their beds they will soon be all over the hospital and it will be impossible to monitor caloric intake, fluid intake, and fluid output. Some estimation of caloric intake can be made by weighing the patient every morning before breakfast. It is very difficult to set up a specific behavioral program in the pediatric hospital unless that hospital can offer recreational therapy programs, school programs, or vocational programs. The anorectic patient can be given increased activity privileges and increased visiting privileges based on weight gain.

The patient should not be discharged from the hospital until she has reached a normal weight and is able to select her own foods to maintain that normal weight. In mild cases this may be a month of hospitalization and in moderately severe cases at least six to eight weeks of hospitalization. If the anorectic patient had a previous hospitalization treatment failure and has been ill for longer than six months, it is likely the patient will need a three- to four-month hospitalization; this should be done in a setting in which the patient can obtain schooling, engage in peer-related activities, and be in a milieu program that has a strong emphasis on training in social skills. Usually this setting just described is an adolescent unit in a psychiatric hospital.

There are times, very rarely, when the anorectic patient's medical condition is so unstable that it is necessary to hospitalize the patient in a pediatric setting rather than in a psychiatric setting.

Family counseling is an important part of a therapy program for an anorectic patient. The family counseling may be time consuming and more efficiently done by a psychiatric social worker or a child psychiatrist. After the patient is discharged from the hospital, she should be followed weekly to be certain that she is maintaining her weight within a normal range. Most patients need continuing psychotherapy and family therapy for several months in an aftercare program. Some patients may need continuing psychotherapy for several years after being discharged from the hospital. There is a great variation in the severity of personality disorders in the anorectic patients. The return of menstruation is usually associated with marked psychological improvement. If the patient has maintained a normal weight for six months, has maintained normal eating behavior, and has had a resumption of menstruation, she is well on her way to recovery and should no longer need frequent pediatric visits. The adolescent should, however, have yearly visits after this to the pediatrician for documentation of weight, height, and menstrual history.

REFERENCES

Bruch, H.: Psychotherapy in primary anorexia nervosa. J. Nerv. Ment. Dis., *150*:51–60, 1970.

Casper, R. C., Eckert, E. D., Halmi, K. A., Goldberg, S. C., and Davis, J. M.: Bulimia: Its incidence and clinical importance in patients with anorexia nervosa. Arch. Gen. Psychiatry, *37*:1030–1035, 1980.

Crisp, A. H., Palmer, R. L., and Kalucy, R. S.: How common is anorexia nervosa? A prevalence study. Br. J. Psychiatry, *128*:549–551, 1976.

Falk, J. R., and Halmi, K. A.: Amenorrhea in anorexia nervosa: Examination of the critical body weight hypothesis. J. Biol. Psychiatr., *17*:799–806, 1982.

Halmi, K. A., Eckert, E., and Falk, J. R.: Cyproheptadine, an antidepressant and weight-inducing drug for anorexia nervosa. Lancet, *1*:1357–1358, 1982.

Halmi, K. A.: Behavior therapy in the treatment of anorexia nervosa. *In* Twentyman, C. T., Epstain, L. E., and Blanchard, E. (Eds.): Progress in Behavioral Medicine. New York, Plenum Publishing Corporation, in press.

Halmi, K. A.: Eating Disorders. *In* Kaplan, H. I., Freedman, A. M., and Sadock, B. J. (Eds.): Comprehensive Textbook of Psychiatry, 3rd Ed. 1980, pp. 2598–2605.

Halmi, K. A., and Falk, J. R.: Common physiological changes in anorexia nervosa. Int. J. Eating Disorders, *1*:16–27, 1981.

Halmi, K. A., Casper, R. C., Eckert, E. D., Goldberg, S. C., and Davis, J. M.: Unique features associated with age of onset of anorexia nervosa. Psychiatr. Res., *1*:209–215, 1979.

Theander, S.: Anorexia nervosa. Acta Psychiatr. Scand., *214* (Suppl.):29, 1970.

COMMENTARY

The pediatrician who has a special interest in the psychosocial aspects of child health has an important role to play in the management of patients with eating disorders. In terms of prevention, if a girl is overweight, the physician should generally provide her the opportunity of raising the question herself about her weight rather than remark that she is obese or is becoming fat. Many anorectic patients report that their eating disorder began after such a gratuitous comment by a parent, a physician, or a peer.

Open-ended questions may provide this chance: "I find that girls (boys) at your age often have some concern about physical development, so this would be a good time to talk about any questions you may have in your mind along that line." "If you could change something about yourself, what would you like to change?" "What kind of physical activity do you do regularly?" If the child is to be offered a weight-control regimen, consultation should be obtained from a nutritionist interested and experienced with adolescents. Each child on a weight-control regimen should be seen by the physician once a week, if only for a few minutes.

Anorexia nervosa is a spectrum of symptoms, etiologies, and responses to therapy. Many of the younger adolescents who are pursuing an overly rigorous weight-control regimen but who do not have a defect in body image can be helped by being seen once a week on an ambulatory basis. In this arrangement, the ideal weight is determined jointly (lean body mass + 20 per cent) and a contract is established to achieve at least that weight.

Those patients who have a distortion in body image, have lost over 25 per cent of their body weight, are adamant about not eating, and have an unsupportive family usually require hospitalization. Such patients under the age of 16 years can be managed in a pediatric hospital, especially if there is a school age or adolescent patient care unit, a tradition of collaboration between pediatrics, child psychiatry, psychology, nursing, social work, child life workers, and occupational and physical therapy, and the availability of school classes, library, occupational therapy, physical therapy, and other opportunities for diversion. Other patients will require referral to a setting such as described by Dr. Halmi. An effective behavioral program can be developed utilizing a series of privileges tied to weight gain. We have not found it necessary to keep these patients in bed or to use nasopharyngeal feeding tubes. Daily schedules and contracts developed between the patient and the pediatrician have been very helpful. A weekly meeting of all the professionals concerned is essential.

Morris Green, M.D.

40

CHILDHOOD PSYCHOSIS

James E. Simmons, M.D.

Serious research and study of psychotic children have occurred only in the past 30 to 35 years. Progress has been handicapped by difficulty obtaining a consensus regarding terminology and specific diagnostic criteria. Etiology and treatment remain enigmatic.

"Psychosis" is no longer accepted as a psychiatric diagnosis or a major category of mental illness in the current psychiatric nomenclature. Rather, psychosis is a generic term associated with the most disabling psychiatric symptom picture seen in both children and adults. Psychotic symptoms may be seen in children with or without obvious brain damage or brain disease.

Significant impairments of personality are present in several areas:

1. Organization of thoughts is unconventional and often incomprehensible.
2. Emotional responsivity is absent or unpredictable and inappropriate.
3. Memory is impaired and/or distorted.
4. Behavior is very inappropriate: strange actions, mannerisms, or repetitive gestures that seem meaningless.
5. Ability to communicate is seriously impaired: muteness to meaningless words and phrases without communicative value; little nonverbal communication.

Signs and Symptoms of Psychosis

1. Social behavior bizarre and unpredictable
2. Inappropriate mood and affect
3. Diminished impulse control
4. Withdrawal
5. Abnormal mental content (delusions and hallucinations)
6. Disturbed forms of thinking (ideas, if expressed, are illogical or meaningless)

When such symptoms occur in normal children they are brief and transitory, but in psychosis the impairments are so severe and so sustained that they interfere with the capacity to meet the ordinary demands of daily life.

The psychoses include (DSM III, 1980, pp. 367–368):

1. Pervasive developmental disorders (autism)
2. Schizophrenic and paranoid disorders
3. Psychotic disorders not elsewhere classified
4. Some organic mental disorders
5. Some affective disorders

These disorders are differentiated on the basis of similarity of symptom clusters within each disorder, degree of functional impairment, and course of the illness. To some extent, these entities can also be differentiated by prognosis and response to different treatments.

Fortunately, most forms of psychosis are relatively rare in children. This is less true for adolescents. These illnesses have attracted much attention because they are usually profoundly disabling and in early childhood carry an extremely poor prognosis.

The term "childhood schizophrenia" has been dropped from the nomenclature. The exact relationship of the adult-onset schizophrenia to psychotic conditions seen in children remains unclear.

AUTISM

Pervasive development disorder (autism) and pervasive development disorder (childhood onset) include those conditions that were previously termed childhood psychosis, atypical children, symbiotic psychotic children, and childhood schizophrenia.

SCHIZOPHRENIA

Schizophrenic disorders and schizophreniform disorders usually have an onset during adolescence or early adulthood but do occur on rare occasions in children. A most important criterion for differentiating a true schizophrenic disorder is that schizophrenia involves deterioration from a previous higher level of functioning, whereas the pervasive developmental disorders are persistent, long-standing aberrations in development. Schizophrenic illness always involves disturbed thought content (delusions and hallucinations).

Delusions and hallucinations along with other psychotic symptoms can and do occur in childhood without the presence of the full criteria for schizophrenia or the history of aberrant development seen in autism. Usually these symptoms have an acute rather than insidious onset. The symptoms may be associated with some type of organic brain disturbance or can be a response to profound psychological and social stresses.

HALLUCINOSIS

Acute hallucinosis with or without delusions occurs in association with brain toxicity or anoxia in children with physical illnesses (near delirium). The symptoms can be associated with a wide variety of drugs or chemicals, degenerative central nervous system diseases, infectious and nonspecific encephalopathies, tumors, and occasionally radiation therapy. In the absence of any demonstrable central nervous system disturbance, acute hallucinosis has been seen following intense psychological and social stresses such as witnessing the murder of a parent or sibling, sexual assault, and other forms of child abuse.

Drug-related psychoses are being seen with increasing frequency in both children and adolescents. A toxic drug screen is indicated as an aid to diagnosis.

It can be nearly impossible to differentiate a true schizophrenic disorder from a drug-related psychosis on the basis of the clinical picture alone. The drug-related psychoses are usually, but not always, acute in onset with florid symptomatology and they rather rapidly, although not always, respond to treatment, in contrast to the schizophrenic disorders, which are insidious in onset and comparatively slower to respond to treatment.

The affective types of mental illness (depression and mania) are being diagnosed with increasing frequency in children and adolescents. However, an affective illness with true psychotic features is relatively uncommon.

Autism and Mental Retardation

Until recently, much time has been spent on differentiating mental retardation from pervasive developmental disorder (autism). Current research indicates that these two conditions are apparently not mutally exclusive and can be diagnosed in the same individual. Those autistic children who are retarded remain so even when social behavior and language improve. Among mentally retarded children without autism the behavior abnormalities are usually not present. Even when some "autistic-like" behavior and mannerisms are present in the retarded child, the full syndrome of infantile autism is rarely present. Whether the child suffers from infantile autism or mental retardation or both, those children with a testable I.Q. above 60 do significantly better in their long-term adjustment than those with very low I.Q.s (below 40).

TREATMENT

The following general principles apply in the management of an *acute onset* psychosis:

1. Treatment is directed at finding and removing the cause(s).
2. When confronted with a child suffering hallucinations and/or delusions of an abrupt onset, this author assumes there is some organic brain condition until proven otherwise.
3. A careful history is taken to pinpoint the actual onset of symptoms and to search for toxic agents or environmental stresses that may have precipitated the symptoms.
4. Care must be taken to differentiate an actual acute onset from a condition that developed insidiously and recently became severe enough to demand attention.
5. Careful physical and neurological examinations and appropriate laboratory studies are essential.
6. The patient usually requires constant attendance by adults who do not become fearful or angry in response to psychotic behavior.
7. There should be protection of the child without chemical or physical restraints if at all possible.
8. Bring the child to a *completely* drug-free or medicine-free state quickly.
9. Use psychotropic medication very judiciously or not at all.
10. If symptoms do not abate in two or three weeks, a more chronic form of psychosis must be considered.

The treatment and management of the child with a *chronic* psychosis is very complicated and time consuming. The diagnostic process as well as long-term treatment can put an impossible burden on the time and expertise of the physician as well as nearly impossible stress upon the psychological and financial resources of the family. The diagnostic and treatment program has two facets: (1) things essential to do with and for the child, and (2) things essential to do with and for the parents.

The initial evaluation procedures, elements of an adequate work-up, and the various treatment possibilities are clearly stated by DeMyer (1982). Many of the elements of evaluation and treatment are not immediately available to the general physician, and referral of a child is necessary. At the same time many things important to assisting the parents are well within the province of the general physician. Some general principles as well as specific techniques for assisting the family are outlined below:

1. The parents need support, reassurance, and a careful explanation from the physician each step of the way.
2. Excluding the parents, blaming them, or giving them pejorative (pseudopsychiatric) diagnoses is never helpful.
3. Research has shown that parents of mentally retarded and psychotic children have fewer and less severe psychiatric symptoms than do parents of children suffering neuroses and behavior disorders and no more psychopathology than parents with other types of chronically ill children.
4. Repeated research in the past 30 years has failed to show a cause-effect relationship between specific parental behaviors or psychological attributes and childhood psychosis.
5. The theoretical concept of the "schizophrenogenic mother" is untrue, has a very pejorative connotation, is never helpful, and can do serious damage to the self-esteem of the parent as well as the psychological equilibrium of the family.
6. The experience of having a psychotic child is often terrifying, frustrating, and emotionally exhausting for the parents.
7. Patience, understanding, and only occasionally psychiatric treatment are needed by the parents.
8. Both false reassurance and nihilistic pessimism are unwarranted before a thorough diagnostic assessment is completed.
9. Most parents want and deserve a diagnosis and a prognosis.
10. Parents can tolerate the lack of finite knowledge about baffling illnesses when such lack is admitted forthrightly fol-

lowed by an attitude of caring and a willingness to guide them toward appropriate resources.

11. The diagnosis and prognosis should not be given to the parents until they are psychologically ready to comprehend, have established a good relationship with the physician, and can believe that a careful, painstaking evaluation has been done.
12. Helping the parents find appropriate resources for long-term care is difficult but not impossible.
13. Treatment is largely special education and rehabilitation or habilitation, which is accomplished in special schools and agencies with trained developmental specialists (preferably day schools rather than residential).
14. Many public schools now have special classes for the mentally ill as well as the retarded child.
15. Local mental health centers and mental health associations can and should provide information on such resources.
16. Lay groups such as Parents and Friends of Retarded Persons or the Association of Parents of Autistic Children are often helpful in guiding new families.

The physician contributes to the treatment by monitoring the child's physical health, prescribing medications as needed, and helping the family in times of crisis. The most common crises during which the physician's guidance is needed are (1) when the symptoms are first noted and a diagnosis is being sought, (2) during the search for a school or agency to provide needed special developmental training and education, (3) at the onset of puberty with its sexual changes, (4) at the end of school age when it is becoming increasingly evident that the child may never be socially and vocationally independent, and (5) when parents become ill or elderly and must plan for the time they can no longer personally care for the child.

Many, perhaps most, physicians believe that childhood psychoses are beyond their knowledge and clinical competence. However, some psychotic reactions can be successfully treated if correctly diagnosed. At present, there are no "cures" for the pervasive developmental disorders. The most we can hope to do is significantly attenuate the deleterious effects of these illnesses on the child's development and on the family's psychological health. A careful, intelligent diagnosis with patient guidance on matters of long-term care can be immeasurably helpful to the families of these unfortunate children.

REFERENCES

MENTAL STATUS AND DEVELOPMENTAL ASSESSMENT

"Examination of Preschool Children," Chapter 6 in Simmons, J. E.: Psychiatric Examination of Children, 3rd Ed. Philadelphia, Lea and Febiger, 1981, pp. 131–163.

"Assessing Developmental Levels," Chapter 2 in Tarjan et al. (Eds.): The Physician and the Mental Health of the Child, Vol. 1. Monograph Series published by the American Medical Association, Chicago, 1979, pp. 15–28.

DIAGNOSIS AND TREATMENT OF CHILDHOOD PSYCHOSIS

DeMyer, M. K.: Infantile Autism: Patients and their Families. XII:4. Chicago, Year Book Medical Publishers, 1982.

Definitions of Psychiatric Illnesses described in the Diagnostic and Statistical Manual of Mental Disorders, 3rd Ed. Washington, D.C., American Psychiatric Association, 1980.

1. Organic mental disorders, pp. 101–128
2. Hallucinogen organic mental disorders, pp. 153–156
3. For mental disorders associated with barbiturates, cocaine, CNS stimulants, phencyclidine, cannabis, etc., see index
4. Substance use disorders, pp. 163–176
5. Schizophrenic disorders, pp. 181–193
6. Affective disorders with psychotic features, pp. 213–215
7. Pervasive developmental disorders (autism and childhood onset), pp. 86–92
8. Mental retardation, pp. 36–41

41

LYING, STEALING, AND FIRESETTING

James E. Simmons, M.D.

Although lying, stealing, and firesetting may have little in common from the standpoint of etiology or psychopathology, they are discussed together because all of them are commonly encountered behavior symptoms. While none of these behaviors is encouraged or even condoned by society, they can occur in otherwise "normal" children. One or all of them also may be the presenting complaints or accompanying symptoms in children with conduct disorders, neuroses, personality disorders, mental retardation, or even psychoses. Such behaviors are also commonly seen in neglected children or those who live in antisocial, criminal-type families.

DIFFERENTIATING "NORMAL" FROM PSYCHOPATHOLOGICAL

These undesirable behaviors occur in children of every age level and from every socioeconomic strata. Such behavior cannot be considered normal. Particularly when the behavior persists, it is an indication that something has gone awry in the child's social and psychological maturation. This "something gone awry" may be of relatively little consequence and self-limiting, so that no action needs to be taken by the physician or the parents; on the other hand, these behaviors may signal serious psychopathology. It can be very difficult to decide which child is urgently in need of intensive professional treatment and which should merely be observed in his development for a few months.

CASE

Eddie, age 7½, was brought to the clinic because of firesetting. At the initial visit his foster mother sighed and said, "I'm so glad we got this appointment. I've been trying to get him here for months. First, the Welfare Department said it wasn't serious enough, and they procrastinated about paying for the visit. Then, last week when I took him to the medical clinic they said Eddie was O.K. and didn't need psychiatry. The young doctor had talked with us a long time and examined him carefully. I told him I didn't see how he could say Eddie was normal. The doctor said, 'Well, I set fires when I was Eddie's age, and I turned out all right.' I replied, 'Doctor, I mean no disrespect, but when a little boy sets his mother's bed on fire, especially while she is sleeping in it, I say he's crazy. Please send us to psychiatry."

After a complete evaluation, it was determined that Eddie was not "crazy" or psychotic, as his foster mother said, but neither was he normal. Fortunately, his firesetting and several other antisocial symptoms did improve after lengthy outpatient psychotherapy for Eddie and some home-management counseling with his foster parents.

Ideally, every child with one or more of the above symptoms should have a complete psychosocial assessment to search for cause(s) and to develop a proper remediation plan; however, in view of the large numbers of children with these problems, the time and the cost required, routine complete assessments on every one of them is unrealistic and often may be unnecessary. Procedures for complete assessment are presented elsewhere in this book (p. 291) and will not be repeated here. Rather, we will offer some guidelines for differentiating those children who must have full psychosocial diagnostic evaluation from those whose development needs only some monitoring and a few suggestions to the parents on home management.

REPETITIVE NATURE OF THE SYMPTOMS

Parents often say, "He *ought* to know better," or "He *should* have better control." The physician's questions properly are, "*Does* he know better?" and "*Is* he showing control?" If serious misbehavior recurs, then the child is not learning control, is not learning right from wrong, or has parents who are unable to teach him, so a full family assessment is needed. The real question is not "What has the child done?" but "Can he learn not to repeat the act?"

SINGLE SYMPTOMS VS. MULTIPLE SYMPTOMS

If the child is well-adjusted in all other areas it is probably safe to reassure the parents that he will "outgrow" it; however, if he has two or more additional psychic, behavioral, or somatic symptoms, a more in-depth evaluation should be done.

WHEN IS "LYING" REALLY LYING?

Many parents label their child a "liar" when he refuses to confess to a misdeed. We remind parents that most people, even socially successful adults, lie when caught. When parents know the child has misbehaved, appropriate disciplinary measures should be taken without having a "trial" or extracting a "confession," even at the risk of the parent being wrong occasionally. The child who purposely fabricates stories, indulges in deceitfulness, or chronically misbehaves does need professional help whether or not he confesses. The parent who accuses a child of lying because he refuses to confess to a crime everyone knows he committed is demonstrating the undesirable, but all too common, game of adult "deceitfulness and entrapment."

AGE-APPROPRIATENESS

The three-year-old who takes other's toys may still have some lessons to learn about property rights; however, the seven-year-old should understand this concept unless he is mentally retarded or psychotic. When the mentally competent seven-year-old takes other's things, he is stealing.

SEVERITY OF THE ACT

If the child has done something that has resulted in serious damage to persons or property, a thorough psychosocial evaluation should be done. Even if the child is mentally normal and the incident a true accident, the psychological sequelae for the child and the family are frequently severe enough to justify an evaluation and some preventive therapy.

SUMMARY

While lying, stealing, and firesetting do occur in psychologically relatively healthy children, all too often the behavior indicates serious psychopathology. Some guidelines for differentiating healthy from mentally disturbed children have been presented.

42

PARENTS WHO SUFFER PSYCHOSIS

James E. Simmons, M.D.

Psychosis is a generic term associated with the most disabling psychiatric symptom pictures. (See Chap. 40 for discussion of childhood psychosis.) The discussion here will be limited to the schizophrenic disorders and the affective disorders (depression and mania) as these conditions may appear in parents. The newer treatments permit most of these patients to avoid prolonged hospitalizations and to live in the mainstream of society. Affective disorders are no longer exclusively illnesses of the middle aged, the elderly, or the hospitalized. Improved methods of diagnosis have revealed these illnesses to be increasing in frequency amoung teenagers and young adults.

SCHIZOPHRENIA

Schizophrenia is not a single illness but rather a group of psychotic disorders which at some phase of the illness always involve delusions, hallucinations, and/or disturbances in thinking. For purposes of this chapter, it is sufficient for the primary care physician to recognize the major signs and symptoms of schizophrenia. Parents suffering this form of psychosis may bring their child to the pediatrician and voice no concern about their own health or well-being; however, the physician may notice or be told by family members or even by the parent of certain significant prodromal symptoms such as social withdrawal, work impairment, peculiar behaviors, deterioration in dress and personal hygiene, flat affect, circumstantial speech, and bizarre or magical ideas. These preliminary symptoms may progress to bizarre delusions, ideas of persecution, auditory or visual hallucinations, incoherent and illogical speech, or marked poverty of speech. The diagnosis is easier if the physician has known the family a long time and has actually witnessed these personality changes take place in a period of months or perhaps years. Even so, the appearance of any of the above symptoms in a parent may well indicate the presence of a serious mental illness and the need for a psychiatric consultation for the parent.

AFFECTIVE DISORDERS

The affective disorders are manifested by a serious disturbance of mood. The emotion is much more intense and prolonged than normal and actually colors the whole psychic and social life. It generally involves either extreme depression and slowed activity or elation and overactivity. While the illness may appear at any time of life, most episodes occur with sufficient severity that a diagnosis can be made before age 30. Although there may be a neglect of personal appearance and an impairment of ability to work, preoccupation with delusions, hallucinations, and bizarre ideas is absent. In a manic episode the person may have a subjective sense of tremendous well-being, but the illness is apparent by extreme overactivity, restlessness, talkativeness, flight of ideas, grandiosity, insomnia, distractibility, and excessive involvement in many activities, with blatantly poor judgment in social and business affairs. During a major depressive episode, the individual feels and looks miserable, speech and movements are slow, and the facial expression appears dejected. There are feelings of hopelessness, worthlessness, and despair. There may be many disturbances of autonomic functions such as appetite, bowels, and sleep. Suicidal ideation is often present, and suicidal risk can be serious.

EFFECTS ON CHILD'S DEVELOPMENT AND FAMILY LIFE

Although few pediatricians are trained to treat the mental disorders of adults, they cannot ignore such illnesses when they are present in one or both parents of a child patient because of (1) possible adverse, sometimes even tragic, consequences for the child and (2) the physician's obligation to assist suffering individuals in obtaining treatment.

Anthony (1969), Anthony and Benedek (1970), and Bolman and Bohien (1979) have studied large numbers of children who have psychotic parents, mostly of the schizophrenic type. Compared with control subjects, these children as a group were found to be significantly at risk for a variety of developmental, emotional, and mental illnesses. Weissman (1979) has similarly studied children whose parents have suffered a significant depressive illness. To date, research has not been sufficient to permit prediction of exactly which children will develop mental disorders themselves, nor the form in which their subsequent problems will manifest. Recognizing that a very large percentage of these "at risk" children do not seem subsequently to suffer adverse consequences at all, Garmezy (1974) is studying the children themselves. He postulates that there may be an inherent vulnerability factor within each child which can account for the fact that some children are less affected than their siblings or other "at risk" peers.

CASE

Twelve-year-old Joseph was brought for psychiatric consultation by his father "to see if he needs help coping with the intense family stress and particularly with his feelings about his mother."

Shortly before his eleventh birthday his mother developed an acute schizophrenic psychosis. During psychotic episodes she had paranoid delusions with religious visions. She required Joseph to pray with her while she expressed fears of dying and confessed various sexual sins she believed she had committed. On one occasion she accused Joseph of being "Antichrist and a child of the devil." She attacked him and attempted to kill with a knife as the "voices" told her. Following her hospitalization, the parents had been unable to re-establish their relationship and were very recently divorced. Custody was placed with the father.

By history from several sources, Joseph was symptom-free. Direct examination failed to reveal any signs of psychosis or neurosis. He revealed an excellent intellectual grasp of his mother's illness and strong affection for her. He denied being "afraid of her anymore," but refused to visit her at her request because "she might get sick and try to kill me again."

The acuteness of the mother's illness, its relatively short duration, Joseph's good understanding of the situation, and the history of a stable premorbid

family adjustment all pointed to a good prognosis for Joe. Rather than offer psychotherapy, it was decided merely to observe his development by periodic check-ups. At the end of three years, Joseph continues to make a good social and academic adjustment and is free of subjective symptoms. The mother has stayed out of the hospital and is employed. Joseph has re-established a relationship with her, visiting weekly and spending one weekend per month with her without anxiety or any particular stress.

In another study Anthony (1970) found some similar developmental and mental problems in children whose parents were not psychotic but were suffering serious chronic physical illnesses. Most investigators agree that the amount of psychiatric risk for children whose parents suffer psychosis depends upon a number of factors such as genetic etiology in certain conditions, the premorbid adjustment of the family, the family's socioeconomic and cultural level, the severity and duration of the parental illness, and possibly the vulnerability of individual children.

Research data at this point are insufficient to permit us to propose specific primary preventive measures for any individual child with mentally ill parents. However, that these children as a group are at risk for future psychiatric problems to a degree much greater than other children, that chronicity of the parental illness seems very significant, and that family suffering is often very great all point to the need for prompt diagnosis and treatment of these parents.

DIAGNOSING AND REFERRING PARENTS

Since helping mentally ill parents may seem so difficult and frustrating, the physician may tend to ignore the parental behavior and hope the matter will somehow resolve itself; however, this is not possible if there is risk of imminent danger to the child or if the parent's mental state is actually interfering with the child's proper treatment. While the management of such situations is seldom easy, the results of careful work and planning with the parents can often be very gratifying.

There are so many variables that no foolproof outline of procedures in these cases can be given, and space does not permit a detailed review of all possible contingencies; however, a few general guidelines are presented in Table 42–1.

1. Be alert to the possibility that a parent may be suffering mental illness.

CASE

Dr. Y, a senior house officer, consulted the hospital psychiatrist. One of his eight-year-old patients was dying. The father expressed concern about his wife. She had been keeping vigil at the bedside without relief for 10 days. She was exhausted. A year ago she had been treated for a serious depression. He feared that if the child died, the mother might commit suicide. The consulting psychiatrist recommended that Dr. Y see both parents, express his concern for the stress they were experiencing, reiterate his knowledge of the mother's past history, recommend they obtain a psychiatric consultation, and offer to telephone the mother's therapist or arrange an appointment with the inhospital psychiatrist.

Unfortunately, a serious emergency occurred and Dr. Y did not get to see these parents immediately. In the meantime the child died, and the father, not the mother, attempted to hang himself. He was rescued and hospitalized on the psychiatric service of a nearby adult general hospital. A routine follow-up of the family at eight weeks revealed the father had been discharged from the hospital to outpatient treatment status and the mother was not receiving treatment. Their grief was still quite severe, but they were going about the work of reintegrating their family in constructive ways.

It was subsequently learned that the father also had a long history of recurring depression. When families are under severe stress, it is often very difficult to determine who, if anyone, in the family needs psychiatric help. The father's contention that the mother was most in need was, of course, incorrect, even though he probably believed it himself. It is quite possible

Table 42–1. GUIDELINES FOR DEALING WITH PSYCHOTIC PARENTS*

1. Be alert to the possibility that a parent may be suffering mental illness.
2. Try to maintain a "helping, nonjudgmental" attitude.
3. Plan the timing and the method of confronting the parents very carefully.
4. When mental illness is suspected, one must include both parents in some of the discussions.

*See text for full discussion and case studies.

that if both parents could have been interviewed together before the child died, this near-tragic incident could have been averted.

2. Try to maintain a "helping, nonjudgmental" attitude.

Most adults in the child-helping professions overidentify with children and from time to time have intense urges to rescue children from their "ignorant" or "evil" or "sick" parents. This may make us act hastily and alienate the parent(s). The parents are inseparable from both the child's psychic life and his reality life. If we fail to form a trusting, workable relationship with the parents, we most surely will fail in our treatment of the child. The physician who himself has had a parent who suffered a psychosis may have extreme difficulty in obtaining enough empathy and objectivity to effectively refer a parent to a psychiatrist. If so, assistance from a trusted colleague may be necessary.

3. Plan the timing and the method of confronting the parents very carefully.

It can be difficult and sometimes impossible to gain the trust of a mentally ill parent. Even so, confrontation must be deferred until the parent understands your true concern for the entire family. Words must be chosen carefully. Parents can usually talk about their own nervousness, sadness, worries, stress, and tension but cannot talk about their ineptness as parents, their bad judgment, their noxious influence on their own child, their mistakes, or their "strangeness" as compared with the community norm. If parents can be brought to talk about their own nervousness, family stresses, etc., it is fairly easy to take the next step and talk about the need for special help.

4. When mental illness is suspected, one must include both parents in some of the discussions.

The ill parent will find such confrontations extremely stressful and needs all the support and understanding the spouse may be able to provide. The physician needs the spouse to make certain his findings and recommendations are understood and carried out. The risk of further alienating an already estranged couple is a very real one and sometimes cannot be avoided. Tact and much patience are required. If neither parent is able to see and accept the fact that the psychotic parent is in need of special help, there is no point in arguing with them. The physician cannot force the parent to seek psychiatric consultation, yet he must make his findings and recommendations as forthrightly as possible without disparagement. If there has been child abuse, one must make the legal reports required by law in most states with the parents knowledge but not necessarily consent. If there is no suspicion of child abuse, one can only hope that one of his colleagues, to whom they most surely will turn, will concur and will also have the courage to confront them. In due time they may come to see the problem and take appropriate action.

When the parent suffers schizophrenia, psychiatric referral may seem nearly impossible; however, one must never underestimate the capacity of the ill parent to have some rational insight and to love his child. The following is an example:

Dear Dr. M.:

I have seen Donald D., your eight-year-old patient, and his parents regularly for the past three months.

At the time of your referral, Donald showed many symptoms of a depressive neurosis of six months' duration. His academic performance had dropped to near failing. The teacher reported decreased attention and poor concentration. He lost interest in many of his play activities, was irritable, had trouble getting along with other children, and cried a great deal.

Donald's father has suffered a major mental illness with strong paranoid trends for more than 10 years. Mr. D. has been in trouble with the law a number of times for angry public outbursts and creating disturbances. Sometime last year he began to develop grandiose ideas, refused to take his medication, and became increasingly delusional. This had happened before, but this time the situation became so acute that he had to be committed to a mental hospital. During and after the hospitalization he filed for divorce and his wife filed a countersuit. On one occasion he took the child without the mother's knowledge and refused to reveal his whereabouts. There has been open fighting in front of the child.

Needless to say, Donald was extremely upset by all of this and his only solution would be for the parents to get back together, although he was not very hopeful that this would happen. He had essentially quit working in school and went around in a rather morose state most of the time.

By the time I first saw Mr. D. he seemed to have recovered considerably from his mental illness, although he is disabled also for some physical condition. He has been disabled since before Donald's birth and has been extremely close to the child, doing much of the day-to-day care as well as helping him with his homework and providing much of his recreation. There seems to be a genuine positive bond between the child and the father. At the time I saw Mr. D., he was on his medication and had some insight into his delusional ideas, realizing that they were part of his illness and were not true,

Because of the disturbances he had raised he was under court order to continue taking his medication. While he seemed to have some insight into his illness and his need for continued medication, his wife was not convinced that he would voluntarily follow the recommended treatment. As Mr. D.'s condition improved, Mrs. D. began permitting visitiation because "Donald cried so hard and begged to see his father." Gradually over the last few weeks, each parent has dropped their legal suits against the other. Mr. D. moved back into the home and they are going to try to resume their marriage. Mr. D. has continued his treatment with Dr. P. and according to him has no intention of stopping treatment as he did last summer. In spite of the seriousness of his mental illness, Donald was never included in the delusions and at this time I do not see Mr. D. as a potential threat to the boy. In fact, his affection for Donald seems to be a positive factor in keeping him on his treatment regimen.

The changes in Donald have been very dramatic in that he has now resumed his school activities and according to both parents he is like his "old self." Naturally, such a family situation can be precarious for the child. However, I think you and I are both in a position to help Donald should sudden chaos break out again.

Signed,

Dr. S.
Psychiatrist

When the parent suffers an affective disorder the technical aspects of a psychiatric referral may be easier, but it can be time consuming and emotionally taxing for the physician. The following is an example:

CASE

Fourteen-year-old Ralph H. was admitted to the burn unit with first and second degree burns over 80 per cent of his body. The family home was completely destroyed by a catastrophic fire in which a younger brother died. A psychiatric consultation was requested to determine if hypnosis and relaxation therapy could reduce the patient's excessive pain and decrease the amount of narcotics required for dressing changes.

The boy's mother, age 34, was obviously grief-stricken and highly anxious. She said her doctor had prescribed Vistaril (hydroxyzine pamoate) to calm her. It helped but she had run out. She asked for and received a prescription for a four-day supply to help her through the younger child's funeral.

Over the next five days Mrs. H. became increasingly agitated and overtalkative. Her speech became loud and rambling. She was unable to sleep even with strong sedatives, and she refused food. She had taken the entire four day supply of Vistaril in the first 18 hours and was still unable to sleep. She was preoccupied with religious concerns over sin and salvation and accosted strangers to pray with her, and her personal grooming deteriorated. Her visits to her son were upsetting to him and disruptive to the entire ward.

Mr. H. contacted the social worker to express concern over his wife's mental state. There was a strong history of affective disorders in Mrs. H.'s family, and she herself had suffered extreme and prolonged mood swings for years but not to the present degree. Arrangements were made for Mr. and Mrs. H. and the social worker to meet in the psychiatrist's office.

Mrs. H. arrived 20 minutes early. She sat on the floor and jumped up frequently to talk loudly and incoherently to any passerby. In the office she produced a 20-page sheaf of papers, which she said she had stayed up all night writing to prove to the doctor "I'm not insane." The handwriting was large and expansive. The content was rambling, disconnected, and incomprehensible. Poems from her childhood and incomplete scripture quotations were randomly inserted throughout. Her speech was very rapid. She berated her husband for "plotting to have me committed," then within a few seconds she would pet and kiss him while loudly proclaiming what a wonderful and loving man he was. She was alternately belligerent and jovial. She admitted she was nervous and possibly needed treatment. When she was told that she needed to come into the hospital for treatment because the attempts to medicate her as an outpatient had failed to help her, she became very angry and verbally abusive. (No mention of her failure to follow treatment direction was made.) She then tried to rationalize her symptoms away, followed by cajoling, pleading, and finally threatening to kill herself if made to go to the hospital. No attempt was made to reason with her, since she seemed so distraught and irrational. The doctor would merely interrupt her rapid-fire speech from time to time and calmly repeat the treatment recommendations. She demanded to talk with her minister. The husband agreed to get him as soon as possible and he would visit her in the psychiatric unit. She then asked him if he would have her committed if she didn't sign herself into the hospital. He said he would but he hoped she would go voluntarily (a courageous man). She then cried loudly for several minutes. She dried her eyes, sighed deeply, and said, "Well, let's go and get this over with." As she left with her husband and social worker, she shouted, "I'm sure going to tell the minister how badly you've treated me. You'll have to answer to him."

Mrs. H. did not respond well to the milieu therapy and several tranquilizer medications during the first two weeks. Changes in medication were made and she began to improve. She was permitted visitation with her son, and both were discharged from their hospitals six weeks later. (It was fortunate that the adult hospital was adjacent to the children's hospital and that a psychiatric bed was available when needed.)

The author has purposely selected cases with good outcomes to offset the general prejudice that psychotic parents cannot be helped. There are many cases that do not have such fortunate outcomes, especially if we cannot obtain cooperation from at least one of the parents. In such instances the physician may be powerless to help. Every effort is made to avoid using the courts. Not only do parents experience court referrals as an insult to their dignity, but some judges rigidly apply old laws pertaining to the rights of parents and cannot comprehend such vague concepts as psychological abuse of children. However, recently more and more courts are accepting the philosophy of "the best interests of the child."

It is important that such psychiatric referrals are clearly made for the benefit of the parents and not just to protect the child. It is important that the physician state his recommendations and his reasons as simply and clearly as possible. He should avoid being judgmental or argumentative while at the same time firmly holding his ground.

REFERENCES

American Psychiatric Association: Diagnostic and Statistical Manual of Mental Disorders, 3rd Ed. Washington, D.C., American Psychiatric Association, 1980.

Anthony, E. J.: A clinical evaluation of children with psychotic parents. Am. J. Psychiatry, *126*:177–184, 1969.

Anthony, E. J., and Benedek, T. (Eds.): Parenthood: Its Psychology and Psychopathology. London, J. & A. Churchill Ltd., 1970.

Anthony, E. J.: The impact of mental and physical disorders on family life. Am. J. Psychiatry, *127*:138–146, 1970.

Bolman, W. M., and Bolian, G. C.: Infants and children in families with psychotic parents. *In* Nospitz, J. D. (Ed.): Basic Handbook of Child Psychiatry. New York, Basic Books, Inc., 1979, pp. 234–235.

Garmezy, N.: The study of competence in children at risk for severe psychopathology. *In* Anthony, E. J., and Koupernik, C. (Eds.): The Child in His Family: Children at Psychiatric Risk. New York, John Wiley, 1974, pp. 77–98.

Weissman, M. M.: Depressed parents and their children: Implications for prevention. *In* Nospitz, J. D. (Ed.): Basic Handbook of Child Psychiatry. New York, Basic Books, Inc., 1979, pp. 292–299.

43

RUNAWAYS

Deborah Klein Walker, Ed.D.

OVERVIEW

The runaway youth phenomenon is not unique to the present period within the United States. In fact, ever since the American society was formed, there have been youth who have run away from home for a variety of reasons. Some popularized examples of runaway youths are Mark Twain's Huckleberry Finn and Tom Sawyer in frontier Missouri, the wandering groups of transient boys of the depression years during the 1930s, and the hippies or "flower children" of the late 1960s.

How these runaways have been viewed by members of our culture has been determined largely by social, political, and economic factors present at the time. "Running away" is difficult to define, explain, and therefore, study, because it is a complex, relatively rare psychological and sociological phenomenon. Thus it is often difficult to distinguish fact from fiction about running away and to make meaningful recommendations for management and treatment of youth who run away from home.

DEFINITION

Some of the key factors included in definitions of a runaway are (1) age, (2) parent's permission or consent, (3) psychological characteristics, (4) inclusion in missing persons records, (5) identification by a juvenile court, (6) child knowledge about consequences of his/her action, (7) time elapsed since youth ran away, (8) where he/she ran from, (9) where he/she ran to, and (10) previous runaway behaviors. Because of a need to have a uniform definition for research and service purposes, the following behavioral definition of running away has been used by most providers, policymakers, and researchers during the past decade: **A runaway is a youth under 18 years of age who is gone from home for at least overnight without his/**

RUNAWAY FACTS

A runaway is a youth under 18 years of age who is gone from home for at least overnight without parental permission or consent.

The majority of runaways
- —leave home only once
- —leave on the spur of the moment
- —leave after an argument or fight at home
- —stay with friends within the community
- —have no contacts with police or social service agencies
- —return home voluntarily

A small minority of runaways (less than 5 per cent) visit runaway shelters or experience sexual or physical victimization while on the run.

Family and parent-child problems are the major causes of runaway behavior.

Primary and secondary prevention strategies should include the family.

her parent(s)' permission or consent. Use of this behavioral definition, which eliminates the intent of the youth's behavior, can be problematic, since some youth—especially older males—fit the behavioral definition but claim they are not running away from home (Walker, 1983).

Related terms such as "throwaway youth," and "street youth" should not be used interchangeably with runaway youth. A throwaway youth is one who is not ready to leave his/her family but is told by word or action that he/she is no longer welcome there. A street youth is a child under 18 years of age who ran away and who has been on his or her own without employment or a stable residence for several months or more. Homeless youth include those who have been thrown out or pushed out, who left home by mutual agreement with their parents, or who for one reason or another cannot go home again.

PREVALENCE OF RUNNING AWAY

Estimates of the prevalence of running away from home vary from 1 to 25 per cent of the youth population, depending on the definition of running away, the source of the estimate (e.g., youth, parent, etc.), the methodology (e.g., telephone interview, class survey, household interview, etc.), and the sample used (Walker, 1983). The higher estimates of running away come from studies of self-reported delinquency behaviors, which have included a question about running away from home. In the two studies that have used random probability samples, estimates from the youth interviews are consistently higher than those from the parent interviews (Brennan et al., 1978; Opinion Research Corporation, 1976).

The most frequently used estimate today comes from a 1975 national statistical survey conducted by the Opinion Research Corporation (1976). Based on telephone interviews with a nationwide probability sample of households containing youth ages 10 to 17, 1.7 per cent of all youth (or 3.0 per cent of youth households) had run away (i.e., been absent from home without parental permission or consent for at least overnight) during the previous year and 8.3 per cent of all youth households had ever experienced such an event. Interestingly, only 47 per cent of the parents considered their youth's reported behavior during the past year to be a runaway event.

PREDISPOSING FACTORS

Two main orientations dominate the literature concerning the causes of runaway behavior. The large majority of older studies (before 1970) use a traditional psychopathological approach that attributes the basic reasons for running away to characteristics within the individual youth. Using this model, runaway youths are described as having psychoneurotic reactions, poor impulse control, uncontrollable acting-out impulses, depression, anxiety, and strong inner tensions. Contrasted with this psychodynamic orientation is the view of runaway behavior as primarily a function of environmental pressures. This orientation, which has dominated the literature during the past decade, describes running away as a reaction to intolerable home situations (e.g., physical abuse, alcoholic parents, poor economic conditions, etc.).

Besides the importance of internal and external factors in determining runaway behavior, findings from in-depth population-based studies support the view that running away also can be a positive and natural step in the normal process of growing up. These studies also show that the majority of runaways—the one-time runners—are not different from their "normal healthy" peers who had never run away, and that a small minority of runaways—the multiple runners—have problems that suggest some psychopathology or severe family disruption. These multiple runners are significantly different on a variety of home, school, and peer variables from both the one-time runners and the nonrunners (Brennan et al., 1978; Walker, 1983).

The one finding that is consistent across all studies—regardless of definition, methodology, and theoretical approach employed—is that runaways experience some type of family problem. Problems with school, friends, or the police are often mentioned and important but are seldom primary.

In conclusion, practitioners and researchers agree that there are several types of runaway youths. Indices that can be used to profile runaway types and to screen for pre-runaway situations include the following: (1) with respect to family—withdrawal of love by parents, parental remoteness and disinterest, disorganized or ineffective discipline practices, and high conflict over freedom and autonomy; (2) with respect to schools—loss of aspiration and involvement, academic failure, perceived denial of access to desirable school roles; and (3) with respect to peer—high levels of antisocial attitudes and behaviors (including running away) among friends, high levels of normative peer pressure toward antisocial behaviors, and large amounts of time spent with friends coupled with minimal time spent with parents (Brennan et al., 1978).

RUNAWAY EPISODES

Most runaways leave home spontaneously after an argument or violent fight with their parents. In the majority of runaway cases, parents did not expect the child to run away and had not sought help for a parent-child or family problem. Most of these episodes are not reported by parents to the police. Traveling by foot with only the clothes they had on when they left home, the majority of runaway youths stay in a friends' home within ten miles of home in their own town. Fewer than 5 per cent of all runaways go to a runaway house or shelter and/or experience violent or sexual victimization. The majority of runaway youth return home voluntarily in less than one week. Most runaways have no contact with the police while on the run; those who do are frequently returned home without arrest. Very few youth and/or families make use of social or health agencies after the youth returns home. The vast majority of runaways are on their first and often only run; the runaway repeater is definitely in the minority of the runaway population. Street youth and homeless youth are part of this selected minority of the runaway youths who frequently get the attention of the media (Brennan et al., 1978; Opinion Research Corp., 1976; Walker, 1983).

MANAGEMENT

Although various treatment recommendations flow logically from what is known about the causes of running away, little evidence about the efficacy of various prevention strategies exists. Because running away is a family and not a court problem, both primary and secondary prevention strategies should focus on the family whenever possible (Morgan, 1982). Primary prevention activities should consist of asking youth and their families about the pre-runaway conditions and other adolescent risk behaviors that tend to be highly associated with running away, followed by referrals to other providers and agencies who specialize in family counseling and therapy. In addition, referral of youth at risk to appropriate school, community, recreation, and employment programs may also help to change the situations that ultimately lead some youth to run away from home.

Secondary prevention strategies should similarly focus on the family. Since most of the youth who run away from home return without contacting any formal agency or professional, the pediatrician should inquire of families with known runaways to determine those at risk for repeated runaway behaviors and refer these families to mental health agencies and professionals for counseling and therapy (Gordon and Beyer, 1981).

A toll-free, 24-hour nationwide telephone number (800-621-4000) can be used by youth away from home who wish to contact their parents and/or need assistance. In the large majority of cases in which the youth does return home, parents and practitioners are advised to handle the situation as one might a serious drug incident or suicide attempt, i.e., focus on the positive feelings of the parents upon the youth's safe return rather than on the anger and amount of hardship the parents have experienced.

The best source of help for the youth who is on the run is often the community's runaway shelter if one exists. These runaway shelters, supported in large part by monies from the Runaway Youth Program (Title III of the Juvenile Justice and Delinquency Prevention Act of 1974), tend to serve a subset of the runaway youth population which includes the most vulnerable runaways—those who are younger, female, and have traveled the farthest (Berkeley Planning Associates, 1982). These programs, staffed by youth professionals trained in crisis intervention, typically provide short-term shelter along with individual and group counseling. Federal law requires that youth stay a maximum of 15 days and that the agency contact the youth's parents within 72 hours. Parents are involved whenever possible with the goal of reuniting the youth with his/her family. Aftercare services should be offered by these programs to the youth and his/her family once the youth returns home. In those cases where returning the youth to the family is not possible, an alternative placement (e.g., foster care, group home, independent living situation) is sought for the youth.

Finally, the legal status of youth with respect to a variety of domains (health care, employment, marriage, driving, alcohol use, etc.) is important to consider in planning services for runaway youth. These legal statutes and related codes vary considerably from state to state. Currently, in most states, running away is considered a "status offense"; the runaway is classified as a "child/person in need of services" rather than as a juvenile delinquent. In order to most effectively help runaways and their families, a pediatrician should be aware of their legal status and of the various services available in the community which can be used to help them and their families. In those cases in which the necessary services are not available, the pediatrician can play an important role as an advocate for the appropriate primary and secondary prevention programs for runaway youths and their families.

The National Fund for Runaway Children is administered by Act Together, a national nonprofit agency that promotes comprehensive services to "high-risk," troubled youth. Its goals are to raise the public's awareness of America's runaway youth; promote the development of runaway prevention and service programs; advocate needed resources and responsive programs at the federal, state, and local levels; and help programs work more effeciently and effectively. For more information, contact the National Fund for Runaway Children, c/o Act Together, 1511 K Street, N. W., Suite 805, Washington, DC 20005 (202) 783–6417.

REFERENCES

Berkeley Planning Associates: The National Runaway Youth Program: Client Services and Outcomes. Berkeley, CA, Berkeley Planning Associates, 1982.

Brennan, T., Huizinga, D., and Elliot, D.: The Social Psychology of Runaways. Lexington, MA, D. C. Heath, 1978.

Gordon, J. S., and Beyer, M. (Eds.): Reaching Troubled Youth: Runaways and Community Mental Health. Rockville, MD, U.S. Department of Health and Human Services, NIMH Publication 81-955, 1981.

Morgan, D. J.: Runaways: Jurisdiction, dynamics and treatment. J. Marital Family Ther., 5:121, 1982.

Opinion Research Corporation: National Statistical Survey of Runaway Youth. Princeton, N.J. Opinion Research Corporation, 1976.

Walker, D. K.: Runaway youth. *In* Moore, P. S., and Gardner, J. (Eds.): Adolescent Health: Issues and Crises. Boston, Appleton-Century-Crofts, in press.

44

ADOLESCENT OUT-OF-CONTROL BEHAVIOR

Stanford B. Friedman, M.D.

"My boy no longer minds—I have lost all control over him."

Frustrated parent of an adolescent

The above remark reflects a frequent fear of parents in our culture—the fear that they will not be able to "handle" the behavior of their child when he or she reaches adolescence. While raising children is usually viewed as a pleasurable task by parents, coping with a teen-ager is not. Why is this so?

First, there are almost always antecedent behavior problems, albeit minor, in childhood, and parents sense that things will only get worse as their child enters adolescence. This generally takes the form of relatively benign disregard of parental requests by the child—refusal to turn off the television set and go to bed or "forgetting" to take out the garbage. Parents battle with children over such issues, which may end in the child *finally* conforming to parental demands. More frequently, the parent "gives in" to the child, feeling that further struggle is not worthwhile and "it is easier to do it myself." Inquiry by the pediatrician regarding this early stage of parent-child interaction is the first step in providing anticipatory guidance to prevent later adolescent out-of-control behavior. When eliciting a history of nonconformance, the pediatrician should determine whether the problem is primarily unrealistic expectations by the parents or inability of the parents to clearly define their expectations *and* communicate to the child the consequences of his disobedience. The pediatrician also should be alert to the common practice among parents of asking their children to do numerous tasks with the hope that at least a small percentage will actually be done. This obviously leads the child to "play the percentages."

Second, parents frequently do not have an understanding of normal teen-age behavior. They find it difficult to view "negativistic" and self-centered behavior as a healthy and desirable developmental process, reflecting the need of the adolescent to establish a greater degree of autonomy and independence. A developmental task for *parents* is to aid in the separation between themselves and their teen-agers. Many parents find this increasing separation distressing and tend to maintain a role of protection and advocacy. For instance, to allow an adolescent, by himself, to resolve a problem at school may actually be guilt-provoking to the parents, who feel that they are derelict in not helping their "child." It is virtually impossible for some parents to experience the transition from "our problem" to "his problem." Obviously this issue is a matter of degree, but the physician should encourage increasing responsibility, independence, and privileges for the young adolescent (Friedman and Sarles, 1980).

Third, parents may not appreciate that adolescence is a period of experimentation. A trial of marijuana should not be equated with drug abuse. Yet, many parents are so fearful that their teen-ager may get involved with drugs—or sex—that they constantly are looking for clues indicative of these behaviors. This parental vigilance frequently leads to violation of the adolescent's healthy need for privacy; no longer is it appropriate for the youngster to share all of his life with his parents.

Lastly, the behavior of their own teen-ager may threaten parents by reminding them of earlier problems they had as adolescents. It is difficult to guide a teen-ager when one's own adolescent conflicts about sexuality were never resolved or views about drugs clarified. Erik Erikson has stated: "The generation gap is just another way of saying that the younger generation makes overt what is covert in the older generation; the child expresses openly what the parent represses."

As mentioned, the pediatrician's optimal approach to adolescent out-of-control behavior is earlier anticipatory guidance. However, the pediatrician often is confronted with this problem only when a crisis has occurred in his teen-age patient, such as a delinquent act, runaway behavior, or parental suspicion of drug abuse. He should first determine to what degree the parents have truly lost "control" over their adolescent's behavior. The question, "Does your girl *ever* mind?" frequently elicits a response that indicates compliance when the parent is firm or loses his temper. This represents "pseudo" loss of control and indicates that the parents might benefit from counseling directed toward techniques for setting limits on their teen-agers behavior. Such counseling should include (1) defining reasonable and realistic parental expectations, (2) advice on how parents should communicate these expectations to their teen-ager, and (3) establishment of reasonable consequences if these expectations are not met.

In evaluating parental expectations, the pediatrician should focus on the common practice of unwittingly *exploiting* an adolescent. Excellent academic achievement or superior athletic performance may be encouraged or demanded, not so much for the benefit of the adolescent as to bring "glory to the family." Such expectations may serve to boost the ego of the parent, but may not be consistent with the teen-ager's priorities or needs. Likewise, high moral standards may be demanded to offer proof that a mother or father is a "good parent." Teen-agers perceive that such demands are not primarily motivated by their best interests and frequently retaliate by engaging in unacceptable behavior. The author heard from one 16-year-old girl from a family influential in their community: "The look of horror on my mother's face when I told her I was pregnant made it all worthwhile!" Parents holding positions of status in the community, such as physicians and members of the clergy, are particularly vulnerable to such behaviors, as the adolescent keenly senses.

A common problem of communication is the difficulty parents have in sharing their concerns with their teen-ager. To be home from a dance early so as to be rested the next day to study for an exam is a *good* reason for a curfew but frequently is not the *real* reason—the true concern of the parent may be the fear that their teen-ager may engage in sexual activity after the dance! Adolescents easily perceive the falseness of the stated reason and rebel, whereas a sharing of true concerns may be the basis of honest and helpful communication between parent and teen-ager. Such discussions allow the teen-ager to have input into limit-setting of his or her behavior—far preferable to the teen-ager merely being told, "Your mother and I decided last night that you must be home by 11:00 o'clock." If the parents differ on issues, resolving them by rational discussion and compromise is a good model for adolescents to observe.

Teen-agers should be aware of the consequences of violating their parent's wishes. Only then can they weigh the pro's and con's of any given behavior. As with the expression of parental expectations, the consequences of unacceptable behavior should be explained in specific, concrete terms. Telling a teen-ager that he "will be punished" if he is not home by a specific time is overly vague. In addition, the consequences or punishment should be enforceable and reasonable. Restricting a teen-ager to the house for a month for a minor infraction only leads to the parents' not following through on the punishment, and their attempt to set limits on their teen-ager's behavior becomes a series of meaningless threats.

In counseling sessions, the pediatrician should *avoid* giving advice based upon a value system devleoped as a result of his own upbringing as an adolescent. Equally important, the pediatrician should not project onto his teen-age patient the goals and values he has for his own child. Finally, the pediatrician should view his patient's behavior both in terms of a theoretical framework of adolescent development and of empirical knowledge of *current* adolescent behavior. A purely intuitive approach to teen-age problems generally is not successful (Felice and Friedman, 1982).

It is imperative to determine if the teen-ager's unacceptable behavior is actually being encouraged by one or both parents, often in subtle ways. Pediatricians frequently cannot accept the notion that parents could possibly be promoting the very behavior they claim they are attempting to control. The answer to this apparent paradox is an understanding that the "encouragement" is unconscious, as is the vicarious satisfaction derived by the parents (Johnson and Szurek, 1954). Indication that such a process exists within the family structure may be elicited by obtaining a *detailed* account of how the parent reacts to the teen-ager's behavior. Does the parent repeatedly request a "blow-by-blow" description of the "unacceptable behavior," and appear to enjoy hearing about these escapades? Are punishments not actually enforced? Is the teen-ager repeatedly put in situations in which the behavior is apt to reoccur? Is the behavior partially excused by statments such as, "Of course, I was like that as a youngster" or "I guess all boys go through this phase"? And lastly, does the parent, while describing the behavior, appear unconcerned or actually smile while relating his concerns to the pediatrician.

If the pediatrician makes the clinical judgment that the adolescent's behavior is truly

Basic Steps in Evaluating Adolescent Out-of-Control Behavior

Is the teen-ager's behavior really a "problem"?
What are the real fears of the parents regarding their teen-ager's behavior?
Is the teen-ager's behavior really out of control?
What are the pre-adolescent out-of-control behaviors?
Is the parent(s) encouraging the out-of-control behavior to meet their own needs?
Is the teen-ager being exploited by the parent(s)?

beyond parental control, a serious problem may exist. In these instances, the vast majority of the adolescents will have a past history of significant deviant or problem behavior. Referral to a mental health facility or professional may be the most appropriate action (Phillips et al., 1980). Also, the pediatrician may wish to advise the parents to file a "Child (Person) in Need of Supervision" (CINS or PINS) petition, enabling the court to provide "surrogate" supervision. However, this approach has been seriously challenged as often being detrimental to the adolescent, and it interferes with more effective family-oriented therapy (Morgan, 1982).

Out-of-control behavior often is exaggerated by parents, and the presenting problem should not frighten off the pediatrician. Indeed, the behavior may represent a "cry for help"—to which the pediatrician can respond.

REFERENCES

Felice, M. E., and Friedman, S. B.: Behavioral considerations in the health care of adolescents. Pediatr. Clin. North Am., *29*:399–413, 1982.

Friedman, S. B., and Sarles, R. M.: "Out of control" behavior in adolescents. Pediatr. Clin. North Am., *27*:97–107, 1980.

Johnson, M. J., and Szurek, S. A.: Etiology of antisocial behavior in delinquents and psychopaths. J.A.M.A., *154*:814–817, 1954.

Morgan, O. J.: Runaways: Jurisdiction, dynamics, and treatment. J. Marital Family Ther., Jan. 1982, p. 121–127.

Phillips, S., Sarles, R. M., and Friedman, S. B.: Consultation and referral: When, why, and how. Pediatr. Ann., *9*:36–45, 1980.

45

TODDLER OUT-OF-CONTROL BEHAVIOR

Morris Green, M.D.

The physician is occasionally consulted about a toddler who is described by his parents as "out-of-control," i.e., disobedient, stubborn, intrusive, resistant, and/or hyperactive. In addition to displaying temper tantrums, the child is reported to cry, scream, fight, swear, bite, hit, disturb, and destroy. Sleeping, eating, and bowel training problems may be prominent.

ETIOLOGICAL CONSIDERATIONS

Inexperienced parents unfamiliar with young children may misinterpret and tolerate poorly normal oppositional or autonomous behavior. Those who are insecure in their parental roles may be ambivalent or reluctant to set limits because of a vague apprehension that firmness may harm their child emotionally. Parents who were harshly reared as children may try to compensate by being overly permissive and overindulgent. Parents of children who are chronically ill or handicapped often find it difficult to set effective limits. Mothers who are depressed or grieving, have low self-esteem, or worry about losing their child (vulnerable child syndrome) have inadequate parenting *presence* authority. A grandmother living in the household may undermine a mother's authority. Working mothers, especially single parents, may be too exhausted at the end of the day to be effective. Disagreement between parents may result in inconsistent expectations. Divorce, illness, or other family crisis may lead to a suspension of parenting. Some children evoke negative feelings and expectations because they consciously or unconsciously remind their parents of themselves or some other relative. Other toddlers may be used as scapegoats for family problems.

Neurological impairment or the attention deficit syndrome with hyperactivity may also account for out-of-control behavior. Some toddlers have been unsupervised, unsocialized, emotionally deprived, and insecure owing to family discord, placement in a succession of foster homes, or frequent moves. Some children are temperamentally more difficult to rear than others, especially those who are extremely irregular in sleeping and feeding, withdraw from new stimuli, cry excessively and frantically, and respond very negatively to changes in foods, routines, places, and activities (Thomas et al., 1963).

The toddler's environment may be disorganized, chaotic, crowded, overstimulating, and/or depriving. There may be frequent exposure to parental fights, alcoholism, violence, sexual activity, hunger, and cold. Children who live in mobile homes or small apartments often have little opportunity for vigorous motor activity, especially in cold or rainy weather.

ANTICIPATORY GUIDANCE

Discipline is an appropriate item for inclusion in health supervision visits. In addition to clarifying that "discipline" means to *teach* and to protect, not to punish, the pediatrician should carefully discuss, at the ninth- and twelfth-month visits, autonomy as an approaching and important developmental achievement of the baby and caution that the infant's emerging independent behavior should not be misread simply as the beginning of an adversarial relationship. Curiosity, initiative, and independence need to be presented as normal stage-related behaviors necessary for the development of a sense of competence. The importance of the parents as models for the behavior of their children should be reinforced. The need for consistency among caregivers should be stressed.

Rules and prohibitions, primarily used to ensure the infant or toddler's safety, should be few, and there should be opportunities for the child to learn what are acceptable and unacceptable behaviors. Desired behaviors should be positively reinforced by approving glances, hugs, kisses, and verbal praise: "I like the way you came right to dinner. You are a very good boy." "Thanks for helping get ready for bed. I am proud of you." "I appreciate your not playing with the stereo. Let's read a story now." "You were very nice when mother was talking on the phone. Let's play one of your records." Reading and playing with each child when he or she is behaving well should be recommended. A brief alert may be given before introducing a change: "You have five more minutes to play, and then we'll eat." "I'll read you one more story, and then it is time to go to sleep." Acknowledging potential objections may help the child cooperate: "I know you want to play with Johnny some more, but it's time for dinner." Potential conflict situations and stimuli to undesired behaviors should be avoided whenever possible.

MANAGEMENT

The management of the toddler with out-of-control behavior depends upon the number and duration of the complaints, the cause, and whether the problem is pervasive or limited to interactions with only one parent. The pediatrician's skill and time, the severity of the symptoms, the number of other problems in the family, the status of the marriage, the level of understanding of the parents, and their ability to follow advice determine whether the problem is to be managed by the physician alone, by collaboration with other professionals, or by referral.

The first step is to define the problem, clarify the etiology, observe the child and family interactions and perform a physical and developmental assessment. Problems primarily due to a misunderstanding of stage-related behavior may respond readily to advice, explanation, reeducation, and support. Behavior that is reactive to specific environmental circumstances, places, persons, objects, or activities may be prevented by minimizing exposure to such provocative stimuli. Schedules and routines for sleeping and eating may help structure the child's environment. Proximal physical presence may be advised so that the parent is immediately available to distract the child or interrupt the process: "If you are going to fight, you'll have to sit over here until you can play nicely with Susie."

Other directive suggestions may include opportunities for the child to run and otherwise expend physical energy, for the mother to have at least one afternoon a week away from the child, for a teen-age baby-sitter to play with the child one or two hours a day while the mother has time for herself, and for the parents to have time out together. Enrolling the child in a well-staffed nursery school may also be helpful.

Behavioral modification or contingency management techniques include rewards (praise, kiss, or hug) for good behavior, ignoring the behavior (extinction), and time out. Corporal punishment is not recommended. Extinction, based on the principle that when behavior is not reinforced it will disappear, is not as easy as it may seem and does not work if there are several behaviors to be changed or the parents cannot follow the protocol. This method should be preceded by positive reinforcement of some other desired behavior. Initially, the undesired behavior may increase in frequency. Time-out or social isolation, which may be tried if ignoring the behavior does not work, is not useful in very young children and inappropriate when the problem is due to parental or environmental factors. In the latter event, the pediatrician may wish to collaborate with a social worker, a psychologist, a marriage counselor, or a family therapist in resolution of the problem. When the child is found to have a moderate or marked emotional disorder, referral to a child psychiatrist is indicated.

REFERENCES

Chamberlin, R. W.: Management of preschool behavior problems. Pediatr. Clin. North Am., *21*:33, 1974.

Drabman, R. S., and Jarvie, G.: Counseling parents of children with behavior problems: The use of extinction and time out techniques. Pediatrics, *59*:78, 1977.

Smith, E. E., and VanTassel, E.: Problems of discipline in early childhood. Pediatr. Clin. North Am., *29*:167, 1982.

Thomas, A., Chess, S., Birch, H. G., et al.: Behavioral Individuality in Early Childhood. New York, New York University Press, 1963.

BOOKS EXPLAINING BEHAVIOR FOR PARENTS

Becker, W. C.: Parents are Teachers. Champaign, Ill., Research Press, 1971.

Patterson, G. R.: Living with Children (Revised). Champaign, Ill., Research Press, 1976.

Schaefer, C. E., and Millman, H. L.: How to Help Children Cope with Common Problems. New York, Van Nostrand Reinhold, 1981.

46

PEDIATRIC PSYCHOTHERAPEUTIC SKILLS

James E. Simmons, M.D., and Morris Green, M.D.

Both as primary care physicians and as consultants, pediatricians are increasingly expected to be concerned with the prevention, early detection, and management of psychosocial problems. In preparation for practice, the pediatrician should

— have a scientific curiosity about human behavior;

— use the pediatric interview skillfully as the basic tool for pediatric diagnosis and as a way to help patients psychologically;

— perform a physical examination that includes physical and mental status findings, provides reassurance for the family, and promotes a constructive physician-patient relationship;

— deal at some level simultaneously with the diagnosis and treatment of both the biomedical and the psychosocial aspects of pediatrics;

— convey to the child and family that, in the doctor's view, social, psychological, and physical health are of equal importance;

— be aware of feelings within himself or herself and his patients;

— give parents and child the feeling that they are understood;

— gain the patient's acceptance, when that is feasible, of the relevance of psychosocial factors to the complaint;

— help the child form a realistic assessment of his capabilities;

— deal with feelings of anxiety, anger, and depression;

— counsel and clarify;

— support the child's healthy adjustment to situations that realistically will not change;

— have the child like and trust him, be

comfortable and friendly, and relate in a strongly positive fashion; and

— gain the patient's cooperation in the therapeutic plan.

THE PSYCHOTHERAPEUTIC ROLE OF THE PEDIATRICIAN

The psychotherapeutic contribution of the pediatrician is utilized in the following clinical situations:

1. The continuing care of well children, including those living in one-parent, adoptive, or foster homes or with working mothers, through anticipatory guidance, early intervention, and management of identified problems.

2. The management of family crises such as separation, divorce, death, suicide, accidents, the birth of an infant with a handicap, child abuse and neglect, and sexual assault. (Most families are reluctant to impose on their physician, but they need to know prospectively of his interest and availability at such times.)

3. Preparation of children for hospitalization and surgery.

4. The care of those disorders for which pediatric diagnostic and *management* skills are appropriate—failure to thrive, rumination, developmental delay, breath-holding spells, feeding problems, temper tantrums, pica, sleep disorders, separation difficulties, tics, school avoidance, school underachievement, anorexia nervosa, enuresis, psychogenic somatic complaints (recurrent abdominal pain, chronic fatigue, headaches, chest pain, and vomiting), and the psychological aspects of long-term illness and handicap.

5. The management of those disorders for which diagnostic and *referral* skills are needed, including infantile autism, failure of maternal attachment, delinquency, gender identity disorders, chronic depression, child custody, parental emotional illness, and the child and family who are resistant to pediatric intervention. Some pediatricians with a special interest and training will manage some of those disorders; others will establish a relationship with psychiatrists and refer those patients needing extended or intensive assistance.

When behavior problems or family crises are identified in health supervision or illness visits and there is insufficient time in the physician's schedule for their proper clarification or management, the patient should be offered a return appointment, depending upon the magnitude of the problem. Likewise, when the pediatrician is asked to see a child in consultation because of a psychosocial problem, an initial visit of appropriate length should be scheduled. In either case, the parent should be advised prospectively of what the fee will be, based on the time involved and comparable to the fee for other pediatric services. Return visits may be as long as 60 minutes or as brief as 20 minutes. (See pp. 5–6 for discussion of Level I, II, and III care.) In those cases in which the physician merely wishes to use periodic positive re-enforcement as part of continuity of care for such problems as enuresis, encopresis, school refusal, anorexia nervosa, or weight control, visits may last only a few minutes. For patients who come from some distance, follow-up may be done by phone. Most pediatricians with a special interest in psychosocial problems schedule these patients at a time when they are less under the pressure of seeing acutely ill children or when an associate is available for that purpose.

The psychotherapeutic role of the pediatrician is integrated throughout this book, especially in the chapters on interviewing and on health promotion and in this section on psychosocial-developmental disorders. The present discussion presents a summary of some of the useful pediatric psychological therapies.

The ability of the pediatrician to assign a precise nosologic diagnosis to a problem or to use a specific psychotherapeutic technique is not as important as his ability to understand and formulate what is going on and to achieve the kind of relationship in which he is perceived as a mature, accepting, sincere, and empathetic physician in whom the patient has confidence, to whom he can relate easily, and by whom he feels understood. In addition to his knowledge base and technical skills, the pediatrician in his psychotherapeutic work with children and families draws upon his feelings, his intuitive awareness, and his clinical judgments as to what may help.

Identification, another important process through which the patient borrows strength from his physician's knowledge, experience, judgment, and attitudes, has been described by Solnit as

> a complex psychologic process through which attitudes and motives are conveyed from one person to another as a result of common experiences which cumulatively lead to characteristic relations of one person to another. In the pediatrician-child and pediatrician-parent relations the common experi-

ences in health care should gradually enable the child and his parents to identify with the pediatrician's attitudes toward the child's physical and psychologic growth and development, the child's resources that enable him to master stress and illness, the child's increasing capacities to care for himself with confidence, and the parents as responsible, developing adults. The physician's partial identifications with the attitudes of the child and his family are, of course, involved in his capacity for empathy.

Identification may develop quickly or require weeks or even months. The physician who has cared for a child since birth has a decided advantage in that the identification so essential for psychotherapeutic work has often been established before the psychological or social problem becomes manifest. A new physician must start to build such a relationship. Some children and some parents will resist such closeness out of fear or anger. If such a mutual identification and trust have not developed with a pediatrician who has cared for the child over many months or years, referral to another physician should be seriously considered. The same caveat applies if the physician-parent relationship is too close, e.g., relatives or other intimate personal ties between families.

PSYCHOLOGICAL THERAPIES AND PROCESSES AVAILABLE TO THE PEDIATRICIAN

The Pediatric Interview

This preeminent psychotherapeutic tool of the pediatrician is discussed in Chapter 28, p. 238, and in several other chapters. The principles cited there will be elaborated upon in this chapter.

There are many good reasons why the clarification of the problem(s) and ventilation that occur in the interview are therapeutic. Surprisingly often, problems such as excessive fears, sleep disturbances, disobedience, sadness, poor school performance, and other behavioral concerns have existed for months or years without the child and *both* parents forthrightly identifying the difficulty, airing their differing views, and discussing possible solutions. Too often, the parents as well as the patient consider the child to be bad or immature or just "going through a stage." Any discussions that may have occurred have been in times of crisis when tempers were out of control and empathic understanding impossible. Parents blame each other for poor handling of the situation. The child may well feel unloved, misunderstood, and even abused. There is an unspoken but obvious demand that each wants the other to change his behavior or personality with essentially no guidance on how that change may be effected or any assurance that such change will really produce any rewards. Some parents zealously search for harsher and more sophisticated forms of punishments and then are confounded that the child does not become happier, less aggressive, and more mature.

In the pediatric interview(s), the child may come to realize for the first time in many years that his parents really do care and they are not just hostile tyrants. Parents may be able to see their spouses in a less judgmental, more understanding light and begin to negotiate and compromise instead of terminating discussion in an angry deadlock. The presence of the physician permits ventilation of feelings with social control and prevents noxious retaliation or endless accusations and counteraccusations. For the very first time, the parents may listen to their child's feelings without interrupting, shaming, or punishing. All of these results can be effective outcomes of ventilation and problem identification through the interview.

Although the pediatric interview can be very therapeutic, the problems and conflicts may be so chronic, deep seated, or unconscious and the individual or family psychopathology so severe that this psychotherapeutic tool, in itself, is not sufficient to effect improvement; nonetheless, it is effective often enough that it must be considered the first step in therapy.

The Physical Examination

The physical examination is necessary not only to detect physical illness or abnormalities but to reassure the child and parents and help establish the functional etiology of the symptoms. Parents and children always have trouble accepting the psychogenic nature of their symptoms, especially the somatic type problems.

CASE

A young mother became very concerned about her three-year-old child's constipation, which she considered very pathological. Physical and laboratory examinations with reassurance failed to relieve her anxiety and she began "doctor-shopping." Only after learning of the recent death of this mother's sister due to cancer could one doctor explain the

difference between the sister's and the child's bowel symptoms. By helping her talk about her grieving over her sister's death, her emotional preoccupation with her child's health was interrupted.

The doctor was aware that several other physicians previously consulted had not found any bowel pathology. After his own careful history and examinations led him to the same conclusion, he carefully explained his lack of positive findings to the mother. She nodded in agreement and thanked the doctor but remained tense and did not seem relieved. The doctor noted aloud that she still seemed worried and, perhaps, anxious about the child. Although this was denied, the physician waited expectantly in silence for a few moments. The mother then giggled nervously and volunteered that the doctor would probably see her as a neurotic, overprotective mother but she did worry about her child's health: "I just can't help it." When she was asked to be more specific about her worries, she again recited the child's symptoms: "sometimes very large stools, may go two days with no B.M., sometimes it's a funny color, child doesn't eat well, sometimes she cries out in the night" (the mother was near tears). In response to the doctor's question: "Can you tell me the worst fear you've had about your child no matter how ridiculous or far-fetched it may seem?" the mother began to cry openly and said she just couldn't stand it if she lost her child. It was a terrible blow when her sister died of cancer seven months ago. Since then, obsessed with the possible death of her child, she had begun sleeping with the child and could no longer leave her with a sitter. Her husband became angry and accused her of being silly, neurotic, and no longer caring for him. When the mother was asked to tell more about her sister's terminal illness, she gave a lengthy account of the illness, its treatment, and the emotional strain on the family. As she talked, her crying diminished. The doctor told the mother he was certain the child did not have cancer; however, he could understand her continued concern. For now, he would not recommend any further "tests" or any medication. She should continue "to observe" the child. (This latter statement may seem countertherapeutic; however, the mother would continue to watch the child closely anyway, and his statement reassured her that he does not criticize or ridicule her for having that "need.")

The doctor invited the mother to return in a few days for further discussions when he had more time in his schedule. He expressed concern that her sister's death might be having an adverse effect upon the mother's relationships with her child and her husband. He asked that the husband accompany her on the next visit so that the doctor could also answer his questions.

At the appointed time, both parents arrived. The mother seemed more relaxed. She said she felt better and the child was doing "O.K." She smiled with some embarrassment, saying she hadn't realized the powerful effect her sister's death had had on her. For months, she had assisted her parents with hospitalizations, home care, and, finally, the funeral arrangements. People had complimented her on her stoicism and efficiency. "I guess I was just holding it all inside," she said. The rest of the interview was spent explaining the findings to the father and discussing with both parents how they could rearrange the sleeping practices and resume a normal social life.

Fortunately, this case responded well to brief psychotherapy with the mother; however, if there had been a pre-existing marital problem or a mental illness in either parent, such prompt improvement would probably not have occurred, and the doctor might have referred the parents for further psychiatric treatment or counseling. It is important that such family crises be resolved quickly before symptoms and undesirable behaviors become chronic and refractory to treatment. Sometimes clinicians have difficulty understanding why such an apparently simple situation could not have been resolved by the family itself, but emotions do not follow logic.

Supportive Measures

Supportive measures such as counseling and education are always more effective if both parents participate. Sometimes a professional parent educator or a group such as "Parent Effectiveness Training" (P.E.T.) is needed. Many intelligent parents, especially those isolated from their own primary families, need much more education and guidance in matters of child development, education, discipline, nutrition, and routine health care than the practitioner can provide alone. Efforts should be made to increase the child's self-esteem by praise from his family and teachers; identification of academic, sports, or vocational roles in which he or she can gain a feeling of competence; training in social and coping skills, grooming, and assertiveness; recognition of personal strengths; and dealing with feelings of anger, disappointment, and fear of rejection and of new situations. Linking the family to social supports and family counselors is another therapeutic measure.

Remedial Education

Any child who is not progressing scholastically needs and deserves a psychoeducational evaluation and, possibly, remedial education. Such evaluations must be performed by a state-certified or otherwise qualified psychologist and in cooperation with the special education section of the child's school.

Possible reasons for the presenting complaint of learning problems are discussed in Chapters 80 and 81, pp. 492 and 497. The physician can best help the child with learning problems by insisting upon and participating in a careful assessment for causes and the formulation of a well-planned remedial program. All too often the parents have guessed at the cause(s) and let the problem compound itself while they use punishments, bribes, tutoring, and other "common sense," shot-gun approaches to solve the problem.

Marriage and Other Counseling

Although this type of therapy is not usually undertaken by the pediatrician, he must make tactful inquiries into the relationship between the parents and help them decide whether or not to seek professional marriage therapy. When parents do reveal their marital struggles, it is often difficult for the physician to remain objective and nonjudgmental and to avoid giving simplistic advice. The physician can give some advice about things they might try, but if the relationship then does not improve, the lack of positive change can be used as evidence that assistance from a marriage therapist is needed. At times, seeking help from their clergyman is more acceptable to parents, and this may be encouraged. One must remember, however, that some clergy have had special training and are skillful in counseling couples, whereas many others are not capable of helping in such situations. Most parents know or think they know that the answer is simply for their partner to change his/her behavior, attitudes, and even personality. It often takes considerable skill to help them see that such simplistic notions do not really resolve the issues.

Although there may seem to be a direct cause-effect relationship between the child's symptoms or emotional status and the state of the marriage, one cannot assume that marriage therapy will automatically cure the child, especially if the situation is chronic. The child may also need therapy. There are some situations in which the child's emotional problems actually seem to be the cause of the parental conflicts. When there are such multiple problems or confusion regarding cause(s) and type of therapy needed, the pediatrician will no doubt advise consultation with a child psychiatrist or other mental health specialist.

In counseling related to other problems, e.g., genetics or chronic disease, the pediatrician's job is to provide reality-based information leading to decision-making by the patient.

Family Therapy

Family therapy consists of directing attention to all the problems of all of the family members and, perhaps, introducing several types of therapy or remedial programs for individual family members. Often, treatment of the whole family requires a team of health and mental health experts.

Family group psychotherapy is a relatively new and still somewhat experimental form of therapy about which some reasonably scientific data are gradually being accumulated. Most professionals agree that in family group psychotherapy the therapeutic focus is on the pathological interaction patterns among family members rather than on the personal psychopathology of the individuals within the family. Specialized advanced training is needed to obtain the skills necessary for family group psychotherapy.

Environmental Changes

Often, making changes in the environment seems to be a logical way to help the child, and parents may ask the physician's advice on such matters. Environmental changes include reassignment of authority roles in the family; rearrangement of bedrooms; increased interactions between a parent and child; changing teachers; changing schools; changing neighborhoods; rearrangement of custody and visitation agreements; foster home placement; boarding school; a short-term psychiatric hospitalization; or referral for more long-term therapy in a psychiatric residential treatment center.

Environmental changes are seldom a panacea, as they always carry the risk of not helping or of making matters worse. Recommendations for environmental change, therefore, must be based upon a thorough understanding of the child and family and not just the vague hope that it might help. Such actions should not be taken hastily and must be made after risk factors have been thoroughly calculated. The risk factors (pros and cons) of such action must be thoroughly discussed with the parents and child. The ultimate decision, the cost, and the responsibility for outcome must, of course, rest with the parents and the child if old enough.

The child must also be aware of the risk in order to avoid a possible devastating sense of failure if the plan does not work out as well as the child and parents had hoped. He must also be given a face-saving alternative plan should a placement or other environmental change not prove to be the best answer.

Re-education of Emotionally Disturbed Children (Hobbs)

Based on the notion that the symptoms of the troubled and troubling child reflect transactions between the child and other significant people in his or her life, the re-education model has developed teacher-counselors as new mental health professionals. Re-education programs utilize a blend of operant conditioning and group process.

Insight-Producing Psychotherapy

"Insight" means self-understanding, which, in turn, helps patients understand the psychological meaning of unwanted or distressing feelings, attitudes, and behavior in such a way that they can bring about lasting changes in themselves. Supportive and all other types of therapy can produce some self-understanding or insight even though the special techniques for producing insight are not used. Insight-producing psychotherapy usually follows the psychoanalytical model, and its primary focus or aim is to bring patients to an understanding of the unconscious elements behind their symptoms or problems in ways that will produce lasting improvement.

By contrast, the supportive therapies are designed to relieve the patient of stressful feelings. Any insight that simultaneously occurs is an incidental bonus. Supportive therapies can and sometimes do result in long-lasting improvement; however, in the case of chronic neuroses stemming from long-existing unconscious conflicts such as phobias, compulsions, and certain kinds of behavioral problems and learning inhibitions, a deeper, more probing type of therapy is needed.

Such treatment is extremely time-consuming. Insight-producing techniques can be used in individual talking therapy, play therapy, peer group therapy, and family group psychotherapy. This type of therapy cannot be adequately learned from books or a brief continuing medical education course alone but rather requires lengthy supervised training as well as intensive reading and study. Some chronic neuroses and personality disturbances are very refractory to any other form of therapy. It may be necessary to see the child for several hours per week over months, even years, while at the same time providing counsel and guidance for the parents. For these reasons this type of therapy requires referral to a child psychiatrist or another mental health professional specifically trained to offer the psychoanalytical type of psychotherapy.

Behavioral Therapy

In contrast to insight-producing psychotherapy, behavior therapy does not concern itself with unconscious mental phenomena but rather with the here-and-now interaction of the individual with his environment. Behavior therapy, also called "behavior modification," is based upon the scientific principles of operant conditioning.

The principles of operant conditioning and the major tenets of psychoanalysis are not contradictory or in opposition to each other, as the popular press and some scientists would have us believe. Both sciences are dedicated to the study and comprehension of behavior. Operant conditioning concerns itself with the external relations between people and environmental factors which affect behavior, whereas psychoanalysis focuses upon the internal factors affecting behavior. Obviously many processes within the psyche as well as within the environment are relevant to how a person acts at any given moment and how his behavior patterns or personality develop.

Behavior modification has long been used to "shape" the behavior of or train animals. Near the middle of this century, some psychologists began using these same principles to study the processes of personality development and as a form of therapy for emotional disturbances in both children and adults. The controversy between advocates of these two disparate theoretical schools of thought has centered on whether operant conditioning principles or psychoanalytic tenets are more relevant to personality development, more effective in producing lasting changes in the personality or in emotional disorders, and more cost-effective and carry fewer hazards for long-term personality adjustment. Although these serious differences of opinion remain largely unresolved, many eclectic-minded clinicians find therapeutic tools from both of these schools useful in different situations.

Space does not permit a full dissertation on the use of behavior modification as a form of psychological treatment. The following principles of operant conditioning can be useful in advising parents in matters of discipline and day-to-day training of their children (see Ferster, 1963, p. 303, and other references listed below):

1. Specific behaviors are influenced by the effect they have upon the individual's environment.
2. Positive stimulation (reward or reinforcement) reinforces or encourages the repetition of specific behaviors. For example, if purely by trial and error, the child finds that certain behaviors produce a desired response (reward) from his parents, he will repeat that behavior until it becomes a more or less fixed part of his behavior repetoire.
3. In a similar fashion, children mold or shape the behavior of their parents.
4. Failure to receive reinforcement (reward or stimulation) tends to extinguish that particular behavior from the individual's behavior repetoire.
5. Negative or aversive reinforcement also tends to extinguish specific behaviors.
6. Behaviors become a fixed part of the personality more easily and much more quickly than they are extinguished.
7. In the context of operant conditioning theory, the stimulus (reinforcer) follows the response (i.e., the environmental reaction acts as a stimulus for a behavior to be repeated).
8. The rate of reinforcement, its intensity, and whether reinforcement occurs continuously or intermittently all have a differential effect upon the degree to which any certain behavior becomes "fixed" into the personality.
9. Different individuals have varying susceptibility to the behavior of others.
10. Susceptibility of individuals to different kinds of reinforcements varies from individual to individual and from time to time in the same individual.

Operant processes occur between and among individuals constantly without much thought or conscious intent on the part of the participants. It is much more complicated than simple reward and punishment, which is the "common sense" approach used by most parents. A simple example is the comedian who repeats his act as long as he receives a positive audience response. However, he may need a long series of poor audience responses before he will rewrite his act. Clinical experience has shown that emotionally overwrought, especially depressed, parents will often inadvertently fail to respond to or reinforce desirable behaviors in their children or their spouses while often reinforcing a host of undesirable behaviors.

The pediatrician who is knowledgeable about operant conditioning may wish to use these principles in advising parents on home management or in the treatment of certain behavior disorders or habit disturbances. Of course, the physician must teach the parents operant principles for them to assist effectively in the therapy. The objective is to change the child's behavior, not necessarily his psychopathology. However, clinical practice has shown that if the underlying pathology is not too chronic or deep, actual personality improvement does occur with changes in behavior. This is especially true for behaviors such as temper tantrums, enuresis, and sleep problems in preschool children, which usually are not due to significant psychopathology. With many of these problems, behavioral modification of the symptom results in more acceptance of the child by the parents and may prevent later disturbances. Behavior modification therapy can be lengthy and tedious and require considerable motivation and sophistication on the part of both the physician and the parents.

In the hospital setting, behavior modification concepts can be incorporated into the ward care plan, with the hospital staff serving as co-therapists, e.g., weight gain tied to privileges. In special schools for the retarded or emotionally disturbed child, behavior modification has been effective in promoting desired behaviors and extinguishing undesirable ones, with all of the staff actively participating in the program. For obvious reasons, knowledgeable participation of the parents in the treatment is still very important in institutional settings. In the outpatient setting, parental participation is crucial. Behavior response patterns are often so resistive to change that appropriate reinforcement must be used by all adults who are attending the child any time of his day. Parents must be made conscious of the fact that the therapy will fail if they inadvertently reinforce a particular behavior that the clinician is trying to extinguish.

Biofeedback

Biofeedback training utilizes an electronic apparatus to train the patient to control the amplitude of the physiological response such as skin temperature, muscle tone, blood pressure, heart rate, or sphincter tone by providing immediate feedback to the subject on the status of that variable. Biofeedback therapy for such conditions as migraine and muscle contraction headaches, cerebral palsy, and encopresis are in an investigational stage.

Hypnosis and Hypnotherapy

In the past 25 to 30 years, hypnosis has been gradually losing its unsavory reputation, owing in part to the success of hypnotherapy as a brief method of dealing with war neuroses or "battle fatigue" during World War II. In 1958 the Council on Mental Health of the American Medical Association recommended that instruction in hypnosis be included in the curriculum of medical schools and postgraduate training centers. There is now some hope that future research in biofeedback, in neurotransmitters, and in brain physiology will further lessen the mystique surrounding hypnosis and provide it with some scientific roots.

Hypnosis is an altered state of consciousness, not a therapy in itself. When combined with various forms of medical and psychological treatments, hypnosis becomes hypnotherapy. Children, even very young ones, can be hypnotized rather easily and many thoroughly enjoy it. Hypnotherapy can accelerate and augment the impact of many psychological and medical interventions. Although abreactions such as portrayed in the treatment of war neuroses can occur in children, more traditional play psychotherapy is probably just as good for relieving the child with an acute post-traumatic stress disorder. Hypnotherapy, however, can be an excellent adjunct with many other physical and psychological problems. No one can be hypnotized against his or her will. When a trance is induced, the hypnotist is not able to produce changes in the patient; however, in hypnotherapy the child is helped through relaxation and imagery techniques to master his own anxiety, stress, or pain.

CASE

Carl, age 14½, suffered second and third degree burns of the right hand and arm plus the right side of his neck and face in a gasoline explosion. During his frequent dressing changes, Carl required large amounts of Demerol. Even with medication, he would scream out in intense pain, struggle against his nurses, and require physical restraint. When hypnotherapy was offered Carl as a method of pain control, he readily agreed and a trance state was rather easily induced. Several techniques for reducing the pain in his arm were practiced. He liked and chose the imagery of a faucet which he could imagine he was turning off while simultaneously turning off the pain and producing numbness in his arm. Although he was taught self-hypnosis so he could use this imagery in the absence of the hypnotherapist, he never felt he could produce a good trance state; nonetheless, he was able to control his pain, an outcome that he and the staff felt was good enough.

One morning during rounds, Carl asked to talk about his bleeding and reported the following experience: "Yesterday afternoon during my soaks and dressing change, I was feeling a lot of pain. When the nurse removed the bandages, I looked at my arm and saw that it was bleeding bad. Blood was just dripping down. I got scared and yelled to the nurse to do something. She said, 'Use your faucet, Carl. Shut off the bleeding.' I brought the faucet into my mind and turned it hard. The bleeding stopped to just oozing and I was O.K."

It is theoretically possible that Carl actually produced vascular constriction in his own arm, but that conjecture cannot be proven. An equally plausible explanation is that there were no objective changes in the vessels or the bleeding. Carl was a highly anxious and suggestible child. The bleeding, perhaps seen for the first time, looked profuse to him in his anxious state. It may have been the level of anxiety and not the rate of blood flow which actually changed. Carl was obviously proud of his mastery of his own body and dynamic explanations of the phenomenon were irrelevant to him. The attending nurse related that Carl was in an agitated state, complaining of severe pain and inability to go into a trance. The arm began to bleed and the blood dripped onto the towel. She said to him, "See, Carl, when you panic like this you make your arm bleed. Now use your faucet and turn off the bleeding." The patient relaxed and in a few seconds the blood stopped dripping. Possibly this represented a coincidence of a normal cessation of bleeding in an open wound or the nurse unknowingly putting pressure on Carl's upper arm. Nevertheless, she had participated in Carl's hypnotherapy sessions and was convinced of his ability to control his pain. Both the nurse and Carl were certain that the trance with its attendant relaxation stopped the bleeding.

Hypnotherapy can be used as part of either supportive or insight-producing psychotherapy. In conjunction with supportive psychotherapy, the goals for hypnosis are to improve relaxation and help the child feel more worthy, more capable, more able to contribute to his own sense of well-being, and more in control of both internal and external circumstances. In addition, the hypnosis exercises can remove, or at least ameliorate, distressing symptoms, as illustrated above with Carl. With insight-oriented psychotherapy, hypnosis can be used to enhance the transference and increase the patient's ability to bring unconscious mental processes nearer to consciousness. Although there is no consensus among dynamic psychotherapists about the benefits or dangers of hypnotherapy, many therapists do use hypnosis in selected cases.

Even though children are relatively easily hypnotized, hypnotherapy is not a treatment modality for the untrained amateur. Rather, the physician must take special training and refresher courses in hypnotherapy which are offered annually in various parts of the country. Gardner and Olness (1981) review nearly 40 different induction techniques that can be used. The therapist must have confidence in himself or herself before he or she can obtain the child's and parents' trust. Poorly trained hypnotists have a high failure rate and, for this reason, soon discontinue offering it to their patients.

Selection of appropriate cases and obtaining high motivation and cooperation from the child and both parents are essential. Prior to any attempt to induce a trance, the specific reasons for utilizing hypnosis need to be reviewed. Misconceptions, fears, and questions must be clarified. No matter how distressing a symptom may be, one must always consider that the child may need to keep that symptom for some unconscious neurotic reason.

In summary, hypnotherapy can be an effective adjunct to medical and psychological treatment of many conditions. Special training in hypnotherapy is very important. Cooperation and confidence from the child and both parents are essential prerequisites for successful hypnotherapy.

Psychopharmacological Therapy

No treatment that can benefit a patient should ever be withheld, but the physician must always weigh the possible benefits against potential dangers. Proper data for making intelligent decisions about the use of psychotropic drugs in children have been seriously delayed because of methodological, legal, and ethical problems in performing research and controlled trials with children. The statement "not recommended for individuals under age 12 years" does not mean that the drug will not help a child or that it is *a priori* dangerous for younger persons. It merely means that the necessary data for such judgments are not available. Research on adult patients cannot readily be extrapolated to children. From clinical experiences we do know that the effective therapeutic dosage of many of these drugs is more variable in children than in adults. Side effects, especially extrapyramidal reactions, can also be more severe and occur with lower dosages in younger patients.

On the basis of current knowledge and experience we know that

1. psychotropic drugs can effectively ameliorate target symptoms but do not cure the mental illness or alter the underlying causes.
2. social measures such as psychotherapy, milieu therapy, family counseling, remedial education, and behavioral modification are usually necessary in addition to medication for long-term benefit.
3. careful monitoring of the child on medication is essential because the long-term effects on cognitive functions and growth have not been adequately studied.
4. the attitude of the physician, the parents, and the child toward the medication can interfere with the effectiveness of the treatment.
5. many psychotropic medications are slow acting and their effectiveness depends upon a sustained blood level; therefore, several days to three or four weeks should be allowed for symptomatic relief to occur, and parents should be cautioned against erratic administration of the prescription.
6. most antipsychotic and antidepressant medications alter biogenic amines and block cholinergic receptors. The resulting autonomic side effects, such as blurred vision, dry mouth, constipation, and urinary retention, are usually temporary but may call for dose reduction and a more gradual increase in dose until therapeutic levels are achieved.
7. extrapyramidal side effects can be very troublesome for children and may require a change to a different drug.
8. drug absorption and rate of metabolism vary from child to child and age to age. Therefore, except in emergencies, start with the lowest recommended dosage and increase gradually over weeks.

Antipsychotic Drugs (Major Tranquilizers)

The major classes of antipsychotic drugs are phenothiazines, butyrophenones, thioxanthenes, dibenzoxapines, dihydroindolones, and rauwolfia alkaloids. Since these agents have little or no abuse potential, they are not classified as controlled substances.

The major tranquilizers are recommended only for severely disturbed, usually psychotic children. They may make it possible for a seriously agitated child to be managed at home rather than to be institutionalized. The common side effects of lassitude and drowsiness usually disappear in a few days. Antipsychotic drugs have also been found helpful in the treatment of severe behavior problems marked by combativeness and/or explosive, hyperexcitable outbursts and in the short-term treatment of hyperactive children. Haloperidol, a butyrophenone, has been effective in controlling the motor and vocal tics of Gilles de la Tourette's syndrome as well as in ameliorating psychotic symptoms.

Major tranquilizers are not recommended for anxiety attacks and other neuroses in which minor tranquilizers or psychotherapy are usually effective.

Minor Tranquilizers

The minor tranquilizers have been extensively used in children managed on an ambulatory basis with a variety of neurotic, behavioral, and psychosomatic symptoms. To date, controlled trials have shown equivocal or only minor benefits. Such findings may be due to very difficult research methodological problems rather than ineffectiveness of the drugs. Careful research must continue, but the indiscriminate use of these drugs is to be discouraged.

The minor tranquilizers (antianxiety drugs) are indicated in the treatment of the neuroses. It seems that the higher the level of obvious anxiety in the child, the more effective the medication. These drugs, which act as sedatives, are hypnotic, produce somnolence, relax muscles, and have anticonvulsive effects. They are habituating. Tolerance develops, and withdrawal symptoms can occur upon cessation after long-term usage. Most of these agents have a depressive effect on the medullary centers and, for that reason, have caused death when taken in suicide attempts. Although they are very effective in reducing anxiety, they have little or no effect on psychotic symptoms. The minor tranquilizers are attractive to many physicians and parents because they are rather quick acting and seem more cost-effective when compared with the various types of psychotherapies; however, they only remove target symptoms without changing underlying causes, and long-term usage has dangers for the child.

A growing number of minor tranquilizers have become available, but there is no definitive evidence that one is superior to the others. The physician is referred to the current issue of the Physician's Desk Reference and to Freedman et al. (1976) for a thorough review of these drugs.

Tranquilizer medications are often used for children when they must undergo frightening or painful diagnostic or therapeutic procedures, especially when these interventions must be done repeatedly. For such purposes, the antianxiety drugs (minor tranquilizers) in adequate dosage are preferred over the antipsychotic drugs. Administration of these drugs orally an hour or two before the scheduled procedure is probably useless, since the child's anxiety usually becomes manifest when he learns of his appointment or prepares to leave for the hospital. As stated above, it takes days to weeks for these drugs to reach therapeutic effectiveness. Therefore, we recommend that children who undergo regular, terrifying treatment for cancer or other conditions either be taught self-hypnosis or be placed on antianxiety medication for a week or ten days before each treatment.

Antidepressants

The monoamine oxidase inhibitors (MAO) are not used for children because of the necessary dietary restrictions and the fact that the tricyclic antidepressants are just as effective, if not more so. While officially the tricyclics are usually "not recommended for children under age 6 or 12 years," they have been used for control of persistent enuresis (see p. 253). Children and adolescents often suffer depression in response to temporary stress or a life crisis. These depressions usually remit spontaneously when the stress is removed or resolved. If a careful examination reveals that the child has true depression, a trial on antidepressant medication may be very helpful. (See also Chapter 36, p. 256.)

Central Nervous System Stimulants

These medications include amphetamine sulfate (Benzedrine), dextroamphetamine sulfate (Dexedrine), methylphenidate hydrochloride (Ritalin), pemoline (Cylert), and deanol acetamidobenzoate (Deaner). Such drugs have been used extensively with hyperkinetic impulse problems (attention deficit disorder). When treatment is successful, the results can be dramatic. For unknown reasons, some children will respond to one of these drugs but not to the others. Methods to predict which drug will be most effective are being developed. (See Appendix C, p. 521.)

Family counseling and some form of special education are usually needed whether or not the child responds to the medication. Controlled trials have shown positive benefits on cognitive and perceptual functions. For children with severely disturbed behavior who do not respond to one of the central nervous system stimulants, it may be necessary to prescribe a major tranquilizer for behavior control.

The central nervous system stimulants currently have an invidious reputation with the public because they are often stolen for resale on the street market as "uppers." Parents usually need much reassurance about their safety and lack of addicting potential when the stimulants are legally prescribed and properly supervised.

Collaboration with Other Disciplines

In most instances, the pediatrician can treat the child without the need for collaboration with other professionals. With more severe psychosocial problems, especially if multiple and lengthy visits over a period of months are required, solo management by the pediatrician is generally not practical. In such instances, collaboration with a social worker, clinical psychologist, or child psychiatrist fits better the style of practice of most pediatricians. Whether to use a child psychiatrist or a child psychologist for consultation and referral should be determined more by the personality and skills of the individual than by academic credentials. A group practice of pediatricians may have a sufficient patient volume to support a full- or part-time social worker and/or psychologist; otherwise, the pediatrician may develop a collaborative relationship with a clinical psychologist or social worker in private practice or on the staff of a community social agency or hospital. In other instances, the child and family should be referred to a child psychiatrist or psychologist. Even though academic credentials do not guarantee expertise, the physician has the obligation to make certain that those persons to whom patients are referred meet the accreditation standards for their profession. All states have licensing boards for physicians, and most states license psychologists. An increasing number of states are establishing licensing procedures for social workers. At the national level, education and training requirements are determined for each respective discipline by the National Association of Social Workers, the American Board of Psychology, Inc., and the American Board of Neurology and Psychiatry, Inc. In some areas, state departments of education maintain lists of qualified or certified social workers and psychologists.

Many, but not all, social workers, psychologists, and psychiatrists have had similar training in one or more of the psychotherapies. Psychiatrists are physicians and are also required to have training in clinical neurology and in pharmacology.

The following variables must be considered by the pediatrician in deciding on the need to refer a child with a psychosocial problem:

1. Severity of the problem(s)
2. Chronicity of the problem(s)
3. The child's premorbid adjustment
4. The ability of the child to engage meaningfully with the physician and/or to work on the problem(s)
5. The ability of both parents to participate actively in the treatment
6. The number of other problems in the family and its overall stability
7. The physician's attitudes toward this child, the type of problem this child has, the family, and his own abilities

Certainly, referral should be considered if (1) the symptoms become worse or remain unchanged for more than 90 days; (2) behavior becomes seriously disruptive to ordinary office routines; (3) the situation becomes increasingly complex, with too many family problems requiring considerable time and attention; (4) suicidal tendencies, physical changes, or custody placement, and other sociological problems become evident; and (5) unremitting discomfort on the part of the physician or the family develops.

Table 46–1 provides a guide to help pediatricians screen children for office treatment of psychosocial problems.

Milieu Therapy

Although most of the psychotherapeutic activities of the general pediatrician are conducted in an ambulatory setting, there is an occasional need to hospitalize a school age child or adolescent because of such psychological problems as persistent anorexia, headache, abdominal pain, fatigue, vomiting, or conversion symptoms. The history of such children is often one of frequent absences from school. The care of the child in the hospital is, thus, part of the continuity of care provided by the general pediatrician.

Table 46–1. PSYCHOSOCIAL SCREENING*

The following chart cannot be quantified in absolutes but is offered as a guide to help pediatricians screen children for office treatment of behavioral or emotional problems.

	Finding Usually Points Toward a Good Outcome	Finding Usually Points Toward a Poor Outcome or Necessity for Long, Arduous Treatment
Severity of problem(s)	Symptoms may be somatic but are not life-threatening	Life-threatening to self or others
	Symptoms uncomfortable to child or family but not incapacitating	Behavior dangerous or illegal; symptoms disrupting usual school or work functioning
	Symptoms in one area only, i.e., school, home, society—including friends, personal well-being	Symptoms in all four areas
Chronicity	Symptoms less than 6 months' duration	Symptoms persisting longer than 6 months or chronically, recurring over several years
	Precipitating stress(es) obvious with clear-cut onset of symptoms	Precipitating stress(es) unclear and onset vague or insidious
Child's premorbid adjustment	Has had good physical health	Many minor or major physical problems since conception
	Developmental milestones within normal range	Development delayed or erratic
	Good relationship with both parents and relatively few discipline problems	Poor relationships with one or both parents—clinging, overcompliant, or rebellious
	Smooth progression in preschool and primary grades, academically and socially	Erratic or chronically poor school performance
	Has friendships with peers Has friendships with adults	No friends or only social deviants Intimidated by or defiant of adults
Child's ability to "engage"	Talks easily about non–emotion-laden topics	Does not talk at all or rattles on and on about superficial matters and this persists for four visits
	With encouragement and time can discuss feelings and other confidential matters	Steadfastly distrusts physician and this persists for four visits
	May blame others but will consider his own contribution to the problems	Projects blame without slightest consideration of own role in the problems
	Can state own views even though they may not be conventional	States only what he thinks examiner wishes to hear and this persists for four visits
	Is serious but maintains a sense of humor	No sense of humor or is inappropriately glib or silly
	May be discouraged but hasn't given up hope	Persists with feelings of hopelessness
	Has the capacity to like himself and others	Has no friends and nothing good to say about himself

Table 46–1. PSYCHOSOCIAL SCREENING* *(Continued)*

	Finding Usually Points Toward a Good Outcome	Finding Usually Points Toward a Poor Outcome or Necessity for Long, Arduous Treatment
Parent's ability to participate in treatment	Both parents are willing to come with child for appointments, if indicated	One or both parents resent giving the time, fail appointments, or make excuses
	Parents seek advice but do not monopolize doctor	Parent(s) monopolizes doctor's time or argues with most suggestions
	Parents pay bills promptly and facilitate child's transportation	Parents are vague about financial arrangements and find transporting child a burden
	Parents share responsibility	One parent has abdicated responsibility
	Parents seek/accept marital counseling, if indicated	Parents persistently use sessions to fix blame on each other
	Parents voluntarily sought help	Parents were *forced* to seek help by a social agency or school
	Both parents are free of serious social and mental problems	One or both parents suffer from mental illness or alcoholism
	Parents are not seriously seeking divorce	One or both parents having an affair or seriously seeking divorce
	If divorced, matters of custody, visitation, and support are relatively settled	If divorced, matters of custody, visitation, and support are a constant battle
Stability of family	Relatively little history of mental illness or serious social problems among grandparents, aunts, and uncles	Family history replete with mental and social problems
	Siblings have few problems	Siblings have so many problems you wonder why only one child was brought to you
	Vocational stability of parents	Frequent job changes
	Residential stability	Frequent family moves
	Family crises are handled quickly and smoothly	Family seems to live in a state of chronic crisis
Physician's attitude(s)	Physician likes the child or believes he will come to like him	Physician dislikes child and has trouble knowing why
	Physician likes or respects most of the family members	Physician dislikes the family or has trouble finding any redeeming features about them
	Physician is not shocked, repulsed, angered, or fearful about child's symptoms	Child's symptoms create considerable inner discomfort in the physician
	Physician would like to try to treat this child (family)	Physician fears he/she is not capable of helping this family

*From Simmons, J. E.: Psychiatric Examination of Children, 3rd ed. Philadelphia, Lea & Febiger, 1981, p. 293.

During the hospitalization, a child care plan—a daily schedule of activities and procedures—may help promote recovery. The child who has been compliant in the past, who is able to share with his doctor both positive and negative feelings, and who believes that the physician understands how he or she feels will usually respond well to this approach. Through active participation in the development of the plan, the child identifies with both the program and the physician. This, or any other, therapeutic plan must be explained to the child and the parents each step of the way. Questions should be encouraged—even, at times, insisted upon.

This process requires from the physician a sizeable time investment. Other professionals (nurse, social worker, occupational therapist, physical therapist, nutritionist, school teacher, and child life worker) should be involved early, either individually or in a group meeting. Weekly group inpatient sessions promote suggestions, observations, clarification, consensus, and staff unity.

The schedule, set as close as possible to the patient's estimated tolerance, should fit the child's style, e.g., high achieving, competitive, passive, compliant, or slow to adapt, and reflect his interests, assets, and needs. Presented as the approach the physician regularly uses for children with similar problems, it will, it is hoped, not be sensed as a punitive personal imposition.

After the daily 24-hour schedule is developed and signed off by the child, the physician, and the child's primary nurse, it is posted in a prominent spot next to the child's bed. Bar graphs, stick figures, symbols, clock faces, and sketches may be used to dramatize the chart. In addition to being fully dressed during the day, the child is scheduled to spend only a minimal amount of time in his hospital room during the day. Developmentally appropriate self-care is expected. All time is accounted for, and the term "rest period" is avoided in favor of "personal time" or "scheduled break."

One or two continuing projects on which the child can do some work each day are included. Group (school, child life, ward rap, meals) and individual (physician, nurse, occupational therapist, physical therapist, peer) experiences are included to promote constructive behaviors. The staff is encouraged to convey that the doctor expects his orders, e.g., the caloric content of a meal or for the child to be out of bed, to be followed precisely ("That's just the way things are done here."), and the doctor's *presence* must convey his firm expectation that the child will follow what has been scheduled.

An attempt is made to select a gregarious roommate who helps keep the patient busy. The staff must be encouraged to enforce the schedule even in the face of resistance, anger, delay, manipulativeness, or deception. These possible reactions should be discussed prospectively with the parents. Such challenges are met with cheerful firmness, and the staff is not misled by the illusion of cooperation, e.g., that the child with anorexia will eat merely because she promises to do so.

Nurses are asked not to reinforce the child's complaints by responding to them directly. Incentives for progress are negotiated, and steps toward recovery are rewarded with privileges such as visitors, telephone use, and canteen or library passes. The schedule is revised daily in order to achieve and demonstrate steady progress. Discharge from the hospital is earned by meeting previously determined weight goals, levels of activity, or symptom improvement.

REFERENCES

Brady, J. P.: Behavioral medicine: Scope and promise of an emerging field. Biol. Psychiatry, *16*:319, 1981.

Chamberlin, R. W.: Management of preschool behavior problems. Pediatr. Clin. North Am., *21*:33, 1974.

Drabman, R. S., and Jarvie, G.: Counseling parents of children with behavior problems: The use of extinction and time out techniques. Pediatrics, *59*:78, 1977.

Ferster, C. B.: Essentials of a science of behavior. *In* Nurnberger, J. I., Ferster, C. B., and Brady J. P. (eds.): An Introduction to the Science of Human Behavior. New York, Appleton-Century-Crofts, 1963, p. 199.

Green, M.: Training the pediatrician in the psychosocial aspects of child health. Zero to Three, *2*:5, 1982.

Hobbs, N.: The Troubled and Troubling Child. San Francisco, Jossey-Bass Publishers, 1982.

Olness, K.: Hypnosis in pediatric practice. Curr. Probl. Pediatr., *12*:5, 1981.

Senn., M. J. E.: The psychotherapeutic role of the pediatrician. Pediatrics, *2*:147, 1948.

Senn, M. J. E.: Emotions and symptoms in pediatric practice. Adv. Pediatr., *3*:69, 1948.

Simmons, J. E.: Psychiatric Examination of children. 3rd ed. Philadelphia, Lea & Febiger, 1981, pp. 293–296.

Solnit, A. J.: Psychotherapeutic role of the pediatrician. *In* Green, M., and Haggerty, R. J. (Eds.): Ambulatory Pediatrics II. Philadelphia, W. B. Saunders Co., 1977, p. 197.

BIOFEEDBACK

Miller, N. E.: Biofeedback and visceral learning. Ann. Rev. Psychol., *29*:373, 1978.

Silver, B. V., and Blanchard, E. B.: Biofeedback and relaxation training in the treatment of psychophysiological disorders: Or are the machines really necessary? J. Behav. Med., *1*:217, 1978.

Whitehead, W. E.: Biofeedback and health care. Behav. Med. Update, *3*:7, 1979.

HYPNOTHERAPY

Gardner, G. G.: Teaching self-hypnosis to children. Int. J. Clin. Hypn., 29:300–312, 1981.

Gardner, G. G., and Olness, K.: Hypnosis and Hypnotherapy with Children. New York, Grune and Stratton, 1981.

PSYCHOPHARMACOLOGICAL THERAPY

Freedman, A. M., Kaplan, H. I., and Sadock, B. J.: Comprehensive Textbook of Psychiatry, 2nd Ed. Baltimore, Williams & Wilkins, 1976.

Physician's Desk Reference. Oradell, N.J., Medical Economics Co., 1982.

47

FAMILY CRISIS AND INTERVENTION

Robert J. Haggerty, M.D.

Recent studies document that acute and chronic stress in families is associated with greater frequency of a wide variety of illnesses and that visits to medical care providers are generally increased by stress, independent of illness (Research on Stress and Human Health, 1981). It is useful to differentiate the stressor (what happens) from stress (the responses of the individual). The nature of the stressor varies but includes death in close relatives, job loss or change, moves, and trouble in school, work, or marriage or with the law. Such events are very common. Families with children experience such upsets on nearly one third of all days (Roghmann, 1973). In the United States, accidents and abuse have been shown to be two to three times more common in families with frequent moves, recent deaths, and evidences of social discord (unmarried mothers, marital problems, unemployment, etc.) (Newberger et al., 1977). Streptococcal infections were seen four times more frequently following stress than during more tranquil times (Meyer and Haggerty, 1962).

Chronic social problems are also correlated with illness. In the Newcastle Study (Spence et al., 1954), children in families with social problems, such as dependency (welfare) or deficiency of care, were twice as likely to have pneumonia in the first five years of life as children from more favored families. Much additional data convincingly demonstrate the association of stress and illness.

Recognizing that such stress is associated with greater risk of illness, several factors have limited the usefulness of this knowledge to clinicians. First, the physiological mechanisms by which stress works are not clear, and logical ways to intervene are not known. In animals and, more recently, in humans a variety of physiological changes have been demonstrated when stress is not mitigated by a supportive environment. Most promising are noninvasive methods to study children, such as pharyngeal secretory IGA (McClelland et al., 1980), which is diminished in certain individuals when they are under stress. Secondly, many children suffer from the same type of social stress without becoming sick. They seem resistant. Some other factor must be involved in addition to the presence of stress. Heredity, coping skills, and social supports seem to be especially important factors in such resistant individuals. Perhaps most important, the clinician asks what he can do practically to help families in stress once they are identified. So much of stress is related to social factors (unemployment, job moves, poverty) that are outside of the individual's control. Even in the more psychologically related stress situations (troubled marriages or delinquency), the ability to solve these problems by the physician is not high.

There are some promising leads, however. Animal and human research shows a widespread biological phenomenon of increased susceptibility to disease when individuals do not receive feedback that their actions are leading to desirable or hoped-for consequences. A key factor appears to be whether one feels able to control the novel situation or not. More stress occurs when the stimulus is unexpected and is unable to be modified or controlled. Teaching children some of the ways to cope with the unexpected may be useful. Lack of a supportive environment, as well as previous life experiences, is a major variable in why some people respond to stress by increased risk of illness or inappropriate use of health services and others do not. This concept provides an avenue through which the clinician can be of help, that is, by enlisting the strength and resources of community support systems to assist families in trouble because their strengths and resources are overwhelmed.

Caplan (1974) points out that in most communities both "generalist" and "specialist" support systems exist. The generalist is more likely a gregarious person who makes human contacts easily. Specialists are frequently people who have personally suffered the same misfortune (i.e., birth of a handicapped child) as indicated in the discussion of family counselors' role in the care of the chronically ill. Group specialists can also be used by the clinician as a support system for his patients, e.g., La Leche League, Parents for Retarded Children, or Parents Anonymous. Peer support groups for students in difficulty, such as the one organized in the public schools of Palo Alto, is another type of endeavor that should be supported in the service of promoting health in one's community.

It may also be possible for children as they grow up to learn to cope with stress more effectively. Innovative educational programs, such as Outward Bound, create controlled crises and stress and then help students to find healthy ways of mastering them. Perhaps, as part of the preparation for marriage or parenthood, educational programs need to be developed to prepare individuals for some of the crises that they must confront. While in the future we may be able to provide children with such skills for mastering crises, it is likely that social support groups will be needed in addition for overwhelming and unplanned crises.

In addition to helping children and adults learn to tolerate stress and engage community support systems for families in trouble, crises offer opportunities for therapeutic intervention. Caplan (1981) has suggested that crises are times when everyday family decision-making, which may have been quite destructive, is more easily changed to a healthier pattern than in more stable times. Since the pediatrician is often the only helping professional involved with families in crises (in part because illness is an acceptable ticket of admission to such help), he can use the crisis as an opportunity to assist families to change some potentially destructive life patterns.

Life-change scales and indices of family risk factors have also been developed, but it is premature to advocate their routine use in clinical practice because of the danger that they may falsely label a family. Since such stress scores are more common in minority and poor families, they could be used inappropriately to label such families as deviant.

The frequency of family crises is high enough in all families to warrant asking about them, especially at times of illness visits, when the severity of the illness seems to be an inappropriate reason for the visit. With such diagnostic alertness and the practice of enlisting social support groups to help families in crises, better health and more appropriate use of services may be the result.

REFERENCES

Caplan, G.: Mastery of stress. Am. J. Psychiatry, *138*:4, 1981.

Caplan, G.: Social Support Systems and Community Mental Health. New York, Behavioral Publ., 1974.

McCelland, D. C., Floor, E., Davidson, R. J., and Saron, C.: Stressed power motivation, sympathetic activation, immune function and illness. J. Human Stress, *6*:11–19, 1980.

Meyer, R. J., and Haggerty, R. J.: Streptococcal infections in families. Pediatrics, *29*:539, 1962.

Newberger, E. H., Reed, R. B., Daniel, J. H., Hyde, J. N., and Kotelchuck, M.: Pediatric social illness: Toward an etiologic classification. Pediatrics, *60*:178, 1977.

Research on Stress and Human Health, Report of a Study. Institute of Medicine, National Academy of Science, Washington, D.C., 1981.

Roghmann, K. J., and Haggerty, R. J.: Daily stress, illness and use of health services in young families. Pediatr. Res., *7*:520, 1973.

Spence, J., Walton, W. S., Miller, F. J. W., and Court, S. D. M.: A Thousand Families in Newcastle-Upon-Tyne. London, Oxford University Press, 1954.

48

HELPING A CHILD COPE WITH THE DEATH OF A LOVED ONE

Morris A. Wessel, M.D.

Parents frequently consult their physician when a child suffers the loss of a loved one through death. They seek advice about how to support and comfort their child at this sad moment. The doctor's guidance during this family crisis can be vital. The manner in which adults care for a bereaved child may determine to what extent the loss remains an overwhelming, unmasterable burden interfering with psychologic development and to what degree it is a stress that he copes with and integrates as he grows and matures. Loss of someone close—uncles, aunts, or grandparents—is a frequent occurrence for most children (in one study such losses occurred once per year for school age children) and offers them opportunities for coping with stress and developing coping skills.

Anyone wishing to help a child during this life crisis must respect his unique way of dealing with the loss. Adults cannot prevent a child from being sad; rather they should seek ways of supporting him in his sadness as he grapples with the loss of someone he loved and who loved him. The physician's task is to help the nurturing adults offer support to the child during his struggle to understand and cope with his feelings about the loss of a loved one.

A child's preparation for understanding death and coping with a loss begins long before the loss occurs. Children of nursery school age can learn that a dead gold fish no longer swims, a lifeless bird lying on the ground cannot sing or fly, and a stiff, motionless dog is unable to romp and play in the fields. The experience of the death of a pet or other animal should be utilized to help a child grasp the concept of *being alive* and *being dead*. Explanations of death using phrases such as "no longer living" and "just resting" are appropriate conceptualizations. Suggesting that the deceased "went to sleep" is unwise. A child may develop fears of going to sleep, wondering if he too might die and "sleep forever."

There is, of course, an enormous difference between the demands placed on a child when an animal dies and those following the loss of a beloved adult or sibling. Prior experience with death of animals, however, provides an opportunity for a child to begin to understand and grapple with the finality of the loss of a human being through death.

The confusion and gloom in a home of a family anticipating a death is bewildering and frightening to a child. Explanations for the disruption of household routines and preoccupation with the care of the sick individual are important. Adults should state the situation in terms of this nature: "Grampa is very sick. The doctors and nurses are doing everything they can to make him comfortable. We're all very sad because he is so sick."

When death is imminent, it is wise to tell a child that the individual may die, even though he may fail to grasp fully the reality of the impending event. The conversation establishes an honest basis for later discussion, when one may say "You remember I said that grandpa was very sick and might die? I'm very sad now to have to tell you that he died a little while ago."

An attempt to protect a child by sending him to the home of relatives or friends is usually a mistake. It postpones the opportunity for dealing with the tragedy immediately. A child suffers not only the loss of the sick person and of his family preoccupied with their own grief, but also the loss of the support of his own bed, toys, and familiar surroundings.

Children experiencing the loss of a loved one wonder whether this could happen to other people who care for them or to themselves. Reassurance must be realistic. None of us knows when we will die. One might say: "I don't think it will happen to any of us for a long time. I (and other relatives) will be here to take care of you." When it is a mother who dies, it is appropriate to say: "We will miss Mommy very much. We will be sad for a long time as we miss her. I will see to it that someone will care for you and do the things for you Mommy used to do."

Adults struggling with their own grief may find it difficult to assume this task, but it is important that they do so. It reassures the child that his nurturing needs will be met, yet at the same time acknowledges his need to express sadness.

If adults cry while discussing the death of a

loved one, it often serves to give the child permission to release his own feelings of desolation. As poignant and heartbreaking as a child's grief may be, he does need to be comforted by those he trusts as he expresses sadness over his loss.

Parents often ask whether or not a child should participate in a funeral. Many children as young as four find the gathering of the family and friends and the ritual a constructive experience. The details of the service should be described and the child should be allowed to choose whether or not to attend. If the child does attend, an adult friend or relative, preferably one who is not deeply involved in grieving, should accompany the child to comfort him and to leave the service with him if necessary. Nothing is sadder than to see a child standing alone at a funeral amidst adults who are so preoccupied with their own grief that they ignore the child completely.

An appropriate way of presenting the choice of attending the funeral would be to say: "We're all very sad because we miss Grandpa so much. I will be sad too. Many grown-ups will cry. There will be music and prayers. Our minister (priest, rabbi) will talk about Grandpa. If you would like to attend with us, I'll ask (a relative or friend) to be with you. Or if you would rather stay at home, that is all right too. Someone you know will be here with you."

It is important to choose one's words carefully when discussing with a child what happens after death. The concept of a life hereafter is difficult for a young child to comprehend. When a family's philosophic belief includes this concept, it can be presented simply: "The body of a dead person is placed in a special box in a cemetery. I will show you where it is. I like to believe that part of the person, their spirit, the part that we love very much, rests in a place called Heaven, where there is no pain or sickness or suffering." It is unwise for parents who have no belief in life hereafter to present this conceptualization, hoping it will help a child cope with his loss. In this instance the child senses insincerity and deviousness, which create confusion and distrust. It is far better to admit, "I really don't know what I believe about what happens after death. All I know is that Grandpa is dead, and he will no longer be with us."

A child who does not wish to attend a funeral may request at a later date to visit the cemetery. It is wise to grant this wish. The fresh grave validates the event. It often helps a child to begin the painful process of adapting to the reality of the loss. The grieving and mourning may continue for many months or years. Although the period of acute grief is usually completed by adults in a year, all human beings experience sad feelings whenever they remember the loss of a loved one. Holidays, birthdays, and anniversaries of deaths are particularly sad moments when families miss loved ones who are no longer present.

Bereaved children often develop a dread of illnesses, even minor ones. A parent's call to a pediatrician concerning a bereaved child's symptoms should evoke a prompt response. This is reassuring to the child, as well as to adults in the family. Furthermore, one must remember that illnesses can occur during bereavement.

Bereaved children who present behavioral symptoms such as clinging, regression, and difficulty in sleeping may be far healthier than the children who deny the loss and present no signs of distress; however, psychological symptoms such as sustained difficulty in sleeping, onset of school difficulties, poor appetite, and weight loss over a period of months suggest a need for psychiatric intervention.

A physician can find professional satisfaction in continuing his relationship with a bereaved family as they grieve, mourn, and regain equilibrium.

All suffering individuals need to know that their doctors care about them. The suggestion that a physician's role is "to cure sometimes, to relieve often, to comfort always" is as true now as when stated by Edward Trudeau more than 50 years ago.

REFERENCES

Furman, E.: A Child's Parent Dies—Studies in Childhood Bereavement. New Haven, Yale University Press, 1974.

Furman, R.: The child's reaction to death in the family. *In* Schoenberg, B., Carr, A., Peretz, D., and Kutscher, A. (Eds.): Loss and Grief—Psychological Management in Medical Practice. New York, Columbia University Press, 1970, pp. 70–86.

Wessel, M.: Death of an adult—and its impact upon the child. Clin. Pediatr., *12*:28–33, 1973.

Wessel, M.: A death in the family: The impact on children. J.A.M.A., *234*:865–866, 1976.

49

THE DEATH OF A NEWBORN

Richard L. Schreiner, M.D.

The effects of the death of a newborn infant are painful and longlasting, whether the baby was stillborn, survived only a few hours, or lived for months. Other than the basic coping skills of the parents, the sensitivity of physicians and the other nursery staff is a major determinant of the outcome of families experiencing a neonatal death. If the infant's physician recognizes that he is uncomfortable working with grieving families, it is important that he arrange for appropriate support for the family from other sources. This is consistent with the principle that one's personal beliefs or reactions should not interfere with a family's need and right to grieve.

Several management techniques have been found useful in providing assistance during this difficult time. Families should always be offered the opportunity to see, touch, and hold the infant prior to and/or after death. Not to have seen their baby deprives the parents of a visual memory of how he or she looked. It is not unusual that their fantasies are much worse than the reality.

Infants who survived only a short period of time may not have been named. It may be helpful in such instances to encourage the family to name the baby, as this adds to the perception of the child as real. A photograph of the baby may be treasured, as may such other tangible remembrances of the child's brief life as nametags, armbands, and locks of hair shaved for IVs.

At the time of death most parents are immobilized in emotional shock, so that information shared with the family at that time may need to be repeated. It may also be helpful to have another family member present during discussions after the baby's death. The option of seeing a chaplain of the appropriate faith should be offered if this service can be readily arranged.

Often it is not what is said but the presence of a caring individual that is remembered by families. A simple, genuine "I'm sorry" or "Can I help in any way?" conveys concern and sympathy. Remarks such as, "You can always have other children" are absolutely contraindicated.

Since parents experience strong reactions at the time of the death and during the weeks and months that follow, it is important that they be prepared. Feelings of shock, guilt, and anger are normal and to be expected. Mothers often report feeling the baby kicking in utero. Other parents awaken thinking they hear their baby crying in another room. Being forewarned of these reactions provides the parents the reassurance that they are not suffering from a mental illness.

Guilt is another normal part of grief. At some point, nearly all parents feel at least partially responsible for the illness and death. Every family can find some event in their lives or the pregnancy itself which they feel might have contributed to the baby's problems: ambivalence about the pregnancy, not following doctor's orders during pregnancy, taking medications or drugs, smoking, previous elective abortions, sexual intercourse late in pregnancy, or lack of prenatal care. We must emphasize to families at the time of death and during later contacts that the illness and death were not their fault.

It would be impossible to overemphasize the need for parental communication. Parents may avoid discussing the baby with each other because of the mistaken but common belief that if the loss is not discussed, the pain will decrease. Although discussions of the dead baby are not without discomfort, attempts to forget the baby will extend unresolved grief and prolong pain. Families who do not anticipate the death and go through grieving have increased illness problems themselves. Parents should be encouraged to talk about the baby, especially between themselves, but also with their family and close friends. In many families, fathers represent a special concern. Some feel they must be "strong." Reassurance that it is appropriate for him to show emotion may ease the father's burden and allow him the freedom to grieve.

Most families have little or no experience in arranging a funeral service, especially for a child, and therefore are unaware that in most cases the cost is much less than a funeral for an adult. The mother should also understand that the funeral can be delayed until she is able to attend.

Each family whose child dies wants to know why. An autopsy may prove useful in answering this question. Families react in a variety of ways to the request for an autopsy. Determining the cause of death may be reassuring for some; other families may feel comfort in knowing that information obtained from the autopsy may benefit other babies. Some families, however, feel their child has "suffered enough already" and choose not to have an autopsy. Another concern is how the autopsy will affect the physical appearance of the baby and whether or not it will necessitate changes in the timing of the funeral.

Before they leave the hospital, it is important to remind the parents to call if they have further problems. They should be given the name and telephone number of the physician or some other person to contact. It may also be helpful to inform them of books and parent groups (The Compassionate Friends, National Headquarters, P. O. Box 1347, Oak Brook, IL 60521). There should be some form of contact with the physician during the next few months. In this follow-up, several goals are appropriate: reinforcing information given to families at the time of the infant's death, ensuring that the grieving process is progressing normally, discussion of future pregnancies, and review of the autopsy report. This follow-up interview or contact may be in person or by telephone. It is ideal to have follow-up contact with the family within a week after the death and once or twice more during the subsequent six months. Programs providing for follow-up may vary widely, but what seems important to families is that some contact with the physician or other medical personnel be made. A note of concern or a phone call can convey the empathy of the physician and lead the way to further contact should the family find that helpful.

Comments which may help:
- I'm sorry.
- I wish there was something I could say.
- Is there anything I can do to help?
- Can I contact anyone for you?

Comments which are not helpful:
- It was God's will.
- You can always have another baby.
- At least you didn't have time to get attached.
- It was for the best.
- I know how you feel.
- He would never have been normal anyway.
- You need to be strong for your wife's/children's sake.

Helpful things the physician can do:
- Be honest but sensitive.
- Provide privacy.
- Provide opportunity to see/touch/hold baby.
- Sit down to talk with the family.
- Discuss guilt feelings.
- Refer to the baby by name and correct gender.
- Provide photograph of baby.
- Bend hospital policies that may interfere with family's needs.
- Discuss funeral arrangements.
- Send a note or card acknowledging the loss.
- Provide follow-up consultation by phone or in person.
- Discuss importance of parental communication.

BOOKS FOR PARENTS

Borg, S., and Lasker, J.: When Pregnancy Fails. Boston, Beacon Press, 1981.

Church, M. J., Chazin, H., and Ewald, E.: When a Baby Dies. Oak Brook, IL, The Compassionate Friends, Inc., 1981.

D'Arcy, P.: Song for Sarah. Wheaton, IL, Shaw Publishers, 1979.

Jensen, A. H.: Healing Grief. Issaquah, WA, Medic Publishing Co., 1980.

Jensen, A. H.: Is There Anything I Can Do to Help? Issaquah, WA, Medic Publishing Co., 1980.

Johnson, J., and Johnson, S. M.: Children Die, Too. Council Bluffs, IA, Centering Corporation, 1978.

Kushner, H. S.: When Bad Things Happen to Good People. New York, Schocken Books, 1981.

Massanari, J., and Massanari, A.: Our Life with Caleb. Philadelphia, Fortress Press, 1976.

McGee J. V.: Death of a Little Child. Pasadena, CA, Through the Bible Books, 1979.

Schiff, H. S.: The Bereaved Parent. New York, Penguin Books, 1977.

Schwiebert, P., and Kirk, P.: When Hello Means Goodbye. Portland, University of Oregon Health Sciences Center, 1981.

REFERENCES

Benfield, D. G., Leib, S. A., and Vollman, J. H.: Grief response of parents to neonatal death and parent participation in deciding care. Pediatrics, *62*:171–177, 1978.

Clyman, R. I., Green, C., Mikkelsen, C., et al.: Do parents utilize physician follow-up after the death of their newborn? Pediatrics, *64*:665–667, 1979.

Kennell, J. H., Slyter, H., and Klaus, M. H.: The mourning response of parents to the death of a newborn infant. N. Engl. J. Med., *283*:344–349, 1970.

Mahan, C. K., and Schreiner, R. L.: Care for the family mourning a perinatal death. *In* Schreiner, R. L. (Ed.): Care of the Newborn. New York, Raven Press, 1980, pp. 203–209.

Schreiner, R. L., Gresham, E. L., and Green, M.: Physician's responsibility to parents after death of an infant. Am. J. Dis. Child., *133*:723–725, 1979.

50

SUDDEN INFANT DEATH SYNDROME AND INFANTILE APNEA

Abraham B. Bergman, M.D.

SUDDEN INFANT DEATH SYNDROME

Sudden infant death syndrome (SIDS) claims about 8000 babies a year in the United States. It is responsible for approximately three deaths of every 1000 live births. After the first week of life, SIDS is the most important single cause of death of infants under one year of age, ranking second only to accidents as the greatest cause of death in children less than 15 years of age. Although much has been learned about SIDS from the increased research efforts of the past decade, the cause or causes remain unknown. Currently there are no means to predict or prevent SIDS.

The tragedy of sudden infant death syndrome, unfortunately, does not end with the death of the baby. Pervasive and long-lasting guilt reactions occurs among family members. The psychiatric morbidity is enormous. The cause of the guilt reactions is lack of information, and prevention of guilt is possible through informed and compassionate counseling.

The parents of a victim of sudden infant death syndrome may have a more difficult time coping with the death than parents of children who die of a better-known disease or whose death is expected. There are three aspects of SIDS that seem to cause an especially profound impact on families: the suddenness of the death, the loss of the child, and the fact that the cause is unknown. The death then causes severe trauma, a grief reaction, and a sense of guilt.

Because a significant relationship between sudden infant death syndrome and socioeconomic class exists, a large number of low-income families who lack personal physicians are unlikely to receive sympathetic support and guidance at a time of great need. These families often feel that this devastating and unexpected loss epitomizes their already existing sense of powerlessness derived from inadequate housing, insufficient food, and poor health. To prevent the psychiatric morbidity accompanying SIDS, programs should exist in each community to ensure that families receive accurate information and compassionate counseling about SIDS.

Management

Immediate. If the clinical picture fits (i.e., previously well infant between one and six months found dead during sleep period), the family can be told: "The cause probably is SIDS, but we must perform a postmortem examination to be sure." Detailed discussions are to be avoided as the shock is too great. Sympathetic listening, on the other hand, is much appreciated.

Autopsy. Autopsies should be performed, if at all possible, both to exclude other causes of sudden death and to provide a desperately sought final answer on the cause of death. Results should be available from the gross autopsy and transmitted promptly to the family.

Certification. The term SIDS on the death certificate, when applicable, helps greatly in the family's resolution of the death.

Information. Besides discussion with an authoritative health professional, written information about SIDS is most helpful, especially in dealing with the questions of relatives and friends. The themes that need to be frequently repeated are "There is no way you could have predicted or prevented the death," and "You are in no way responsible."

Counseling. A visit should be made two to three weeks after the death. At this time, the physician should stress the normality of the characteristic grief-guilt reaction and answer the parents' questions about SIDS. Serious or persistent adjustment reactions warrant referral to a mental health professional.

Special attention should be focused on the reactions of the siblings. These are often veiled. Children are especially vulnerable to guilt feelings about the death of a sibling. Painful as it is, open discussion of the death among family members should be encouraged. Often a good indication of parental coping mechanisms in relation to grief is determined by what parents tell their children about the infant's death. A health professional's visit to the home and interaction with the parents and children quickly reveals areas of need and the probability of future counseling sessions by mental health workers.

Referral or contact with voluntary agencies working with sudden infant death syndrome can be most supportive. Many families gain comfort and support from contact with other families who have lost children to this syndrome. The National SIDS Foundation, Inc. (2 Metro Plaza, Suite 205, 8420 Professional Pl., Landover, MD 20785), an organization with chapters around the country, provides authoritative information about sudden infant death syndrome to both health professionals and parents.

INFANTILE APNEA

Concomitant with the acquisition of more knowledge about SIDS, there has been an explosion of interest in a related problem, infantile apnea, otherwise known as "near-miss" or "aborted" SIDS. The latter two terms are inappropriate, because they imply a close relationship which has not, as yet, been proven.

Whatever the connection between apnea and SIDS, infants who cease to breathe for 15 seconds or longer, or who have briefer episodes associated with cyanosis, brachycardia, or pallor, should be evaluated.

The major known causes of apnea are infections (especially sepsis, meningitis, pertussis, and interstitial pneumonia), anemia, metabolic disturbances, seizure disorders, cardiac rate abnormalities, and gastroesophageal reflux. A careful history and physical examination, including evaluation of neurodevelopmental status, often provide clues that may be confirmed by appropriate laboratory studies. If answers are not forthcoming from a traditional work-up, consultation with a center specializing in evaluation of apnea is advisable. Such centers perform sleep studies consisting of simultaneous monitoring of an electroencephalogram, electro-oculogram, electrocardiogram, electromyogram, and respiration monitoring. Naturally, appropriate intervention is provided when specific lesions are identified. More often than not, however, no etiology for the apneic episodes is found.

Home Monitors

The emotionally charged question of when to employ a home apnea monitor is never easy to answer. The physician must be content to use his clinical judgment and knowledge of the family until further research provides more definitive guidelines.

The author recommends home monitors (a) when the sleep studies corroborate significant apnea without an apparent cause; (b) for the subsequent sibling of an SIDS victim who demonstrates apneic episodes as previously defined; and (c) for subsequent siblings of the SIDS victims when the parental anxiety is so great that the benefits of an "electronic babysitter" might outweigh the psychological costs of life with a monitor.

Apnea monitors should be prescribed only by personnel experienced in their use and capable of providing continuous supervision. This means 24-hour-a-day availability to the family.

Parents should be trained in use and care of the monitor, as well as in cardiopulmonary resuscitation. Local emergency medical personnel should be available for back-up services.

Finally, with more research being conducted on SIDS and recurrent apnea, enthusiastic claims of prevention appearing in the lay media are inevitable. Physicians will be hard pressed to convince anxious parents that the truly significant advances in medicine emerge only after critical peer-review has taken place.

REFERENCE

Beckwith, J. B.: The sudden infant death syndrome. Curr. Probl. Pediatr., 3:8, 1973.

51
PHYSICAL ABUSE

Barton D. Schmitt, M.D.

Physical abuse (or nonaccidental trauma), defined as injuries inflicted by a caretaker, can range in severity from minor bruises to fatal cerebral contusions. Physical punishment that causes bruises or leads to an injury that requires medical treatment is included. Such bruises imply hitting without restraint and punishment outside normal limits. Physical abuse is the most common type of child abuse seen by physicians, accounting for about 75 per cent of the total.

Physicians have three main responsibilities toward abused children: detection, reporting, and prevention. Case finding is especially important in the first six months of life, because the risk of a fatal outcome is high if the diagnosis is missed at this age. In all 50 states the law requires that physicians immediately report all suspected cases of child abuse to the local child protection agency. He should be certain that the telephone number is on his emergencies list. Reluctance to report can lead to a recurrence of injuries or even death. The laws protect physicians from liability if their suspicions should prove unfounded.

EPIDEMIOLOGY

During childhood 1 to 2 per cent of children in the United States are abused. The incidence of abuse, based on number of cases reported, is approximately 900 new cases per million population per year. If physical neglect cases were included, these figures would be much higher. Approximately 10 per cent of injuries seen in a hospital emergency room in children under five years of age are inflicted. The mortality is about 3 per cent, or 2000 deaths per year. The victims of physical abuse are estimated to be one third under one year of age, one third from one to six years of age, and one third over six years of age.

ETIOLOGY

The abuser is a related caretaker in 90 per cent of cases, a male friend of the mother in 5 per cent, an unrelated babysitter in 4 per cent, and a sibling in 1 per cent. Parents who abuse their children come from all ethnic, geographic, religious, educational, occupational, and socioeconomic groups. Groups living in poverty may have an increased incidence of child abuse because of the increased number of crises in their lives (e.g., unemployment and overcrowding) and because they have limited access to resources. An increased incidence of physical abuse has been noted on military bases. Abusive parents tend to be lonely, unhappy, angry individuals who are currently stressed by loss of a job, eviction, marital strife, birth of a child, or physical exhaustion. Less than 10 per cent of these individuals are psychotic or have criminal records. Abusive parents often report that they were physically abused as children. They are most apt to injure their children after being provoked by some misbehavior such as intractable crying, wetting, soiling, or spilling.

HISTORY

Many cases of physical abuse are first suspected because the injury is totally unexplained; others will give a vague explanation such as, "She might have fallen down." More commonly an explanation is offered, but it is implausible. Inconsistencies are common between the history offered of a minor accident and the physical findings of a major injury, or between the history given and the child's developmental level. Stories of babies rolling over on their arms and breaking them or getting their heads caught in the crib and fracturing the skull are fabrications. Also, seeking of medical care is often postponed. While normal parents contact a physician immediately following trauma, some abused children with major injuries are not brought to medical care for hours or days.

PHYSICAL EXAMINATION

Bruises, welts, lacerations, and scars identify physical abuse. Bruises confined to the buttocks and lower back are almost always related to punishment. Finger and thumb prints may be found on the arms where a child has been forcefully grabbed. Hard pinching leaves two circular or curvilinear bruises. A slap mark leaves a bruise on the cheek with two or three parallel lines running through it. Attempts to silence a screaming child with impatient, forced attempts at feeding may lead to bruising of the upper lip and frenulum. Human bite marks are distinctive, paired, crescent-shaped bruises facing each other. When a blunt instrument is used in punishment, a bruise or welt will often resemble it in shape. Loop marks or scars on the skin are secondary to a doubled-over cord or rope. Lash marks are seen after beating with a belt, tree branch, or hard-edged ruler. Choke marks may be seen on the neck, and circumferential tie marks may be seen around the ankles or wrists. The most common sites of accidental bruises are over the forehead, anterior tibia, and bony prominences. A mongolian spot may be mistaken for a bruise, but the color is blue-grey without any red hue.

Burns comprise approximately 10 per cent of physical abuse. Hot solid burns are the easiest to diagnose. The shape of the burn is pathognomonic if the child is held against a heating grate or electric hot plate. Cigarette burns give circular, punched-out lesions of uniform size and are often found on the hands or feet. Bullous impetigo can cause confusion with these. Hot water burns are the most common type of inflicted burn. A dunking burn occurs when a parent holds the thighs against the abdomen and places the buttocks and perineum in scalding water as punishment for enuresis or resistance to toilet training. This results in a circular type of burn restricted to the buttocks and genitals. The hands and feet are spared, which is incompatible with falling into a tub or turning the hot water on while in the bathtub. Forcible immersion of a hand or foot as punishment can be suspected when a burn goes well above the wrist or ankle.

Subdural hematoma is a dangerous inflicted injury, often causing death or serious sequelae. In the classic case, the subdural hematomas are associated with skull fractures, secondary to a direct blow to the head. Over half of the cases of inflicted subdural hematomas have no skull fracture or swelling of the scalp. The mechanism is violent, whiplash-type shaking which leads to tearing of the bridging cerebral veins. Retinal hemorrhages are nearly always present and help to establish this diagnosis. Grab mark bruises of the upper extremities or shoulders may support this diagnosis, as do radiological findings at these sites.

Intra-abdominal injuries are the second most common cause of death in battered children. Affected children present with recurrent vomiting, abdominal distention, absent bowel sounds, localized tenderness, or shock. The abdominal wall is often free of bruises. In order of frequency, the findings are a ruptured liver or spleen, intestinal perforation, traumatic pancreatitis, intramural hematomas, and ruptured blood vessels.

LABORATORY DATA

Tests for a bleeding disorder in an abused child, although rarely indicated, should be performed when the parents deny inflicting the injuries and claim "easy bruising" or the case is a severe one that will definitely be going to court. The tests for bleeding tendencies obviously are not necessary when the parents admit to causing the bruises.

RADIOLOGICAL FINDINGS

When physical abuse is suspected in a child under two years of age, a radiological bone survey consisting of films of skull, thorax, and long bones should be made. Pelvis and spine films can be ordered if any of the preceding films are positive. Between two and five years of age, most children also receive a bone survey unless the child has very mild injuries or is in a supervised setting (e.g., preschool). Over age five, x-rays need to be obtained only if there is bone tenderness or a limited range of motion on physical examination. Clinical findings of a fracture can disappear in one week even without orthopedic care, whereas they persist on radiograph for four to six months. Bone trauma is found in 10 to 20 per cent of physically abused children.

DIAGNOSIS

Most diagnoses can be based solely on the physical findings (Table 51–1). Certain bruises,

Table 51–1. DIAGNOSTIC CRITERIA FOR PHYSICAL ABUSE

1. Child accuses adult
2. Adult admits causing injuries
3. One parent accuses another
4. Pathognomonic physical findings
5. Pathognomonic radiological findings
6. Unexplained subdural hematomas with retinal hemorrhages
7. Injuries incompatible with explanation offered

burns, and scars are pathognomonic. Radiographic findings of metaphyseal chip fractures or multiple bony injuries at different stages of healing are also diagnostic. A child over the age of three or four years will often confirm that a particular adult hurt him. Accusations by one parent against the other are also usually true, except in custody disputes. A tentative diagnosis of physical abuse can be made if an injury is unexplained or inadequately explained.

MANAGEMENT

When a physician sees a child whom he or she suspects of being abused or neglected, the following steps are recommended:

Treat the child's injuries. The child's medical and surgical problems should be cared for in the appropriate manner. The parents should be reassured that excellent medical care for their child is the first priority.

Hospitalize selected cases. In most metropolitan areas, child protective service caseworkers are on call 24 hours a day. No abused child should be discharged from a clinic setting without consulting them or hospital social workers. Usually they will come to the hospital and evaluate the family regarding the safety of the home. The 20 per cent or so of children that are at risk for serious reabuse can be placed in emergency receiving homes. The others can be sent home with services and close follow-up. Under these circumstances, the only patients requiring admission are those with major trauma requiring ongoing medical care, those from an outlying county, or young children in whom the diagnosis is unclear. If in doubt, it is better to err on the side of protecting the child.

Inform the parents of the diagnosis and the need to report it. The physician should tell the parents his or her diagnosis and inform them of the need to report suspicious findings. One can state: "Your explanation for the injury is insufficient. Even though it wasn't intentional, someone injured this child and that person needs counseling. I am obligated by state law to report suspicious injuries to child protective services." The physician should do this, since the case is reported on the basis of his medical findings. In fact, after all diagnostic studies are completed, the physician should review his interpretation of the actual cause of each specific injury in as supportive a way as possible. This convinces the parents that the physician knows what actually happened and permits them to turn their attention to therapy. The over-all outlook should be positive, with emphasis that this problem is treatable and everyone's goal is to help them find better ways of dealing with their child (not to punish the parents).

Make a telephone report to the child protective services agency immediately, unless they accompany the patient. This agency is made up of specially trained social workers. Reporting should secure evaluation, treatment, follow-up, and access to the juvenile court when necessary.

Complete an official written report of the incident within 48 hours. The official medical report is required by law; it should be written by a physician and contain the following brief but accurate data: (1) *History:* Date and time the patient is brought in; name of professional(s) who accompany the patient; the informant(s) (parent, child, other); date, time, and place of the abuse incident; how the injuries occurred (verbatim); who allegedly injured the child; and any history of past abuse. (2) *Physical examination* (description of the injuries): List the injuries by site (e.g., head, arms, legs, back, buttocks, chest, abdomen, genitals); describe each injury by size, shape, color; if the injury identifies the object that caused it, always say so (e.g., strap mark, cigarette burn); use nontechnical terms like "bruise" instead of "ecchymosis." (3) *Laboratory tests:* Roentgenograms, bleeding tests, etc. (4) *Summary:* Concluding statement on reasons why these findings are believed to be inflicted.

Request a hospital social worker consultation. The hospital social worker provides an in-depth evaluation of the parents of all inpatients to determine the danger or safety of the home. In complex cases, he or she will request psychiatric evaluations. In general, the psychosocial evaluations in outpatient cases will be done by child protective services.

Maintain a helping approach toward these parents. While feeling angry with these parents is natural, expressing this anger is very damaging to parent cooperation. Confrontation and accusation must be avoided. Keep the parents informed of what is happening to their child at all times.

Examine all siblings within 12 hours. Although it is unusual to have multiple children abused in the same family at the same time, it does occur (20 per cent). Parents can be told this is "child protective services policy" or "hospital policy."

Provide medical testimony for court cases. Child abuse cases are usually heard in juvenile court rather than criminal court. Most of the less serious cases are settled out of court. If the physician keeps precise medical records, reviews them before the hearing, and confers with the protective agency's lawyer about the points to be stressed, the court hearing can have an appropriate outcome for the safety of the child. The physician should bring a copy of the typed medical report to court and refer to it during testimony.

Child protective services will provide psychosocial follow-up and treatment. Child protective services are legally responsible for coordination of the family's therapy. Some innovative types of therapy that have been successful when designed for individual families include Parent Aides, Homemakers, Parents Anonymous groups, telephone hotlines, marital counseling, and childrearing counseling. Child protective services also make home visits and attempt to locate any families who become lost to follow-up. The treatment needs of the child should not be overlooked; consider infant stimulation program, day care, therapeutic preschool, or psychotherapy. A pediatrician can contribute to the therapeutic process by coordinating the child's health care and giving the parent his telephone number as an additional lifeline.

PREVENTION

The pediatrician is in a strategic position to detect dysfunctional or precarious families. Child abuse is one of the common manifestations of family breakdown in this group. These families can be identified early if more attention is paid to unwanted pregnancies; a newborn in a family with previous abuse of a child; drug addiction, serious psychiatric illness, or aggressive tendencies in a parent; derogatory comments about the newborn infant; lack of evidence of maternal attachment or infrequent visits to a newborn whose discharge is delayed owing to prematurity or illness. Extra services can be provided for these families without labeling them in any detrimental way. Intervention includes prenatal classes, arranging for contact between mother and baby in the delivery room, a rooming-in maternity ward, increased parental contact with premature infants, extra help with the crying infant, more frequent office visits, ongoing counseling regarding discipline, visits of public health nurses, lay health visitors, crisis nurseries, close follow-up of acute illnesses, telephone lifelines, arrangement for day care, and assistance in family planning. These helping, reaching-out, supportive services can often prevent abuse and serious neglect.

PROGNOSIS

With comprehensive, intensive treatment, about 80 per cent of these families can be rehabilitated and thereafter provide adequate care for their child. Approximately 15 per cent can only be stabilized and require indefinite services until their children are old enough to leave home. Termination of parental rights and release of the child for adoption is required in 1 to 2 per cent of cases.

If an abused child is returned to his or her parents without any intervention, 5 per cent will be killed and 25 per cent will be seriously injured. The child with repeated injuries to the central nervous system may develop mental retardation, an organic brain syndrome, seizures, or hydrocephalus. Common emotional traits of abused children are fearfulness, aggression, and hyperactivity. Further, untreated families tend to produce children who become the violent members of our society, and the next generation of child abusers.

REFERENCES

Altemeier, W. A., O'Connor, S., Vietze, P. M., Sandler, H. M., and Sherrod, K. B.: Antecedents of child abuse. J. Pediatr., *100*:823, 1982.

Bernat, J. E.: Bite marks and oral manifestation of child abuse and neglect. *In* Ellerstein, N. S.: Child Abuse and Neglect: A Medical Reference. New York, John Wiley and Sons, 1981, p. 141.

Bittner, S., and Newberger, E. H.: Pediatric understanding of child abuse and neglect. Pediatr. Rev., *2*:209, 1981.

Caffey, J.: The whiplash shaken-infant syndrome. Pediatrics, *54*:396, 1974.

Feldman, K. W., Schaller, R. T., Feldman, J. A., and McMillon, M.: Tap-water scald burns in children. Pediatrics, *62*:1, 1978.

Leake, H. C., and Smith, D.: Preparing for and testifying in a child abuse case. Clin. Pediatr., *16*:1057, 1977.

McNeese, M. C., and Hebeler, J. R.: The abused child. CIBA Clinical Symposia 29(5):1–36, 1977.

Pascoe, J. M., Hildebrandt, H. M., Tarrier, A., et al.: Patterns of skin injury in non-accidental and accidental injury. Pediatrics, *64*:245, 1979.

Schmitt, B. D.: The child with non-accidental trauma. *In* Kempe, C. H., and Helfer, R. E. (eds.): The Battered Child, 3rd Ed. Chicago, University of Chicago Press, 1980, p. 128.

Swischuk, L. E.: Radiology of the skeletal system. *In* Ellerstein, N. S.: Child Abuse and Neglect: A Medical Reference. New York, John Wiley and Sons, 1981, p. 253.

52

SEXUAL ABUSE (INCEST)

Barton D. Schmitt, M.D.

Incest refers to any sexual activity between persons too closely related to marry. Adopted and step children are included in most legal codes. The most common type of sexual mistreatment of children is family-related. Sexual abuse by friends and acquaintances of the family is the second most common type. Least common is sexual abuse perpetrated by strangers. This section will not deal with extrafamilial child sexual abuse, although the steps in medical evaluation of both types are similar. Intrafamilial sexual abuse is more difficult to manage because the child must be protected from additional abuse at the same time that attempts are made to preserve the family unit.

Incest can be divided into three types: molestation, sexual intercourse, and family-related rape (Table 52–1). Child molestation includes fondling the genitals of the child or asking the child to fondle or masturbate the adult's genitals. Non-touching offenses such as genital viewing and deliberate exposure to sexual acts or pornography also fall into this category. Without detection and intervention, over time molestation almost always progresses to full sexual intercourse. Sexual intercourse includes vaginal, oral, or rectal penetration (or attempted penetration) on a nonassaultive basis. Less than 10 per cent of incest is of the assaultive, forced intercourse type (family-related rape). The level of physical examination and laboratory investigation depends on the type of incest.

INCIDENCE

At least 0.2 to 0.3 per cent of children have been involved in incestuous relationships for an average period of five years. Brief sexual encounters occur more frequently. Sexual abuse constitutes 15 to 20 per cent of child abuse. Eighty-five per cent of victims are female and 15 per cent male. Male victims experience more violence and physical injuries. No age group is exempt. Approximately one third are less than six years of age, one third six to twelve, and one third twelve to eighteen. The process is often repeated with successive daughters. Ninety-nine per cent of offenders are males. Incest cuts across all socioeconomic groups to a greater degree than physical abuse.

ETIOLOGY

Most incest is of the father-daughter type. Sexual relationships usually begin gradually and without any violence. The father brings to the relationship a need for sexual gratification, and the daughter brings a need for affection and nurturance. The father is usually rigid, patriarchal, and emotionally immature. He is unlikely to engage in extramarital relationships. The mothers are usually chronically depressed, unavailable to their husbands because of work or illness, and aware of the incest but seemingly able to overlook it on any conscious level. Many were sexually abused as children. The child victim tends to be pseudo-mature and has taken on many of the housekeeping tasks. The families are often closely knit and socially isolated. In the violent cases of family-related rape, the father is usually a sociopath and his sexual abuse extends outside the family circle.

CLINICAL HISTORY

Sexual abuse victims may present to the physician in several ways. The child may disclose the incestuous relationship to her mother and be brought to a physician at that time. If the mother does not believe the child, the child may later tell a girlfriend, friend's mother, or school counselor and be brought in. Some adolescents will disclose their secret to a physician during a private interview. At other times the physician must elicit the history of incest based on his suspicions. His suspicion should be aroused when a prepubertal child is brought in with vaginal bleeding or other unexplained genital symptoms (e.g., vaginitis). A pregnant adolescent who has not dated and offers no information regarding the baby's father should be suspected of being an incest victim. The main cause of any venereal disease in the pre-pubertal child is sexual transmission from adults. Other suspicious behaviors or findings are com-

Table 52–1. TYPES OF INCEST

1. Molestation—touching or non-touching
2. Sexual intercourse—vaginal, oral, rectal
3. Family-related rape

pulsive masturbation, precocious sexual behaviors, adolescent prostitution, running away, a rectal or vaginal foreign body, proctitis, and recurrent urinary tract infections.

Incest cases require careful history-taking, because less than half of the victims have any physical or laboratory findings. A detailed explicit account of sexual experiences by a prepubertal child should be considered hard evidence in these cases. Interviewing should proceed gently and at the child's pace. Pictures or anatomically correct dolls can be used to clarify body parts and the child's vocabulary should be elicited and used. Content of the interview should be focused on "what" and "where" questions, rather than "why" or "when" questions. If a social worker has performed an in-depth interview, the physician can review this material and repeat only the parts relating to sexual activities. Corroboration of the history is helpful in court.

PHYSICAL EXAMINATION

Most female victims prefer a female physician to examine them, but the sensitivity and gentleness of the physician are of greater importance. A body surface examination should be carried out for any signs of nongenital trauma, especially bite marks or grab marks of the face and neck. An abdominal and pelvic examination should assess the possibility of pregnancy. The mouth should be examined for signs of acute trauma such as redness, abrasions, and purpura. The rectum should be examined for signs of trauma such as anal fissures or swelling/hematoma of the anal verge. The external genitals should be visually examined (with the girl in the frog-leg position) for signs of trauma, laxity, or vaginal discharge. Most acute genital injuries occur between the 4 and 8 o'clock positions. The labia minora and posterior fourchette are damaged first, followed by tears of the posterior hymenal ring. A speculum examination of the vagina is rarely needed except in the presence of nonmenstrual vaginal bleeding or major trauma of the external genitals.

Acute trauma (i.e., swelling, bruises, abrasions, or tears) of the genitals, rectum, or mouth usually heals completely in four to seven days. Laxity of the anal sphincters is usually temporary and changes to spasm within a few hours after penetration. However, dilatation of the hymenal ring causes a permanent change to this structure. In prepubertal girls, a hymenal ring of 5 mm or greater to inspection is abnormal. With repeated penetration, the opening will usually be greater than 10 mm. Following the onset of puberty, hymenal laxity must usually be assessed by palpation.

LABORATORY DATA

The amount of laboratory evidence sought depends on the history (Table 52–2). (1) *Molestation* victims should receive a genital washing or urinalysis for sperm. (2) *Sexual intercourse* victims receive tests for sperm if less than 96 hours have passed since the last sexual contact (also tests for acid phosphatase if less than 24 hours have passed). In the vagina, sperm are motile for 6 hours and nonmotile for 72 to 96 hours. Acid phosphatase persists for 24 hours. Sperm and semen can also be recovered from the mouth and rectum when these sites are involved. Rimsza found evidence of semen in 30 per cent of the patients in whom it was looked for. While the the presence of semen substantiates the victim's history, its absence does not contradict the history of vaginal intercourse (consider vasectomy, azospermia, or withdrawal before ejaculation). Cultures for gonorrhea are taken from the throat, vagina, and anal canal in all victims. About 5 per cent of the victims have positive cultures. Occasionally tests are found to be positive at sites initially denied by the child because of embarrassment (especially the throat). Tests for syphilis are not routinely indicated.

In addition to the preceding tests, a forensic examination collects specimens that help to determine the identity of the perpetrator. These specimens include pubic hair, scalp hair, fingernail scrapings, blood samples, and sperm type. The specimens are usually transferred to the police laboratory in sealed, signed, and dated envelopes. While this extensive evidence is collected mainly in cases of third-party sexual

Table 52–2. LABORATORY DATA TO COLLECT

1. Molestation cases
   Urinalysis or vulva washing for sperm
2. Sexual intercourse
   GC cultures from three sites (all patients)
   Sperm tests (if less than 96 hours since sexual contact)
   Acid phosphatase tests (if less than 24 hours since sexual contact)
3. Family-related rape
   Forensic specimens (see Table 52–3)

abuse, it is also indicated in family-related rape cases. A gynecologist or emergency room physician may be consulted to provide this examination. Table 52–3 summarizes the specimens to collect in a rape evaluation.

DIAGNOSIS

The diagnosis of child molestation and most sexual intercourse rests on the graphic history offered by the victim (Table 52–4). False accusations are rare. Laboratory findings are usually normal because of the long delay before the victim feels safe in confiding in someone.

The finding of a dilated hymenal ring is supportive of the patient's history of vaginal penetration and may precipitate an admission of guilt by the alleged perpetrator. Obviously, such laxity could also be caused by a foreign body or a finger. Also, the hymenal ring would be normal in attempted (unsuccessful) intercourse or in simulated intercourse between the girl's thighs. In family-related rape cases, the victim is usually brought to an emergency room immediately. The diagnosis is then confirmed by evidence of recent genital and nongenital trauma as well as positive laboratory findings. Overall, however, a normal physical and laboratory examination is compatible with most types of sexual abuse and never disproves it.

MANAGEMENT

Evaluation and management of sexual abuse cases is more complex than physical abuse

Table 52–3. RAPE EVALUATION: SPECIMENS TO COLLECT

1. Soiled clothing (for blood or semen)
2. Plucked scalp hair*
3. Plucked pubic hair*
4. Foreign hair
5. Vaginal secretions (wet-mount) for motile sperm and Trichomonas
6. Vaginal secretions (air-dried for sperm, sperm typing, and acid phosphatase) (the same with suspicious secretions from any site)
7. GC cultures (× 3)
8. Blood of victim for syphilis serology and blood type
9. Saliva of victim for typing
10. Foreign blood (for typing)
11. Fingernail scrapings (for typing)
12. Toxicology—blood or urine specimens, if patient was drugged

*Defer if no foreign hair is detected.

Table 52–4. DIAGNOSTIC CRITERIA

1. Molestation cases—positive history
2. Sexual intercourse
   a. With no contact in 96 hours
      Positive history
      Dilated hymenal ring
   b. With recent contact
      Above plus sperm/acid phosphatase
3. Family-related rape
   Acute genital trauma
   Acute extragenital trauma
   Positive laboratory tests

cases. This process can begin in the physician's office if extensive laboratory evidence is not needed. A child protective services caseworker must be called as soon as possible. Larger communities will often have a designated emergency room where sexual abuse evaluations are completed.

All victims of sexual abuse require psychological support. Often both parents deny the girl's accusation and turn on her for reporting the incident. Victims of a single, nonviolent episode (e.g., some child molestation cases) may only need reassurance and a chance to ventilate about the event on one or two occasions. Usually they are less distressed about the incident than their mothers. In a single, violent episode case (e.g., family-related rape), the patient is usually in serious emotional distress and requires the immediate services of a child psychiatrist and/or rape victim advocate. Most of these patients make a good adjustment after several months in age-appropriate psychotherapy. The victims of multiple episodes of sexual abuse almost always need long-term psychotherapy. The victim can return home if the father is out of the home or has confessed and is in therapy. The girl must be placed in foster care if she prefers it, the mother does not believe her story, family life is chaotic, or all evidence has not yet been collected. Medication to prevent pregnancy can be given to girls who are postmenarchal and mid-cycle and have experienced vaginal intercourse within the previous 72 hours.* At a minimum, all victims should revisit their primary physicians within two weeks to assess their psychological functioning and the services that have been implemented.

Most incest offenders are treatable. The fathers require a psychiatric evaluation and the

*The prophylactic drug currently of choice is Ovral, 2 tablets immediately and repeated once in 12 hours if the pregnancy test is negative.

mothers should at the very least be evaluated by a social worker. Both parents usually need psychotherapy, marital therapy, and group therapy. Offenders are always investigated by the police, and commonly criminal filing and prosecution occur. Sentencing is usually deferred if the father becomes earnestly involved in his therapy. The offender in family-related rape cases has much more serious psychopathology. These offenders are usually placed in jail and subjected to full criminal prosecution and sentencing. Sociopaths, sadists, and pedophiles are generally untreatable with present techniques.

PROGNOSIS

With intervention, most incest victims can lead a normal adult life. Without intervention, many of them run away from home and become adolescent prostitutes and drug addicts. Those who stay at home manifest depression, suicidal gestures, and conversion reactions. As adults most of them have difficulties with close relationships and need psychiatric help.

REFERENCES

Cowell, C. A.: The gynecologic examination of infants, children and young adolescents. Pediatr. Clin. North Am., *28*:247, 1981.

Ellerstein, N. S., and Canavan, J. W.: Sexual abuse of boys. Am. J. Dis. Child., *134*:255, 1980.

Jones, G. J.: Sexual abuse of children. Am. J. Dis. Child., *136*:142, 1982.

Nakashima, I. I., and Zakus, G. E.: Incest: Review and clinical experience. Pediatrics, *60*:696, 1977.

Orr, D. P., and Prietto, S. V.: Emergency management of sexually abused children. Am. J. Dis. Child., *133*:628, 1979.

Paul, D. M.: The medical examination in sexual offenses against children. Med. Sci. Law, *17*:251, 1977.

Rimsza, M. E., and Niggemann, E. H.: Medical evaluation of sexually abused children: A review of 311 cases. Pediatrics, *69*:8, 1982.

Soules, M. R., et al.: The forensic laboratory evaluation of evidence in alleged rape. Am. J. Obstet. Gynecol., *139*:142, 1978.

Tilelli, J. A., et al.: Sexual abuse of children. N. Engl. J. Med., *302*:319, 1980.

Woodling, B. A., and Kossoris, P. D.: Sexual misuse: Rape, molestation, and incest. Pediatr. Clin. North Am., *28*:481, 1981.

53

CHILDREN AND DIVORCE

Morris Green, M.D.

Since parental divorce represents one of life's most disruptive changes, the physician's role in helping families master this stressful process warrants exploration. Children of divorce constitute a highly vulnerable population.

Occurring in approximately one out of each three families, divorce affects over one million children for the first time each year. Thirty to 45 per cent of the nation's children have experienced either a separation or a divorce. Most family breakdowns occur in the first five years of marriage, so young children are predominantly affected. Like death, separation and divorce lead to losses: little or no continued contact with the father, return of the mother to work, a move from a familiar environment and friends, and a lower general standard of living. Even the re-establishment of a new family—for most divorced persons do remarry—can be very stressful.

Although it is hoped that in the future pediatricians will be consulted prospectively before divorce in relation to its impact on children, that is not a common practice today. Rather, children of divorce are now seen because of sequelae. These depend upon the parents, their ability to segregate their feelings toward each other from those toward their children, the emotional support available, the amount of parental conflict, custody and visiting arrangements, and the age of the child.

In infants and young children, associated symptoms may include regression in developmental achievements (bowel training), separation anxiety, sleep disorders (awakening, nightmares, or night terrors), irritability, whining, fearfulness, anorexia, increased oppositional or aggressive behavior (hitting, biting, temper tantrums), fear of abandonment, and "hyperactivity."

In addition to feelings of grief, guilt, anger, resentment, low self-esteem, and rejection, school age children may demonstrate scholastic underachievement, school refusal, urinary frequency, enuresis, moodiness, whininess, encopresis, tantrums, somatic complaints, and aggressive acting-out. They may agonize over divided loyalties. Adolescents may feel depressed, lonely, anxious, powerless, and ashamed. Forced to give up denial of their parents' sexuality, they may be much troubled by parental dating or a live-in boy or girl friend. In addition to somatic complaints such as abdominal pain, headache, or backache, teenagers may have an exacerbation of a chronic illness, e.g., asthma or diabetes, or may fail to cooperate in its management. Antisocial activities may include lying, stealing, delinquency, substance abuse, sexual acting-out, and other aggressive behavior.

Preoccupied with their own difficulties, experiencing considerable personal stress, and largely unaware of their child's feelings, the parents may not spontaneously relate the child's symptoms to the divorce. Especially in the first year after separation, parents find it difficult to be understanding and emotionally supportive of their children. If the mother moves in with her parents, she confronts intergenerational conflicts, loss of her parenting *presence*, and blurring of generational boundaries.

When the physician's advice is sought before the divorce, he should ask to see both parents so that he can help the parents prepare the children over time for what is about to happen, to emphasize the importance of their providing opportunities for questions, to underline the critical need to perserve or achieve as much stability as possible, and to familiarize the parents with the concerns of children of divorce: Where will I live? Will I have to go to a new school? When will I see my father (mother)? Why are my parents doing this?

The physician may suggest that the parents, in addition to their answering such questions, emphasize that the children's needs will be met, that the relationship with both parents will continue (if true), that the separation is final, that every attempt was made to avoid the divorce, that the children were not responsible, that they cannot reunite them although they might wish to do so, and that they are not expected to take sides.

Both the mother and father should be encouraged to continue as close a relationship with the children as is feasible. If direct contact with either the father or the mother is to be seriously disrupted, the importance of some other male or female role model should be mentioned. Other resources such as books about divorce, mental health centers, psychiatrists, psychologists, women's centers, and groups for single and divorced parents may be noted.

In addition to identifying strengths in the child's life that may help him cope, the physician should encourage the child to share his feelings about the divorce. Recognizing that children commonly believe that they caused their parents' separation, the doctor should flatly state that this is simply not the case. He may also state that he is the *child's* doctor and that he will not take sides between the parents.

Although most children show the effects of divorce for a long time, others compensate well, particularly those who do not feel responsible for the divorce, who ask questions and receive thoughtful parental answers, who distance themselves from the parents' conflicts, who have a support network, and who come to accept the fact that their parents will not reunite.

REFERENCES

Anthony, E. J.: Children at risk from divorce: A review. *In* Anthony, E. J., and Koupernik, C. (Eds.): The Child and His Family. Children at Psychiatric Risk. New York, John Wiley and Sons, 1974, p. 461.

Derdeyn, A. P.: Children in divorce: Intervention in the phase of separation. Pediatrics, *60*:20, 1977.

Divorce, Child Custody and the Family. Committee on the Family. Group for The Advancement of Psychiatry. Vol. 10., No. 106. N.Y. Mental Health Materials Center, 30 East 29th Street, NY, NY 10016, 1980.

Jellinek, M. S., and Slovik, L. S.: Divorce: Impact on children. N. Engl. J. Med., *305*:557, 1981.

Rofes, E. (Ed.): The Kids' Book of Divorce By, For and About Kids. Lexington, MA, The Lewis Publishing Co., 1981.

Wallerstein, J. S.: Children and divorce. Pediatr. Rev., *1*:211, 1980.

Wallerstein, J. S., and Kelly, J. B.: Surviving the Breakup: How Children and Parents Cope with Divorce. New York, Basic Books, 1980.

54

THE PEDIATRICIAN AND ADOPTION

Morris A. Wessel, M.D.

Adoptive placement provides a home for a child who would otherwise be deprived of parental love and family life. It also allows adults to experience the satisfactions of parenthood.

Pediatricians offer professional services in many aspects of adoption: adults seeking information regarding appropriate ways to adopt an infant or child turn to a pediatrician for advice; social agencies, or parents planning to adopt independently, often request a pediatric evaluation of an infant or child prior to placement; adults or social agencies may seek consultation concerning the adoption of a child with a physical handicap or the advisability of a transracial adoption; and adoptive parents may seek routine pediatric care with special emphasis on the unique aspects of normal life crises in adoptive familes (Academy of Pediatrics, 1973; Wessel, 1960).

The primary goal of adoption is to arrange for the optimal placement of a child whose biological parents are unable to provide for his care. Successful adoptive placement is more likely to occur when specialized social agencies arrange the placement than when physicians, lawyers, or other individuals act as the intermediary (Academy of Pediatrics, 1973; Bernard, 1974).

Preadoptive interviews with a staff member of an agency specializing in adoptive services provide an opportunity for applicants to consider what it means to become adoptive parents. Once adults considering adoption clarify their feelings about the process, they are ready to begin to look at what is involved in assuming parental responsibilities.

An agency adoption also provides the opportunity for the natural mother and father to consider alternative plans before concluding that the relinquishment of their parental rights is in the best interests of themselves and the infant. In later years, biological parents are less likely to feel that they have been pressured into releasing their infant unwisely when they come to this decision after careful deliberation.

There are many family situations that may preclude successful adoptive placement. A husband and wife unhappy in their relationship to each other, who seek to create a family through adoption, are unlikely to resolve their marital difficulties, and the child, in most instances, will have an unsatisfactory experience. A couple's infertility should not be the sole basis for adoptive placement. While grieving for a child who has died recently, parents may consider adoption in order to alleviate their loss. Although at first consideration this may appear to be an adequate basis for adoption, the child who is adopted can never "be just like" (replace) the one who died. He may suffer continuously from a failure to live up to the parents' idealized memory of the deceased child. It is important to evaluate such parents in relation to adoption after they have had time to work through their grief.

Transracial adoption of children, often from war torn areas, is currently a frequent occurrence. Couples considering this specific arrangement need to explore with agency case workers the complex ramifications of adopting a child different from oneself, for such adoptions can result in many unanticipated difficulties, including a risk of illnesses rarely seen in the United States (Grow and Shapiro, 1975). Placement of children arranged by unlicensed individuals or organizations frequently fails to provide the appropriate services necessary for the protection of the biological parents, the child, and the adoptive parents. A "proxy adoption," i.e., the adoption of a child residing in one country sight unseen by parents residing in another country through the intermediary of a third independent party is hazardous for both parents and children.

Both couples planning independent adoptions and adoption agencies often seek a pediatric evaluation of an infant or child prior to placement. The pediatric examination should be comparable to that of any initial visit. The most important need is to establish that the baby or child is healthy and presents a normal potential for growth. The pediatrician should review available genetic data and the obstetrical history as well as examine the child. When the history and the examination appear within normal limits, the physician should state that there is no evidence to suggest any other than a potential for normal development. It is wise to emphasize that no one can predict "normal" development—only the potential for such. If adoptive parents show great concern over the risk, which is considerably smaller than that taken by biological parents, it may be wise to delay the process until they clarify their reasons for the adoption. When there are indications for considering the child to be in a "high-risk" category or specific problems are identified, the pediatrician should share his clinical impressions fully with the adopting parents or the social agency as the case may be.

The adoption of "hard-to-place" children, that is, those with handicaps such as congenital heart disease, clubfoot, cerebral palsy, cystic fibrosis, deafness, or blindness, is increasingly common. The pediatrician should discuss fully with the social workers and the adoptive parents the exact nature of the problem, the prognosis, and the anticipated costs of treatment. Subsidized adoptions in which voluntary or public agencies underwrite the cost of medical care are increasingly available and enable the placement of a child in an ideal home which would be unavailable without financial support (Hornecker, 1962).*

Adoptive parents are deprived of the meaningful experience that biological parents may have before the birth of a baby. Pregnancy, starting with conception and ending with labor and delivery, are highly significant biological and psychological life experiences that serve as a springboard for parenthood. The bodily changes during pregnancy, the labor and delivery, the initial glimpse of the newborn infant, the first feeding, and the mutual participation of husband and wife in the experience are important events which help to propel human beings through the transition from "coupleness" to parenthood. Adoptive parents become parents under vastly different circumstances. Whatever the motivations are for adoption, there is often a detailed agency evaluation process which, although it offers an opportunity for professional counseling, is something of a hurdle that adults wishing to adopt either "pass" or "fail." Having passed, there is always a delay until a suitable infant or child becomes available. Then, often at a few days' notice, the couple must abruptly assume total parental responsibilities.

Adoptive parents sometimes place considerable importance on their "success" in caring for a child. They often interpret rashes, colds, sleeping problems, and other normal common vicissitudes of life as personal failures. Various developmental stages may have special meaning. The year-old infant, for example, who with a teasing expression on his face crawls off to explore the world just when his mother calls him, is reflecting the security required for independent action—a result of good parental care. To insecure adoptive mothers, however, this may be considered an indication that "he doesn't love me or need me any more."

Telling a child of his adoption is an important process that parents and the pediatrician should discuss from time to time. There is no easy way to share this information, but it is important that this discussion take place early in a child's life before he learns it from outsiders. To withhold information from a child about his origin denies him the opportunity of hearing this important fact from his trusted parents. It will come as a shock to learn it in later life from friends or relatives, which is so often the case when the information is hidden from him.

Current controversy regarding the interest and right of adoptive children to have access to court records leading to identification and possible finding of natural parents is a new phenomenon with which child welfare workers, pediatricians, and parents will have to deal. The rights of the biological parents who have terminated their relationship to a child in good faith, never anticipating that at some unpredictable future time the child might appear, need to be considered. The complications of recent court decisions in this area and in establishing some rights of the unmarried father of a child demand a careful re-evaluation of agency practices.

Adoptive parenthood, like all parenthood, is a continuous process. The pediatrician who develops a warm and effective relationship with parents and children is in a position to provide counseling and support at critical moments of a child's development.

*Adoption Resource of North America (ARENA), 67 Irving Place, New York, N.Y. 11003 provides appropriate information and advice concerning the availability and adoption of "hard-to-place" infants and children.

REFERENCES

American Academy of Pediatrics: Adoption of Children, 3rd Ed. Evanston, IL, 1973.

Bernard, V.: Adoption. *In* Arieti, S. (Ed.): American Handbook of Psychiatry, 2nd Ed. New York, Basic Books, 1974, pp. 513–534.

Grow, L. J., and Shapiro, D.: Transracial Adoption Today. New York, Child Welfare League of America, Inc., 1975.

Hornecker, A.: Adoption opportunities for the handicapped. Washington, D.C., Department of Health, Education and Welfare, pp. 149–152.

Sakoloff, B.: Adoption and foster care—the pediatrician's role. Pediatr. Rev., *1*:57, 1979.

Wessel, M. A.: The pediatrician and adoption. N. Engl. J. Med., *262*:446–451, 1960.

Wessel, M. A.: A pediatrician views adoption and unwed parenthood. Child Welfare, *45*:334–337, 1966.

55

SCHOOL ABSENCE

Michael Weitzman, M.D., and Joel J. Alpert, M.D.

Children who are frequently or persistently absent from school tend to perform poorly academically and are likely not to graduate (Lloyd, 1976). Excessive school absence is associated with maladaptive behaviors, wasted opportunities, and unemployment and dysfunction during adulthood. It may also signify important health issues of concern to the physician. Despite epidemiological information that demonstrates that physical and mental health problems of students or their family members are often contributing factors in absenteeism, it is unusual for physicians to focus on this aspect of child functioning and rare for schools to involve them in its prevention and management (Weitzman et al., 1982). Excessive school absence may signal such health problems as poor coping with or management of chronic illness in the child or family members, teen-age pregnancy, substance abuse, depression or other emotional problems, inappropriate response to minor illnesses, or severe family dysfunction. Specific attention to this area of child behavior as part of routine health care will frequently uncover previously unrecognized health problems of major importance to the child's development and adjustment. Since children tend to establish their patterns of school attendance early in their academic careers, it is important to monitor this area of their functioning so that aberrant patterns and deviations from their own norms will be promptly identified.

EVALUATION

In general, the pediatrician should be concerned about the health and functioning of students whose school absences meet the following criteria: (1) absence of six or more consecutive school days; (2) frequent, short absences of less than six consecutive days, but a total of 10 or more days in an academic quarter; (3) patterned absences of less than six consecutive school days in a quarter but exhibiting a systematic pattern such as repeated absences on a specific day of the week.

The determination of the reason for absences in these cases should commence with a history from multiple sources—student, parents, and school personnel. Each may have his own perception of the problem and its causes. Information obtained from school personnel should focus on the pattern of the absences: Longstanding or of recent onset? Prolonged or repeated short absences? Only on certain days of the week? Repetition of grades, school achievement, evidence of learning disabilities, school adjustment problems, and previous evaluative steps should also be reviewed. It is also important to obtain a detailed history of the child's home environment, including recent moves, moves of close friends or relatives, or changes in friendship patterns.

Approximately 75 per cent of all school absences are attributed to illness by student and/or parent (Rogers and Reese, 1965). Many students with an absence problem appear healthy on examination but report multiple minor or psychosomatic complaints, such as frequent upper respiratory infections, headaches, stomach aches, and menstrual cramps. In some cases, these explanations represent inappropriate health beliefs, such as the perceived need to keep a child out of school for a cold or a headache. In other cases, these complaints signal children whose parents perceive them as being excessively vulnerable. Nonspecific physical complaints may also indicate depression or other serious psychological problems such as school phobia. It is unusual for children to state directly that they are depressed or that their sadness is interfering with their daily activities. Depression in school age children is likely to present as angry or rebellious behavior, excessive school absences, underachievement in school, running away, drug abuse, or early sexual activity (Malmquest, 1971).

For the child with chronic illness, absence behavior may be an important indicator of adaptation. Regular school attendance and success in school suggest overall satisfactory adjustment, invulnerability, and an ability to compensate for his problem and utilize residual skills without succumbing to a sense of futility.

When the amount of school absence cannot be explained by the severity of the child's condition, it may mean that the parents, seeing their child as excessively vulnerable, overreact by keeping the child home unnecessarily. When children with chronic illness begin to miss school without physical reasons, both the child and family may be emotionally endangered. Children with chronic illness and their families often rely on medical treatment and schooling as symbols of hope, and the breakdown of their commitment to this routine has implications for all areas of the child's and family's life.

There are also situations in which the child's medical problem or its treatment interferes with regular school attendance. Some drugs, such as antiseizure medications, may make the child drowsy so that there is difficulty waking in the morning or concentrating in school. The school nurse may be reluctant to administer particular medications, or regulations may prohibit the dispensing of certain medications on school premises. In other situations, school personnel may not know how to manage acute exacerbations of the underlying condition such as seizures or acute asthma attacks, how to help the child make up missed school work, or when the child should be kept home. In these situations, school personnel may inadvertently give students messages that encourage excessive absences.

In children who have a sudden increase in their school absences without a history of chronic illness, certain rare but exceedingly important medical conditions should be ruled out, e.g., brain tumors, neurodegenerative conditions, and endocrine abnormalities such as hyperthyroidism. If there is a strong history of malaise, easy fatigability, or loss of appetite, a complete evaluation should be done to rule out serious organic problems. More commonly, sudden changes in school attendance signal problems such as depression, drug abuse, or a change in the health status of other family members.

Abnormal school attendance patterns in children with ill family members may suggest that the student feels neglected and rejected or is excessively preoccupied with his own well-being. This behavior may be a response to parental withdrawal, unavailability, lability of mood, or altered expectations or disciplinary tactics. Whenever a physically healthy child with a family member with a serious illness begins to miss school frequently or develops nonspecific complaints leading to school absences, it is useful to explore the meaning of the illness to the student and its effect on his daily routine. Frequently children will miss large amounts of school because they stay home to care for ill family members, to accompany them to medical appointments, or to carry out household chores.

If students with absence problems do not have recognizable physical or emotional problems, the child may have an attention deficit disorder or a specific learning disability. Too often these problems are undetected for years while the child, labeled as lazy or rebellious, falls further and further behind. Often the child will appear bored or agitated in school, complain of a dislike of school, or focus on psychosomatic complaints as the explanation for excessive absences. If there is reason to believe that a particular student has a learning disability, the child should be referred for appropriate evaluation.

Students and parents may, at times, overreport health problems because of misperceptions or because they have learned that they can legitimize absences if they are labeled as health related. Some students choose not to attend school because they or their parents do not believe that it is an important activity. Some families do not believe that schools are meeting their children's needs and may encourage nonattendance as a reaction to racism, busing, crowded classrooms, or school policies. Many children, especially those living in poverty, are subject to peer group pressures that do not support success in school and will miss large amounts of school to avoid censorship of peers. Overreporting, for whatever reason, should be viewed as maladaptive behavior not in the child's best interest.

MANAGEMENT

The physician can do a number of things to impact significantly on the child and family when the child is missing excessive amounts of school. First, he can rule out serious organic problems, deal with inappropriate health beliefs, and screen for social and emotional causes of this problematic behavior. Some of the socioemotional problems may be amenable to counseling by the physican. The physician can also facilitate and coordinate referrals for specialized tests or treatments.

The majority of children with excessive school absence will present with multiple minor or psychosomatic complaints without evidence of serious organic pathology. Efforts should be directed to correcting student's and parents' unfounded health concerns and inappropriate health behaviors. Counseling should be directed both toward relieving anxiety and toward providing the student and parents with problem-solving skills related to the physical complaints. Instructions concerning when it is appropriate to keep the child out of school with a cold, headache, stomach ache, or menstrual cramps may prove helpful. It may also be useful to tell the family to call the physician or school nurse before they decide to keep the child home. Similarly, if the school is asked to notify the physician whenever the child is absent for long periods or in a repetitive pattern, the physician can intervene shortly after significant absences by contacting the family and reviewing the guidelines for keeping the child at home. Significant absences are those that meet the criteria already mentioned, or, in the case of students who have already been identified as meeting these criteria, may actually be any subsequent absences.

In many cases multiple minor complaints are suggestive of underlying depression. If the physician suspects this but has little success with counseling, a referral to a mental health professional is indicated. Often both the child and other family members will need psychotherapeutic intervention. Any indication of school refusal requires immediate attention, since successful intervention appears related to the length of time between onset of the problem and the institution of treatment. Possible learning disabilities should be brought to the attention of the school and a thorough psychological evaluation undertaken.

When the child's absence is a direct result of poor management of a health condition such as frequent acute asthma attacks, drowsiness due to overmedication, or exclusion from school, a change in medication or dosage schedule may solve the problem. The physician should also allay the anxiety of school personnel by sharing information with them or helping change school policies. More often, however, the amount of the child's absence from school will be out of proportion to the severity of his medical problem and in these cases the possibility of depression, inappropriate expectations, and altered disciplinary tactics must be investigated.

Success in school for children with chronic illnesses often requires the collaboration of parents, physicians, and school personnel. Parents of children with chronic illnesses may be reluctant to collaborate with schools because of previous painful experiences with human service providers, and they may fear that disclosing the details of their child's medical problem will result in preferential or prejudicial treatment. The physician may contribute by making initial telephone calls to the school, attending meetings with school personnel, or supervising the parents' effort to work with the child's school. A visit to the school by the physician is often very useful in clarifying issues and in devising school-based interventions. Most schools will schedule conferences at the physician's convenience. In the vast majority of cases the physician should encourage and support parents' efforts to work with school personnel themselves.

When illness in a family member appears to be the cause of the child's excessive absence, efforts should be directed toward normalizing the child's home experiences. This may require counseling the student and/or family members, collaboration with the physician caring for the ill family member, or providing home services via social services agencies so that the child can be freed from home care responsibilities.

Children or parents frequently indicate that the excessive school absences are due to the fact that they do not believe in the importance of schooling. This is a difficult situation to change. It is sometimes helpful in these cases to identify a person in the child's school who will serve as the child's advocate and attempt to motivate the child by encouraging success in school. If parental dissatisfaction with a particular school or peer pressure is causing the child to miss excessive amounts of school, the physician should consider contacting the school system to facilitate the student's transfer to another school.

REFERENCES

Lloyd, D. N.: Concurrent prediction of dropout and grade withdrawal. Educ. Psychol. Measurement, *36*:983, 1976.

Malmquest, C. P.: Depression in childhood and adolescence. N. Engl. J. Med., *284*:887, 1971.

Rogers, K. D., and Reese, G.: Health studies—Presumably normal high school students. Am. J. Dis. Child., *109*:9, 1965.

Weitzman, M., Klerman, L. V., Lamb, G. A., et al.: School absence: A problem for the pediatrician. Pediatrics, *69*:739, 1982.

56

ALCOHOL AND DRUG ABUSE

S. Kenneth Schonberg, M.D.

The three leading causes of death among older adolescents—accidents, homicide, and suicide—are all behavioral. Other behaviors that have a major impact upon adolescent and, eventually, adult health include school performance, sexuality, social relationships, delinquency, and drug use.

Within our society the use of mind-altering drugs has long been a frequent feature of the passage from adolescence to adult status. The use of alcohol has always been an aspect of adolescent and adult behavior, and concerns regarding its social and medical effects are longstanding. Recent events, however, have dramatically increased the level of concern among health professionals regarding drug use by teen-agers. The past two decades have witnessed a marked expansion of the types of chemicals used by adolescents. Newer drugs of abuse have different, often more dangerous side effects, some of which are only now coming to light. The age of onset of drug use has dropped below adolescence, and substance abuse is encountered even within the elementary grades. There has been an increasing awareness not only of substance abuse as a concomitant of major behavioral disruption during the teen years but also the chance that young people, otherwise doing well, may suffer a tragedy during an episode of recreational intoxication.

The role of the pediatrician regarding drug use is complex. The clinician must be able to recognize and treat the somatic consequences of drug abuse; obtain a history of drug use behavior from an adolescent who may at times be reluctant to divulge such information; offer counsel when frequently no such counsel has been requested; and serve as a consultant to schools and other community agencies concerned with youth. A knowledge both of the complications of substance abuse and of the interviewing and counseling skills required to bring that knowledge to bear have of necessity become a part of pediatrics.

CHANGING PATTERNS OF DRUG USE

The late 1960s and early 1970s were characterized by the abuse of dangerous drugs by large numbers of adolescents. Opiate, barbiturate, and inhalant use, previously rarely encountered in young people, became common during the teen years. Such drug use was responsible for widespread morbidity and significant mortality. Rising rates of delinquency and antisocial behavior were seen as concomitants of such drug abuse. The war against drugs was joined by physicians, educators, politicians, law enforcement officials, parents, and community agencies.

The use of heroin, and later methadone, was responsible for an epidemic of drug-related illnesses, hospitalizations, and deaths. Intravenous opiate abuse became an initial consideration in the adolescent presenting with jaundice, and death from hepatic coma was far from rare. Chronic persistent hepatitis was now described in teen-age opiate abusers. Cellulitis, brain abscess, and subacute bacterial endocarditis were among other serious infections seen in those teen-agers abusing via the intravenous route. Menstrual irregularities, infertility, and severe constipation, although not life-threatening, were frequently encountered complaints (Litt and Cohen, 1970). The ability to manage opiate overdose and addiction became a required skill for those who cared for teen-agers.

In the early 1970s, it was unclear how many adolescents would eventually be involved in this behavior. By the early 1980s, opiate abuse has become an uncommon, if not rare, phenomenon among teen-agers (Hein et al., 1979). A similar pattern of rise and fall has been experienced for both barbiturates and inhalants. Concurrent with the epidemic of opiate abuse were major problems with barbiturate dependence and the inhalation of volatile hydrocarbons. Hospitalization for barbiturate overdose or dependence was not infrequent, and the detoxification of the barbiturate addict was an often-encountered and difficult clinical problem (Smith and Wesson, 1971). Both acute hepatitis and sudden death were experienced by adolescents, often very young adolescents, who chose to become intoxicated by inhaling a variety of volatile hydrocarbons, including cleaning fluid and glue (Litt and Cohen, 1969). Although drug use surveys continue to report that some 15 per cent of high school seniors have had some experience with sedative or inhalant abuse, frequent use and related clinical sequelae are now rarely seen.

The most prevalent concerns regarding adolescent substance abuse no longer relate to the opiates, barbiturates, and inhalants. Rather, the use of alcohol and marijuana, with their potential for both tragedy secondary to intoxication and disruption or illness from abuse, is now a major source of distress. The repetitive emergence of new hallucinogens into the adolescent drug scene and the increasing use of cocaine by young people are additional sources of anxiety.

HEALTH CONSEQUENCES OF DRUG USE

Somatic illness represents but a portion of the difficulties encountered by the adolescent drug user. The effects of intoxication upon education and socialization, the expense of a drug habit, the life style of the drug abuser, the legal entanglements involved in using illicit drugs, and the family turmoil that any drug use may cause all impact upon well being. For some drugs such as the opiates and barbiturates, physiological disturbance and serious illness are so common as to be by themselves condemning. For other substances, immediate medical complications may be infrequent or minor, and adequate counsel cannot be given without a broader understanding of the less tangible but nonetheless important impacts of drug use upon adolescent activities and development.

The Intoxicants

Alcohol and marijuana are now the psychoactive drugs most frequently used by adolescents in the United States. Prior to graduation from high school, over 90 per cent of teenagers will have used alcohol, and over half will have tried marijuana (Johnson et al., 1980). Such drug use often begins in early adolescence. Before entrance into the ninth grade over 30 per cent of students will have tried alcohol, and approximately 15 per cent will have smoked marijuana. Although these two drugs are markedly different in their pharmacology, somatic consequences, and legality, they have much in common. In addition to being the most commonly abused drugs, they are both intoxicants, are used as recreational drugs at adolescent social gatherings, and have major ill effects beyond direct somatic insult.

Alcohol remains the most commonly used psychoactive agent in our society. Experimentation with alcohol often begins early in adolescence, and nearly half of ninth graders have had at least one experience with drinking. By the time of graduation from high school, nearly 95 per cent of teen-agers have used alcohol, with over two thirds reporting drinking at least once a month. The easy availability, legality, and tacit approval by many adults contribute to the extent of alcohol use.

The somatic consequences of alcohol use during adolescence are in the main restricted to episodes during which large amounts are ingested at one time. Coma, respiratory arrest, aspiration pneumonia, and death all may result from an alcohol overdose. The treatment of overdose is in the main supportive. Particularly for mixed ingestions with alcohol, barbiturates, other sedatives, or tranquilizers, the depth of respiratory depression may require mechanical ventilatory assistance. The prevention of aspiration pneumonia, another acute consideration, may necessitate the insertion of a cuffed endotracheal tube. Acute gastric hemorrhage and acute pancreatitis may also follow from a large ingestion. Hemorrhage, profuse vomiting, and severe abdominal pain may mandate hospitalization. Such complications of chronic alcoholism as cirrhosis, polyneuritis, and Korsakoff's psychosis are not observed in teen-agers. Similarly, delirium tremens, the major withdrawal syndrome from alcohol, is rarely, if ever, seen in that age group. In contrast, a more benign withdrawal syndrome consisting of tremors, diaphoresis, agitation, disorientation, and, rarely, brief seizures may occur in adolescents who have drunk heavily over weeks or months. Teenagers whose drinking history suggests the possibility of a minor withdrawal syndrome should be hospitalized for observation if they become abstinent. Adolescents who drink to this extent are clearly at great risk of becoming adult alcoholics. Of more immediate concern are the behavioral consequences of repetitive or even occasional intoxication during the teen years. Those concerns are similar regardless of the intoxicant involved, applying to both alcohol and marijuana.

During the past 20 years marijuana has become a most popular intoxicant for both adolescents and young adults. Currently, over 55 per cent of high school seniors have tried marijuana; nearly 10 per cent use it on a daily basis and fully a third at least once a month. Over 20 per cent of young people report a first experience prior to entrance into high school. Over 50 million Americans have used marijuana at least once.

As most parents and older adults have had

little or no personal experience with marijuana, dispassionate discussion of its use has been difficult. Concerns regarding illegality, potential physiological consequences, and seduction into the use of more dangerous drugs often introduce both anxiety and hostility into any attempt at thoughtful discussion. Frequently such discussions focus on poorly documented and exaggerated claims of physiological danger without emphasis on the risks involved in the use of any intoxicant by young people, even one that would be physiologically safe. Society continues to have difficulty in finding a comfortable way of coping with a phenomenon that now involves over half of its young adults.

Marijuana is neither pharmacologically benign nor among the more dangerous drugs used by adolescents. Despite much recent research, a total picture of the effects of marijuana on humans is not available; however, definitive effects upon brain, cardiovascular, pulmonary, endocrine, and psychological function have been demonstrated. Placing these effects in a proper perspective in order to address the impact of marijuana use upon young people is not easy. The more important concerns regarding marijuana use may lie outside physiological consequences and within behavior while intoxicated.

The effect of marijuana upon brain function is of great concern. Although the most common acute effect is euphoria and intoxication, anxiety, panic, and confusion may occur. Particularly with high doses, hallucinations and loss of contact with reality may ensue and last for several hours to several days. Although no definitive information exists to suggest that marijuana causes permanent psychosis, young people with pre-existent mental instability may be at risk of becoming psychotic with marijuana use. No permanent changes in brain cell morphology or gross changes in brain structure have been demonstrated. Acute effects also include an impairment of short-term memory and the ability to learn; however, there is no evidence that even prolonged use of marijuana by humans causes any permanent or sustained impairment of brain function. Prolonged use has, however, been associated with a permanent deleterious effect upon behavior—the amotivational syndrome—but it is unclear whether marijuana is a cause or a concomitant of that life style (Relman, 1982).

Although acute marijuana smoking causes transient bronchodilation, chronic use has been associated with mild and reversible airway obstruction. As with the smoking of tobacco, respiratory tract infection and irritation is a concomitant of chronic use. Preliminary information would suggest that marijuana smoking may be carcinogenic. That marijuana smoking increases the heart rate and raises blood pressure represents a potential risk to individuals with hypertension and cerebrovascular or coronary artery disease. In young people, the clinical significance of such effects is minimal.

Marijuana can lower gonadotropin secretion and decrease both sperm number and motility. No link has been established with male infertility. Although effects upon gonadotropins, menstrual patterns, and ovulation have been reported in females, these studies remain unconfirmed and without demonstrated relationship to fertility. Similarly, there is no evidence that marijuana is teratogenic. Information regarding the effect of marijuana upon the immune system is conflicting. At present, there are no data to suggest that marijuana smokers have an increased risk of infection. In sum, marijuana affects multiple organ systems but most of these changes are transient and of little clinical impact.

The effect of marijuana upon motor and learning functions may be of greatest clinical importance. Marijuana impairs motor coordination, sensory and perceptual functions, tracking (the ability to follow a moving stimulus), and reaction time—all important components of driving skills. Tests of driving ability after the administration of marijuana using both simulators and actual driving on closed courses have demonstrated impaired driving ability, occasionally lasting for four to eight hours after feelings of euphoria had disappeared. Accidents, especially automotive accidents, are now the leading cause of death among older adolescents and young adults. Although the relationship between drinking and automotive accidents has been well-established, it has been more difficult to demonstrate a direct relationship between smoking marijuana and automotive accidents and fatalities. The detection of marijuana use requires a blood sample, and hence the permission of the driver, whereas demonstrating alcohol use requires only a breath analysis. It would appear, however, that the combination of either of these intoxicants and driving is a major contributor to fatalities among young people. While other somatic consequences of marijuana or alcohol use by adolescents may be unconvincing, such is not the case for injury and death secondary to intoxication while driving or engaged in other potentially hazardous recreational or vocational activities.

Cocaine

Over 15 per cent of high school seniors have used cocaine, with approximately one third of these students reporting use at least once per month. The number of young people using cocaine has gradually and consistently risen over the past decade. Despite this degree of exposure, complications from cocaine do not commonly come to medical attention (Johnson et al., 1980).

The drug produces an intense but short-lived euphoria, often lasting no longer than 10 minutes. On occasion, anxiety reactions, paranoid thinking, and hallucinations may occur, rather than euphoria. Violent behavior may be encountered, but as with the other dysphoric effects, episodes are transient and disappear before medical care can be sought. Other side effects include elevation of the heart rate, increase in blood pressure, and tachypnea. As cocaine is a vasoconstrictor, irritation and ulceration of the nasal mucosa can occur if the drug is sniffed ("snorted") over prolonged periods (Cohen, 1975). Those who use cocaine intravenously are subject to the same infectious risks as heroin users. Overdose reactions can occur characterized by tremors, delirium, and convulsions. Death may rarely result from either respiratory failure or cardiovascular collapse (Wetli and Wright, 1979).

Although addiction does not occur, dependence upon the drug with depression upon abstinence has been reported. The great expense of the drug (up to a thousand dollars per ounce for high-quality cocaine) serves as a deterrent to its frequent use by most adolescents.

The Hallucinogens—Phencyclidine

Over the past two decades, a variety of drugs capable of producing hallucinations have waxed and waned in popularity among adolescents. Included within this category are lysergic acid diethylamide (LSD); 2,5-dimethoxy-4-methylamphetamine (DOM); peyote (mescaline); and, most recently, phencyclidine (PCP or angel dust). Phencyclidine is among the most toxic of these agents.

Phencyclidine appears in multiple forms including a crystalline powder, tablets, and capsules. Originally investigated as a possible anesthetic agent during the 1950s, its use in humans was abandoned because of postoperative side effects which included agitation and delirium. As a drug of abuse, it can be swallowed, injected, or smoked (often sprinkled on marijuana). PCP is used because of its ability to cause euphoria, disinhibition, feelings of power, and hallucinations. Unfortunately there is a thin line between desired effect and unpleasant or, at times, dangerous side effects.

Toxic reactions to phencyclidine include psychosis, coma, and death. Psychotic reactions, which may be indistinguishable from schizophrenia and include elements of paranoia, agitation, or catatonia, may last for days and, rarely, weeks (Cohen, 1976). With high-dose ingestions, convulsions, opisthotonus, respiratory arrest, coma, and death may ensue. Treatment of overdose reactions includes anticonvulsants for seizures, support of respiration, and enhancement of drug excretion by gastric lavage with half normal saline, the administration of furosemide, and the acidification of the urine by administering ammonium chloride in conjunction with ascorbic acid (Aronow and Done, 1978). Fortunately, the number of adolescents being brought to emergency rooms with phencyclidine overdoses has decreased dramatically during the past few years. Although nearly 10 per cent of high school seniors report some use of PCP during their lifetimes, the number who have used it during the past year appears to be declining rapidly.

DETECTING THE DRUG USER

It is the task of the pediatrician to detect both those adolescents who are abusing dangerous drugs or suffering a major life disruption as a concomitant of drug use and those who are placing themselves at risk through the occasional recreational use of intoxicants. Infrequently, an adolescent will present for medical attention specifically for remediation of drug abuse. In these instances the presence or fear of addiction, the detection of drug use by parents, or legal difficulties provide the motivation necessary to address a drug problem. More frequently the adolescent will seek care because of a drug-related illness that requires medical attention. The physician needs to be aware of the somatic consequences of substance abuse so that the use of drugs as a possible etiology for the presenting symptoms will not be overlooked. The role of drugs may be obvious, as in the adolescent with hallucinations, or far more subtle, as in the teenager with fever of unknown origin.

Most frequently, however, the adolescent who is using drugs will be seen not for a specific drug problem or a somatic consequence of substance abuse, but rather for a non–drug-related problem or for routine health supervision. Including a question regarding drug use as part of the history from every adolescent is the only way to detect and address drug use in these young people.

A drug use history is a natural part of the assessment of other areas of psychosocial and behavioral adjustment, such as school performance, dating behavior, and relationships with family and peers. The exploration of these areas of behavior requires that the interview take place in a setting that offers privacy, with parents absent, and with some assurance that answers will be held in confidence. It is often best to initiate the questioning with inquiries about the extent of drug use within the adolescent's environment rather than directly probe the teenager's personal behavior. As the use of alcohol and marijuana is now universal within secondary schools and common at adolescent social events, inquiries regarding the practices of peers at school and parties almost always yield positive answers. The response of the physician to such positive answers will in large part determine whether the adolescent will be truthful about his or her own drug experience. If the pediatrician responds with dismay or disgust, it is less likely that accurate statements will be forthcoming when the questioning becomes more personal. In contrast, if such information does not evoke alarm or condemnation, most adolescents will, when asked, relate their own experiences with alcohol, marijuana, and other less commonly utilized substances.

Having learned that an adolescent is using alcohol, marijuana, or other drugs, the physician needs to determine the degree of risk or disruption the drugs are causing. Not all teenagers who are using psychoactive drugs suffer disruption from such behavior. In fact, the majority of young people continue to carry on productive and worthwhile lives despite recreational substance use. To determine which adolescents are at greatest risk, information will need to be gathered on not only the drugs being used but also how often, in what quantity, in which settings, and toward what desired end. An assessment of the extent of disruption attributable to or concomitant with substance abuse should be a part of the evaluation of every teenager, not only those using drugs. This appraisal should include inquiry about problems in school, difficulties with family or friends, episodes of delinquency or arrests, sexual promiscuity or maladjustment, and evidence of depression or other psychopathology.

It is unusual to find a teen-ager who is evidencing marked disruption in only one sphere of behavior. Significant substance abuse, delinquency, school failure, promiscuity, family problems, and depression almost always coexist. Addressing one area of difficulty while ignoring others is not often successful. Clarification of the degree and nature of disruption will not only allow appropriate attention to young people who are having difficulty concomitant with substance use but will also help identify those areas of difficulty in the teen-ager's life which will need to be addressed.

The teen-ager who is found to be using drugs but experiencing few or no consequences from this behavior will also be in need of counsel. The risks of accidents, injuries, and physiological side effects are not confined to adolescents who are deeply involved with drugs. The vast majority of teen-agers who are using alcohol or marijuana are neither drug addicts nor delinquents, school drop-outs, or sociopaths. Rather, they use drugs on a recreational basis at parties and with friends, at times subjecting themselves to the risks inherent in intoxication.

MANAGEMENT

The adolescent who is abusing any of the more dangerous drugs and, as is often the case, doing poorly in other spheres of performance, urgently needs intense therapeutic intervention. A somatic illness requiring treatment may motivate the teenager to confront a drug abuse problem. Other professionals, including psychiatrists and social workers, may be required for evaluation and management. Since the physician may not be familiar with community facilities for the treatment of addiction and serious drug abuse, consultation with individuals who specialize in dealing with such problems can be most helpful. The role of the pediatrician in these instances includes identification of the problem, convincing the adolescent and the family of the need for help, and directing the teen-ager toward professionals or community agencies with expertise in substance abuse.

A far more common role for the pediatrician is counseling adolescents who are using recreational intoxicants. Such counseling includes not only an honest recital of the possible medical complications but, probably of greater importance, a discussion of the potential risks involved in intoxication. Were there instances in the past when the teen-ager was intoxicated and at risk? Does the teen-ager drive while intoxicated? Does the adolescent have a plan for dealing with a situation in which he or she will have the car and become intoxicated, or, alternatively, be in an automobile when the driver is intoxicated? Does the family have a plan for dealing with such eventualities? Is that plan so punitive as to discourage the teen-ager from asking for help at a time of risk? Does the adolescent use intoxicants at inappropriate times such as school or work? Does the teen-ager consider such behavior inappropriate? All such inquiries and counseling should be viewed as a necessary part of preventive health care for adolescents. Considering the extent of alcohol and marijuana use among adolescents, instances of risk while intoxicated should be regarded as an almost certain probability rather than a remote possibility.

REFERENCES

Aronow, R., and Done, K.: Phencyclidine overdose: An emerging concept of management. J. Am. Coll. Emerg. Phys., 7:56, 1978.

Cohen, S.: When friends or patients ask about cocaine. J.A.M.A., *231*:74, 1975.

Cohen, S.: Angel dust: The pervasive psychedelic. Drug Abuse Alcohol. Newsletter, 7:1, 1976.

Hein, K., Cohen, M. I., and Litt, I. F.: Illicit drug use among urban adolescents: A decade in retrospect. Am. J. Dis. Child., *133*:38, 1979.

Johnson, L. D., Bachman, J. G., and O'Malley, P. M.: Highlights from student drug use in America 1975–1980. Rockville, MD, National Institute on Drug Abuse, 1980.

Litt, I. F., and Cohen, M. I.: "Danger. . . Vapor Harmful": Spot remover sniffing. N. Engl. J. Med., *281*:543, 1969.

Litt, I. F., and Cohen, M. I.: The drug-using adolescent as a pediatric patient. J. Pediatr., 77:195, 1970.

Relman, A. S. (Ed.): Marijuana and Health. Washington, D.C., National Academy Press, 1982.

Smith, D. E., and Wesson, D. R.: Phenobarbital technique for treatment of barbiturate dependence. Arch. Gen. Psychiatry, *24*:56, 1971.

Wetli, C. V., and Wright, R. K.: Death caused by recreational cocaine use. J.A.M.A., *241*:2519, 1979.

57

FAILURE TO GAIN; FAILURE TO THRIVE; WEIGHT LOSS

Morris Green, M.D.

Weight gain during early infancy is relatively rapid, amounting to 5 or 6 and sometimes up to 10 ounces a week. In the latter half of the first year the gain becomes slower, 3 to 5 ounces a week. During the first year of life, infants should demonstrate a steady weight gain. Failure to do so calls for a careful investigation. *As a general rule, if an infant fails to gain on a formula that is quantitatively and qualitatively correct, there is something wrong with the infant or with the environment and not with the formula.* Alterations in the formula or changing to other preparations will usually not correct this problem. Breast fed infants may not gain because of a quantitatively inadequate supply but not because of a qualitative deficiency. (See p. 42 for discussion of breast feeding.)

During the second year of life the rate of weight gain continues to diminish, the child gaining 2½ ounces a week. Instead of a steady weight gain each week, the weight may remain constant for two or three weeks at a time. This pattern of periodic rather than constant weight gain becomes more pronounced in older children.

DIAGNOSIS

Table 57–1 presents an etiological classification of failure to thrive. Psychosocial factors represent the most common cause for this symptom. The pediatric interview, the physical and developmental examination, and observation of the interaction between the mother or other caretaker and the infant, especially in a feeding situation, may provide the data base for the diagnosis of a mothering disability, an inadequate caloric intake, or an organic disorder.

The diagnosis and management of mothering disabilities are discussed in Chapter 29, p. 240. Breast-fed babies may fail to gain adequately simply because the mother's milk supply is inadequate. Some of these babies will demonstrate hunger by crying, but others will not. In addition to efforts to increase the mother's milk

Table 57–1. ETIOLOGICAL CLASSIFICATION OF FAILURE TO THRIVE: WEIGHT LOSS

- I. Psychosocial; Environmental
  - A. Mothering disability
  - B. Rumination
  - C. Inadequate caloric intake
  - D. Anorexia
  - E. Child neglect
- II. Inadequacy of Food Intake
  - A. Calorically inadequate formula or diet offered
  - B. Quantitative deficiency of breast milk
  - C. Organic feeding difficulties
  - D. Anorexia
  - E. Economic privation; starvation
- III. Defective Assimilation of Food
  - A. Inadequate digestion, e.g., cystic fibrosis
  - B. Inadequate absorption, e.g., gluten-induced enteropathy; giardiasis
  - C. Crohn's disease
- IV. Loss of Food Substances
  - A. Vomiting
  - B. Diarrhea
- V. Failure of Utilization or Increased Metabolism
  - A. Systemic acute or chronic infections
    - 1. Prenatal viral infection
    - 2. Tuberculosis
    - 3. Histoplasmosis
    - 4. Parasites
  - B. Malignancy
  - C. Cardiac disease
  - D. Chronic pulmonary disease
  - E. Renal disease, e.g., chronic renal insufficiency or renal tubular acidosis
  - F. Idiopathic hypercalcemia of infancy
  - G. Chronic anemia
  - H. Hyperthyroidism; hypothyroidism
  - I. Diabetes
  - J. Inborn errors of metabolism
- VI. Neurological
  - A. Cerebral damage, mental retardation, cerebral palsy
  - B. Subdural hematoma
  - C. Diencephalic syndrome
  - D. Leigh's syndrome

supply, the breast feedings may need to be supplemented by formula preparations. In non–breast-fed infants who do not gain, the mother may exaggerate in the history the actual caloric intake of the infant. In these instances, the infant will gain rapidly in the hospital.

Failure of an infant to gain in spite of a large food intake may be an early symptom of cystic fibrosis. Failure to thrive is not an early symptom in patients with celiac syndrome but may follow vomiting and diarrhea. Unexplained loss of weight in older children may be an early manifestation of Crohn's disease. Infants with congenital infections or cardiac defects may gain weight poorly. Inborn errors of metabolism, including galactosemia, may present as poor feeding, lethargy, and failure to thrive.

Infants with cerebral damage, mental retardation, or cerebral palsy often do not thrive. Although children who demonstrate excessive muscular activity may have caloric needs considerably above the average, their caloric intake is often less than that of normal children because of their feeding difficulties. The diencephalic syndrome, caused by intracranial neoplasms in the region of the hypothalamus and third ventricle in infants and children under two years of age, is characterized by a paradoxical alertness, euphoria, and hyperactivity in the presence of emaciation.

LABORATORY EVALUATION

If diagnostic uncertainty remains after the interview and physical examination, selected laboratory evaluations may include a CBC, urinalysis, serum electrolytes, calcium, BUN, serum creatinine, and T4 and T3. Other studies, e.g., urine for genetic screening, bone age, skull films, sweat chloride, carotene, etc., may be obtained as clinically appropriate.

REFERENCES

Berwick, D. M.: Nonorganic failure to thrive. Pediatr. Rev., *1*:265, 1980.

Fischhoff, J., Whitten, C. F., and Pettit, M. G.: A psychiatric study of mothers of infants with growth failure secondary to maternal deprivation. J. Pediatr., *79*:209, 1971.

Goldbloom, R. B.: Failure to thrive. Pediatr. Clin. North Am., *29*:151, 1982.

Rosenn, D. W., Loeb, L. S., and Jura, M. B.: Differentiation of organic from nonorganic failure to thrive syndrome in infancy. Pediatrics, *66*:698, 1980.

Sills, R. H.: Failure to thrive. The role of clinical and laboratory evaluation. Am. J. Dis. Child., *132*:967, 1978.

Whitten, C. F., Pettit, M. G., and Fischhoff, J.: Evidence that growth failure from maternal deprivation is secondary to undereating. J.A.M.A., *209*:1675, 1969.

58

HYPERACTIVITY; ATTENTIONAL DEFICIT

Morris Green, M.D.

Hyperactivity is a nonspecific term that is applied to a cluster of behavioral symptoms. Attentional deficit disorder (ADD) with hyperactivity, the most recent label applied to this grouping of symptoms, includes developmentally inappropriate inattention, impulsivity, and motor hyperactivity.

The child seen because of "hyperactivity" may, in fact, have normal behavior that has been misinterpreted as abnormal. Occasionally, the complaint may come from a very inexperienced teacher who cannot maintain discipline in the classroom, especially an open classroom. Others have constitutionally high levels of motor activity, perhaps due to a genetic predisposition. Commonly, "hyperactive" or overactive behavior is a manifestation of anxiety and/or depression secondary to environmental and situational stresses such as not doing well in school, having a sibling who is handicapped or ill with a serious disorder such as leukemia, family financial problems, marital discord, divorce, parental illness including alcoholism, maternal depression, death of a relative, crowding, a chaotic living situation, and developmentally inappropriate care with too little or too much stimulation. Possible organic etiologies include brain damage secondary to infection, injury, hypoxia, or lead intoxication. Hyperactivity, distractibility, headache, vertigo, difficulty in controlling anger, and sleep problems may be part of the post-traumatic syndrome after a head injury. Children with what may be termed the "little bit" syndrome, a clinical picture that consists of hyperactivity, developmental retardation, brain damage, and autistic-like behavior, present difficult diagnostic and management problems and require longitudinal observation, preferably in a nursery school, by an interdisciplinary group. Hyperactivity may occur in children with neurofibromatosis and may be an early manifestation of hyperthyroidism. More rarely, increased motor activity may be seen in a gifted child who is bored in school. Finally, there are those children who have the attentional disorder of unknown etiology.

CLINICAL MANIFESTATIONS

I. The child is unable to sit still. He may constantly move about, aimlessly pick up objects, open drawers, climb on chairs, touch everything in sight, and bother others. He may be unable to sit through a television program or a story. Disorders of sleep and eating may have been present since infancy. When maternal depression is present, the child's hyperactivity is often worse on those days when the mother is most depressed.

II. The short attention span and easy distractibility cause failure to complete tasks, sloppy school work, disorganization, and inability to remember instructions and assignments. The child does not seem to listen. All these complaints seem to be less marked in one-to-one or structured situations and relatively stimulus-free environments.

III. The child shows impulsive motor and verbal behavior: interrupts others, blurts out in school, has trouble waiting his turn.

IV. The child exhibits overexcitability. Stimulating or exciting situations such as parties, guests, shopping centers, amusement parks, crowds, other children, and Christmas activities tend to make the behavior worse. Temper tantrums or crying occurs over trivial matters.

V. There are socialization problems. The child often bothers or comes crashing in on other children as well as adults. He has poor peer relations, fights frequently, and is overly aggressive and demanding.

VI. Other emotional and behavioral symptoms may include fire-setting, disobedience, defiance, destructiveness, and mood swings.

VII. School problems may be secondary to

the child's short attention span and distractibility or to learning disorders.

THE PHYSICAL EXAMINATION

Many children seen because of hyperactivity or the attention deficit syndrome do not display abnormal behavior in the one-to-one office setting. On neurological examination, a number of nondiagnostic "soft" signs may be present. Since they usually represent a maturational lag in motor development, these signs in time disappear. Occasionally there is hyperreflexia or asymmetry of the deep tendon reflexes and extensor plantar reflexes.

APPROACH TO DIAGNOSIS

The diagnosis of hyperactivity is a matter of clinical judgment, since there is no specific test or array of diagnostic studies. Reports of the parents and teachers regarding the child's behavior in a variety of settings and a review of possible environmental contributing factors are diagnostically helpful. The assessment of the family should include recent deaths, other acute stresses (e.g., marital discord and divorce), and long-term family vicissitudes, such as alcoholism, mental illness, and chaotic, crowded living arrangements. An electroencephalogram is indicated only if the history or physical examination suggests a convulsive disorder. Psychoeducational and language evaluation is indicated in children thought to have a learning disorder. A variety of parent and teacher rating scales are available for evaluation of the child's attention span and social adjustment. Electronic devices being developed to be worn by the child during observation periods may permit a quantification of motor activity.

MANAGEMENT

Many parents, inclined to assume responsibility and guilt for their child's disorder, feel frustrated, angry, and helpless. They should be told that the problem is not their fault and helped to participate in the process of assessment, planning, and working with the school. Special education approaches and tutoring are indicated in the presence of a learning disorder. When hyperactivity is caused by other problems in the family or anxiety in the child, appropriate counseling and therapy should be pursued.

In terms of behavioral therapy, the parents should tell the child patiently and repeatedly what they expect. These rules should be few in number and clearly defined. Consequences of breaking them should be clearly stated prospectively. Discipline should be firm, unequivocal, and invoked at the time of the infraction. Incessant nagging should be avoided. Time-out or isolation should be used instead of physical punishment. The child's environment and schedule, e.g., meals and bedtime, should be heavily structured. Since fatigue and crowds may excite the child, shopping centers and other public places in which the child is expected to sit still, e.g., church, restaurants, or athletic events, should be avoided. Socially acceptable behaviors should be promptly rewarded and, if not too intrusive, inappropriate behaviors ignored. The parents should identify activities in which the child's attention span may be lengthened, i.e., reading stories, playing board games, drawing, and block building. Daily opportunities should also be provided for the child to run and otherwise discharge energy. The mother also will need respite periods away from the child.

Most children improve with changes in the family or school, so that medication is not usually indicated. Even when appropriate, pharmacotherapy is not the sole treatment for hyperactivity. When prescribed, the stimulant drugs should be started at a low dosage and the teacher and parents asked to rate the child's response. If little or no improvement is observed after a few days to a week with methylphenidate or dextroamphetamine, the dose should be increased over similar intervals of time. Anorexia and insomnia, the most common side effects, may subside even if the same dosage is maintained over a one- to two-week period. Crying and irritability may require discontinuation of the drug. If the patient has motor tics or Tourette's syndrome, stimulant medication is contraindicated. One of these conditions in a member of the family is a relative contraindication to their use in the hyperactive child. Medication may be periodically discontinued over weekends and during vacation periods to determine whether it is still needed. It does not need to be tapered. Methylphenidate and dextroamphetamine usually achieve their maximum effect on the day of administration, occasionally within an hour or so. Improvement in handwriting may be one objective evidence of a positive drug effect.

The initial dose of methylphenidate may be 5 mg twice a day (before breakfast and lunch), with increments of 5 to 10 mg weekly. The total dose should not exceed 60 mg. Methylphenidate should not be used in patients under six years of age. If there is no response in a month, the medication should be discontinued. The initial dose of dextroamphetamine in children between three and five years of age is 2.5 mg daily. The dosage may be increased by increments of 2.5 mg weekly until a clinical response is obtained. In children six or more years of age, the initial dose may be 5 mg once or twice a day, followed by increments of 5 mg at weekly intervals, to a maximum of 40 mg per day. This drug is available in a long-acting spansule form.

The only major known adverse effect of the prolonged use of stimulant drugs may be delay in linear growth. Regular height and weight measurements are, therefore, of special importance.

Premoline, another drug available for use in children with the attentional deficit syndrome, is administered as a single oral dose each morning. The recommended starting dose is 37.5 mg per day. This dose may be gradually increased at one-week intervals, using increments of 18.75 mg until the desired clinical response is obtained. The mean daily effective dose ranges from 56.25 to 75 mg per day. Clinical improvement is gradual, and significant benefit may not be seen for three or four weeks. Insomnia is the most frequently reported adverse reaction. Anorexia, nausea, abdominal pain, skin rash, irritability, and headache have also been reported.

Defined diets which seek to eliminate foods that contain high levels of naturally occurring salicylates or artificial colors and flavors have been advocated for use in the treatment of hyperactivity; however, controlled trials demonstrate a positive association in only a few patients between the diet and a decrease in hyperactivity.

The ultimate prognosis in severe forms of hyperactivity is not as uniformly good as had been heretofore believed. Although hyperactivity diminishes with age, some of the basic problems, especially learning difficulties, when present, tend to persist into adolescence. A poor self-image and depression, along with academic failure and occasionally antisocial behavior, may occur.

REFERENCES

Bax, M.: Who is hyperactive? Devel. Med. Child. Neurol., *20*:277, 1978.

Cantwell, D. (Ed.): The Hyperactive Child—Diagnosis, Management, Current Research. New York, Spectrum Publications, Inc., 1975.

Clements, S. D.: Minimal Brain Dysfunction in Children: Terminology and Classification. NINBD Monograph No. 3, PHS Publication 1415. Washington, D.C., U.S. Department of Health, Education and Welfare, 1966.

Eisenberg, L.: Hyperkinesis revisited. Pediatrics, *61*:319, 1978.

Lerer, R. J., Lerer, M. P., and Artner, J.: The effects of methylphenidate on the handwriting of children with minimal brain dysfunction. J. Pediatr., *91*:127, 1977.

Lowe, T. L., Cohen, D. J., Detior, J., Kremenitzer, M. W., and Shaywitz, B. A.: Stimulant medications precipitate Tourette's syndrome. J.A.M.A., *247*:1729, 1982.

Miller, J. S.: Hyperactive children: A ten-year study. Pediatrics, *61*:217, 1978.

Sandberg, S. T., Rutter, M., and Taylor, E.: Hyperkinetic disorder in psychiatric clinic attendence. Devel. Med. Child Neurol., *20*:279, 1978.

Schmitt, B. D.: The minimal brain dysfunction myth. Am. J. Dis. Child., *129*:1313, 1975.

Schmitt, B.: Guidelines for living with a hyperactive child. Pediatrics, *60*:387, 1977.

Weiss, G., and Hechtman, L.: The hyperactive child syndrome. Science, *205*:1348, 1979.

59

TICS

E. Lawrence Hoder, M.D., and Donald J. Cohen, M.D.

Habit spasms, or tics, are stereotypic involuntary movements of individual muscle groups. Disorders involving tics are divided into four categories according to age of onset, duration of symptoms, and the presence or absence of vocal tics (DSM III, 1980). Although an exact incidence is not known, most people, especially children between 7 and 8 years of age, experience transient tics that last only a short time and up to 10 per cent of the population will experience a tic lasting a month or more.

Sniffing, swallowing, throat clearing, coughing, eye blinks, facial grimacing, and neck stretching are frequently seen motor tics; however, any part of the body may become involved, e.g., shrugging movements of the shoulders or shaking movements of the trunk. Although motor tics are most common, repetitive vocalizations and even repetitive thoughts are variably seen in certain tic disorders. The tic disorders described below must be differentiated from other abnormal movement and seizure disorders (athetosis, chorea, hemiballismus, dystonias, dyskinesias, and myoclonic seizures) and from stereotyped behaviors and tics that may be seen as a consequence of drug ingestion (in particular amphetamines) or degenerative diseases of the CNS (in particular Wilson's disease and subacute sclerosing panencephalitis).

TRANSIENT TIC DISORDER

Diagnostic criteria for a transient tic disorder include an age of onset during childhood or early adolescence, the presence of motor and occasionally vocal tics, the ability to suppress these tics for minutes to hours, a variation in the intensity of the symptoms over weeks or months, and a duration of at least one month but less than a year (DSM III, 1980). Facial tics, especially eye blinking, are most common. At least three times as many boys as girls suffer from a transient tic disorder, and there is a greater likelihood for occurrence among family members.

CHRONIC TIC DISORDER

The chronic tic disorder differs from the transient form in its duration for greater than one year, a more unvarying intensity of tics during its course, and by an age of onset either during childhood or after the age of 40 years (DSM III, 1980). More men than women develop a chronic tic disorder.

ATYPICAL TIC DISORDER

Tics that do not fit well into the other categories because of age of onset, course, or nature of the movement involved are designated as atypical (DSM III, 1980).

SYNDROME OF GILLES de la TOURETTE

Tourette's syndrome (TS) is the most debilitating of the tic disorders. Diagnostic criteria for Tourette's include an age of onset between 2 and 15 years of age, the presence of motor as well as multiple vocal tics, the ability to suppress these tics for minutes to hours, variation in the intensity of symptoms over weeks or months, and a duration of symptoms for more than a year or throughout life (DMS III, 1980). The prevalence of TS ranges from 0.1 to 0.5 cases per thousand (DSM III, 1980). A clear genetic contribution to TS and multiple tic syndromes has been revealed in family studies (Pauls, 1981). A high incidence of nonspecific abnormalities on EEG and "soft" signs on neurological examination support a neurological basis for TS. Neurochemical studies, as well as the response of TS to neuroactive medication, have suggested that the neurotransmitters, dopamine, serotonin, and noradrenaline, may be involved in the expression of TS (Cohen, 1978). Stimulant medications, in particular methylphenidate, dextroamphetamine, and pemoline, have precipitated tic syndromes and TS in children being treated for attentional disorders (Lowe, 1982).

Clinically, TS in children follows a typical natural history. Attentional, behavioral, and learning problems are found in up to 60 per cent of children with TS and often precede motor and phonic symptoms by many years. While psychometric testing fails to reveal specific learning disabilities, the children generally have difficulty in focusing attention, particularly in unstructured situations or when on their own (e.g., doing homework). Motor tics involving the eyes, face, neck, and/or shoulders eventually develop, and vocal tics, such as grunts, barks, yelps, throat clearing, or coughing, subsequently appear. Echolalia (a repetition of one's own last words or phrases) and echokinesis (a repetition of another person's movements) may develop. Coprolalia, an irresistable urge to utter profanities, occurs in 40 per cent of cases. Mental coprolalia as well as obsessive thoughts and compulsive acts or rituals may appear. In severe cases, self-abusive behavior may be seen.

The expression of TS varies considerably; at its most severe, children may feel they are going crazy—the tics come in rapid succession and are impossible to control or to disguise. Although physical disabilities may ensue as a result of repetitive self-abusive behavior, TS imposes primarily a social disability on those affected, a disability that often evolves into a social ostracism by family and friends as well as strangers.

The severity of TS is usually manifest early in its course. While the symptoms of TS may periodically wax and wane, it is unlikely that the disorder will continue to worsen after the child has had symptoms for several years. Those children with serious attentional, behavioral, and learning problems will tend to have the most severe problems throughout life. Although long-term remissions or a marked attenuation in the severity of symptoms may occur as children reach adolescence and young adulthood, there is no way of predicting which patients will have this fortunate outcome.

TREATMENT

Central to the evaluation of a tic disorder and the decision for or against treatment is a review of the affected child's overall development. Developmental assessment of a child with a tic must include a careful evaluation of the child's cognitive and motor development, psychological functioning, and role in the family. Specific pharmacological therapy is indicated only when a child's normal development is at risk, e.g., when his self-esteem is threatened, when his family cannot tolerate the symptoms, or when physical danger is possible. The process of thorough evaluation is often therapeutic in improving a child's social difficulties.

Transient and atypical tic disorders resolve over time, and thus reassurance is probably the best approach to treatment. Since anxiety and stress often aggravate the tics, efforts to identify the causes of anxiety may be useful. Psychotherapy, biofeedback, and other behavioral techniques have been used, but critical comparisons of these techniques or even definitive evidence of effectiveness is lacking. Negative reinforcement by teasing or punishing a child are of little value in the treatment of tics and may precipitate concomitant psychosocial difficulties.

Because of the more dramatic and overwhelming nature of TS, the pressure to begin treatment for this type is usually much greater. However, careful evaluation of the child's overall social and cognitive development is here particularly crucial, since the long-term adjustment of children with TS is more a function of school achievement and social learning than of the severity of the motor and phonic symptoms. Family-oriented therapy and an innovative school program are often required for a child to achieve this full potential.

When drug therapy is elected, haloperidol is the initial drug of choice and will relieve symptoms initially in up to 80 per cent of patients with TS. Low doses of haloperidol, 1 to 3 mg/day, are generally best. Children who require higher doses usually experience disturbing side effects—cognitive blunting, decreased motivation, weight gain, dysphoria, and school phobia. These side effects usually preclude long-term therapy, and only a minority of patients remain on haloperidol. Newer pharmacological approaches include clonidine hydrochloride and pimozide. Clonidine is not yet specifically approved for use in TS and thus remains investigational (Cohen, 1980). It is begun at 0.05 mg/day and is slowly titrated up to 0.15 to 0.30 mg/day. Six to eight weeks of treatment may be required before any effect is seen, usually an initial calming, then a decrease in motor and phonic symptoms and an increased attention span. While the effects on motor tics may not be as dramatic as with haloperidol, the absence of cognitive and emotional side effects make it a more desirable medication for some patients. Pimozide achieves amelioration of tics similar to haloperidol but with less sedation. Although abnormal EEG patterns (resembling temporal lobe or paroxysmal disorders) may be seen in some patients with TS, there is no evidence that treatment with anticonvulsants is of any use.

When pharmacological treatment is begun, the pediatrician must focus on the child's overall functioning and not simply on the control of the tics. Overmedication that interferes with normal functioning may occur if tic suppression alone is taken as the end point of therapy. Because of the likelihood of concomitant emotional problems in TS, when family or psychiatric problems become evident, referral should be made to a center skilled in the treatment of TS, which includes medical and psychiatric management of the tic disorder, family counseling, and school placement if necessary.

Genetic counseling for parents and their families is unfortunately quite limited. General guidelines can be offered. Boys are at greater risk, as are the children of women with TS or multiple tics. While there is a definite increase in risk to first degree relatives of patients with TS, the majority will not be affected and there is, as yet, no specific genetic model that can accurately predict who will be affected. Prenatal diagnosis is not yet available.

REFERENCES

Chase, T., and Friedhoff, A.: Tourette's Syndrome. New York, Raven Press, 1982.

Cohen, D. J., Detlor, J., Young, J. G., and Shaywitz, B. A.: Clonidine ameliorates Gilles de la Tourette syndrome. Arch. Gen. Psychiatry, *37*:1350–1357, 1980.

Cohen, D. J., Shaywitz, B. A., Caparulo, B., Young, J. G., and Bowers, M. B.: Chronic multiple tics of Gilles de la Tourette's disease. Arch. General Psychiatry, *35*:245–250, 1978.

Diagnostic and Statistical Manual of Mental Disease, DSM III. Washington, D.C., American Psychiatric Association, 1980, pp. 73–79.

Hoder, E. L., and Cohen, D. J.: Repetitive behaviors of childhood. *In* Levine, M.D. (Ed.): Developmental-Behavioral Pediatrics. Philadelphia, W. B. Saunders Co., 1983.

Lowe, T., Cohen, D. J., Detlor, J., Kremenitzer, M., and Shaywitz, B. A.: Stimulant medications precipitate Tourette's syndrome. J.A.M.A., *247*:1729–1731, 1982.

Pauls, D. L., Cohen, D. J., Heimbuch, R., Detlor, J., and Kidd, K. K.: Familial pattern and transmission of Gilles de la Tourette syndrome and multiple tics. Arch. Gen. Psychiatry, *38*:1091–1093, 1981.

Sharpiro, A. K., Shapiro, E., Brunn, R., and Sweet, R. D.: Gilles de la Tourette syndrome. New York, Raven Press, 1978.

SECTION

V

THE MANAGEMENT OF CHILDREN WITH CHRONIC DISEASE

The care of children with long-term disorders has been an underemphasized aspect of pediatric education and practice. In the past, inadequate educational preparation, underdevelopment of supporting services, and lack of adequate reimbursement for comprehensive management of chronic disease have limited the primary clinician's participation in the care of these children.

PRINCIPLES OF MANAGEMENT

In a chronic illness the child and family need professional allies on whom they can depend to be their vigorous advocates to enlist the best help available, to communicate closely with other professionals, and to coordinate or be aware of all that is going on. Although children with long-term disorders and their families are vulnerable to many secondary problems, especially those of a psychosocial nature, many are able to contain these risks. The following principles may contribute to such an optimal outcome (see also Table 1).

Competence

Competent, conscientious, continuing care is a basic need for the personal health care of these children. Although the pediatrician's training and daily clinical experiences permit him to remain comfortable about the developmental needs of the child with a long-term disorder, he may be less secure about the current management of many of the major chronic illnesses that are uncommon in his practice. He will generally not have readily available in the office setting the medical and allied professionals required for consultation and interdisciplinary care; therefore, collaboration with other professionals in regional centers or in the community is required.

Continuity and Time

Time is required to make a comprehensive diagnosis, assess the results of treatment, and arrive at new recommendations. Management of the psychological aspects of the illness requires the kind of trusting relation with the physician that can usually evolve only over time. House officers and fellows should tell their patients at the onset about the duration of their rotation. Preparation for the physician's leaving must start long before it occurs. If possible, the new house officer should be introduced by the departing physician in person or by name.

The interpretation of a chronic illness is accomplished in segments attuned to the readiness and willingness of the parents to know. Confronted with serious diagnostic realities, parents need time to gain an understanding of

Table 1. THINGS TO REMEMBER IN CARING FOR A CHILD WITH A CHRONIC ILLNESS

1. Without an effective plan for continuity of care, the initial evaluation makes but a limited contribution.
2. Time and regularly scheduled visits are needed to clarify the illness and to permit the formation of a trusting relationship between patient and doctor.
3. While planning for the future, concentrate on the present.
4. Try to alleviate guilt, a feeling always present.
5. Include the father.
6. Be interested in how the mother and siblings are getting along.
7. Help the parents understand the identity of their child.
8. Understand that parents may initially feel overwhelmed and inadequate.
9. Promote communication.
10. Help the parents and child avoid social isolation.
11. Encourage the early and active participation of the parents in the care of their child.
12. Increase parental competence in the care of the child.
13. Help the child understand his illness.
14. Enhance the child's sense of competence and his active role in management of his illness.
15. Prepare the child for what is going to happen.
16. Be comfortable in sharing the care of the child with others.
17. Work with the child's and parents' strengths and resources rather than exclusively with their problems and weaknesses.
18. Be experienced by the child as a long-time friend as well as a physician.
19. Make the family and the child feel that you are glad to see them.
20. If there is hope, be hopeful.

the physician's explanation and to participate in an effective and organized manner. Parents do best with the structure of definable tasks and short-term goals. Frequent, even though brief, visits should be scheduled rather than left for the parents to arrange. An office or home visit one to two weeks after birth is advisable for infants born with a congenital anomaly.

What Happens in Return Visits

The *parents* and the *child* have a chance:

1. To talk about how things are going, the impact the illness has on their daily life, relations, and plans.

2. To develop a trusting relationship with the physician, which permits a sharing of problems and worries.

3. To ask questions about daily care, such as feeding, colic, constipation, diaper dermatitis, teething, weaning, use of walker, baby sitters.

4. To clarify the nature of the illness or handicap.

5. To ask questions about development such as responsiveness, crawling, talking, bowel training, separation problems, day care, toys, tantrums, masturbation, school, aggression, menstruation, sexuality.

6. To receive feedback from the physician on how the child is doing.

7. To ask for information, e.g., his opinion of other therapies or special diets that have been suggested to them or they have read about and to clarify the conflicting advice they receive.

8. To share their successes.

9. To ask questions about the cause and prognosis of the disorder.

10. To ask what the future holds.

The *physician* (see Table 2) is provided with opportunities:

1. To provide continuing treatment and health promotion.

2. To assess the parents' adjustment to the illness in terms of the realism of their perceptions; the appropriateness of their expectations; their concern with current rather than distant problems; their ability to meet the child's needs; the degree of their preoccupation with what might have been; the pertinence of their questions; their ability to utilize advice; the quality of their relations with the child and each other; and their decreasing need for denial.

3. To provide advice about child care. In general, this should include answering questions that reflect current concerns, providing anticipatory guidance for what parents may expect before the next visit, and offering practical recommendations for day-to-day problems of child care, such as feeding, suggestions for

Table 2. WHAT THE PHYSICIAN DOES IN CONTINUING CARE FOR CHILDREN WITH LONG-TERM DISORDERS

1. Provides continuing treatment and health promotion.
2. Assesses the parents' and child's adjustment to the illness.
3. Provides advice about child care.
4. Encourages sharing of feelings of loss.
5. Clarifes the nature of the disorder.
6. Alleviates guilt.
7. Contributes to the quality of the family's life.
8. Helps parents understand their child.
9. Talks with the child.
10. Helps identify strengths and resources.

alternate modes of stimulation in the presence of sensory handicaps, methods of motivating mobility in the child with motor difficulties, and assistance in training for self-care.

4. To encourage parents to share their conscious feelings of loss, frustration, and disappointment. This ventilation of feelings may be facilitated if the physician verbalizes his understanding that all such parents at times feel trapped, very much alone, resentful of the unrelenting burdens of child care, and tempted to just walk away from it all.

5. To clarify and reinterpret the nature of the child's handicap or illness until the parents are able to encompass the explanation. For some this requires little time; others never achieve this degree of adaptation.

6. To alleviate guilt. It is often helpful if, at some time, the parents are able to express their self-blame openly and to be reassured by the physician that what they did or failed to do had no bearing on the illness or its outcome.

7. To be aware of family interactions and practices and to contribute to the quality of the family's life: the effects of the baby on the family; the extent of the father's participation; whether the family goes out together; and whether the mother has some time to herself each day or a regular free afternoon. Helping the family find a resource for respite care may make a major contribution to family health and stability. Because of the major stressors they experience, family disruption and alienation are not infrequent. Sensitive recognition of this common aftermath may be coupled appropriately with referral for marital counseling or family therapy.

8. To help the parents understand the *identity* of their child.

9. To talk with the child, demonstrate interest in his school work and play, help him understand and accept his problem, seek his active participation in what needs to be done, prepare him for changes in treatment, and support him in times of depression and self-doubt.

10. To validate the parents' ability to care for their child and to help the parents and child identify and use effectively their strengths and invulnerabilities.

Even after a "cure" has been achieved in patients with a malignant disorder, the child and the parents need regular follow-up because of their worries about recurrence and the long-term side effects of the treatment. Although inconvenient and, at times, painful, the treatment protocols that led to the "cure" had provided a well-defined and supportive structure. The previously required periodic visits, in themselves supportive, may be missed.

Availability

The child and his family should have prompt access to their physician, should the need arise, either through a phone number or immediate access to substitute coverage. Continuous care by one physician and regular, not too widely spaced, return appointments permit the physician to be psychologically as well as physically available to the child and his family. It is a source of great comfort for the parents of chronically handicapped or sick children to know that their physician is available in time of emergency as well as for regular care. A research project conducted in relation to a family support and treatment unit at Honeylands in Essex, United Kingdom, impressively demonstrated the importance of a resource, including provisions for scheduled or emergency respite care, to which parents could always turn at any time of the day or night.

A Family Focus

The birth of a handicapped infant or the onset of a serious long-term illness in a previously healthy child is followed by the parents' mourning the "loss" of the healthy expected baby or older son or daughter. The reaction is more gradual and usually less intense if the handicap or illness occurs after the child has been in good health for a period of months or years. In the case of anomalies noted at birth, resolution of this grief reaction is a prerequisite to adequate parental investment in the "unexpected" handicapped infant.

Whether the family arrives at a healthy or a maladaptive resolution of this crisis and whether the child eventually achieves a maximal adaptation within the limits set by his illness may be influenced positively by the intervention of physicians and other health professionals; otherwise, a number of secondary problems may ensue:

1. The parents may feel inadequate. Otherwise resourceful parents may seem surprisingly uncertain about steps in growth and development and day-to-day care of their sick or handicapped child: "I just don't know how to take care of a child with this problem." The extent of parental lack of information and misinformation is frequently great.

2. Child-rearing practices may be distorted

because of parental depression, anxiety, ambivalence, inability to cope, and undue focus on the child's handicap without seeing the child as a child. Since the parents may be unable to perceive accurately the child's developmental needs, they may not know what to expect or what to do.

3. The striking lack of communication in many of these families is often not considered. The father may detach himself by being away much of the time, participating neither in the child's physical care nor in play, implying or actually stating to the mother, "He's your child. You take care of him."

4. The family may become socially isolated. Many parents of chronically ill children never go out together socially. The preoccupation of the mother with the sick or handicapped child may leave little time for her other children or her husband. Siblings, receiving little or no help with their feelings of depression, anxiety, and guilt, may attempt to compensate by being too good or by developing somatic symptoms. They may not be able to understand why the patient is receiving what seems to them undue attention.

5. The handicapped child may have low self-esteem.

Visits in which parents have a chance to express anxieties to a physician who listens, is empathetic, and has their confidence are of great therapeutic value. Because of its duration and the peculiar stresses and vicissitudes involved, the relation between physician and family in long-term disease differs from that in episodic illness or health supervision. Since the family necessarily is heavily dependent upon the doctor, they carefully scrutinize not only his actions and statements, but also those of his associates. Although most parents and children will show confidence in his care and gratitude for his help and support, they may also have feelings of disappointment that the physician is not able to cure the patient.

Some families are able to express these dissatisfactions openly; others do this indirectly in their questions, comments, changes in behavior, disinclination to talk, or by canceling, failing to keep, or lengthening the interval between appointments. As a reaction to their feelings of ineffectiveness, some parents may be openly skeptical or critical of physicians. When the family suddenly has little to say, it may be helpful to take notice by a statement such as "You seem bothered. Is there something on your mind . . . something I've done or not done that you're unhappy or disappointed about?" The thoughtful physician keeps in mind that it is easy to spend time with families who seem to be appreciative, to be cursory with parents who are unresponsive, and to be affronted by those who are hostile.

Long-term illnesses are psychologically as well as physically upsetting. The parents of a chronically ill child experience a number of psychological reactions, prominent among which are denial, guilt, and anger. In the case of a serious long-term illness, denial initially prevents the complete parental disorganization that might ensue were it necessary to face immediately the full reality. It helps to explain why parents may report observations strikingly different from those of the physician; why they cling to the belief that everything will be all right; why they may not raise many questions; why they may deny that they have been told anything; why they may distort what they have been told; why they may not wish regular appointments; and why they may shop for a magical solution or a physician who agrees with their perceptions. Denial seems to be more prominent with intellectual than physical defects. Although both the mother and the father may give up denial about the same time, when they do not, the results are distorted communication, inconsistent child care, and marital discord. Denial may also break down when the baby's developmental achievements clearly are delayed, e.g., walking in the case of the blind infant, or when entrance to school illuminates the cognitive differences from peers in the case of the mentally retarded child.

The seemingly unending demands of frequent visits to the physician, expensive medications, repeated laboratory procedures, preparation of the child for recurring hospitalizations, and special diets, injections, or inhalation therapy may bring physical and psychological fatigue and economic hardship. They disrupt the family's independence and privacy. Resentment, anger, guilt, and fear, or simple lack of information, lead to worrisome, demanding, and querulous parental behavior in which blame is projected on the child, the spouse, or the physician. Although some families are strengthened, many are severely strained. Those with marginal personal or marital adjustments break down. One parent may take, or be forced to assume, all responsibilities, while the spouse, seemingly unconcerned or critical of the time and cost involved, distances or disengages himself from the family.

Since even the most mature parents find it difficult to cope with both their own feelings and the needs of their child, the illness almost always alters their relations, the change being dependent, in large part, on what has gone before. Some parents, abandoning all discipline, are overprotective and overindulgent; others redouble control or become punitive and distant. A mother who has successfully reared other children may be unable to foster healthy child development, e.g., acquisition of self-help skills, and may uncharacteristically fail to prepare her child for procedures or hospitalization. Fearful for the child, she may resort to threats about his becoming worse in order to gain his cooperation. Siblings may envy the patient's extra attention and privileges and resent the expectation that they help provide care, but they may also be depressed about his disease and the chance that they are "next."

Rather than be consigned to a side-line role as passive observers totally reliant on professionals, the parents should be encouraged to be active participants and collaborators under the supervision of therapists. The enhancement of parental competence, self-confidence, and coping abilities are important aspects of management. Although pamphlets and books may be used selectively if followed by a chance for discussion of what the parent has read, they are no substitute for personal communication. The physician needs to contribute to the mother's ability to take care of her child without reinforcing her tendency to be self-sacrificing. It may be helpful to discuss with the father his ideas of what he can do to help, e.g., bring the child for some of the visits to the physician, or help take care of the child at home. The doctor's insistence that both parents, especially the mother, reserve time to themselves away from the child may help promote parental effectiveness and communication.

Seeing the Child as a Child

In time, most children accept and adapt to the reality of their illness, although they do so with varying degrees of success and comfort. Anxiety, usually the primary response in patients with long-term illnesses, may be evident even in very young children. Those with an inadequate understanding of their disease may overestimate its seriousness. Children with covert diseases such as diabetes find it difficult to comprehend what they cannot see. Repeated hospitalizations, bone marrow aspirations, and corrective operations engender chronic anxiety and anger with the parents, especially the mother, for not protecting them from those ordeals. Because their disease makes them feel more vulnerable, failure and disappointment may be built into their anticipation of many new experiences. Thus, they may be very sensitive to environmental events, e.g., changes in school, moves of the family, discord between parents, illness or death of relatives or friends, separation experiences, medical procedures, hospitalization, and changes in symptoms, medication, or physicians. Even mild and self-limited illnesses or injuries may be poorly tolerated. Anxiety contributes to regression and an increase in dependency. When coupled with pain, restriction of body movement, or isolation, symptoms such as anorexia, apathy, thumb-sucking, masturbation, restlessness, sleep disturbance, and uncooperativeness are readily understood.

Whether told or not, the child with a serious chronic illness knows that the disease is life-threatening. A feeling of special risk is kept alive by the necessity for frequent visits to the physician, special diets, warnings about side effects, daily medications, blood transfusions, and repeated hospitalization. The child may attempt to reduce this threat by converting the danger symbolically and displacing it to a limited part of the body as abdominal pain, headache, or concern about a small skin nevus. The child and the parents thus have a definable symptom to take to the physician for reassurance, in this way avoiding to some extent the painful awareness of the fear of dying prematurely. The expectation of a premature death may also cause the child to be hyperactive and unable to learn in school.

Denial is frequently used by the child with a chronic illness to help cope with the limitations and discomfort imposed by the illness. Failure of patients to cooperate in medical regimens may represent denial of the illness.

Chronic illness poses a direct threat to the integrity of the child's body. Physical weakness, weight loss, scars, growth retardation, alopecia, cushingoid appearance, or edema changes his body image. Besides potentially or actually compromising his independence from his family, his sexuality, and his ability to compete, the disease may cause the child to be excluded from peer activities. The adolescent's self-concept reflects not only his own perceptions of his problem but also how he is regarded by others, both within and outside the family. He is especially worried about being different from his friends.

The adolescent with such problems as mental

retardation, cystic fibrosis, or cerebral palsy may suddenly one day, in a flash of insight, consciously recognize fully for the first time that he has a major problem that he will not "outgrow." If the child believes that all his growth has been "used up," this poignant moment of truth may cause him to be engulfed by feelings of inadequacy, shame, and a sense of losing out in life. He may become dejected about his ability to achieve success in school, vocation, marriage, and society and appear disorganized in knowing what to do or plan next. On the other hand, if the child believes that his potential for growth and mastery of his handicap remains open, this moment of truth may be incorporated into a continuum of healthy adaptation.

The patient may be angry at the world for being dealt an unfair blow, at his parents for "causing" the disease—especially if it is hereditary, and at physicians, first for finding a disease which the child reasons would not otherwise have been present, second for not effecting a cure, and third for prescribing restrictions, deprivations, injections, and procedures. He is troubled by the repeated invasions of his privacy created by the treatment of his disease. He needs the opportunity to express his fears, angers, and worries. These reactions may be expressed in a variety of ways, e.g., rebellion, overdependence, passive resignation, or manipulativeness. Parents are usually not well prepared for the problems related to aggression or sexuality that may become prominent in adolescence. Some may ask questions about such behavior directly, but all appreciate the physician's interest and inquiry in these important areas.

When parental coping patterns are functioning well and the parent-child relation is characterized by mutuality, the child may be expected to achieve a high degree of physical, intellectual, psychological, and social development notwithstanding all the potential problems. Many invulnerable children with long-term problems do make excellent psychological, social, and vocational adaptations.

The physician who cares for a child with a long-term illness sees his patient frequently over months or years. He gets to know him well and shares many vicissitudes of life. Personalized care, based on the kind of seasoned experience that leads to an empathetic responsiveness to the needs of the patient, contributes greatly to the child's comfort and security. The physician's attentiveness is demonstrated by the kind and thoughtful way in which he talks to and examines the child; remembering birthdays, holidays, and other special dates; spontaneous conversation about things of interest to the boy or girl, e.g., school, sports, play, movies, television programs, trips, books, pets, and hobbies; alertness to the child's feelings of depression ("You seem kind of discouraged today"), discomfort, or fear of death—*and of life;* an occasional phone call, especially if the child has missed an appointment; appropriate compliments; encouraging him to talk about his strengths; encouraging the development of new strengths; asking the receptionist or nurse to welcome each child by name; introducing the child to the physician's associates; talking to him alone as well as to his parents; an open invitation to call the doctor between visits; understanding of his fearful reaction to new or painful procedures; granting permission for an occasional relaxation of the medical regimen; patience in understanding why the child may be uncooperative; avoidance of criticism, sermons, threats, or exhortation; and acceptance of the negative feelings that he may express. All of this is important whether or not the child seems to respond overtly to the physician's interest.

The child's sense of competence and his active role in the management of his illness are enhanced by unhurried, honest explanations of the disease and both the promise and limitations of its treatment. Diagrams and other visual aids may be helpful. Whereas this is especially true of the adolescent, the approach also applies to younger children who need to be informed at their level of understanding. These discussions need not be complete in every detail but should be sufficient for the child to feel that he has an active role in his own destiny. Such open presentations, adapted to the cognitive level of the patient, are reassuring rather than upsetting.

As soon as feasible, the child should be permitted to regulate his own diet, take his own medicine, and give his own injections. Since social, recreational, and educational activities are essential to the child's sense of well-being, achievement, and self-esteem, restriction of activity and other restraints and prohibitions should be prescribed only when clearly indicated. The parents and the child should be specifically cautioned against imposing needless restrictions of their own.

Patient compliance or cooperation with the therapeutic plan is an imperfectly understood process (see also Chapter 2, p. 18). Achieving a therapeutic alliance remains, in large part, an art that draws heavily upon the physician's warmth, sincerity, and empathy. Patients who feel positively evaluated are likely to accept their doctor's recommendations. One may expect positive compliance when the patient's and the physician's perceptions of the problems and what needs to be done are congruent, and when the patient believes that he receives adequate attention for his problem. Mothers of children with persistent problems are extremely sensitive to the slightest implication that they have been at fault.

Ordinary courtesies that promote patient compliance include seeing the same doctor each time, scheduling visits so as to minimize waiting, being gracious, and sitting down for discussions. Parental factors that contribute to a positive therapeutic alliance include faith in the physician's treatment, positive attitudes about health, high expectations for the child, concern about being a good mother, ability to mobilize family resources, belief that they have an important role in the child's health, interest in being an active participant in the child's care, accurate perception of the illness and its consequences, ability to communicate with the physician, knowledge of what to do, and belief that the prescribed medication is safe or that its benefits outweigh its possible side effects.

Even with a physician's best efforts, cooperation is not always forthcoming, especially with long-term regimens, asymptomatic disorders, and preventive medications. A history of prior noncompliance, frequent broken appointments, suspicion, distrust, or a disappointing medical experience in the past is a reliable predictor of noncompliance. Compliance may also be compromised in the presence of family discord, separation, or divorce or with an indifferent, preoccupied, or depressed parent.

It is part of the competence of the physician to minimize pain and discomfort, important contributors to psychological distress. A few children tend to suffer in silence, but the chronically ill patient is no more able to tolerate pain than a healthy child, although this seems to be frequently assumed.

The pediatrician sees the total child as well as the illness. His growth and development, physical health, nutrition, immunization, psychological adjustment, outside interests, maturation, sense of self responsibility, school progress, ability to acquire and keep friends, and vocational plans are all of interest. Every effort should be made to keep the child in school. Children with chronic illness, especially asthma or malignancy, tend to miss many more school days than their healthy peers. Such absences should be carefully monitored and avoided whenever possible.

Although concerned with matters of the moment, the physician recognizes the eventual goal to be a socially competent adult. Opportunities for socialization and for education in playgroups, nursery school, and kindergarten, as well as elementary, high, and vocational schools, are important steps in the achievement of this goal.

Preparation for What is Going to Happen

A child's trust that he will always be told what is going to happen greatly fosters his perception of the physician as truthful, predictable, and safe. Anticipatory discussion of changes in medication and treatment or need for hospitalization or procedures helps prevent undue anxiety. Preparation for procedures includes a truthful explanation of their nature. What may seem minor to the physician, e.g., an intravenous pyelogram or a bone marrow aspiration, may loom as a major event to the child. In the preparation for the procedure, questions should be answered honestly without discounting discomfort or pain. The child should be comforted by the person doing the procedure. If this is to be done by another doctor and the child's physician believes the experience may be upsetting, he should try to be there.

Open Communication

Openness is essential in the management of children with long-term illness, including communication between health providers, with the family, and between the parents and child. Continuing care provides the opportunity to enhance such interchange.

To a considerable extent, one can sense what the child understands and how he feels about his illness by the nature of his questions. While some questions are asked immediately, those that engender the most anxiety ("Will I grow up? Will I be cured? Will I die?") can be communicated only in the freedom of a secure and close relationship. This takes weeks or months. Although one cannot neutralize realistic anxieties, one can utilize the opportunity of the question or the statement that fronts for a question to clarify misconceptions, alleviate guilt, and emphasize that a doctor can and will do much to control the disease.

Since questions are more commonly and freely asked of parents, especially the mother, they should be prepared to answer. Indeed, the doctor should stress the importance of creating a climate in which the child feels free to ask questions. Such openness is less oppressive than what may appear to be a conspiracy of silence.

Collaboration

Since the individual physician does not have immediately available in the usual office setting all the services which these children and families require, collaboration and communication are frequently required between physicians, allied health specialists, and community hospitals and other institutions where such services are available. Parenthetically, the ability of the parents, assisted by their doctor, to mobilize needed resources contributes significantly to their own self-esteem and helps the child to see them as effective, invested, and caring persons.

Although most effective, face-to-face collaboration between professionals is often not possible; as a substitute, letters and telephone calls are a continuing responsibility of both the general care physician and the consultant. The latter may be requested to provide care limited to the area of their specialization, with the former responsible for the child's personal health care, or the total health care may be delegated to the systems specialist. Whatever the arrangement, the responsibility of each person is often not defined early for the family and for each doctor, leading to confusion, duplication, gaps in communication and services, e.g., immunization, or abdication of care of the chronic illness by the practitioner. Although it takes considerable effort to establish effective lines of communication between the providers of the services required, the generalist pediatrician should play the central role in the management of many chronic disorders of children, using subspecialists as consultants rather than relinquishing care entirely.

Promoting a Positive Identity

It is important that an accurate diagnosis of the illness or handicap be established as soon as possible and that the parents and the child have this clearly explained. Whereas the discussion of the diagnosis—the *identity* of the illness—must be straightforward and reflect the exact state of affairs without overstatement or understatement, the physician should temper truthfulness in order to inform the parents and the child at a time and in a manner that is helpful and understandable rather than overwhelming. Although some persons seem to do best if they are given the information all at one time, others benefit more from a gradual presentation. An exhaustive discussion is generally inappropriate at the initial visit.

Questions commonly raised explicitly or implicitly by the parents at the time of diagnosis include: What caused this? Why did this happen? What can be done? What will be done next? Where can this be done? How soon? How much will this cost? Will this affect our other children?

In the case of the child born with a congenital anomaly, the parents' expectant notion of the baby's identity—what the infant would be like—is abruptly and strikingly modified. The unusual replaces the familiar. The baby is different from what might have been. The growing mutuality between mother and infant seems suddenly extinguished. The parents feel apart, cheated, faulted, deprived, and isolated ("Where is everyone?"). Especially vulnerable are single mothers who confront this crisis alone. There are few times when support is more needed and sophisticated care that attends to the parents' minds and hearts more appropriate. The parents' vulnerability and receptivity create a special bond with the doctor who is with them at this critical time.

The clinician needs to help the parents refashion the baby's ill-defined identity in a constructive manner so as to see clearly the child's strengths and potentialities as well as problems and vulnerabilities. One simple but useful technique is to examine the baby in front of the parents. This shared examination permits the doctor to emphasize normality while delineating deviations from the normal, clarifies for the parents the nature of their baby's difficulties, conveys to them something of the baby's personality, encourages them to ask more questions than they otherwise might, and facilitates communication between the parents while they are both focused on the baby. Demonstration of the baby's responsiveness and the physician's regard for the infant as a person rather than as a malformation importantly promotes the parents' positive acceptance of the baby as well as the reality of the malformation.

Repeated explanations of the baby's status and development, with a special emphasis on normality but without a denial of the long-term problems, in return visits over time, help the parents clarify further the baby's identity. Both normality and difference need to be integrated and accepted as simultaneously as possible by the parents and eventually by the child. Not only does the parents' perceived identity of their baby or an older child change at the time of the diagnosis of a congenital or acquired long-term illness or handicap, but the parents' self-identities and how they perceive their spouse are no longer the same. The physician has a central role in the reconstruction of the identities of the child, of his parents, and of the family by promoting open communication and discouraging the kind of isolation that invites identity diffusion. The adaptation achieved eventually by the parents—either accepting, realistic, and confident, or rejecting, angry, and denying—will obviously have a major impact on the child's own identity.

Support, Encouragement, and Advocacy

Once the diagnosis, treatment, and prognosis have been explained to the child and family, the physician should maintain an optimistic, encouraging outlook without, of course, promising too much. The parents should be helped to identify and mobilize supporting persons. The steady nurturing of an atmosphere of hope and encouragement is a cardinal principle in the care of children with long-term illnesses. This climate is created both by what the physician says and by what he does in terms of aggressive care with meticulous attention to detail, personal interest in the child and parents, suggestions of things which parents and child can do, and counseling in relation to immediate questions and concerns. Parent groups may both provide considerable support and increase the parents' understanding, management, and participation.

The pediatrician can be an important opinion leader in promoting the local availability of the services that a community's handicapped children need for their continuing care, including therapeutic services in the home. Such planning requires a community census of the children with long-term disorders, their ages, and the nature of their handicaps. The determination of the scope of services the community needs may be facilitated by consultation with the various therapists at the regional center. Two-way communication of this type in the service of network development permits the services at the center (Level III) to be *coupled with* those available (or to be implemented) in the child's home community (Levels I and II). In relation to an individual child, the pediatrician may serve as a knowledgeable advocate in helping ensure that the specific needs of that boy or girl are being met in the individual educational plan prepared in accord with PL 94–142.

Family strengths and resources need to be identified. These include a supportive marital relationship, relatives and friends to whom the parents can turn for support, the parents' ability to articulate their feelings and needs, their ability to regard their baby as a person, a healthy older sibling, and the opportunity to talk with "pilot" parents who have mastered a similar crisis.

Chronic illness and handicaps confront the physician with problems of uncertain outcomes and potential feelings of inadequacy and ineffectiveness. Unless he is secure as to his competence, the physician may be vulnerable to undetected feelings of guilt and self-criticism that impair his self-esteem to the point that his diagnostic and therapeutic effectiveness is reduced. Although the reality is that reimbursement is often limited for much of what the doctor does in the care of children with long-term problems, he should not be hesitant to charge for the personal services he provides in Level I, II, or III care.

Since caring for large numbers of chronically and seriously ill children is emotionally demanding, the physician may feel psychologically drained. In order to protect his feelings the doctor may become impersonal and see the chronically ill child infrequently, perhaps not scheduling return visits. Believing he has little to offer, he may make the family uncomfortable about taking his time or even returning. On the other hand, the physician who recognizes his own competence, eschews unrealistic goals, and is comfortable in sharing the care of the child with others is able to maintain an active, supportive interest. He is in a unique position to provide the support and encouragement children with chronic disorders and their families need. Such skilled physicians have a way of evoking the strengths and invulnerabilities of their parents—accentuating the positive; while managing their vulnerabilities and illnesses—limiting the negative.

REFERENCES

Alpert, J. J.: School absence: A problem for the pediatrician. Pediatrics, 69:739, 1982.

Bibace, R., and Walsh, M. E.: Development of children's concepts of illness. Pediatrics, 66:912, 1980.
Breslau, N., Weitzman, M., and Messenger, K.: Psychologic functioning of siblings of disabled children. Pediatrics, 67:344, 1981.
Brimblecombe, F. S. W.: An Exeter project for handicapped children. Br. Med. J., 4:706, 1974.
Bywater, E. M.: Adolescents with cystic fibrosis: Psychosocial adjustment. Arch. Dis. Child., 56:538, 1981.
Drotar, D., Doershuk, C. F., Stern, R. C., Boat, T. F., Boyer, W., and Matthews, L.: Psychosocial functioning of children with cystic fibrosis. Pediatrics, 67:338, 1981.
Featherstone, H.: A Difference in the Family: Life with a Disabled Child. New York, Basic Books, 1980.
Green, M.: Care of infants and children with long-term handicaps. Bull. N.Y. Acad. Med., 55:832, 1979.
Hayden, P. W., Davenport, S. L. H., and Campbell, M. M.: Adolescents with myelodysplasia: Impact of physical disability on emotional maturation. Pediatrics, 64:53, 1979.
Lavigne, J. V., and Ryan, M.: Psychologic adjustment of siblings of children with chronic illness. Pediatrics, 63:616, 1979.
Lichstein, P. R.: The resident leaves the patient: Another look at the doctor-patient relationship. Ann. Intern. Med., 96:762, 1982.
Litt, I. F., and Cuskey, W. R.: Compliance with medical regimens during adolescence. Pediatr. Clin. North Am., 27:3, 1980.
Millstein, S. G., Adler, N. E., and Irwin, C. E.: Conceptions of illness in young adolescents. Pediatrics, 68:834, 1981.
Perrin, E. C., and Gerrity, P. S.: There's a demon in your belly: Children's understanding of illness. Pediatrics, 67:841, 1981.
Pless, I. B., and Pinkerton, P.: Chronic Childhood Disorder—Promoting Patterns of Adjustment. London, Henry Kimpton Publishers, 1975.
Pless, I. B., and Satterwhite, B. B.: Health and illness. Chronic illness. *In* Haggerty, R. J., Roghmann, K. J., and Pless, I. B. (Eds.): Child Health and the Community. New York, Wiley Interscience Publishers, 1975.
Rosenbloom, A. L.: Chronic illness in children and adolescents seen in private practice. 67th Ross Conference on Chronic Physical Disease in Children, June, 1974.
Rosenbloom, A. L., and Ongley, J. P.: Who provides what services to children in private medical practice? Am. J. Dis. Child., 127:357, 1974.
Shope, J. T.: Medication compliance. Pediatr. Clin. North Am., 28:5, 1981.

Morris Green, M.D.

60

CEREBRAL PALSY

Lawrence T. Taft, M.D.

Cerebral palsy is a disorder affecting posture and movement due to a static encephalopathy, with the insult to the brain occurring prenatally, perinatally, or in early childhood. Although the term *cerebral palsy* refers to a "motor disorder," the majority of patients are additionally handicapped with seizures and cognitive, sensory, visual, and auditory impairments.

Reported to occur in 1 to 2 of every 1000 births, cerebral palsy is of relatively low frequency but high severity. It is a lifelong handicap that requires many adaptations for living by the child, parents, extended family, and society. These adaptations are not only continuous but also must take account of the growth and development of the handicapped individual.

CLASSIFICATION

Classification of cerebral palsy has proven difficult. An "etiological" classification has not been used, since causative factors are inapparent in over 50 per cent of patients. Specific location and extent of the pathological findings are rarely ascertained even after extensive and sophisticated evaluation. Out of necessity, a "clinical" classification based on the description of the movement disorder has evolved (Table 60–1), but this has not been entirely satisfactory. The clinical picture associated with damage to the nervous system changes dramatically with growth and maturation, especially in the first years of life. In fact, the fully developed movement disorder that can be classified may not appear until two to three years of age. Many patients with cerebral palsy have two or more disorders of involuntary movement, e.g., spastic and athetoid components. With maturation of the brain, the clinical manifestation of the motor abnormality may not only change but even disappear, especially in infants who weigh less than 1500 grams or are small for gestational age.

In the past, a hemiparesis was reported as the most common type of cerebral palsy; however, in recent years, spastic diplegia may be more common. Monoparesis is very rare. In fact, if the examiner is convinced that one extremity is involved, he must examine the other ipsilateral extremity carefully for similar impairment. Premature infants may manifest an "atonic" diplegia during the first one to two years of life which then evolves into a classic "spastic" diplegia. Full-term babies may be atonic at birth and remain so throughout their lifetime. These youngsters are usually severely retarded.

EARLY RECOGNITION

Early recognition of cerebral palsy and early therapeutic intervention have been shown to optimize the ultimate functioning of the cerebral palsied child so far as his motor, cognitive, and social competences are concerned, and to facilitate the family's adaptation to their child's handicap.

ETIOLOGICAL RISK FACTORS

A high index of suspicion that cerebral palsy may develop in a baby should result from "high-risk" factors in the history. Factors which should alert the physician to do a very careful neurodevelopmental examination during each office visit include low birth weight infants, especially below 1500 grams; small-for-gestational-age babies, especially preterm babies; reproductive complications such as threatened abortion, toxemia, rubella during the first trimester of pregnancy; postmaturity; abnormal presentation of the fetus, especially breech; evidence of abnormalities in fetal heart rate as noted by fetal monitoring; meconium staining of the amniotic fluid; mid- or high forceps delivery or the need for emergency cesarean section; neonatal complications such as hyperbilirubinemia, convulsions, apnea, cyanosis, very low one-minute and moderately low five-minute Apgar scores, meningitis or sepsis, and postnatal events such as encephalitis, meningitis, head trauma, lead encephalopathy, and reactions to vaccination and immunization procedures (Walker, 1967).

Prematurity remains one of the most common causes of cerebral palsy. It has been estimated that 27 per cent of occurrences of cerebral palsy could be avoided if low birth weight were eliminated. The relative risk of having a baby with cerebral palsy is 25 times greater in babies weighing under 1500 grams at birth than in those weighing over 2500 grams. Contemporary newborn care has increased the survival rate of preterm infants, but whether the prevalence of neurological morbidity has actually decreased remains undetermined.

Certain etiological factors are causally related to the development of specific clinical types of cerebral palsy. If a preterm infant develops cerebral palsy, it has been estimated that 80 per cent will have a spastic diplegia (lower extremities more involved than upper extremities). Small-for-gestational-age preterm infants with relatively small head circumferences and low one-minute Apgar scores are especially predisposed to spastic diplegia. With the advent of the CT scan, it has become apparent that low birth weight infants are prone to develop subependymal hemorrhages. The pyramidal tracts to the lower extremities are situated in this area, and their destruction results in spastic involvement of the lower extremities. More widespread hemorrhage may also involve the more peripherally located pyramidal tracts, resulting in a spastic quadriparesis.

Athetosis is usually secondary to bilirubin encephalopathy or to birth anoxia. The basal ganglion nuclei are especially sensitive to hyperbilirubinemia and anoxia. Traumatic deliveries may result in cerebral hemorrhage and in hemisyndrome. Hydrocephalus causes stretching of the pyramidal tracts, especially those adjacent to the ventricles, resulting in spastic diplegia with ataxia.

Congenital hypoplasia of the cerebellum has been associated with the congenital ataxia syndrome and its variant, the "disequilibrium syndrome." The disequilibrium child does not have signs of tremor or dysmetria but has marked difficulties in postural adjustment. This problem in equilibrium makes the achievement of gross motor milestones difficult. Independent walking may not occur until nine years of age. Hypotonia and mental retardation are usually associated with this syndrome.

DEVELOPMENT RISK FACTORS

Qualitative differences (e.g., sucking and swallowing difficulties; early handedness; prolonged drooling; asymmetrical crawl; buttocks crawl or "hitching"; bunny hop crawl; persistent toe walking; tendency to fall easily when ambulating; delayed motor milestones) must also be regarded with suspicion.

Difficulties in sucking may be the first manifestation of a problem in neuromotor integration and competency. The sucking problem may be due to incoordination of the tongue, as a result of which the nipple is pushed out of the baby's mouth. Also, poor neuromotor coordination causes variations in the rate and strength of the sucking and does not permit strong lip closure around the nipple. Observation of the baby's sucking may permit recognition of these patterns. Unfortunately, the difficulty in feeding is often attributed to the shape or size of the nipple or to the formula. Rather than being due to changes in these, improvement in sucking may be due to maturation of the central nervous system with a resultant lessening of the motor dyspraxia and incoordination.

Problems with swallowing should also be an alerting factor. Many babies with poor neuromotor control of the muscles used in swallowing gag on coarse foods if they are given too early. Improvement usually occurs with maturation.

Infants who roll over at an exceptionally early age may appear to be developing precociously, but one must be suspicious that this achievement may be due to increased extensor tone. With the reinforcement to extensor tone that accompanies crying, the baby may arch his back and "flip over." These are the same babies who will show advanced head and neck control when they are in the prone position. Their increased extensor tone is due to an abnormal tonic labyrinth reflex which, if functioning normally, would be accentuating a flexor posture in babies under two months of age.

Unusual crawling patterns should always be suspect. An asymmetrical crawl in which the baby pushes off with one arm and the ipsilateral leg indicates a hemiparesis of the contralateral extremities. An early onset of handedness is also an alerting finding. Most normal babies do not show hand preference until about 12 to 18 months of age. The mother should be asked if she thinks her five- or six-month-old infant is left-handed or right-handed. If she is convinced that handedness has been established, the baby requires careful assessment for a hemisyndrome.

The buttocks crawl, "hitching" or "scooting" on the buttocks with the feet or hands or both being used for movement, is not an uncommon finding in babies who develop a cerebral diplegia. This means of locomotion is utilized by the infant who cannot develop a reciprocating movement pattern of the lower extremities. A caveat is that 10 per cent of normal infants reportedly may "bunny hop" as an early method of locomotion. This is an inherited trait with dominant transmission. These babies do not like to lie prone and are frequently hypotonic. At approximately six to seven months of age, the same normal infant, held in vertical suspension, will flex his hips and extend his legs while seemingly resistant to extending his hips and bearing weight on his lower extremities. Because there is also a delay in motor development until 17 to 18 months of age in these children, an erroneous diagnosis of cerebral palsy may be suggested. The buttocks crawl may be considered an early finding of spastic diplegia in the absence of a family history of shuffling, tightened hamstrings, and hyperactive deep tendon jerks in the lower extremities. Also, a low birth weight baby should be especially suspect. A bunny hop crawl in which babies jump up and down on their knees without using an alternating pattern is frequent in infants who will later develop cerebral palsy.

Although an infant may walk at the expected age, the stability and character of his gait are important. A normal infant, on first attempting independent ambulation, will frequently be up on his toes, walk with his legs spread apart, and keep his arms flexed beside his head in order to achieve better balance. Over a period of a month or two, the normal infant will gradually lower his arms to a position beside the trunk and assume the plantigrade position of the feet with the legs closer together that is characteristic of a more mature gait pattern. Babies with a motor handicap affecting the lower extremities will, however, persist in toe walking and a wide-base gait. Those who are spastic will gradually lose their wide base and move to a scissoring pattern while the babies who are ataxic will maintain their wide base. Both groups will stumble more often than normal.

TEST FOR CEREBRAL PALSY

A delay in achievement of a motor milestone should alert the physician to the possibility of a motor handicap and evoke a more complete neuromotor examination. In young infants, the developmental screening tests are of limited value in judging the competence of the motor system, since there are so few assessable skills in their motor repertoire. In addition, the screening tests are quantitative estimates of motor development and do not meausure its quality or style. Inclusion of a few neurodevelopmental tests that are especially valuable in identifying a motor abnormality only adds a minute or two to a routine office evaluation.

Infants Under Six Months of Age

Key Points

The neuromotor assessment of infants below six months of age.

1. Evaluation for asymmetry of movement.
2. Assessment of primitive reflexes.
3. Evaluation of abnormalities in tone.
4. Evaluation for the presence of hyperreflexia.

Asymmetry of Movement

Observation for asymmetry of movement is indicated if the baby is older than three or four months of age. Asymmetry of movement under two months of age usually indicates a lower motor neuron disorder of the brachial or sciatic type. Occasionally, the limitation of movement may be secondary to pain caused by a fracture. In babies four months of age or older, the physician should note if one hand remains fisted more than the other or if the infant seems to reach out preferentially with one hand. Such behavior may be the earliest manifestation of a hemiparesis. The absence of classic confirmatory neurological signs at this early stage should not negate the possibility that the baby has a motor handicap.

Assessment of Primitive Reflexes

Asymmetrical Tonic Neck Reflex. Passively turn the head of a supine infant first to the left and then to the right and maintain each posture for a minimum of 30 seconds. If an infant of any age, especially one who is crying, appears unable to break down the "fencing" posture noted in the extremities, the test is considered abnormal (Fig. 60–1). Normal babies under four to five months of age may not demonstrate an asymmetrical tonic neck reflex. If present, it will not be obligatory, in that the imposed patterns of the extremities will be quickly broken down when the baby cries or becomes agitated. After four to six months of age, any vestige of an asymmetrical tonic neck reflex is abnormal. Abnormalities in the maturation and disappearance of this primitive reflex are fairly good predictors of a motor handicap. The absence of the asymmetrical tonic neck reflex when the head is turned to one side in contrast to the other does not indicate the side of the hemiparesis, but it may demonstrate the presence of a hemisyndrome. The obligatory tonic reflex will be especially prominent if a baby is to develop athetoid cerebral palsy or spastic quadriparesis.

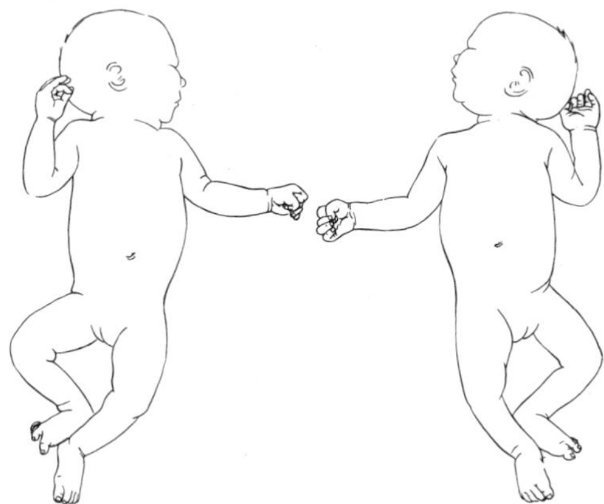

Figure 60–1. Asymmetrical tonic neck reflex.

Crossed Extensor Reflex. If a noxious stimulus is applied to the sole of an extended lower extremity, the reflex response is flexor withdrawal of the contralateral extremity immediately followed by extension and then adduction. A crossed extensor reflex is not always apparent, but if easily elicited in a baby over four months of age, it indicates spastic involvement of the lower extremities.

Assessment of Tone

Hypotonia. Andre-Thomas et al. have attempted to provide a more rigid definition of hypotonia with range of motion of joints as the frame of reference. Measurements of shoulder and hip joint mobility appear to be reliable indicators in infants and should be assessed routinely.

The anterior scarf sign (Fig. 60–2) is elicited with the infant supine, head in midline, and shoulders held against the examining table. Normally, an attempt to pull the arm anteriorly around the neck results in an ability to draw the elbow past the chin. If the elbow can be drawn past the chin, this is interpreted as an increased range of motion of the shoulder joint. When doing the test, it is important that the scapula not be lifted off the examining table when the hand is being pulled to the opposite side.

The posterior scarf sign is tested by pulling the hand directly posterior, keeping the forearm parallel to the head. This should be done with

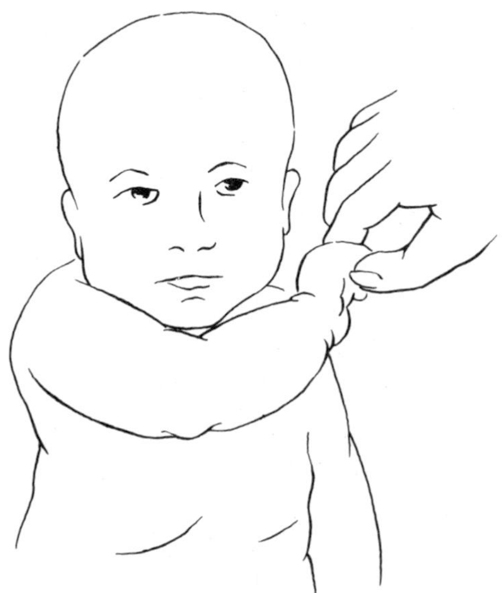

Figure 60–2. Anterior scarf sign.

the baby in the sitting position and the head should be in line with the trunk. If the arm is pulled straight back and the elbow can be pulled past the ear, this "positive" posterior scarf sign indicates an increased range of motion of the shoulder joint.

In the lower extremities, a simple test to judge range of motion of the hip joint is to abduct the hips of a supine infant while keeping the knees and hips extended. Abduction to 170 degrees or more is considered significant. Most tests of abduction are usually done with the hips flexed in order to judge congenital subluxation of the hips. Abduction of the hips when both they and the knees are being extended should also be checked.

An increased range of motion of joints does not necessarily indicate an upper motor neuron lesion. A lower motor neuron abnormality or a collagen disorder (e.g., Ehlers-Danlos syndrome) must be excluded.

Hypertonia. Although many babies who go on to develop hypertonus are initially hypotonic, there are exceptions, and some infants under six months may be hypertonic. Since formal signs of spasticity or rigidity such as clasp-knife, plastic, or cog-wheel responses are difficult to elicit in an infant, an attempt is made to judge abnormalities in the tonic labyrinth reflexes. Quite active in infants, these adjust the tone of the agonist and antagonist muscles according to the position of the head in space. The specific sequential maturational changes that occur permit a judgment as to appropriate muscle tone relative to the infant's age. For example, in the newborn baby, the tonic labyrinth reflexes cause the baby to assume a fairly marked flexor posture and to "double up like a ball" when in the prone position. This same baby, when placed in the supine position, shows relaxation of the flexor posture but not enough to extend trunk or extremities. However, with maturation, there is a gradual change so that the tonic labyrinth reflex in the prone position results in less of a tendency toward a flexor posture with gradual domination of the extensors. In fact, a prone infant over three months of age whose buttocks are higher than the chest because of marked flexion at the hips and knees should be suspected of developing cerebral palsy.

With these factors in mind, it is worthwhile to do the following routine evaluation for hypertonia in babies under six months of age:

1. The baby should be held in ventral suspension by placing the examiner's hands under the abdomen. Most infants under a few months of age cannot keep their head and neck extended in line with the trunk for more than a few seconds. A tendency for excessive arching suggests hypertonus of the neck extensors. Further evidence for increased tone of the extensor muscles may be apparent when the baby is lifted from the supine position and an excessive head lag occurs.

2. A normal tendency for the baby when pulled up from the supine to a sitting position is flexion of the hips and knees. It is abnormal when the infant comes up with the hips and knees extended to almost a standing position (Fig. 60–3).

3. The baby should then be held in vertical suspension. Hip adductor hypertonus will cause the baby to scissor. The same baby in the supine position might keep the lower extremities abducted, externally rotated, and flexed at the hips and knees (frog position). Scissoring after two to three months of age, even in a baby who was delivered from the frank breech position, should be an alerting sign of increased tone of the lower extremities.

4. An attempt to dorsiflex the ankles should be made. For the first few months of age, it should be possible to dorsiflex the ankles of an infant so that the dorsum of the foot touches the shin. Any limitation of this full range of motion suggests hypertonus of the gastrocnemius muscle. In eliciting this sign, it is preferable to dorsiflex the ankle passively by pulling on the toes in the direction of the shin. Pushing on the sole of the foot may cause a normal

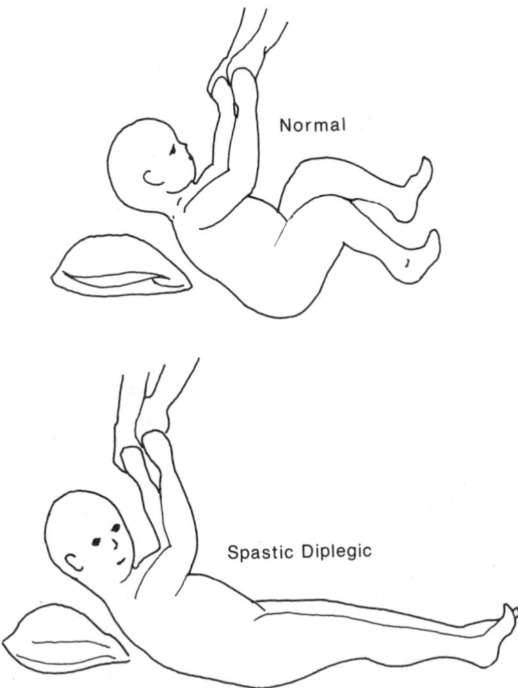

Figure 60–3. Evidence of spastic diplegia.

positive supporting reaction with reflex plantar flexion.

Hyperreflexia. The patellar reflex is difficult to judge. If a hyperactive response is obtained, it is suggested that the examiner percuss over the dorsum of the leg, working gradually up from the lower third toward the patellar tendon. The elicitation of a knee jerk response with a sensory input distant from the primary area confirms that the reflex response is pathologically exaggerated. Ankle jerks are frequently difficult to obtain because of the lack of relaxation of the baby. Ankle clonus should be considered significant only if it is sustained. A few beats of clonus are seen in many normal infants but are uncommon after a few months of age.

An abnormality of any one of these neuromotor tests must be considered significant. Although a recent prospective study indicates that there are no clear-cut signs of symptoms present at one year of age which offer conclusive evidence of cerebral palsy, the children who seemingly outgrew significant motor abnormalities may end up with mental retardation, learning disabilities, dysarthria, and/or seizures. Many of the signs that make an infant at risk for a neuromotor disability may also be indicative of other manifestations of cerebral dysfunction.

As the infant matures, a number of other observations should be routinely made to rule out a neuromotor disability:

1. Observe the baby crawling to see if there is an asymmetrical crawl.
2. Offer the baby an object to see how he reaches out. Although involuntary movements will not be apparent until after one year of age, the physician may be able to judge whether there is increased posturing of the fingers as well as clumsiness (e.g., absence of a pincer grasp in a 10-month-old who is still using an immature raking movement).
3. In a six-month-old baby, a cover should be placed over the infant's face to see which hand he uses to remove the cover (Fig. 60–4). Most babies will use both hands simultaneously. If the hand used initially is restrained, similar dexterity will be displayed in the other. Babies with a hemisyndrome will prefer one hand and become very agitated when that hand is restrained. Babies with normal intelligence will attempt to remove a cover placed over the face by six months of age.
4. A six-month-old infant will have lateral propping reactions (Fig. 60–5). When the baby, supported by the trunk, is then pushed to one side, the arm on that side will extend with the fist opening up and the fingers abducting as if to prevent a fall. This test should be done bilaterally and responses compared. Asymmetry in response could suggest a hemisyndrome. A delay in the appearance of these responses could also suggest a hemisyndrome or a primary motor difficulty. In fact, delay in the protective reactions is thought to reflect more a motor difficulty than a cognitive problem.
5. At around seven to nine months, normal infants develop a parachuting response (Fig. 60–6). Held by the trunk and propelled forward

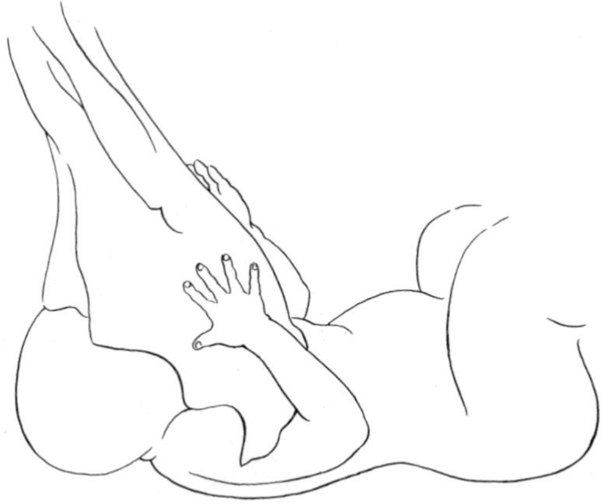

Figure 60–4. Cover test.

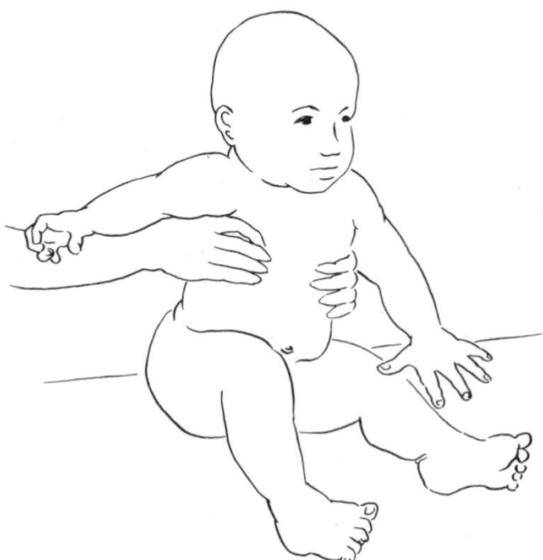

Figure 60–5. Lateral propping.

and downward, the infant will extend the extremities (as in the lateral propping reactions) to prevent the fall. Both extremities should respond symmetrically. Asymmetry of the response points to a hemisyndrome. Delay in achieving this reaction is also of concern.

6. At 10 months of age, babies will demonstrate posterior propping. The examiner approaches the sitting infant from behind, places his hands on the baby's shoulders and suddenly pushes him backwards. The baby's response is to extend both arms posteriorly in order to prevent falling in that direction. Once again, asymmetry in response is significant.

It should be emphasized here that the existence of a functional disturbance as demonstrated by any one of these tests may not be accompanied by tone or reflex asymmetries. In fact, in the immature nervous system, tone or reflex asymmetries in babies who have congenital hemisyndromes are not easily apparent. Therefore, one must recognize the functional disturbance as a true neuromotor deficit and not disclaim the findings because of the absence of reflex or tone changes. Classic neurological signs may not be observed until a later date.

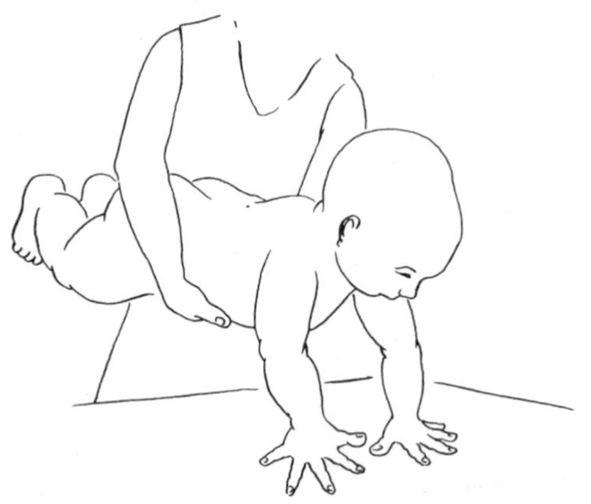

Figure 60–6. Parachuting.

COURSE OF HEMIPARETIC CEREBRAL PALSY

Suspicion of a spastic hemiparesis will rarely occur prior to six months of age. It is unusual to note asymmetry of movement or to find abnormal signs on neurological evaluation prior to four months of age. The first awareness that something may be wrong is the mother's observation that her infant tends to keep one hand fisted in contrast to the other. When the physician is asked to evaluate the infant, the asymmetry may not be evident if the baby is crying and, therefore, fisting both hands. Tone or reflex changes may not be apparent at this early stage. However, when the baby reaches five months of age, the physician may be able to confirm a functional deficit by using the "face-cover" test, even if the infant is irritable. When the baby is six to seven months of age, tightness of the elbow flexors and the wrist pronators may become apparent, as well as slightly exaggerated reflexes. Lateral propping can be helpful if these tests are equivocal, since the state of the baby (active, crying, etc.) will not interfere with this response.

A disability in the ipsilateral lower extremity may not be demonstrable in an infant less than 10 months old if tone or reflex changes are used as criteria. Observation will reveal an asymmetrical crawl. It may also be possible to demonstrate unilateral tightness of the gastrocnemius muscle when passive dorsiflexion is attempted.

The spasticity and tightness of the antigravity muscles become more apparent during the next two years. The toddler gradually develops a hemiplegic posture of the upper extremity with flexion at the elbow, pronation of the wrist, and flexion of the fingers. The lower extremity will reveal equinovarus posturing of the foot with slight knee flexion and hip abduction.

During infancy it is very difficult to predict the functional and cosmetic outcome of a hemiparetic cerebral palsy; however, it can be stated unequivocally that if there is only unilateral motor abnormality, the child will eventually walk. For the majority of spastic hemiparetic infants, independent ambulation will usually be accomplished by 17 to 18 months of age. If the youngster with hemiparetic cerebral palsy is of normal intelligence, he usually becomes completely independent for all activities of daily living.

The main complication is related to flexion contracture at the wrist and to heel cord contractures. Fifty per cent of hemiparetic children will have a cortical sensory deficit and, in many of these same children, there will be a relative shortening of the extremities as compared to the normal side. Since the shortening of the lower extremity rarely will exceed 2 inches after full growth is obtained, orthopedic procedures will usually not be required in order to equalize the leg length discrepancy.

COURSE OF SPASTIC DIPLEGIA

A majority of the babies with spastic diplegia secondary to prematurity usually show hypotonia in the lower extremities with exaggerated reflexes. The initial manifestation of their problem might be delayed sitting or walking. When they do walk, they show a tendency to be up on their toes. Scissoring may also soon become apparent. Increased and typical spasticity with classic hyperreflexia is manifested by one or two years of age.

The extent of the motor handicap varies greatly. Notwithstanding the severity of disability of the lower extremities, if the upper extremities are functionally usable, community ambulation may be achieved with the aid of crutches and lower extremity bracing. If an ataxic component to the diplegia is present, independent ambulation will be more difficult to achieve.

COURSE OF SPASTIC QUADRIPARESIS

A quadriparetic baby has more involvement of the upper than the lower extremities. Occasionally the involvement is asymmetrical, and not infrequently there will be a triplegia with one leg or one arm less involved.

Because of bilateral cerebral involvement, quadriparetic individuals are more often retarded than those with other types of cerebral palsy. Although they may initially be hypotonic, they develop spasticity at 1 to 2 years of age.

Functional competence is difficult to predict early. Motor achievements depend not only on the extent of the neuromotor damage but also on the presence and amount of the cognitive deficit. Prognosis as to community ambulation is especially guarded if an infant has not achieved independent sitting by two years of age. This is especially true if infantile primitive reflexes (e.g., asymmetrical tonic neck reflex) persist.

COURSE OF ATAXIC CEREBRAL PALSY

The ataxic cerebral palsied child usually will be hypotonic and have normal deep tendon reflexes. There may be a marked delay in the achievement of postural control. A wide base is used on standing, and there is a tendency toward hyperextension at the knees with pronation of the feet. Depending on whether limb ataxia is present, an intention tremor may or may not be noticeable. Titubation of the head and trunk may exist when the dysfunction is severe.

There is a natural tendency for the balance problem to improve and for independent ambulation to occur, although this may not be achieved until three, four, or five years of age. If the ataxia is combined with a spastic diplegia or quadriplegia, the prognosis for achieving independent ambulation is guarded.

COURSE OF ATHETOID CEREBRAL PALSY

Development of athetoid cerebral palsy after kernicterus is a dramatic example of the changing clinical picture that may occur with maturation of the brain in spite of the presence of a static encephalopathy. During the period of kernicterus, the infant will show hyperextensibility of the neck and back, increased deep tendon reflexes, and extensor rigidity of the extremities. At two weeks of age, there will be a gradual change to relatively normal muscle tone. The only manifestation of a disorder in tone may appear when the infant cries, at which time excessive arching of the back may be seen. On formal neurological examination, an obligatory tonic neck reflex may be the only evidence of central nervous system dysfunction.

As the baby approaches the third month of life, a gradual change occurs from normal muscle tone to hypotonia. The presentation will be that of the "floppy infant" syndrome. The anterior and posterior scarf and hip signs are positive. The deep tendon reflexes are normal, but the tonic neck reflex remains obligatory.

With further growth, the baby will show delayed motor accomplishments, although, during the first year of life, involuntary movements may not be seen. For example, at 10 months of age, the baby will not have developed a pincer grasp but will persist with the less mature digit-palmar grasp. This maneuver will be done without evidence of involuntary movements. The deep tendon reflexes will be normal. The prime indicator that a motor disability exists will be the persistence of the asymmetrical tonic neck reflex, probably nonobligatory at this stage.

Babies under one year of age who demonstrate delayed motor accomplishments, hypotonia, normal reflexes, and no gross involuntary movements are frequently diagnosed as retarded. This is a classic pattern seen in Down's syndrome and, for that matter, in many non–motor-handicapped retardates. The clue that a motor deficit may be present is the presence of an abnormal asymmetrical tonic neck reflex pattern, not usually a finding in a primarily retarded infant.

Between 12 and 18 months of age, the hypotonia gradually changes to hypertonus. At about this same period, athetoid movements become obvious. The typical cog-wheel or plastic rigidity and the classic choreoathetotic movements may not be fully manifested until two to three years of age.

ASSOCIATED HANDICAPS AND COMPLICATIONS

In a child with cerebral palsy, a number of complications and associated handicaps must be considered during routine office visits, since these may prove more disabling than the primary motor disability. Many of these handicaps are preventable, and others respond favorably to treatment.

Approximately 50 to 75 per cent of cerebral palsied youngsters are retarded. Many with normal intelligence have learning disabilities. Cognitive growth in children with potential for normal intelligence may be seriously compromised because the motor handicap may not allow the infant to obtain optimum sensory stimulation. Therefore, the physician must be careful not to label as retarded a motor-handicapped youngster simply on the basis of his delayed developmental adaptations. Developmental assessments should be done periodically.

More than two thirds of children with cerebral palsy have ophthalmological difficulties, especially strabismus. Careful routine evaluation for the presence of phorias or tropias is important. Nearsightedness and hearing loss are also common.

Normal babies should begin to localize sound between four and six months of age. The examiner should routinely attempt to elicit this response by ringing a bell or by crinkling tissue paper (a high frequency sound). If the baby does not orient toward the sound, a referral to an audiologist is indicated.

More than half the youngsters with hemiparesis have a cortical sensory deficit on the involved side. If a child has a mental age of four years, cortical sensory testing may be possible. Stereognosis, position sense, and two point discrimination should be tested. Absent cortical sensation may explain why a child with a seemingly minor motor handicap shows very little voluntary use of the extremity involved.

The tendency for the development of fixed contractures of joints is relatively common, especially in children with spasticity. Many children with cerebral palsy are susceptible to severe dental decay, since enamel defects are quite frequent.

MANAGEMENT

If the physician suspects or confirms the presence of cerebral palsy, he should be honest and direct with the parents. Even though unable to make a diagnostic or prognostic statement, he should express his concern. If they wish another opinion, he should help the parents find an expert consultant. Parents with handicapped children express confidence in and respect toward those physicians who candidly, but sympathetically, inform them of their child's problem.

If a developmental delay is recognized, referral to an "early intervention center" ("early infant stimulation centers," "infant centers," or "developmental infant programs") is indicated. Referral to an early intervention program is especially timely after the parents first learn that their baby has a neurodevelopmental problem. Most parents, after hearing this devastating news, are not satisfied to "sit back and let nature take its course." They usually display angry denial and begin to "shop around," hoping to prove the physician wrong.

Referral to an early intervention center encourages the parents to participate actively.

Most programs, either center or home based, begin by educating the parents to understand their youngster's limitations and strengths and to be therapists. The "infant curricula" is of the multisensory stimulation type that attempts to improve the cognitive ability of the cerebral palsied youngsters who cannot explore their environment as normal youngsters do. The mothers are informed as to how to work with the infant's present level of functioning rather than at the level expected for his chronological age. Counseling parents, either individually or in a group, is an important aspect of these special programs.

Specific intervention strategies ease the burden the mother may have in feeding, bathing, or dressing a spastic baby. For example, many of these infants have trouble sucking because of a tongue thrust. That the feeding times become quite distressful, for both infant and mother, has the potential of causing disturbed maternal-infant interaction patterns. Therapists may recognize that the sucking problem can be minimized if the head and trunk are held slightly flexed during bottle or spoon feeding. If this maneuver proves helpful, the parents are taught the technique.

Cerebral Palsy Treatment Centers

Since the diagnosis and management of cerebral palsy require the expertise of many professionals, the physician should refer the toddler to a multidisciplinary cerebral palsy treatment center if one is available in the community. Because so many specialists are involved, the parents may become confused and disillusioned if plans and treatment are not coordinated. The lack of a well-planned, integrated rehabilitation program causes anxiety for the child and his family, whereas a specific goal-oriented approach tends to give confidence and security.

Physical and Occupational Therapy

There is no universally accepted therapeutic regimen. Rather, there are many doctrinaire approaches to treatment, each with its followers and believers and no controlled clinical studies to prove or reject the benefits claimed.

Orthopedic Surgery

Orthopedic surgery is frequently necessary for the spastic equinovarus deformities of the foot, for hip and knee flexion deformities, and for hip internal rotation deformities and adduction deformities. The success rate of surgery is estimated to be relatively high for the spastic group. Orthopedic procedures for children with the athetoid type of cerebral palsy are usually contraindicated.

Muscle Relaxants

The use of medication to improve motor control of cerebral palsied children has had limited success. Diazepam, dantrolene sodium, and baclofen have been used, but these medications should be reserved for severely motor handicapped children with excessive hypertonus. Although benefits may be slight in these children, management by the caretaker may become easier. For example, if the drug helps relax the adductor spasms in an incontinent child who scissors, it will be easier for the parents to change the diapers.

Bracing

The use of bracing for cerebral palsy to provide stability and, therefore, improve function is becoming less popular; however, short-leg braces will permit the child with a spastic equinus foot to walk plantigrade and improve his balance.

Neurosurgery

A number of neurosurgical approaches have been explored for correction of the motor abnormality. There are indications that an implant for constant cerebellar stimulation improves function in hypertonic cerebral palsy individuals, at least many parents have been pleased with the results in spite of the negative findings by formal assessment. Cerebellar stimulation should be limited to those children whose severe motor difficulty may justify the risk of surgery.

The parents should be informed that there is no evidence that any one neurosurgical treatment regimen significantly improves motor control. If the physician is not knowledgeable about these regimens, he should refer the patient to a colleague or multidisciplinary center for a more informed opinion.

Primary Care Physician Responsibility

The primary care physician should not abdicate complete responsibility for the care of the child to the cerebral palsy center but should continue to be responsible for supportive guidance, general health supervision, diagnosis, and management of acute illnesses. When he sees the child and parents on routine visits, he should ask the parents how they are managing and facilitate their talking about the handicap or asking questions about the welfare of their child.

Many parents report that their primary care physician does not seem interested in children with chronic handicaps. The physician may rationalize that since the child is being handled effectively by the treatment center, his participation may complicate matters. In addition, a physician may fear that, if he asks "How are things going?" he may be bombarded by many questions that he cannot helpfully answer because of the limitations of his knowledge and experience.

The physician should be candid and explain to the parents that he lacks the experience needed to offer sophisticated advice about some of their highly technical questions. Nevertheless, he should encourage the parents to verbalize their problems and worries, as this process, in itself, can be very helpful to distressed parents.

Good communication between the treatment center and the primary care physician would be ideal. If time permitted, it would be advantageous to have the physician attend team conferences when his patient's rehabilitation program is being reviewed. All the disciplines usually report their findings and recommendations before treatment plans are formulated. If the physician participated, he would learn firsthand of the plans and goals of the treatment team, and his input would also be helpful. Regretfully, practical limitations of time and financing make this difficult.

Another useful technique is to have the office nurse call the treatment center before the patient makes a routine visit. By speaking to the center's coordinator or social worker, information can be obtained on the child's progress, problems, and recommended therapies.

Primary care physicians are in a good position to explore some of the vital issues. Parental guilt that leads to overprotection and infantilization of the handicapped child can be a detriment to the rehabilitation process. The physician should be alert to this possibility if the parents continue to call about minor illnesses and if the concerns they express seem to be out of proportion to the symptoms.

Inquiries should be made as to whether the parents find it difficult to discuss their child's chronic illness with friends and family. Feeling that there is a social stigma in having a handicapped child, some parents may avoid and deny any type of association with such a youngster using all covert mechanisms to get this message across. Ideally, it is hoped that parents would try to maintain their conventional social roles without hiding their relationship to their handicapped child. On the other hand, they may also completely identify with the handicapped person, letting everyone constantly know that this is their plight in life.

It is important that the primary care physician try to make sure that the handicapped youngster is not leading a home-bound existence and that he is receiving all the advantages the community has to offer. Some parents feel that a handicapped child does not need the same social and intellectual stimulation as normal children. They make few demands on the child "because he is sick." This is a self-fulfilling prophecy.

A cerebral palsied adolescent may unfortunately still be considered a child because of his appearance. When he reaches sexual maturity, his normal physiological, psychological, and developmental needs should not be disregarded simply because he is handicapped. The reaching out for independence that occurs in adolescence causes many conflicts for the teenage motor-handicapped individual. It would serve the adolescent cerebral palsy patient well if the physician would freely discuss with him privately his feelings about his handicap, dependency, career plans, and sexuality.

The family physician should suggest to the parents that they contact local cerebral palsy organizations. Involvement with these organizations is especially helpful when the disability is first recognized. When a person is assigned a new and unexpected role, that of a parent of a handicapped child, the availability of other parents "who have been through it" appears to make the transition easier.

PROGNOSIS

During childhood, there usually is an unfortunate tendency for parents and professionals to focus primarily on the motor disability, with emphasis on the achievement of independent ambulation. The physical and psychological energies of the child and even the family for motor independence may detract from meeting the social, recreational, and cognitive needs of the child. Professionals and parents alike are often ambivalent in their feelings as to when to make a decision that independent ambulation will be an unattainable goal and to allow the child the comfort and mobility of a wheelchair. From recent studies it appears that if a child does not develop independent sitting balance by four years of age, especially if some of the primitive reflexes persist, community ambulation, that is, the ability to walk outdoors with or without the aid of braces or crutches, is unlikely.

The Federal Legislation in 1975—PL 94–142, The Education for All Handicapped Act—guarantees the right of every handicapped child to a free and appropriate education. In most states, for children between the ages of 3 and 21, there are educational programs. Many states are now offering educational programs for the 0-to-3 age group.

For handicapped adults, depending on the physical and intellectual competence of the individual, there are a number of opportunities for living outside of the home part of the day or permanently. Sheltered workshops that offer a noncompetitive environment are available to the majority of physically handicapped. Group homes that have a few adults with cerebral palsy living in a communal "family" are now increasing in number. These group homes allow the handicapped adult to be independent in the sense that he can live outside his own home. They also offer more opportunities for socialization and recreation. Independent, adult functioning in a competitive society is achieved by relatively few cerebral palsied adults. If the motor disability does not negate independent functioning, the associated cognition, language, hearing, and vision disabilities prove to be the main obstacles.

REFERENCES

André-Thomas, Cherni, Y., and Sainte-Anne Dargarssies, S.: The Neurological Examination of the Infant. Little Club Clinic in Development Medicine, No. 1. London, Spastics Society, 1960.

Bax, M. C. O.: Terminology and classification of cerebral palsy. Devel. Med. Child Neurol., *6*:295, 1964.

Birenbaum, A.: On managing a courtesy stigma. J. Health Soc. Behav., *11*:196, 1970.

Breakey, A. S.: Ocular findings in cerebral palsy. Arch. Ophthalmol., *53*:852, 1955.

Byers, R. K.: Evolution of hemiplegia in infancy. Am. J. Dis. Child., *61*:915, 1941.

Crothers, B., and Paine, R. S.: The Natural History of Cerebral Palsy. Cambridge, Harvard University Press, 1959.

Denhoff, E., and Robinault, P. P.: Cerebral Palsy and Related Disorders. New York, McGraw-Hill Book Company, 1960.

Hagberg, B., Sanner, G., and Stern, M.: The disequilibrium syndrome in cerebral palsy. Acta Paediatr. Scand., (Suppl.) *61*:226, 1972.

Haynes, U.: Comprehensive services for atypical infants and their families. Pediatr. Ann., 2:68, 1973.

Ingram, T. T. S.: Paediatric Aspect of Cerebral Palsy. Edinburgh, E. & S. Livingston Ltd., 1964.

Marquis, P.: Therapies for cerebral palsy. Acad. Fam. Pract., *19*:101, 1979.

Molnar, G. E.: Clinical aspect of cerebral palsy. Pediatr. Ann., 2:10, 1973.

Nelson, D. K., and Ellenberg, J. H.: Children who "outgrew" cerebral palsy. Pediatrics, *69*:529, 1982.

Paine, R. S., Brazelton, T. B., Donovan, D. E., Drorbraugh, Y. E., Hubbel, J. P., and Sears, E. M.: Evolution of postural reflexes in normal infants and the presence of chronic brain syndromes. Neurology, *14*:1036, 1964.

Paneth, N., Keily, J. L., Stein, Z., and Susser, M.: Cerebral palsy and newborn care. III. Estimated prevalence rates of cerebral palsy under differing rates of mortality and impairment of low birth-weight infants. Devel. Med. Child Neurol., 23:801, 1981.

Perlstein, M. A.: Kernicterus and Its Importance in Cerebral Palsy. Springfield, IL, Charles C Thomas, 1957.

Prechtl, H. F. R.: Prognostic value of neurological signs in the newborn infant. Proc. J. Soc. Med., *58*:3, 1965.

Simeonson, R. J., Cooper, D. H., and Scheiner, A. P.: A review and analysis of the effectiveness of early intervention programs. Pediatrics, *69*:635, 1982.

Soboloff, H. R.: Surgery in cerebral palsy. *In* Lewis' Practice of Surgery, Vol. II, Chap. 12. Hagerstown, MD, Harper and Row, 1969.

Solomons, G., Holden, R. H., and Denhoff, E.: The changing picture of cerebral dysfunction in early childhood. J. Pediatr., *1*:113, 1963.

Taft, L. T., Delagi, E. F., Wilkie, O. L., and Abramson, A. S.: Critique of rehabilitative techniques in treatment of cerebral palsy. Arch. Phys. Med. Rehabil., *43*:238, 1962.

Walker, R. G.: An Assessment of the Current Status of the "At-Risk" Register. Scottish Health Service Studies, No. 4. Edinburgh, H.M.S.O., 1967.

61

SEIZURES

John F. Griffith, M.D.

A seizure is the clinical expression of abnormal, excessive neuronal discharges within the central nervous system (CNS). It is a symptom of a number of different disease processes that cause transient disturbances of brain function. When these recur, the condition is referred to as epilepsy or a seizure disorder.

The typical seizure is characterized by a brief episode of altered consciousness, frequently associated with some motor, sensory, or behavioral manifestations. The variability is dependent upon the functional units of neurons involved and the stage of nervous system development. It may be simply a fleeting change of expression or fluttering of the eyelids, or the entire body may become rigid and shake repeatedly, accompanied by drooling, tongue-biting, incontinence, and postictal stupor lasting several hours. When a seizure is very brief, it may not be recognized for prolonged periods and may subsequently pose problems in management because the end-point of effective seizure control is difficult to identify.

At the cellular level a seizure begins with depolarization of the neuronal membrane. When this spreads to involve adjacent nerve cells, an excessive discharge results which either stimulates or inhibits a number of body functions controlled by these neurons. This process requires additional energy, which in turn is dependent upon an increased availability of oxygen and glucose. Prolonged seizures may deplete the available energy stores and result in neuronal exhaustion and irreversible damage. To prevent this, seizures should be recognized promptly and treated effectively, especially in the young when the nervous system is particularly vulnerable to injury due to impaired cerebral energy metabolism.

The type of seizure does not identify the nature of the underlying disease process nor the location of the primary disturbance. Focal cerebral lesions occurring as a result of trauma or tumor may cause generalized rather than focal seizures. Generalized brain dysfunction resulting from hypoglycemia or hypoxia may be associated with discrete focal or partial seizures. The latter are thought to arise from epileptogenic foci in the cerebral cortex. Generalized seizures reflect widespread electrical discharges originating from subcortical neurons with secondary spread to the cortex and brain stem structures. As the nervous system matures, the seizure pattern may change without any alterations in the underlying disease process. Similarly, the seizure focus that was active in the infant or small child may spontaneously disappear in later childhood and not recur; or a relapse may occur after many seizure-free years in a patient who is presumed to have "outgrown" the problem.

The prevalence of seizures in the child under age two is estimated to be approximately 2 to 4 per cent. The majority of these are benign, self-limited, generalized seizures associated with fever and often not requiring anticonvulsant therapy. Knowing the type of seizure sometimes provides a clue to both the etiology and prognosis and is helpful in decisions regarding therapy. The international classification, which is now in common usage, provides a means to diagnose and manage seizures based on clinical features and correlative electroencephalogram (EEG) findings (Table 61–1). The term "focal seizure" was previously used to describe partial seizures with elementary symptomatology. Psychomotor or temporal lobe seizures are now classified as partial seizures with complex symptomatology. Seizures in the neonatal period are not discussed in this chapter because they are largely diagnosed and managed in the hospital.

PARTIAL SEIZURES

With Elementary Symptomatology

The classic expression of this is the Jacksonian seizure, originating in the motor strip and progressing to involve adjacent neurons. Usually it begins on one side (i.e., corner of the eye, mouth, or thumb) and progresses in a "march-like" fashion to involve the rest of the face, arms, trunk, legs, and sometimes the other side of the body. Frequently these attacks are abortive in children and only fragments of this progression are evident. A focal sensory seizure may progress in a similar manner, or there may be mixed elements of motor and sensory symp-

Table 61–1. CLASSIFICATION OF SEIZURES

I. Partial Seizures (seizures beginning locally)
  A. Partial seizures with elementary symptomatology (generalized without impairment of consciousness)
    1. With motor symptoms (includes Jacksonian seizures)
    2. With special sensory or somatosensory symptoms
    3. With autonomic symptoms
    4. Compound forms
  B. Partial seizures with complex symptomatology (temporal lobe or psychomotor seizures—generally with impairment of consciousness)
    1. With impairment of consciousness only
    2. With cognitive symptomatology
    3. With affective symptomatology
    4. With "psychosensory" symptomatology
    5. With "psychomotor" symptomatology (automatisms)
    6. Compound forms
  C. Partial seizures secondarily generalized
II. Generalized Seizures (bilaterally symmetrical and without local onset)
    1. Absences (petit mal)
    2. Bilateral massive epileptic myoclonus
    3. Infantile spasms
    4. Clonic seizures
    5. Tonic seizures
    6. Tonic-clonic seizures (grand mal)
    7. Atonic seizures
    8. Akinetic seizures
III. Unilateral Seizures (exclusively or predominantly)
IV. Unclassified epileptic seizures (due to incomplete data)

Abstracted from Gastaut (1970).

toms. Sensory seizures in children are probably more prevalent than the available literature suggests, because of the unreliability of reporting in this age group. The symptoms may include peculiar paresthesias, numbness, or symptoms referable to the visual, auditory, or olfactory systems. Small children will often become frightened by sensations produced by the seizure of flashing lights, unusual sounds, or peculiar smells and not be able to describe the experience in enough detail to permit conclusions. Unless there is a motor component to the seizure, the entire episode may be overlooked and remain untreated for a prolonged period. Unusual, unexplained behavioral features should suggest the possibility of a seizure disorder, and the EEG usually confirms that suspicion.

Seizures may be associated with significant changes in heart rate, skin color, pupillary size, sweating, and intestinal motility. These autonomic manifestations may be the predominant feature of a seizure, particularly in newborns and small infants. Occasionally a discrete focal disturbance, such as unilateral pupillary dilatation, is the only sign indicating a seizure. The diagnosis is frequently one of exclusion under these circumstances. Fortunately, most seizures are recognized early because of the bizarre involuntary motor and behavioral disturbances that are obvious even to an uninformed observer.

With Complex Symptomatology

A significant percentage of seizures that are difficult to completely control are of this type. They may begin at any time, but the diagnosis is usually difficult to establish before the age of four to five years. A typical seizure may begin with a sudden change of consciousness, manifested by staring followed by purposeless automatic activity, such as lip-smacking, chewing, repetitive swallowing, or grimacing. These are referred to as *automatisms*. The entire spell may last a few seconds or one to two minutes and promptly subside or progress to a more generalized motor seizure. Occasionally more complicated automatic behavior, such as running or repetitive pulling at clothes or body parts, is evident, but this is unusual in children. Older patients sometimes experience peculiar symptoms of fullness, emptiness, dizziness, etc., which may be expressed as fear or anxiety, or in bizarre behavior. Autonomic vasomotor disturbances such as salivation, vomiting, flushing, and pallor may also be features of this type of seizure.

The etiology of complex partial seizures remains unclear, despite extensive clinical studies. They are usually not due to a mass lesion or an antecedent diffuse cerebral insult such as hypoxia or hypoglycemia. Some have considered previous prolonged febrile convulsions to be important in their pathogenesis; others have favored the idea that these seizures occur as a result of incisural sclerosis, occurring from herniation of the medial temporal lobe through the tentorial incisura at the time of birth. An heredofamilial basis for this type of seizure has also been suggested, but in most patients this cannot be documented. These patients usually have a normal physical examination, although a higher percentage have behavioral problems and intellectual impairment than in the general population.

GENERALIZED SEIZURES

Absence (Petit Mal)

These are brief (5 to 30 seconds) seizures, consisting of frequent staring or blinking. Mild motor manifestations, particularly twitching about the eyes or mouth, are sometimes present. They may be difficult to distinguish from brief complex partial seizures because both can have repetitive, automatic behavior or automatisms. Absence seizures can sometimes be precipitated by hyperventilation and at times will recur uninterrupted for a prolonged period (absence continuing or status). This may be interpreted as daydreaming or disinterest by the uninformed observer, and the patient may be initially referred for evaluation of deviant behavior or school problems. The electroencephalogram is helpful in this situation because well-organized spike–slow wave complexes are characteristically seen with absence seizures.

Generalized Tonic-Clonic Seizures

This type of seizure was formally referred to as *grand mal.* The clinical features usually include an aura, followed by tonic contraction of muscles, rolling of eyes, tongue-biting, drooling, cyanosis when the muscles of respiration are tonically contracted, and sometimes urinary and fecal incontinence. The onset of tonic spasms usually coincides with loss of consciousness. This is followed by a state of violent, clonic movements involving extremities and trunk, lasting for a few seconds to several minutes. The clonic movements gradually subside and the patient may sleep for minutes to hours before regaining full consciousness. Occasionally there are transient postictal focal neurological signs, but complete recovery is usual and the patient remains well between convulsions.

Tonic Seizures

Tonic seizures, as the name implies, have as their major clinical manifestations tonic contractions of major muscle groups with little or no clonic component. Manifestations are similar to those seen during the tonic phase of tonic-clonic seizures. Postural deformities, loss of balance, and cyanosis are frequently associated when the state of tonic contraction is prolonged.

Atonic and Clonic Seizures

Occasionally muscle tone is suddenly lost rather than increased. This is referred to as an *atonic seizure.* A motor seizure may also have only clonic features, without a tonic phase. The clinical course of *clonic seizures* is like those of tonic and generalized tonic-clonic symptoms. Focal spike or polyspike cortical discharges are the EEG abnormality most frequently seen in this type of seizure.

Myoclonic Seizures

This seizure is characterized by sudden, rapid forward jerking of the head, often with associated outward movements of the arms. When the child is standing, this frequently looks like "head-nodding," with sudden extension of the arms. These patients frequently fall and incur abrasions, contusions, and lacerations to their face and head. As a result, protective headgear is usually worn.

This is one of the most difficult types of seizure to completely control. Like most seizures, the etiology varies, but the prognosis for normal psychomotor development is not as good as with most seizures. The reason for this is probably a combination of factors, including the underlying process affecting brain function and the secondary effects of long-standing seizures that are difficult to control. The EEG is usually grossly abnormal, with irregular bursts of spikes and slow waves superimposed on a poorly organized background.

Akinetic Seizures

This type of seizure was previously grouped with myoclonic seizures and typical petit mal, because they shared similarities on EEG and all were difficult to control with conventional anticonvulsant agents. Although they are no longer classified in this way, akinetic and myoclonic seizures have some similarities, both clinically and electrographically. The akinetic spell is characterized by sudden loss of postural tone with rapid recovery. Usually the patient falls or becomes abruptly unsteady. Although this pattern differs from that usually seen with myoclonic seizures, both are characterized by sudden falling, rapid recovery, and minimal postictal depression. Despite their brevity, they are frequently difficult to control with conventional anticonvulsants.

Infantile Spasms (Flexor Spasms, Massive Myoclonic Spasms, "Salaam" Seizures)

These seizures classically occur between the ages of six months and three years. They usually begin suddenly and are characterized by symmetrical flexion of the head or trunk, with synchronous clonic movements of arms and legs. The eyes may roll upwards or inwards, and there is usually little or no loss of consciousness. Frequently they occur in clusters of eight to ten or more, and these may recur many times daily.

Infantile spasms may be symptomatic of a developmental or acquired CNS disorder or may occur in normal, healthy infants without previous evidence of cerebral disease. The latter, idiopathic form is particularly tragic because it is frequently followed by delayed motor and mental development. Some have no further seizures and subsequently develop normally after a course of corticotropin (ACTH) or high dosages of corticosteroids. Unfortunately, there is no way to predict this, nor are there effective treatment alternatives to ACTH or corticosteroids. The EEG in all forms of myoclonic epilepsy is usually poorly organized. In infantile spasms, the typical pattern is called *hypsarrhythmia*. This is characterized by chaotic, multifocal spike and slow wave activity. It is not always a feature of infantile spasms and occasionally is seen with other types of seizures.

An identical seizure pattern may be seen with a number of diseases affecting the brain. Metabolic disorders, particularly cerebral hypoxia, aminoacidurias, hypoglycemia, cerebral lipidosis, and developmental defects (i.e., holorosencephaly), have been associated with massive myoclonic seizures. The prognosis in these instances is particularly poor, because the underlying disorder has usually irreversibly injured the brain by the time the seizures occur.

Febrile Seizures

Despite the many studies and publications on the subject, there is still controversy regarding the classification of febrile seizures and the indications for treatment. The traditional view is that most febrile seizures are benign, self-limited, brief, generalized seizures that recur infrequently and usually require no therapy. This type of patient differs from the one with a predisposition to develop recurrent afebrile seizures or epilepsy and requires extensive evaluation and usually long-term therapy.

A consensus statement published recently by Kendig et al. on this subject, provides a practical schema for classifying and managing this problem. A febrile seizure was defined as one occurring between the ages of three months and five years, associated with fever but without evidence of intracranial infection or other defined cause. The risk of recurrence following the first seizure in children who are untreated is 30 to 40 per cent. The risk of developing subsequent nonfebrile seizures is insignificant, unless at least two of three high-risk factors are present. These are (1) family history of nonfebrile seizures, (2) abnormal neurological or developmental status prior to the first seizure, and (3) an atypical febrile seizure that is exceptionally prolonged or has focal features. If none of these is present, the risk of developing nonfebrile seizures is only 2 to 3 per cent, which is not significantly increased over the risk in the population at large. The latter group requires no therapy unless the seizures recur, because the therapy does not change the prognosis, although it does reduce the number of seizures during the period of treatment. When high-risk factors are identified, treatment with phenobarbital is indicated for at least two years in dosages adequate to maintain a minimum therapeutic blood level of 15 μg per ml (Table 61–2).

Table 61–2. FEBRILE SEIZURES*

	A LOW-RISK GROUP (no risk factors†)	B HIGH-RISK GROUP (2 or 3 risk factors†)
Subsequent epilepsy:	2–3%	13%
Treatment:	None (unless recurrent)	Phenobarbital: 3–5 mg/kg/day for 2–4 yr

*Adapted from Censensus Statement on Febrile Seizures. Pediatrics, *66*:6, 1980

†Risk Factors:

a. Family history of nonfebrile seizures
b. Abnormal neurological or developmental status
c. Prolonged or focal seizures

Status Epilepticus

Status epilepticus refers to a state of continuous seizure activity lasting at least 30 minutes. They may be in the form of a prolonged single seizure or a series of seizures between which the patient does not regain consciousness. Convulsive or tonic-clonic status is the usual and most serious clinical type, but absence, complex partial, and other types of status also occur. Absence status is often interpreted by the parents or a schoolteacher as "daydreaming," and the patient with repetitive, complex partial seizures appears to be in a "twilight" state.

This is an important problem because the mortality and morbidity figures for children with prolonged tonic-clonic status are significant. Discharging nerve cells have heightened metabolic activity and increased energy requirements and may be irreparably injured by a cascade of toxic-metabolic events. Acidosis, hyperthermia, dehydration, impaired ventilation, cerebral edema, and altered perfusion eventually interfere with the availability and utilization of oxygen and glucose. For this reason, treatment should be instituted as soon as possible and continued for several days or until the risk of recurrent status is eliminated.

An adequate airway, supplemental oxygen and glucose, maintenance of cerebral perfusion, reduction of elevated intracranial pressure and hyperthermia when present, and prompt and effective anticonvulsant therapy are the treatments needed. There is an ongoing debate concerning the preferable drug combinations to use, but all agree that whatever regimen is employed, it should be started promptly, using correct drug dosages and with full awareness of their major side effects. The two different approaches that are summarized in Table 61–3 presume that the patient is treated in an intensive care facility by personnel who can recognize and properly manage the major complications of therapy.

Table 61–3. ANTICONVULSANT THERAPY OF STATUS EPILEPTICUS

PLAN A	PLAN B
- Immediate -	
Diazepam (Valium) 0.3-0.5 mg/kg; I.V. slowly (2 min) (10 mg max); can be repeated in 10-15 min and again in 30-45 min	*Phenobarbital* 8-10 mg/kg; I.V. slowly; repeat in 2-4 hr; total dose for 1st 24 hr 20-30 mg/kg; maintenance 5-10 mg/kg/24 hr
+ *Phenytoin* 10 mg/kg; I.V. slowly (10 min); then 5-10 mg/kg q 4-6 hr as required (total dose 20-30 mg/kg 1st 24 hr); maintenance dose 5-8 mg/kg/24 hr P.O.	+ *Phenytoin* 10 mg/kg; I.V. slowly (10 min); then 5-10 mg/kg q 4-6 hr as required (total dose 20-30 mg/kg 1st 24 hr); maintenance dose 5-8 mg/kg/24 hr P.O.
- Later -	
Phenobarbital If seizures are not controlled after 2-3 dosages of diazepam, I.V. phenobarbital can be added, providing blood pressure, respiration, and consciousness are monitored and techniques for resuscitation are available.	*Paraldehyde* 150 mg/kg per rectum (as required) in infants and small children until major anticonvulsants are effective.
- Comments -	
Diazepam Rapid anticonvulsant effect, usually within 1 minute; duration of 20 minutes to 2-3 hr; may cause respiratory depression and/or persistent drowsiness.	*Phenobarbital* May cause respiratory depression requiring assisted ventilation; seizure control not as rapid as with diazepam, but more sustained once control is achieved.

ETIOLOGY AND PATHOGENESIS OF SEIZURES

Since seizures are symptomatic of an underlying brain disorder, it is imperative to identify the nature of the underlying disease early. The majority of seizures in children have no identifiable etiology but can be completely controlled with medications. Despite this, it is best to view the seizure as an expression of disordered brain function and proceed to localize the lesion and define the cause as precisely as possible. Early in the course of disease, a seizure may be the first clue that something is wrong. The classic example of this is meningitis in the infant or an arteriovenous (AV) malformation or brain tumor in the older child. When the investigation fails to define any cause for the seizure and the patient is otherwise well, it is sometimes assumed that it is the result of antecedent, unrecognized cortical injury from trauma occurring either at the time of birth or subsequently during the early years of life. Seizures following cranial-cerebral trauma may occur at any time following the injury, although the cause and effect relationship is speculative when the trauma was mild and the seizures occurred many years later. The reason for the spontaneous onset of seizures is usually not clear, although stress, fatigue, and other stimuli known to activate seizures may be precipitating factors.

Every patient with an initial seizure should be considered to have a treatable lesion until proven otherwise. Prompt treatment of inflammatory lesions of the brain and meninges (meningitis, encephalitis, abscess) or correction of a metabolic imbalance (hypoglycemia, hypocalcemia, hypomagnesemia, amino and organic acidemias) is mandatory for effective seizure control and prevention of permanent cerebral injury. Although focal mass lesions do not usually present with seizures in an otherwise well patient, they need to be considered because the success of treatment is dependent upon early surgical intervention before secondary complications develop from increased intracranial pressure.

Seizures occur frequently with chronic subdural hematomas in infants. The same is true for mass lesions involving the cerebrum. Arteriovenous malformations, aneurysms, intracerebral hematomas, cerebral abscesses, and benign or malignant neoplasms may have seizures as a presenting sign or later feature, depending on the location and growth characteristics of the mass. Clues to the presence of these lesions are usually provided by symptoms and signs of raised intracranial pressure and focal neurological signs, particularly weakness, gait disturbance, visual field defects, reflex asymmetry, and personality changes. Most brain tumors in children are localized below the tentorium and, as a result, seizures are not common, except when the intracranial pressure is increased to a level that interferes with cerebral perfusion.

Seizures may also occur in families as an expression of a genetic disease such as tuberous sclerosis. In this condition, seizures may be seen before skin manifestations or mental retardation are recognized. Seizures may also occur in successive generations of families without other stigmata of a genetic disorder. However, a hereditofamilial or genetic basis for the problem should not be assumed simply because a number of family members have been affected. Without other disease markers, an acquired seizure disorder cannot be excluded without very careful study. This is essential before genetic counseling is undertaken.

Nonepileptic Spells

A number of brief spells, characterized by changes in behavior or peculiar sensory symptoms, may be confused with seizures, particularly if they are not observed by the examiner. One of these, *atypical migraine*, may result in transient alteration of consciousness or disturbed motor function. An awareness of the entire spectrum of this disorder and a positive family history for migraine will usually be sufficient to make the diagnosis.

Breath-holding spells, which may mimic atonic seizures in the infant and young child, occur typically following an episode of frustration resulting in vigorous crying. There is frequently a concern about seizures because the sequence of events usually includes cessation of respiration, pallor or cyanosis, falling to the floor, limpness, and transient confusion before complete recovery. *Syncopal spells* from vasovagal discharges or episodic cardiac asystole, although rare in children, must be differentiated from akinetic or atonic seizures. The EEG in this situation helps to differentiate the entities causing sudden syncope (breath-holding attacks, vasovagal attacks, cardiac syncope) from atonic seizures. *Paroxysmal gastroesophageal reflux* in infants is frequently characterized by sudden pallor, tonic posturing, and brief apnea mimicking tonic seizures. A careful history relating this activity to food ingestion is almost diagnostic and can be confirmed with sophisticated radiological, pneumographic, and electrochemical studies. *Night terrors* may suggest nocturnal seizures because they are episodic and associated with the type of automatic behavior and amnesia that may be seen with abortive complex partial seizures. Another confusing clinical picture that may suggest seizure to some is the unusual *conversion reaction* which may be seen, particularly in the adolescent female. This can be suspected when there is a history of anxiety, guilt, or social maladjustment and the spells are characterized by asynchronous motor activity or peculiar, inconsistent sensory symptoms.

Epileptic equivalent is the term used by some to describe episodic attacks of either headache, abdominal pain, or unusually aggressive behavior in patients who are subsequently shown to have abnormalities on the EEG. Although these symptoms are occasionally components, they are rarely the sole expression of a seizure. If there are paroxysmal discharges on the EEG coinciding with these symptoms or episodic, bizarre behavior, the diagnosis of seizure disorder needs to be considered and appropriate investigation and treatment initiated.

INVESTIGATION

History and Physical

The etiology of most seizures should be suspected following a careful history and physical examination. Initially it is important to obtain a clear description of the seizure, including its duration, pattern of progression, and any associated postictal phenomena. Specific questions should be asked to exclude recent infections, trauma, intoxications, hypoglycemia, fluid and electrolyte disturbances, and other metabolic and endocrine dysfunctions. Specific questions should be asked regarding headache, diplopia, motor incoordination, unusual sensory disturbances, and weakness. A family history of seizures or paroxysmal activity of any kind should be sought. If the patient is known to have seizures, inquiry concerning drug compliance is mandatory.

The physical examination in infants and small children should always include careful evaluation of the head and the anatomical structures contiguous to the brain. Careful examination of the fontanelles, sutures, and scalp provides clues relative to intracranial pressure and the state of hydration. Palpation of the cranium is important in order to exclude significant asymmetries or bony defects. It is important to transilluminate the head in all infants. Hydrocephalus as well as intracerebral or extracerebral cystic lesions may be discovered if this is done properly. The head should be measured on a regular basis, especially if it appears large or the sutures and fontanelle suggest the possibility of raised intracranial pressure. The initial clue to the presence of an arteriovenous malformation is often a bruit heard on routine auscultation of the head. The ears, paranasal sinuses, face, and scalp are sites of infection that can spread to the nervous system. Normal optic fundi, extraocular movements, and visual fields help to exclude a mass lesion producing raised intracranial pressure. Careful examination of the cardiorespiratory system is always indicated, because both acquired and congenital heart or lung disease can result in cerebral embolization or chronic hypoxemia causing seizures. Kidney or liver dysfunction can cause altered consciousness, but this is an unlikely explanation for seizures unless there are other clinical signs indicating organ failure. Hypertension is important to exclude because seizures may occur with hypertensive encephalopathy. Skin lesions, i.e., depigmented nevi, adenoma sebaceum, and café-au-lait spots, provide important clues to the presence of cerebral defects sometimes associated with seizures. The midline spine and cranium also deserve careful scrutiny in order to exclude skin defects, e.g., sinus tracts, hemangiomas, hair tufts, which occur with anomalies of the CNS. A capillary hemangioma (port-wine stain) involving the face and/or the scalp is a feature of the Sturge-Weber syndrome, which is frequently associated with difficult-to-control seizures.

Table 61–4. RECOMMENDED INVESTIGATIONS OF PATIENTS WITH SEIZURES

Following the Initial Seizures	On Subsequent Office Visits*
CBC	CBC
Urinalysis	Serum drug level
Serum electrolytes	EEG
Glucose, calcium	CT scan†
Skull x-ray and/or CT scan†	Liver function (SGOT, bilirubin)
EEG	Renal function (urinalysis, creatinine)
L.P.	

*Choice of study depends on effectiveness of seizure control, type of anticonvulsants, signs of toxicity, concern about compliance, etc.

†If there are focal neurological signs or raised intracranial pressure.

Laboratory Investigation

General Laboratory

The appropriate laboratory studies to be done are usually obvious, assuming a careful history and physical examination are performed at regular intervals. Certain studies are indicated almost routinely following an initial seizure, and others should be reserved for patients being treated with anticonvulsants, particularly when the seizures are not completely controlled (Table 61–4). If the patient is well and seizure-free, laboratory tests are usually not indicated. When drugs that are known to produce bone marrow, liver, or renal toxicity are being used, laboratory studies of these functions are recommended, particularly early in the course of treatment.

A complete blood count (CBC) and urinalysis should be done routinely. A CBC is important to do because infection, hemoglobinopathy, and drug toxicity are important considerations in patients with suspected or proven seizure disorders. A concentrated urine with a high osmolality, in the absence of significant dehydration, is seen in inappropriate antidiuretic hormone (ADH) secretion. This occurs in association with a number of intracranial conditions, particularly infection and tumor. The resultant fluid retention can affect neurons and precipitate severe seizures requiring fluid reduction for effective control. Serum electrolytes and osmolality should be obtained whenever inappropriate ADH secretion or fluid imbalance is suspected. This should be requested whenever patients are dehydrated, hyperthermic, or acidotic, or if there is impaired consciousness that is not well understood. Abnormal serum glucose or calcium concentration is rarely the cause for seizures in an otherwise well older child with an initial or recurrent seizure. However, these parameters should be tested routinely in neonates and small infants, because seizures may be the sole presenting feature of hypoglycemia or hypocalcemia in this age group.

Neurodiagnostic Studies

Skull x-rays provide valuable information in a select number of patients following the initial seizure, especially when there is a question regarding raised intracranial pressure, cerebral malformation, antecedent head trauma, or congenital infection. However, the computerized tomography (CT) scan, when available, provides more precise information and is the preferred diagnostic procedure when increased intracranial pressure or a focal mass lesion is suspected. Skull x-rays are not indicated in the routine work-up of an uncomplicated initial febrile or afebrile seizure.

The electroencephalogram (EEG) is most helpful when the patient is having atypical spells that are difficult to categorize as seizures. It provides valuable information, not only about the presence of paroxysmal discharges but about their location, frequency, and pattern. Knowing whether the type of epileptic discharges are single or mixed and especially their relationship to sleep and activating procedures such as photostimulation and hyperventilation aids in decisions regarding therapy. Prolonged waking and sleeping EEGs are indicated when insufficient information is provided by standard tracings to effectively manage the patient. Intravenous pyridoxine (vitamin B_6) infusion during EEG recording excludes the rare seizure problem due to a deficiency of this substance. A dramatic improvement or normalization of the EEG occurs during infusion when this is the problem. Pyridoxine infusion should always be considered when seizures are refractory to drug therapy, especially in very young infants.

Some patients may report recurring symptoms suggesting seizures when therapy seems appropriate and the standard EEG is normal. Under these circumstances alternatives include strict monitoring of the treatment regimen and careful clinical follow-up and possibly extended EEG recordings. Since the EEG reflects only a sampling of brain activity at one point in time, it may be normal when the seizures are incompletely controlled. The EEG should be obtained during the interictal period because when done in the early hours or days after seizure, excessive slowing is often present which obscures the seizure complexes and makes meaningful interpretation difficult. It should be repeated as often as necessary when problems arise, but when seizures are well-controlled, it is unnecessary except possibly at the time of discontinuing anticonvulsant therapy.

The examination of the cerebrospinal fluid (CSF) is always indicated when infection of the nervous system is a concern. If raised intracranial pressure is suspected, the lumbar puncture should be done with a small (No. 22) needle and only enough fluid should be removed (approximately 1 to 2 cc) to establish the diagnosis. Most lumbar punctures are done following an initial febrile seizure when the explanations for the fever are not obvious. Although the CSF is usually normal, it is a sound practice because a seizure may be the first sign of meningitis in a patient who may not appear acutely ill. It is not recommended following an initial afebrile seizure unless subsequent investigations indicate the possibility of a degenerative or unusual infectious process.

Computerized tomography (CT) scan is not indicated in the routine investigation of children with seizures but should be requested whenever the clinical data suggest raised intracranial pressure or the possibility of a mass lesion. If the patient's neurological picture is worsening, and especially if consciousness is affected, a CT scan should be obtained in order to exclude an evolving focal mass lesion. Intracranial hemorrhage or progressive hydrocephalus are examples of lesions that may become obvious only after repeat CT scanning. All patients with prolonged unconsciousness or residual focal findings after a seizure should have a CT scan unless there is an obvious metabolic explanation.

TREATMENT

General

The diagnosis and management plan should be reviewed in detail with the parents and the patient at the time the initial diagnosis is made and subsequently during the course of treatment. The disease process should be discussed in enough detail for the patient to appreciate what is happening at the cellular level. Factors influencing seizure susceptibility such as fatigue, anxiety, stimulant drugs, or intercurrent infections should be stressed. If this is successful, the patient with seizures will usually assume more responsibility for his or her condition and be more attentive to the drug regimen and less concerned about society's reaction to this diagnosis. Understanding the problem also permits the patient to recognize abortive seizures and treatment complications early before serious problems arise. Part of the educational process should include instruction about first aid for the patient who is having a seizure, particularly the importance of ensuring a clear airway while avoiding the placement of metallic or loose objects in the mouth.

The mainstay of therapy is long-standing oral anticonvulsant medication. This assumes a knowledge of the various drugs, including their specificity for certain types of seizures and the symptoms and signs of both idiosyncratic and toxic side effects.

Anticonvulsants do not alter the biological basis for the seizure disorder, only the seizure frequency and sometimes their clinical manifestation. The seizure per se is not considered harmful to the brain, except when prolonged or complicated by an obstructed airway, cranial-cerebral trauma, or metabolic derangements. When seizures remain uncontrolled for extended periods, secondary epileptogenic foci may develop. This makes a strong case for instituting drug therapy early and the complete elimination of all seizure activity whenever possible.

Medication is not always indicated following the first seizure. In certain clinical situations it is reasonable to withhold drugs because the probability of a second seizure is not great. Prophylactic anticonvulsants are unnecessary following an initial "simple" febrile seizure not associated with any high-risk factors. They are usually unnecessary following a brief, generalized seizure in an otherwise well child with a normal physical examination and laboratory investigation. This may occur under circumstances of major stress, excitement, or fatigue or with transient metabolic disturbances such as those which occur with inappropriate ADH secretion. If the seizure is questionable because the history was unclear or unavailable, treatment is usually withheld until the diagnosis can be established. Anticonvulsants that are initiated to control seizures occurring as a result of acute inflammation, i.e., meningitis, can usually be withdrawn following complete recovery, assuming no further seizures in the interim. This is usually after six to eight weeks in the child without any neurological sequela following meningitis.

When seizures are not controlled with anticonvulsant therapy, it is important to consider whether the seizure problem was correctly classified and appropriate drugs are being given in adequate dosages and for sufficient periods of time. Drugs have variable half-lives and, as a result, the time required to reach a steady state in the blood and tissues differs significantly, depending on the drug and rate of administration. In general, steady state is reached five half-lives after drug initiation or dosage change. Complete seizure control may not be achieved when drug therapy is modified prematurely, and suboptimal seizure control will persist despite what might appear to be adequate dosages. Compliance with the treatment program is a concern in every age group and deserves special consideration when problems are encountered in seizure control. The seizure problem may worsen despite optimum therapy if the clinical diagnosis is incorrect, especially if a progressive CNS disease is accounting for the seizures. If excessive amounts or certain combinations of drugs are used, it may become worse because toxic levels of some drugs are known to induce seizures.

Drug Levels

The optimal dosage of drug for any patient is the least amount that will completely control seizures without producing undesirable side effects. This will vary with patients of the same sex and age who are having similar types of seizures. Serum anticonvulsant levels provide a means to help evaluate the relationship between drug dosage and seizure control. It is now clear that tissue levels of a drug may vary in patients given similar dosages based on weight or surface area, and that seizures may be completely controlled with subtherapeutic blood levels in some, whereas in others they may recur despite levels that should be effective. These apparent paradoxes point out how little is known about the action of most of these compounds and underscores the importance of clinical observations in order to accurately gauge the success of therapy. As a general rule, however, therapeutic blood levels of a drug (Table 61–5) correlate well with effective seizure control with no toxic side effects. It is important to obtain drug levels whenever there is a question of toxicity or inadequate seizure control despite what seems to be adequate dosages of drugs.

Specific Drug Therapy

In recent years a number of anticonvulsants have become available, significantly improving the outlook for seizure control in children. Carbamazepine (Tegretol), Valproate (Depakene), and clonazepam (Clonopin) have joined Dilantin, phenobarbital, Zarontin, and Mysoline as the first-line drugs for most seizure problems in children. ACTH remains the drug

Table 61–5. CHARACTERISTICS OF SEVERAL ANTICONVULSANTS IN CURRENT USAGE

Drug	Indications	Dosage (mg/kg/day)	Therapeutic Blood Level μg/ml	Time to Reach Steady State (days)
Carbamazepine (Tegretol)	*Complex partial Tonic-clonic Simple partial	15-25	6-12	4
Valproate (Depakene)	*Absence Myoclonic Atonic Akinetic Infantile spasms	30-60	50-100	2-3
Clonazepan (Clonopin)	Absence Akinetic Myoclonic	0.02-0.2	0.02-0.05	4
Phenobarbital	*Neonatal seizures *Febrile seizures Tonic-clonic Simple and complex partial	3-5	15-40	10-18
Phenytoin (Dilantin)	*Tonic-clonic *Simple partial *Complex partial Myoclonic	5-8	10-20	5-7
Ethosuximide (Zarontin)	*Absence	20-25	40-100	2-5
Primidone (Mysoline)	Complex partial Tonic-clonic	15-25	8-15	2-3
ACTH	*Infantile spasms	40-80 units/day		

*Drugs of choice

of choice for massive spasms of infancy but is not effective in other types of seizures (Table 61–5).

Carbamazepine (Tegretol) is now considered by many to be the drug of choice for partial seizures with complex symptomatology and an effective agent for other types of partial and generalized tonic-clonic seizures. The major side effects are drowsiness, dizziness, rash, and occasionally diplopia or ataxia. Bone marrow depression and hepatopathy are reported but considered rare. The drug has a relatively short half-life (12 hours), making it necessary to administer it three to four times daily in order to ensure optimal tissue concentration.

Valproate (Depakene) is a short-chain fatty acid with important anticonvulsant properties. It has proven valuable in all forms of childhood epilepsy but is considered most effective in absence seizures. Generalized seizures of the myoclonic and tonic-clonic type frequently respond to this drug used alone or in combination. Its major toxic side effects include gastrointestinal disturbances (anorexia, nausea, vomiting), altered behavior, sedation, and elevated SGOT and SGPT, although the hepatic dysfunction is usually asymptomatic. Fatal hepatopathy has been reported. It has also been associated with coagulation defects, alopecia, anorexia, tremor, and, more rarely, other nervous system disturbances including diplopia, incoordination, headache, insomnia, hallucinations, and other disturbances of mentation. Since the half-life is brief (10 hours), it should be administered on the average of three to four times daily.

Clonazepam (Clonopin) is effective in a number of seizure states, including partial, myoclonic, absence, and generalized tonic-clonic, as well as in infantile spasms and status epilepticus. The mean duration of action is 24 hours. This is significantly longer than that of diazepam, which is another of the benzadiazepam group of drugs used to control seizures. Its major side effects are sedation, ataxia, and hypotonia.

Phenytoin (Dilantin), used alone or in combination with other drugs, is effective therapy for most seizures with significant motor manifestations. It is not effective for the control of absence seizures nor currently recommended for febrile seizures. Chronic administration of the drug results in cosmetic side effects that are significant, particularly for adolescent females. Hirsutism, acne, and gingival hyperplasia occur often; less frequent complications include bone marrow depression, allergic rash, lupus-like reaction, hepatopathy, and a pseudo-lymphoma picture. These are considered idiosyncratic reactions and can occur at any time following the initiation of therapy. Because the metabolism of phenytoin by the liver is activated by phenobarbital, higher dosages of Dilantin are usually required when this drug combination is used. It is also important to appreciate that its absorption is variable, making it necessary to carefully monitor blood levels if seizures recur on what seem to be therapeutic dosages of the drug. It can be given twice daily because it has a half-life of 24 hours. When infants or children are receiving the liquid form of phenytoin, it is important to vigorously shake the bottle in order to ensure a uniform dosage of drug per unit volume.

Phenobarbital remains the most widely used anticonvulsant to treat most forms of seizures because it is safe and effective. Because of its long half-life, it can be administered once daily in older children. It is the standard anticonvulsant for most seizure problems in neonates, infants, and preschool children; in older children and adolescents other drugs are preferred. The reason for this is that the behavioral side effects which occur, particularly hyperkinesis, drowsiness, and personality changes, frequently interfere with school performance.

Phenobarbital is the drug of choice for the prophylactic treatment of febrile seizures and, in combination with phenytoin, is one of the recommended therapies for status epilepticus. It is usually not recommended for the control of absence or partial seizures with complex symptomatology, but it is effective therapy for generalized tonic-clonic seizures and sometimes for partial seizures with elementary symptomatology.

Ethosuximide (Zarontin) is an excellent drug for typical absence seizures (petit mal) but is less effective for other types of seizures. It is the traditional drug of choice for absence seizures but can be reserved for those situations in which valproate is either ineffective or poorly tolerated. Therapy with this drug should begin with small amounts and gradually be increased over the course of several weeks. Since one of the major side effects is gastrointestinal irritation, the drug should be taken with meals. It may also cause lethargy, dizziness, ataxia, leukopenia, agranulocytosis, and allergic skin rashes. Periodic liver function studies, blood counts, and urinalyses are recommended for patients, particularly in the early months after the initiation of therapy. Ethosuximide may increase the frequency of generalized tonic-clonic seizures in certain patients with mixed seizure disorders. If this is observed, supplemental therapy with carbamazepine or phenytoin is indicated.

Primidone (Mysoline) is a barbituate anticonvulsant that is used primarily for the control of complex partial seizures. One of its biotransformation products is phenobarbital. As a result, it has major behavioral and sedative side effects, making it suboptimal therapy for older children. Side effects can be minimized by increasing the dosage slowly over a number of weeks. In contrast to phenobarbital, primidone has a short half-life (6 to 12 hours), making it necessary to administer it at least twice daily to maintain effective blood levels.

ACTH therapy should be started immediately once the diagnosis of massive spasms is made. Its anticonvulsant actions are not understood nor is the pathophysiology of the myoclonic seizures, which are sometimes completely controlled with this medication. When it is effective, the seizures are dramatically reduced in number or eliminated entirely within a few days. Daily therapy is continued for four to six weeks and then gradually discontinued because by that time the maximum benefit will have been realized. It is also important not to prolong therapy, because the side effects in growing children are potentially very serious and usually reversible once the medication is discontinued. Diabetes mellitus, hypertension, demineralization of bone, and growth failure are infrequent unless the therapy extends over several months. Acne, hirsutism, and obesity are less severe but more frequently encountered.

Duration of Therapy

This is a controversial subject, but most agree that medications can be gradually withdrawn in children after four seizure-free years. Approximately 70 per cent of patients will remain seizure-free after this, regardless of the nature of the seizure problem. The risk of recurrence is increased if there were many seizures before control was achieved or if there are associated neurological abnormalities. If these patients are excluded, the prognosis for the remaining group to remain seizure-free is significantly improved over the 70 per cent figure. For this reason, some advocate discontinuing medication after three or possibly two seizure-free years in the low-risk group with onset of seizures after the age of two and a normal EEG while on treatment.

Intractable Seizures and Surgery

A small percentage of seizures recur despite comprehensive drug therapy and careful attention to every detail that is known to effect seizure control. This often includes a ketogenic diet which, although temporarily effective for some atypical absence or akinetic seizures, is usually not well-tolerated by children for prolonged periods. When it is apparent that seizures cannot be controlled with medication, surgery may be helpful if the cortical discharges are well-lateralized. Under these circumstances, cortical resection of the epileptogenic focus or partial lobectomy will sometimes produce dramatic reduction or cessation of seizures.

Complex partial seizures with electroencephalographic evidence of discharges from one temporal region is the type of problem most frequently considered for surgery. Unfortunately, by the time most patients have proven resistant to therapy, secondary epileptic foci will have developed, making surgery less effective or impractical to undertake. The younger patient is the best candidate for surgery, but there is an understandable reluctance to recommend major surgery until all medical therapies have been tried and proven unsuccessful. With the many anticonvulsants currently available, it is usually years before the child with intractable seizures is considered for surgery and by then most are not acceptable candidates because of the multifocal nature of the seizure activity.

REFERENCES

Brill, C. B., et al.: Seizures and other paroxysmal disorders. Adv. Pediatr., *18*:441–489, 1981.

Dodson, W. E.: Pharmacology and therapeutics of epilepsy in childhood. Clin. Neuropharmacol., *4*:1–29, 1979.

Emerson, R., et al.: Stopping medication in children with epilepsy. N. Engl. J. Med., *314*:1125–1129, 1981.

Griffith, J. F., et al.: Diseases of the Nervous System. St. Louis, The C. V. Mosby Co, 1980, pp. 717–763.

Johnston, M. V., et al.: Pharmacologic advances in seizure control. Pediatr. Clin. North Am., *28*:179–194, 1981.

Kendig, E. L., Jr., et al.: Febrile seizures: Long-term management of children with fever-associated seizures. Pediatrics, *66*:1009–1012, 1980.

Lenn, N. J.: Nonepileptic spells in children. Devel. Behav. Pediatr., *2*:54–60, 1981.

Mikkelsen, B., et al.: Clonazepam (Rivotril) and carbamazepine (Tegretol) in psychomotor epilepsy: A randomized multicenter trial. Epilepsia, *22*:415–420, 1981.

Penry, J. K.: Complex partial seizures and their treatment. Adv. Neurol., *11*:1–449, 1975.

Sherard, E. S., Jr., et al.: Treatment of childhood epilepsy with valproic acid: Results of the first 100 patients in a 6-month trial. Neurology, *30*:31–35, 1980.

Thurston, J. H., et al.: Prognosis in childhood epilepsy. N. Engl. J. Med., *306*:831–836, 1982.

Van Buren, J. M., et al.: Temporal-lobe seizures with additional foci treated by resection. J. Neurosurg., *43*:596–607, 1975.

62

SPEECH AND HEARING PROBLEMS

Carl W. Fuller, Ph.D.

Speech and language development begin with the random vocalizations of early infancy and proceed at a rapid rate through the preschool years. By his eighth birthday the average child will have mastered the prosodic features (rate, rhythm, duration, inflection) and virtually all of the grammatical structures of his native language and will have acquired mature articulation skills.

School age children with communication disorders ordinarily will be identified and treated through the school system. The primary care physician must assume major responsibility for identification of communication disability in children of preschool age. When developmental lag is evident, prompt initiation of remedial treatment will help minimize the social penalties of inadequate communication and will enhance the child's readiness to cope with the linguistic demands of the academic curriculum when he begins formal schooling.

ASSESSMENT OF LANGUAGE

Successive steps in language acquisition are highlighted by the major milestones below (Lilywhite, 1958):

1st birthday — one to three words

2nd birthday—two to three word phrases

3rd birthday—routine use of sentences

4th birthday—routine use of sentence sequences; conversational give-and-take

5th birthday—complex sentences; extensive use of modifiers, pronouns, prepositions

Vocabulary—20-50 words by 18 months, 100-200 by 24 months; size doubles each year through the preschool years

Formal tests suitable for office practice include the Peabody Picture Vocabulary Test, Revised (Dunn, 1981), the Utah Test of Language Development (Mecham et al., 1967), and the Denver Developmental Screening Test (Frankenburg and Dodds, 1969). If a child is unwilling or unable to cooperate in a formal test procedure, an approximation of language level may be determined by interviewing the parent or other informed caretaker, utilizing a standardized questionnaire like the Developmental Profile (Alpern and Boll, 1972) or the Verbal Language Development Scale (Mecham, 1971). Any of these tests can be used by office personnel appropriately trained in testing and interviewing techniques.*

These tests may single out the child who is doing poorly, but they will not explain the cause of his difficulty. A virtue of the Developmental Profile, the Denver Developmental Screening Test, and the more complex battery described by Hartlage and Lucas (1973) is that they allow the clinician to compare language status with other parameters of developmental progress, thus highlighting language deficiency as an isolated disability on the one hand or as a component of more pervasive developmental delay on the other.

Estimates of developmental *level* should be accompanied by estimates of developmental *rate*. Thus, a child who seems immature in language development but who has made marked gains in recent months is of less concern than the child who has recently made few gains even though he meets the screening criteria. A preschool child who is not steadily improving his language skills should always be considered at risk for language disorder regardless of his present status.

Differential diagnosis must consider specific language learning disability, subnormal intelligence, hearing impairment, childhood psychosis, infantile autism, the effect of severe or prolonged illness early in life, and psychosocial disturbances such as environmental neglect, inappropriate teaching procedures used by parents, chronic maternal depression, and instability of the home environment, notably in the case of children in foster care. In most cases it is imprudent to expect a language-disordered child to "grow out of it" when the conditions

*For a more detailed discussion of screening tests, see the chapters by Northern, pp. 346–388, and Drumwright, pp. 439–476, in Frankenburg, William K., and Camp, Bonnie C.: Pediatric Screening Tests. Springfield, IL, Charles C Thomas, 1975.

that allowed him to "grow into it" are unrecognized or unaltered. Waiting for growth to cure what growth has not prevented is a poor substitute for direct action.

Indications for more detailed investigation by a speech and language specialist, listed below, imply that intervention will be required, either as intensive parental counseling or as remedial teaching, or both.

Failure to say recognizable words by the age of 20 months

Failure to combine words into phrases by 30 months

Failure to speak in sentences by 36 months

Failure to comprehend the speech of others at an age-appropriate level

Conspicuous echolalia after the age of 24 months

Vocabulary below the 10th percentile at any age after 24 months

Vocalizations devoid of consonants after 15 months

Regression in language output or in skill of usage

Word transpositions in sentences, frequent transpositions of sounds or syllables in words, word-finding difficulty after 3 years

Parental exasperation and worry over the child's slow rate of language acquisition

ASSESSMENT OF SPEECH

The term *speech*, as used here, refers to the acoustic characteristics of spoken language. These include loudness, pitch, and quality of the voice; rate and rhythm of utterance; and articulation of speech sounds. Children usually have normal rate, rhythm, loudness, and inflection patterns by the time they begin to use sentences. Articulation skills have a slower maturational rate and may not match the adult model until the child is eight years old.

Faulty articulation is the most prevalent disorder of speech. The detailed analysis of articulation patterns is a task for speech pathologists; a preliminary assessment of articulation skills may be made by using the Denver Articulation Screening Test (Drumwright, 1971) or the 50-Item Screening Articulation Test (Templin and Darley, 1960), both of which have norms related to chronological age. The average listener's judgment is probably best guided by the intelligibility of the child's utterance. As a rule, the two-year-old's speech should be intelligible to the mother most of the time; the three-year-old's should be intelligible to the mother all of the time and to the father most of the time; and a four-year-old's to strangers most of the time. A five-year-old's speech may contain recognizable articulation errors, but it should be easily understood by all listeners.

Most children undergo a period of mild dysfluency, typically appearing as uneven flow of speech without other manifestations of disturbance, some time between the ages of three and four-and-a half years. This transient phenomenon should not be labeled stuttering. Parents who are unduly alarmed about this behavior should be counseled to accept it calmly and casually and to avoid admonishing the child to "relax," "slow down," "think before you speak," and so on.

In contrast, the patient who truly stutters usually resorts to a variety of behavioral devices intended to aid the initiation of speech and the maintenance of continuing utterance. These devices include such mannerisms as waving or tapping the extremities, changing the breathing rhythm, avoiding feared words or sounds, peculiar postures of the face, and so on. These so-called "secondary" accompaniments of dysfluent speech indicate a need for intervention by a speech specialist.

The primary care physician can usually determine whether speech or voice disorders have a biomedical basis, e.g., tongue paralysis, laryngeal polyps, cleft palate. He should request a speech pathologist to assist in analyzing the speech behavior itself and in planning a program of speech correction. The following conditions suggest a need for diagnostic speech examination:

Speech unintelligible to both parents after two years of age

Speech unintelligible to the father after three years of age

Speech unintelligible to strangers after four years of age

Persistent hoarse, husky, or breathy voice quality, or voice marked by conspicuous hypo- or hypernasality

Tics, grimaces, or stereotyped hand or head movements accompanying disordered speech rhythm

Voice pitch inappropriate to age or sex

Failure of the child to correct articulation errors after continued intensive stimulation by the parents

Structural or functional anomalies that obviously will impair speech or voice, e.g., cleft palate, cerebral palsy, hearing loss, and so forth.

Anxiety in the child because of dysfluent or misarticulated speech or peculiarity of voice

Similar anxiety in the parents

ASSESSMENT OF HEARING

Pure tone audiometry is the method of choice for screening purposes and for threshold determination. Testing can be conducted by a nurse or other trained office assistant. Air conduction threshold testing must be supplemented with bone conduction audiometry, tympanometry, or both to identify hearing loss, if present, as conductive, sensorineural, or mixed. Air conduction audiometry by itself will not identify the locus of pathology.

Ambient noise levels tend to be relatively high in average office environments. Consequently, threshold audiometry at very low stimulus intensities requires isolation of the patient in a sound-proof room. In its absence, testing should be performed in the quietest room available, where externally generated (wind, traffic, lawn mowers) and internally generated (ventilation, plumbing, waiting room) noises are at a minimum. In general, the stimulus intensity for screening audiometry should be the lowest level permitted by the acoustic environment.

Screening audiometry may rule out hearing impairment of significant severity, but it does not necessarily rule out middle ear disease. For detection of middle ear dysfunction, tympanometry is the method of choice.

In simplified terms tympanometry is an indirect measure of the efficiency with which acoustic energy in the ear canal is transduced into mechanical energy in the vibrating middle ear system. The equipment consists of an air pump and associated manometer, a pure tone generator, and a sensing mechanism to measure the intensity of sound reflected from the tympanic membrane. A probe surmounted by a plastic or rubber cuff is inserted in the ear canal; the cuff is chosen of appropriate size to insure a hermetic seal of the canal. The air pressure in the canal is then systematically varied, and the resulting changes in the compliance of the tympanic membrane can be recorded either manually or automatically on a graph in which the abscissa represents ear canal pressure relative to atmospheric pressure, and the ordinate represents compliance amplitude. This graph is called a tympanogram.

Typically the tympanic membrane has maximum compliance when air pressure in the canal equals air pressure in the middle ear; ordinarily this will be atmospheric pressure, arbitrarily designated on the tympanogram as 0. After the probe is firmly seated, the air pressure is increased to a positive pressure of 200 mm H_2O and is then gradually reduced to a negative pressure of as much as 400 mm H_2O. The normal ear will show minimal compliance at 200 mm H_2O positive pressure, steadily increasing compliance to a peak at or near 0 as the air pressure is reduced, and then steadily decreasing compliance to a second minimum as the pressure is further reduced to create a partial vacuum in the canal. Abnormal conditions in the middle ear will be revealed in the tympanogram as (1) abnormal compliance amplitude, (2) abnormal shape of the compliance curve, and (3) abnormal pressures at which maximum compliance is reached.

The test procedure does not require the active cooperation of the patient other than to sit still, preferably, although not necessarily, without vocalizing. It is simple and quick, and it can be performed with patients of any age, whether awake, asleep, or sedated.

Space does not permit a detailed discussion of tympanogram interpretation here. In practice, a normal tympanogram may exhibit a variety of compliance curves within a range of pressures above and below 0. Equipment manufacturers supply charts that indicate the pressure-compliance relations considered normal for the instrumentation in use. Pressure-compliance curves that differ from these "templates" imply middle ear abnormality.

As stated earlier, normal ears yield tympanograms having compliance peaks at or near 0. Apparently only acute otitis media produces a compliance peak at greater than 0 pressure. Compliance peaks appearing at negative pressures exceeding 100 mm H_2O represent middle ear dysfunction, since, by definition, they indicate abnormal negative pressure in the middle ear. A "flat" tympanogram, one in which compliance is constant regardless of pressure change, indicates an immobile tympanic membrane.

The fact that a tympanogram exhibits maximum compliance at 0 pressure does not rule out a dysfunctional ear. Very high compliance amplitude at 0 pressure may result from an abnormally flaccid tympanic membrane or from a disarticulated ossicular chain. Very low amplitude at 0 pressure can be produced by stapes fixation or by ossicular adhesions. Dome-shaped compliance curves are more frequently associated with middle ear effusions than are curves with sharply defined peaks (Paradise et al., 1976).

These are but a few of the tympanogram variations resulting from middle ear pathology. Accuracy of tympanogram interpretation derives largely from the skill and experience of the examiner in synthesizing tympanometric data with information gained from audiometric and otoscopic examination and from the case history.*

Despite its appealing simplicity of administration, tympanometry is not without pitfalls. The ear should be inspected otoscopically prior to testing to insure that the canal is free of impacted cerumen and foreign bodies. The canal should be cleaned, if necessary; dirt, cerumen, and flakes of skin can occlude the probe tip, resulting in a false positive flat tympanogram. Care must be taken not to seat the probe tip against the canal wall or to collapse the canal—a particular hazard in the case of infants. If tympanostomy tubes are present, the interpretation of the tympanogram is paradoxical: a normal tympanogram means that the tubes are occluded, i.e., nonfunctional (if the ear is otherwise normal). Patent tubes should produce a flat tympanogram, which, under other circumstances, would suggest otological intervention. A flat tympanogram should not be discarded as invalid simply because the drum is seen to move under pneumatic otoscopy—the pneumatic otoscope may generate three to four times as much air pressure as is used in tympanometry.

Finally, it must be remembered that tympanometry is *not* a test of hearing sensitivity. A patient with an abnormal tympanogram may have hearing within the normal range. A patient with profound deafness may have a normal tympanogram. Tympanometry and audiometry are complementary, not interchangeable.

Children who are hard to test and children known to have hearing loss should be referred for detailed audiological assessment. There is *no* age at which hearing tests cannot be performed. Competent pediatric audiologists can use conditioning procedures for behavioral testing of children as young as six months of age. The advent of evoked response audiometry permits testing of neonates and of all other patients who cannot, or will not, respond reliably to a test by more conventional means. Postponing audiological assessment by a specialist when auditory integrity is in doubt cannot be justified. Referral for comprehensive audiological evaluation is indicated:

When hearing loss is detected by office testing

When the child persistently responds to the speech of others with "What?" or "Huh?"

When language delay or distorted speech is present and hearing loss cannot be ruled out by office testing

When the child has failed a hearing test administered by school personnel

When abnormal tympanograms persist despite treatment (except when the tympanic membrane is perforated)

In the case of infants, when the child fails to babble or fails to localize the source of sound by the age of 12 months

*The theory and practice of tympanometry are discussed in detail in Feldman and Wilber, 1976. Some of the practical problems of clinical assessment of children are reviewed in Harford et al., 1978.

SUMMARY

Screening procedures are available to the primary care practitioner for early identification of communication disorders in children. Children who fail screening tests in the physician's office should be referred to speech and hearing specialists for further examination and for recommendations for treatment.

Communication disorders in children are developmental handicaps, as real as, and sometimes more disabling than, organic disease. They deserve the same sympathetic attention as their physical counterparts.

REFERENCES

Alpern, G. D., and Boll, T. J.: Developmental Profile. Indianapolis, IN, Psychological Development Publications, 1972.

Drumwright, A. F.: Denver Articulation Screening Exam. Denver, University of Colorado Medical Center, 1971.

Dunn, L. M.: Peabody Picture Vocabulary Test, Revised. Minneapolis, MN, American Guidance Service Inc., 1981.

Feldman, A. S., and Wilber, L. A.: Acoustic Impedance and Admittance—the Measurement of Middle Ear Function. Baltimore, the Williams and Wilkins Co., 1976.

Frankenburg, W. K., and Dodds, J. B.: Denver Developmental Screening Test. Denver, Ladoca Foundation, 1969.
Harford, E. R., Bess, F. H., Bluestone, C. D., and Klein, J. O. (eds.): Impedance Screening for Middle Ear Disease in Children. New York, Grune and Stratton, 1978.
Hartlage, L. D., and Lucas, D. G.: Mental Developmental Evaluation of the Pediatric Patient. Springfield, IL, Charles C Thomas, 1973.
Lillywhite, H. J.: Doctor's manual of speech disorders. J.A.M.A., *167*:850–858, 1958.
Mecham, M. J.: Verbal Language Development Scale, Revised. Minneapolis, MN, American Guidance Service, 1971.
Mechan, M. J., Jex, J., and Jones, J. D.: Utah Test of Language Development. Salt Lake City, Communications Research Associates, Inc., 1967.
Paradise, J. L., Smith, C. G., and Bluestone, C. D.: Tympanometric detection of middle ear effusion in infants and young children. Pediatrics, *58*:198–210, 1976.
Templin, M., and Darley, F. L.: The Templin-Darley Tests of Articulation, 2nd Edition. Iowa City, University of Iowa Bureau of Educational Research and Service, 1960.

Preparation of this paper was supported in part by DHHS, Maternal and Child Health Training Grant #924–13 (UAF), and by Office of Human Development Grant Award 59–P–25293/5–10 (Indianapolis—UAF).

63

ASTHMA AND ALLERGIC RHINITIS

Asthma

Howard Eigen, M.D., and Peter H. Scott, M.D.

Definition

The definition of asthma is a difficult one on which to find general agreement. To the physiologist asthma can be defined as hyperreactive airways; to the pathologist, mucosal edema and smooth muscle hypertrophy; and to the clinician, wheezy dyspnea. Asthma is characterized by episodic airflow obstruction that results in wheezing and breathlessness along with cough and increased sputum production. The obstruction is reversible by the use of medication to relax spasm of bronchial smooth muscle. "Extrinsic" asthma is generally defined as pure atopic asthma, provoked by allergens for which a wheal and flare hypersensitivity exists; "intrinsic" asthma, on the other hand, is neither allergic nor IgE-mediated and is characterized by exacerbations that may not be seasonally related. Most patients, however, have neither purely extrinsic nor purely intrinsic asthma, but rather mixed disease in which the patient's hyperreactive airways can be triggered into spasm by a variety of irritants and allergens.

Pathophysiology

Whatever the initiating event, the response of the airways is similar and contains three essential elements: (1) contraction of bronchial smooth muscle leading to airway obstruction and eventual hypertrophy of these muscle cells; (2) hypersecretion consisting of a thick, abnormal mucus along with mucous gland hypertrophy resulting in airway obstruction; and (3) edema of the respiratory mucosa with infiltration of inflammatory cells and eosinophils.

The traditional teaching has been that the onset of an asthmatic attack is heralded by an audible expiratory wheeze and that disappearance of the wheeze implies successful therapy. This is, of course, true, since the bronchospasm associated with bronchial asthma is reversible. However, bronchoconstriction, although it may be the most noticeable clinical feature of asthma, is only part of a complex syndrome that physiologically has four interacting parts: (1) bronchospasm and wheezing, (2) air trapping, (3) changes in lung mechanics, and (4) hypoxemia. The pathophysiology of asthma involves both the large (greater than 2 mm) and small (less than 2 mm) airways. Knowledge of the pathophysiology facilitates an understanding of the physical findings associated with asthma and the specific goals of therapy.

Wheezing, the symptom most commonly associated with asthma, is secondary to obstruction of the large airways from any of the three mechanisms cited above and a subsequent increase in airway resistance. Sufficient air close flow past the obstruction creates air turbulence, heard by the examiner as a wheezing or whistling sound. Understanding that these two elements, obstruction and air turbulence, must both be present to produce wheezing is essential. If either element is absent, the wheeze will disappear. Clinically, this means that wheezing may disappear either if the patient improves (because airway resistance is reduced) or if he gets worse (because flow past the obstructed airway becomes so low that turbulence is not created).

While wheezing is the most dramatic feature of asthma, many characteristic clinical features are related to air trapping rather than increased resistance of the large airways. Air trapping is not caused by increasing large airway resistance, such as by breathing through a narrow tube, but by closure of the small airways at increasingly higher lung volumes. The mechanism of such closure is still controversial but probably involves mucosal edema and obstruction of the airway lumen by secretions. Air trapping forces a patient to breath at high lung volume, which reduces pulmonary compliance, increases the work of breathing, and puts the respiratory muscle at a mechanical disadvantage; thus, the asthmatic struggles as much to inspire as to expire. This added work increases oxygen consumption and cardiac output at a time when gas exchange is already compromised. A further consequence of breathing at high lung volume is that the highly negative pleural pressures increase transmural pressure on the pulmonary vessels, causing exudation of fluid out of the pulmonary circulation into the interstitial spaces of the lung. The resultant fluid, which further decreases pulmonary compliance, has to be considered when treating a patient with intravenous fluids. Gas trapping also creates marked abnormalities of ventilation-perfusion ratios in the lung, with a consequent decrease in arterial oxygen tension. These changes in breathing mechanics, which are responsible for many of the physical findings apparent during an acute asthma attack, are also present between acute exacerbations. Blood oxygen tensions in asymptomatic asthmatic children have been shown to be less than 80 mm of mercury in nearly one fourth of patients. In addition, air trapping in those who are apparently well is seen in 40 per cent of patients. These clinically occult abnormalities are exaggerated during acute episodes.

The changes in arterial blood gases during the acute episode follow a characteristic pattern. With worsening obstruction, further mismatching of ventilation with perfusion occurs. Arterial oxygen tension falls immediately and continues to drop steadily as the attack continues. Changes in arterial carbon dioxide tension follow a more complex pattern. Initially the $PaCO_2$ is low, owing to hyperventilation from excessive respiratory drive, probably the result of stimulation of vagal pulmonary receptors either mechanically or by chemical mediators. As the severity of the attack increases, it becomes mechanically impossible to maintain sufficient minute ventilation, so $PaCO_2$ starts to rise. As it does, the $PaCO_2$ crosses into the "normal" range of 35 to 45 mm of mercury. Thus a hypoxic patient with an apparently normal $PaCO_2$ is, in fact, showing signs of impending respiratory failure.

Relationship to Physical Findings

Knowledge of the pathophysiology of asthma can help the physician interpret the physical signs associated with acute episodes of wheezing. The time-honored, subjective dyspnea, wheeze, and prolonged expiration are the least useful indices of severity of disease in children (Commey and Levison, 1976); however, sternocleidomastoid contraction and superclavicular retractions closely correlate with the severity of airway obstruction. These physical signs are evidence of increased *inspiratory* rather than expiratory effort and result from poor pulmonary compliance due to breathing at high lung volume. Pulsus paradoxus, also a useful index of severity, is the result of the negative pressures created in the chest during inspiration. The hyperinflation noted on inspection and the hyperresonance to percussion are signs of air trapping secondary to small airway involvement during the acute asthmatic episode. It is especially important to recognize that the disappearance of wheezing heard on physical examination does not herald improvement in oxygenation, since wheezing is a large airway phenomenon, and hypoxemia is caused by small airway involvement. Patients can be severely hypoxemic and yet appear comfortable and be free of wheezes.

CLINICAL CONSIDERATIONS

Triggers

In early childhood, irritants such as cigarette smoke, strong odors of soaps and perfumes, and viral respiratory agents are important triggers of asthma symptoms. This is also true in older children, although to a lesser extent. These wheezing episodes do not result from IgE-mediated allergy to virus protein or to the irritants, but rather they represent a neurologically and chemically mediated response to these nonspecific airway irritants. Bacterial infection of the respiratory tract rarely, if ever, results in exacerbations of symptoms in asthmatic patients. Certainly, there is no evidence that allergy to bacterial products is involved. The tendency of an asthmatic child to have bronchospasm after exposure to irritants or strong odors should not be mistaken for IgE-mediated allergy. In some children with asthma, it appears that emotional distress will lower the threshold at which other irritants can trigger a wheezing episode, while in others it can cause wheezing without additional triggering mechanisms.

It is very common for asthma symptoms in asthmatic children to be induced by exercise. A large proportion of, if not all, asthmatic children develop wheezing after sufficient exercise, but the response depends upon the type and intensity of the exercise. Children with and without allergically mediated asthma may have exercise-induced bronchospasm. When measuring peak flow as the response to exercise, we typically see an immediate increase in peak flow of about 20 per cent, followed by a precipitous fall during the first five minutes following the exercise. The degree of bronchospasm induced by exercise is directly related to the amount of heat lost from the airway during exercise, which seems to explain the different degrees of airflow obstruction induced by different types of exercise. Swimming, typically carried out in a warm, moist environment, causes little heat loss from the airway and is easily tolerated, whereas running, especially in cold weather, causes bronchospasm at low levels of exercise. Asthmatic children who play competitive sports may wheeze during a game but may be able to tolerate the same amount of exercise during practice, demonstrating the linkage of emotional stress with exercise in causing bronchospasm.

Nonwheezing Manifestations

The clinical spectrum of asthma has been broadened in recent years with the recognition of the many nonwheezing manifestations of asthma, chiefly chronic cough. Coughing has been shown to occur in persons who react positively to bronchial challenge with either exercise or methacholine inhalation. Bronchodilator therapy in these patients leads to a relief of the cough and reversal of pulmonary function abnormalities. Nonspecific episodic dyspnea, unrelated to exercise, may be another initial manifestation of asthma. Patients who present in this fashion often have abnormal pulmonary function or increased airway reactivity and respond to oral bronchodilators.

Several types of antigen-antibody reactions have been shown to be involved in the pathogenesis of asthma. While there is little question that allergens trigger asthma, the exact role of allergens and their treatment remain to be clarified. The most frequent of these reactions is the result of minor exposures to small amounts of antigen. Type I allergens combine with surface receptors on the mast cell to release mediators of tissue reaction (histamine, slow reacting substance of anaphylaxis, SRS-A), which affect capillary permeability, cause smooth muscle contraction, and increase production of secretions. The antibodies involved are the IgE immunoglobulins.

Type III allergic reactions activate complement that both causes histamine release and acts as a chemotactic factor for neutrophils. These reactions result in a delayed bronchospastic reaction that occurs from 3 to 5 hours after the inhalation of the offending substance.

The clinical history provides the most helpful information as to the identification of causal allergens. Environmental conditions, both at home and at school, must be reviewed. Care must be taken to distinguish the effects of true allergens from those of direct irritation after inhalation of various agents. Inquiry should be made as to seasonal and environmental variations. Symptoms related to allergens such as grass, tree pollens, and molds may overlap, making distinction difficult. A history that symptoms are provoked by specific allergens is a clinical feature of asthma in atopic patients; however, some children who have negative skin tests also have a history of allergen-provoked asthma. In one study, 77 per cent of skin test–positive patients give positive histories of allergy to one or the other tested allergens, while a full 47 per cent of the skin test–negative asthmatics gave allergic histories suggestive of provocation. Problems in interpretation include the fact that the allergen extracts are not yet standardized and that the size of the wheal and the level of specific IgE antibodies do not necessarily correlate with the clinical severity of the disease. Positive tests serve primarily to guide the allergic management of the patient, and overall results should not be taken as an absolute indication for injection treatments (immunotherapy). Furthermore, the correlation between the bronchial provocation test sensitivity to an antigen and skin test hypersensitivity does not demonstrate a one-to-one relationship. A patient may be positive by skin test and negative by bronchial provocation test with the same antigen.

Hypersecretion plays an important role in asthma. Asthmatic patients secrete abnormal respiratory tract mucus having an increased protein content and excessive cellular constituents. These patients clear secretions from the respiratory tract more slowly than normal subjects, i.e., have a reduced tracheal mucus velocity, and respond to allergenic challenge with further reductions in tracheal mucus clearance that persist beyond the allergen-induced bronchospasm. Thus, alterations in secretion clearance can contribute to the clinical picture of asthma. Chronic bronchitis in children overlaps with asthma in etiology, pathophysiology, and treatment (Taussig). Children with asthma demonstrate recurrent chest infiltrates and atelectasis, with a predilection for the right middle lobe. Another presentation of asthma is with what appears to be recurrent pneumonia but is probably recurrent atelectasis. The majority of children who present with recurrent pneumonia have bronchial hyperreactivity, as demonstrated by a response to methacholine, and are improved with bronchodilator therapy.

Differential Diagnosis

The differential diagnosis of wheezing in childhood includes cystic fibrosis, foreign body aspiration, congenital malformations, and infections.

Cystic Fibrosis

This disease often presents with wheezing or a clinical picture similar to bronchiolitis. On the physical examination the child will appear more chronically ill than can be explained by his pulmonary disease alone. Digital clubbing may suggest bronchiectasis. Other chronic pulmonary diseases, such as those associated with immunological deficiencies and Kartagener's syndrome, may result in bronchial hyperreactivity because of airway injury from chronic infection.

Foreign Body Aspiration

Although most aspirated foreign bodies in children are not radiopaque, they can be detected by radiological examination. An aspirated foreign body may cause generalized wheezing, often without a recent history of a choking episode.

Congenital Malformations

Congenital malformations, such as a vascular ring or intrathoracic tracheal stenosis, may mimic the signs and symptoms of asthma by causing partial airway obstruction.

Infections

Viral infections of the respiratory tract often cause bronchial hyperreactivity and wheezing. Even in normal children, bronchial reactivity may be increased for 6 to 8 weeks following a viral respiratory infection. Bronchiolitis may be indistinguishable from asthma in infants and young children; however, rarely does an infant have more than one or two episodes of infectious bronchiolitis. Not all children with bronchiolitis wheeze during the acute episode, but over half can be expected to have repeated wheezing episodes later in life and to have airway abnormalities even after 10 years. Fifty-seven per cent of children with previous bronchiolitis have been found to have bronchial hyperreactivity demonstrable on methacholine bronchial challenge (Gurwitz et al., 1981). Since there is a high incidence of asthma in first degree relatives of infants who have bronchiolitis with wheezing, this response to RSV infection may reflect a genetic predisposition to bronchial hyperreactivity, especially if the infant has wheezing initially or repeated episodes of so-called bronchiolitis.

EVALUATION

Physical Examination

Even in the absence of glucocorticoid therapy, asthmatic children tend to be smaller in height and weight than normal children. Some severely asthmatic patients have a retarded bone age. The degree of growth retardation is related to the severity of the asthma. Despite this, ultimate height is usually normal. While it is important to understand that asthmatics may be undergrown, children with both wheezing and growth retardation should be investigated for cystic fibrosis, bronchiectasis, or other chronic destructive pulmonary diseases.

Examination of the child with respiratory disease starts with the fingers. Digital clubbing occurs in less than 4 per cent of asthmatic patients, so a child with episodic wheezing and digital clubbing should have a quantitative sweat test for cystic fibrosis.

Inspection of the chest in patients with asthma may reveal an increase in the anteroposterior diameter, retractions, or use of the accessory muscles of inspiration or expiration. The percussion note may be hyperresonant. During mild exacerbations, light palpation may reveal contraction of abdominal muscles with each exhalation. These contractions demonstrate that exhalation, usually passive, has now become active due to expiratory airway obstruction. This "pushing" on exhalation, which becomes obvious long before other physical signs of obstruction, is an especially useful sign in infants.

Auscultation of the chest should be done carefully, comparing homologous bronchopulmonary segments and attempting to localize any abnormalities. It is critical to evaluate air entry, as this may indicate the degree of obstruction more accurately than the presence of wheezing. Wheezing itself may be heard on either inspiration or expiration. We interpret inspiratory wheezing to be the result of airway secretions. The sounds are less musical, usually coarse, and change with coughing. Expiratory wheezing tends to be musical and polyphonic and does not change as readily with respiratory manuevers. In the mildly obstructed child, expiratory wheezing may not be heard unless a forced expiration is obtained. We routinely ask children to blow out hard during the examination to determine if they wheeze during forced expiration, even if they are clear during quiet breathing. Many children with asthma, especially infants, have excessive nasal secretions that make examination of the chest more difficult. Gently pinching the nose closed is often helpful in forcing the child to breathe through his mouth in order to separate nasal noise from lower airway findings. Other physical signs of allergy may be evident, e.g., allergic shiners, a transverse nasal crease, the typical allergic gaping of the mouth from nasal obstruction, or the so-called fourth turbinate sign consisting of heaped up mucosa along the floor of the nasal passages.

PULMONARY FUNCTION TESTING

In children able to cooperate (generally those over six years old), pulmonary function testing is an invaluable part of the initial diagnosis, continuing assessment and evaluation of response to medication. Such testing also helps parents guide home therapy.

Some of the most important tests, such as simple spirometry and the measurement of peak expiratory flow rate (PEFR), can easily be performed in a pediatric or general medical practice office. One of the goals of therapy should be to normalize the spirometric tracing of each patient. From spirometry one can measure the FEV_1 (forced expiratory volume in one second) and FVC (forced vital capacity). The FEV_1, which measures flow over a large range of lung volume, is a relatively sensitive measure of airway obstruction. It may be normal during asymptomatic periods, but decreases as airway obstruction progresses. The FVC is usually normal in asthmatic children and decreases during severe episodes. As small airway obstruction worsens and air trapping increases, the residual volume rises and impinges upon the vital capacity. Thus, a decrease in forced vital capacity indicates severe air trapping. An especially useful calculation is that of the FEV_1/FVC ratio, which compares the amount of gas exhaled in one second to the total forced vital capacity. In normal persons, this ratio is 85 per cent. As obstruction increases, the FEV_1 falls while the FVC remains constant, causing a reduction in the FEV_1/FVC ratio. Caution is necessary, however, because if both FEV_1 and FVC fall, as in severe obstruction, the ratio may be unchanged. Both FEV_1 and FVC can respond to inhaled bronchodilators. Another measurement that can be made from a spirogram is the MMEF or (maximum mid-expiratory flow), also known as the FEF25-75%. This determination, which demonstrates flow over the midportion of the vital capacity, cannot be improved by increasing patient effort or by training and so is a good indication of small airway function.

Static lung volumes and capacities also reflect the physiological abnormalities of asthma. These measurements are calculated from a measurement of FRC (functional residual capacity), which is determined by either body plethysmography or gas dilution. This evaluation requires equipment that is more sophisticated and expensive than is practical for the physician's office. As air trapping increases, FRC and one of its components, RV (residual volume), increase. At first, the entire chest can expand, increasing TLC (total lung capacity) as well, but TLC is limited by the ability of the bony thorax to increase in size. When TLC reaches its maximum, RV may continue to increase, impinging on the vital capacity. Airway resistance, which reflects primarily large airway disease, can be measured directly by body plethysmography.

Use of Pulmonary Function Testing

The diagnosis of asthma can be confirmed by the appropriate use of pulmonary function testing. The simplest among these tests assesses a patient's response to an inhaled bronchodilator. If the patient shows a spirometric picture of airway obstruction (a decrease in FEV_1 or a decrease in FEV_1/FVC ratio), an inhaled bronchodilator may be given in an effort to increase airflow. In our laboratory we have the patient inhale several breaths of isoproterenol sufficient to raise the heart rate 10 beats per minute as an indication of an adequate dose. Responsiveness to inhaled bronchodilators is consistent with the reversible airway obstruction characteristic of childhood asthma; however, since reversible obstruction is not diagnostic of childhood asthma, other pulmonary diseases, such as cystic fibrosis, which can result in reversible obstruction, should be ruled out.

In the event that the patient has normal baseline pulmonary function, in the presence of a history suggestive of asthma, an airway challenge test can be performed. Bronchial challenge testing is especially useful in patients who do not have a history of wheezing, but have complained of such symptoms as chronic cough, nocturnal dyspnea, or recurrent pneumonia. During challenge testing, the airway is irritated by a stimulus, either chemical, such as methacholine or histamine; physical, such as exercise or the inhalation of frigid air; or allergenic. The FEV_1 is measured before and after the stimulus. A significant fall in FEV_1 (usually 20 per cent from baseline), which indicates airway sensitivity to the challenge agent, is diagnostic of bronchial hyperreactivity. Because these tests start with a small dose of the trigger agent and work up to large doses, they are safe as well as effective. It is important that bronchial challenge testing is done according to standard protocols and in a pediatric pulmonary center that performs these tests routinely. Exercising patients in the office by having them run or jump briefly and then listening for wheezing or checking simple spirometry may be more misleading than informative. For example, in asthmatic patients, exercise results first in mild bronchodilation followed by constriction. This lability of the airways can be detected only during formal exercise testing.

Laboratory Investigations

The judicious use of a few simple laboratory tests can add greatly to patient management. Radiographic findings include air trapping, atelectasis, pulmonary hypertension, and pulmonary edema. Air trapping, one of the most common findings in the patient during an acute episode and usually bilateral and symmetrical, is diagnosed when flattened diaphragms, increased retrosternal air space, vertical heart, and hyperlucent lung fields are noted on the radiograph. Pneumothorax, pneumomediastinum, and pneumopericardium are uncommon but potentially serious complications that can be diagnosed by chest radiographs.

Abnormal shadows are seen frequently on chest radiographs and may be difficult to evaluate. Although infiltrative processes, such as pneumonia, can occur, asthmatic children are not at higher risk for bacterial pneumonia. On the other hand, atelectasis due to mucus plugging of the airways is a common finding in pediatric asthmatic patients. The degree of atelectasis can be inconsequential, as when the patient has mild subsegmental atelectasis, or significant, with atelectasis of an entire lung. More commonly, however, the chest film of an asthmatic patient merely shows mild perihilar accentuation due to an increase in bronchovascular markings secondary to airway wall edema and excess bronchial secretions in the central airways. Antibiotics are rarely indicated for the patient with asthma whose chest radiographic findings are abnormal. Rather, they should be reserved for the patient who has persistent fever and leukocytosis and shows progression of an infiltrative process on chest radiograph.

Pulmonary hypertension leads to a fullness of the main pulmonary artery segment, a prominence of the right and left pulmonary arteries, and an abrupt decrease in the caliber of the vessels at the secondary or tertiary divisions. Pulmonary hypertension is usually transient and occurs in the acutely severely obstructed patient. Similarly, pulmonary edema, secondary to elevation of the pulmonary transmural vascular pressure, is seen exclusively in the acutly ill asthmatic patient. Pulmonary edema is characterized by bronchial cuffing with fluid in the perivascular and peribronchial interstitial spaces and the intralobar and intralobular septa. The propensity of the acutely obstructed asthmatic patient to develop pulmonary edema must be kept in mind when considering intravenous fluid management. Unless the patient with status asthmaticus is dehydrated at the time of admission, we routinely administer only maintenance fluid. Administration of 1½ to 2 times maintenance intravenous fluids may be potentially harmful.

The most useful blood tests are the white blood cell count (WBC), the differential, and the total eosinophil count. The WBC can help identify infectious processes in the evaluation of the wheezing child with fever. Since epinephrine moves mature marginated white cells into the circulatory pool, thereby raising the white count but not increasing the fraction of immature polymorphonuclear cells (bands), the differential count is of clinical importance.

The esopinophil count (obtained as a total count and not estimated from the WBC and differential) is elevated above 250 cells/cu mm in both allergic and nonallergic asthma, especially if there has been a recent wheezing episode. Corticosteroid treatment can be monitored by serial assessment of total eosinophilia, using the dose necessary to suppress the eosinophil count.

Sputum in asthmatics, abnormal even between wheezing episodes, is tenacious, stringy, and white in color and often causes the child to gag. It contains such abnormal cellular constituents as protein spirals, casts, eosinophils, sloughed ciliated epithelium, and Charcot-Leyden crystals. It is not necessary to stain sputum for microscopic examination, as these elements can be seen by examining a thick wet-prep of sputum under a coverslip. Sputum cultures are generally not helpful, as bacterial superinfection is rare in asthmatic children.

The RAST (radioallergosorbent test) method can identify allergen-specific IgE in the serum. However, this expensive test does not improve significantly on the accuracy of a good allergic history and selected, properly done allergy skin tests.

Intradermal prick testing to specific, commonly encountered inhalant allergens, which may identify substances to which the patient is likely to react, are best used judiciously to confirm the history or to clarify the patient's reactivity to specific substances that overlap seasonally.

Arterial blood gas analysis is an essential part of the evaluation of the patient during an attack. Moderate hypoxemia is frequently present even if the child does not appear very ill. Although wheezing may respond to therapeutic measures, patients with severe hypoxemia (PaO_2 less than 60 mm Hg) often require hospital admission.

In the office, routine assessment of pulmonary function by spirometry is helpful to assess the adequacy of therapy and to be sure that prescribed therapy maintains the child's pulmonary function at optimum levels. This is important because children may be symptom-free but remain mildly obstructed. Such children often modify their activities to prevent further episodes of wheezing or chest tightness rather than participate fully in normal school and play activities. Rapid assessment of peak expiratory flow in the emergency room is helpful in judging the severity of an acute asthmatic episode and the response to emergency room therapy. Often, subjective sensations change without a signficant increase in expiratory flow rate, giving the false impression of improvement. The decision on whether to admit a child can be aided greatly by the use of a peak flow meter.

Peak expiratory flow measurements can be used at home to give the physician and the parents objective data on which to base therapeutic decisions. Peak flow can be measured daily by parents using an inexpensive peak flow meter. If the child becomes symptomatic the values from symptom-free and symptomatic periods can be compared to judge the severity of the obstructive episode. We often provide parents of problematic asthmatics with guidelines based on changes in peak flow. For example, if pulmonary function is 25 per cent below the child's normal state, the mother is instructed to give an inhalation treatment of a beta agonist drug. If function drops 30 to 40 per cent, she is instructed to call the physician and if more than 50 per cent, to seek medical attention immediately. These instructions vary with the patient, his past history, and distance from our hospital. Use of the peak flow meter can help decide if the child complaining of respiratory symptoms has acute airway obstruction, an upper respiratory illness, or a behavioral cause for his complaints.

Certain patterns of asthma become clear with the use of a home peak flow meter. Measurement of peak flow can discern the pattern of obstruction known as "morning dipping," in which flows drop during the early morning hours, causing the child to awaken with shortness of breath. Flows then rise during the day so that by the time the child is seen, the physician finds no abnormal physical findings. This form of asthma is difficult to diagnose without home pulmonary function monitoring and is peculiarly resistant to therapy.

THERAPY

Chronic Therapy

The goals of therapy in chronic asthma are outlined in Table 63–1. An aggressive approach to treating childhood asthma can be justified from a number of standpoints. Although the cost of treatment at home is sometimes high, if one hospital admission is averted, many health dollars are saved and school absence is decreased.

Although exercise is a trigger of airway obstruction in many asthmatic children, we stress participation in normal daily activities, including unrestricted physical activities, as an important goal. There are now many more ways to treat exercise-induced bronchospasm than there were several years ago. In the child who is unable to tolerate certain forms of exercise despite maximum therapy, a change in the type of activity is sometimes necessary; however, the asthmatic child rarely must live a sedentary life. He should always be encouraged to participate in some form of activity.

The first goal of chronic therapy for asthma is to eliminate acute episodes, especially those that require emergency visits to the hospital or physician's office. To deal with the broad spectrum of severity of asthma in children, we use a graded or staged approach to management as depicted in Table 63–2. Not all patients are

Table 63–1. GOALS OF THERAPY

Prevention of acute asthmatic episodes and school absence
Maximum possible control with minimum medication and treatments
Participation in normal activities including unrestricted physical education and sports
Normalization of pulmonary function tests
Normal growth and social development

Table 63–2. OUTPATIENT THERAPY

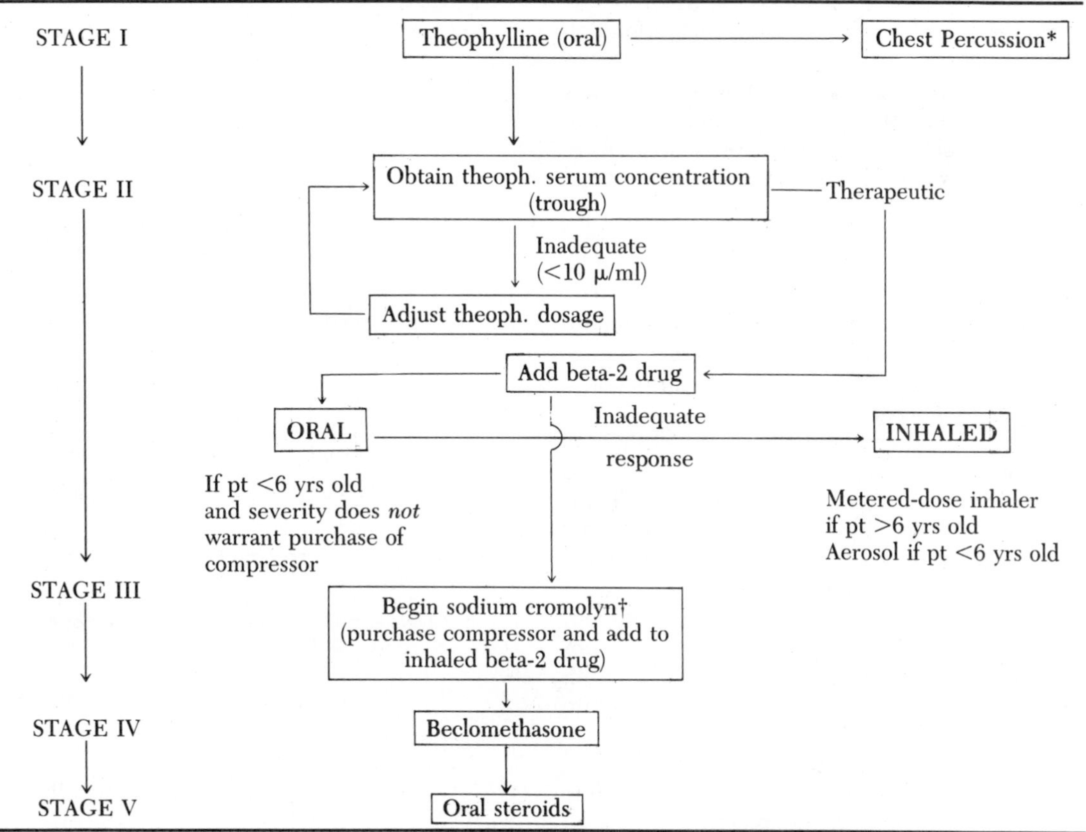

*May be added at any stage if clinical condition warrants.

†We have found the Intal nebulizer solution to be tolerated better than the capsule form.

started at Stage I, but this approach offers an orderly therapeutic guide.

Stage I

Theophylline, the mainstay of asthma therapy in the mildly to moderately affected patient, is used to initiate therapy in the Stage I patient. It is relatively inexpensive, provides good long-term bronchodilation, and has pharmacological properties that are well-known. As a phosphodiesterase inhibitor, theophylline and other methylxanthines retard the destruction of cyclic AMP within the bronchial smooth muscle cell. With increased levels of cyclic AMP, bronchodilation is effected. Other drugs that raise the level of intracellular cyclic AMP, e.g., the beta agonists, can be used additively to theophylline.

There are many theophylline products from which to choose. Within the last eight years it has become apparent that timed-release drugs offer significant advantages over their rapid-release counterparts (Table 63–3). This is especially the case in children aged one to nine years, an age group in which, on the average, the very rapid metabolism of theophylline results in wide fluctuations in serum theophylline concentrations. Timed-release preparations allow for tighter control of the theophylline concentrations and can be given on an eight-hourly or twelve-hourly schedule, thus enhancing compliance. Children on timed- or sustained-release theophylline have fewer symptoms than those on rapid-release drug.

There are now many dosage forms and strengths that make timed-release theophylline useful in all but the youngest patients. The physician should choose several brands whose dosage forms fulfill his requirements and use them singly or in combination to attain the dose required by his patient.

Because of altered absorption, theophylline concentrations during the night-time hours tend to be lower than during the daytime. As this is the period of time during which airway obstruction is often most marked in asthmatic patients, the physician should be cautious as to whom he elects to treat on a 12-hour dosing regimen. Every-12-hour dosing and the attendant improvement in medication compliance is often very useful for the child with mild to moderate asthma.

The patient's age, underlying diseases, and other medications all can affect the theophylline dose requirements. As theophylline is cleared principally (90 per cent) by the liver, hepatic or cardiac disease can markedly reduce theophylline metabolism and necessitate a lower

Table 63–3. ORAL THEOPHYLLINE PREPARATIONS

Sustained Release

Dosage (Anhydrous Theophylline)	*Name*	*Form*
50 mg	TheoDur Sprinkle	Beads[1]
	Somophyllin CRT	Beads
60 mg	Slophyllin GC	Beads
65 mg	TheoSpan SR	Beads
75 mg	TheoDur Sprinkle	Beads
100 mg	TheoDur	Tablet[2]
	Somophyllin CRT	Beads
125 mg	Slophyllin GC	Beads
	TheoDur Sprinkle	Beads
	Others	
130 mg	TheoSpan SR	Beads
200 mg	TheoDur	Tablet[2]
	TheoDur Sprinkle	Beads
250 mg	Slophyllin GC	Beads
	Somophyllin CRT	
	Others	
260 mg	Theospan SR	Beads
300 mg	TheoDur	Tablet[2]
	Quibron-T/SR	Tablet[3]

Rapid Release

Dosage (Anhydrous Theophylline)	*Name*	*Form*
100 mg/5 cc	Elixicon	Liquid
90 mg/5 cc	Somophyllin	Liquid
64 mg/5 cc	Choledyl	Liquid[4]
80 mg/15 cc	Theostat	Liquid
	TheoClear	Liquid
	Elixophyllin	Liquid
86 mg	Aminophylline	Tablet
300 mg	Quibron-T	Tablet[5]

[1]Bead-filled capsules can be opened and given with food if child is unable to swallow capsule. Beads or sustained-release tablets should not be chewed. We do not recommend giving partial doses from bead-filled capsules, as children can be adequately dosed by using appropriate combinations of whole capsules. All are single ingredient products.

[2]TheoDur tablets are scored.

[3]The Quibron-T/SR Dividose tablet is scored so that 100, 150, 200 and 300 mg doses can be obtained from the 300 mg tablet.

[4]Choledyl is oxtriphylline.

[5]The Quibron-T Dividose tablet is scored so that 100, 150, 200 and 300 mg doses can be obtained from the 300 mg tablet.

theophylline dose compared with other children of similar age. Commonly used medications that affect theophylline metabolism are phenobarbital, which by microsomal enzyme induction enhances theophylline clearance, and erythromycin, which reduces theophylline clearance. Thus, the theophylline dose of patients who require treatment with erythromycin may need to be reduced.

Mechanical means of loosening pulmonary secretions have been advocated in children with asthma, although no clinical study of their effectiveness has been done. However, patients in whom hypersecretion of mucus rather than bronchospasm seems to be the more significant component of airway obstruction may benefit from percussion and postural drainage therapy. A trial of postural drainage is indicated, as adverse effects are rarely, if ever, seen. A strict, anatomically sound plan for percussion and postural drainage must be followed. We use the techniques and positions published by the Cystic Fibrosis Foundation, which have been shown to be of proven effectiveness in patients with bronchiectasis.

Stage II

Many patients do well on theophylline, so further therapy is often not required. However, when patients do not respond to theophylline at the calculated dose we move to Stage II. Here we optimize theophylline therapy by measuring serum concentrations, and adjusting the dose accordingly, to obtain a stable concentration between 10 and 20 μg/ml. If the patient does poorly while receiving a dose of theophylline that is documented to maintain therapeutic theophylline concentrations, a beta-adrenergic receptor agonist is added.

Sympathomimetics given by inhalation are more effective than their orally administered counterparts (Table 63–4). Because they are unable to use metered-dose inhalers, children less than about six years of age must be treated with a compressor/nebulizer system if inhaled bronchodilators are to be used. In order to avoid the initial expense of the compressor, it is useful, in these young patients, to start a trial of an oral sympathomimetic, usually metaproterenol. Although oral beta agonists are not available in sustained release forms and should be administered four times a day, we frequently instruct families to administer the oral sympathomimetics every eight hours if that is the theophylline dosing schedule.

A significant advance in the treatment of asthma has been the introduction of safe and effective inhaled sympathomimetics. When used appropriately, metered-dose inhalers are very effective in controlling chronic asthma and in treating the acute episodes of bronchospasm. Three different drugs are available: isoetharine, metaproterenol, and albuterol. Since albuterol has the most specific beta-2 action, it gives the greatest effect with the fewest side effects. The usual dose is two inhalations separated by five minutes and given three to four times a day. The method of inhalation or administration should be demonstrated carefully to the patient and his parents when it is started (Fig. 63–1).

Patients who cannot use a metered-dose inhaler often can be treated effectively with an inhalant solution of a beta-2 drug. We use nebulized metaproterenol with normal saline. The aerosol treatment should last 10 to 15 minutes and be given two to four times daily, depending on the patient's needs. Other sympathomimetics that have a longer duration of action are albuterol and fenoterol, a drug that may soon be available in the United States.

Stage III

If the patient is poorly controlled despite implementation of Stage II therapy, and we are convinced that compliance with the medication schedule is reasonably good, we move on to the use of other drugs. In patients not already receiving them, inhaled beta agonist drugs are

Table 63–4. ADRENERGIC AGENTS FOR INHALATION AND INJECTION

Generic Name	Trade Name	How Supplied*	Onset (min)	Peak (min)	Duration (hr)
Isoproterenol	Isuprel	MDI/Solu	5–15	60	2–3
Isoetharine	Bronkosol	MDI/Solu	5–15	60	3
Metaproterenol	Alupent Metaprel	MDI/Solu	5–30	60	4
Albuterol	Ventolin Proventil	MDI	5–15	60–90	4–6
Fenoterol	Berotec	MDI	5–15		

*MDI = metered-dose inhaler.

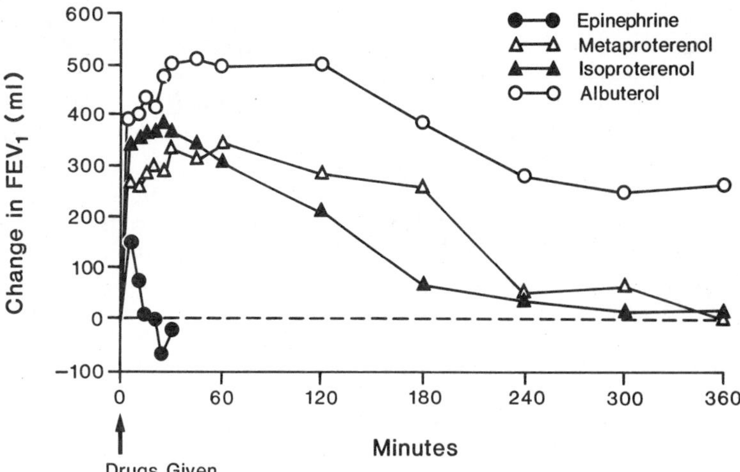

Figure 63–1. This comparison of three commonly used inhaled bronchodilators to epinephrine demonstrates the greater efficacy of the beta-2 specific drugs in increasing flows (FEV_1). The longer duration of action provides a clinical advantage in daily therapy and when used in the emergency room. (Adapted from Riding, W. D., Dinda, P., and Chatterjee, S. S.: The bronchodilator and cardiac effects of five pressure-packed aerosols in asthma. Brit. J. Dis. Chest., *64*:37, 1970.)

instituted. Depending on age, the child is taught to use the compressor and nebulizer or the metered-dose inhaler.

If inhaled drugs by nebulizers have failed to control wheezing in a given patient, we add sodium cromolyn to the drug regimen. For the child who has been using a metered-dose drug, a compressor and nebulizer are prescribed and the dose adjusted. After this is accomplished and sometimes concurrently, we institute therapy with cromolyn sodium. A dose of 20 mg per treatment is used initially. Cromolyn now is available in a 2-cc ampule of liquid containing 20 mg and requires no mixing or dissolving as had been the case with cromolyn powder. Although sodium cromolyn is not a bronchodilator, it does stabilize mast cell membranes, preventing degranulation when the mast cell is stimulated by an allergen. In addition, sodium cromolyn is effective in nonallergic forms of asthma, especially exercise-induced bronchospasm. When it is used in combination with beta-2 agonists, one can continue to give cromolyn in spite of airway obstruction.

Stage IV

At this stage we are dealing with a patient who has failed to respond satisfactorily to maximum bronchodilator therapy and to the addition of a membrane-stabilizing agent such as cromolyn sodium. In this case, we must resort to the use of corticosteroid preparations. In order to minimize systemic side effects from the use of steroids, we begin by using beclomethasone dipropionate (Beclovent, Vanceril). In recommended doses this topically active drug provides corticosteroid action with minimal absorption and without adrenocortical suppression. As with any metered-dose inhaler, proper technique should be emphasized. After administration of the drug, the patient should rinse his mouth with water to remove residual drug, thus reducing the risk of developing monilial infections.

Stage V

Should the inhaled corticosteroids fail, one is forced to use oral steroids. The principle here is to use the minimum dose that will keep the patient wheeze-free and to change to an alternate-day schedule of steroids as soon as possible. It is important to continue the inhaled beclomethasone while using oral corticosteroids. The inhaled drug has a corticosteroid-sparing effect, and one may use a lower dose of oral steroids than would otherwise be possible. The patient should be reassessed frequently in an effort to move from daily to alternate-day corticosteroids and to discontinue oral corticosteroids at the earliest date.

Immunotherapy

The role of immunotherapy ("allergy shots," desensitization) in asthma is not clear as yet. One should consider immunotherapy as one of the potentially helpful modalities in asthma therapy but should weigh its cost, discomfort, dangers, and modest degree of proven efficacy with that of drug therapy.

The response to immunotherapy depends on the disease being treated, the correct identification of specific allergens and their presence in the extract, the total dose given to the patient, and the ability of the antigen to induce antibody response. One cannot extrapolate from the proven efficacy of immunotherapy in hay fever to that in asthma, nor should it be assumed that because one allergen is effective other antigens will be. Since skin test reactivity to given antigens does not correlate directly with bronchial reactivity, there is a problem in selecting which antigens to use during immunotherapy. Aas (1971) has been able to reduce symptoms of house dust–sensitive children but only after 2½ to 3 years of treatment with house dust extract. Immunotherapy may be helpful in selected children as part of an overall program of management.

Treatment of the Acute Attack

Although a better understanding of the pathophysiology of asthma and improved medication have led to better control of its symptoms, every physician who cares for children must still deal with the child who has an acute asthma attack. Acute episodes of wheezing should not be viewed as an unavoidable part of asthma but as a failure of the basic treatment program. A child with frequent wheezing should have adjustments made to daily therapy so that these are avoided. Early recognition and prompt, appropriate treatment of the wheezing child will not only decrease severity and duration of acute asthma but may also be life-saving.

When a patient arrives at the office or the emergency room with an acute obstructive asthma episode, a quick evaluation must be done prior to treatment (Table 63–5). The most important things to evaluate are (1) air entry on auscultation and (2) the degree of respiratory distress as manifested by the use of the accessory muscles of inspiration and retractions in the intercostal and supraclavicular spaces. Severe respiratory distress with poor air entry and few wheezes is an ominous sign. In the mildly or moderately ill patient, measurement of peak expiratory flow rate is helpful in judging the extent of airway obstruction, especially if previous test data are available. A theophylline blood concentration, even if the results are not immediately available, can be helpful in guiding therapy if the patient needs to be hospitalized and acts as an assessment of patient compliance and the adequacy of the theophylline dosage that has been prescribed. A chest radiograph for signs of pulmonary infection, atelectasis, or extrapulmonary air should also be obtained.

Hypoxemia is the first problem to treat during an asthma attack. One fourth of all patients will be hypoxemic even when asymptomatic. All wheezing patients should be assumed to be hypoxemic. Hypoxemia may cause pulmonary

Table 63–5. TREATMENT OF ACUTE ASTHMA

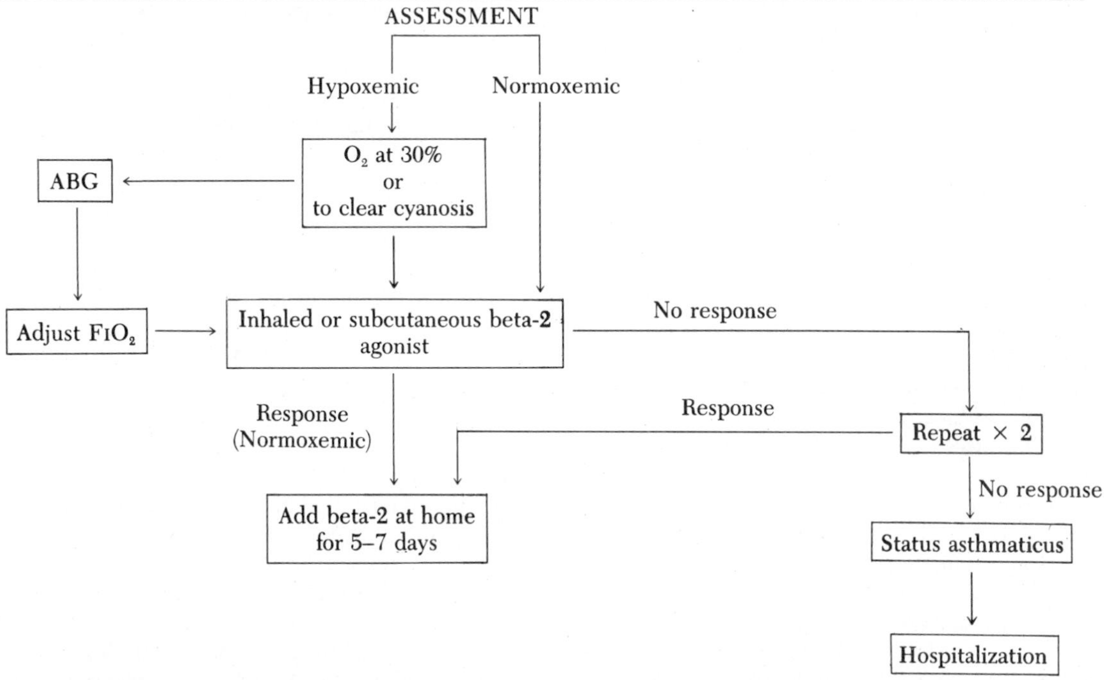

ASSESSMENT

Hypoxemic → O_2 at 30% or to clear cyanosis → ABG → Adjust FIO_2 → Inhaled or subcutaneous beta-2 agonist

Normoxemic → Inhaled or subcutaneous beta-2 agonist

Inhaled or subcutaneous beta-2 agonist → Response (Normoxemic) → Add beta-2 at home for 5–7 days

Inhaled or subcutaneous beta-2 agonist → No response → Repeat × 2

Repeat × 2 → Response → Add beta-2 at home for 5–7 days

Repeat × 2 → No response → Status asthmaticus → Hospitalization

Table 63–6. DRUGS USED TO TREAT ACUTE ASTHMA IN CHILDREN

Drug	Route	Dose	Max. Dose*	May Repeat
Metaproterenol†, ‡	Aerosol	0.01 ml/kg (mouthpiece) 0.02 ml/kg (mask)	0.30 ml	q 20 min × 2
Isoetharine†	Aerosol	0.01 ml/kg (mouthpiece) 0.02 ml/kg (mask)	0.30 ml	q 20 min × 2
Terbutaline‡	Subcutaneous	0.01 ml/kg	0.25 ml	q 20 min × 2
Epinephrine HCl (1:1000)	Subcutaneous	0.01 ml/kg	0.30 ml	q 20 min × 2
Epinehrine susp. (1:200)	Subcutaneous	0.005 ml/kg	0.15 ml	None

*Maximum recommended dose should not be exceeded until patient demonstrates tolerance of this dose without toxic side effects.

†Aerosol medications diluted with 1.0 to 2.5 ml normal saline. Treatment should last 10 to 15 minutes.

‡FDA recommended for children to 12 years and older.

hypertension, increased airway resistance, altered cerebral function, and decreased cardiac contractility. Initiation of oxygen therapy should not be withheld until cyanosis, a late sign of hypoxemia, is evident. To prevent drying of the airway, which may potentiate wheezing, oxygen should be humidified (have water vapor added to it), but one should not give water in the form of mist (particulate water). While injectable medications have been the stand-by for acute treatment in the past, the development of newer sympathomimetic agents has enabled us to treat patients with more precision by using inhaled drugs in the treatment of the acute attack. The newer drugs offer a considerable advantage over the injectable ones in that they provide greater bronchodilation for a longer time with fewer side effects.

The beta-2 agonists provide the most rapid bronchodilation for the acute asthma attack and should be the primary pharmacological agents in the emergency room. A summary of these agents and recommended doses are presented in Table 63–6.

Sympathomimetics are most effective when they are administered by aerosol. The time-honored approach of giving up to three subcutaneous injections of aqueous epinephrine at 20-minute intervals until there is a good response is no longer optimal treatment. More specific beta-2 agents are now available and may be used safely and with fewer potential side effects in children.

Nebulized metaproterenol may be given and repeated in 20 to 30 minutes if the patient's response is inadequate and the heart rate is less than 180 beats per minute. The long-term efficacy of metaproterenol and its safety have been well-documented in clinical studies and years of clinical experience in Europe and Canada. Alternatively, isoetharine inhalation solution may be given; however, this agent is less beta-2 specific and has a shorter duration of action. The approximate dose of aerosol can be calculated on the basis of the patient's weight and the method of aerosol delivery. Compressor-generated aerosol administered with a mouthpiece delivers roughly twice the total dose of medication to the lower airway as with a mask. A mask must be employed for the infant and toddler and the older child who is too ill to use a mouthpiece.

Aerosol beta-2 drugs should be delivered by air compressor–driven continuous-flow nebulizers. Administration of aerosol medication by continuous nebulization air is as effective as with intermittent positive pressure breathing (IPPB), less patient cooperation is required, and potential side effects of positive pressure administration are avoided.

Inhaled albuterol and metaproterenol are safe even at high doses. In one study of side effects, these drugs caused no significant change in heart rate, blood pressure, electrocardiogram, or arterial oxygen tension. Higher-than-recommended doses of these drugs were, however, no more effective in increasing FEV_1 than recommended doses. The dose may be repeated in 20 to 30 minutes if the initial response is unsatisfactory.

It is rare to encounter a patient who is "too tight" to benefit from inhaled bronchodilators; however, in such a case terbutaline by injection may be given followed by inhaled drugs. Most such patients, however, will need to be admitted to the hospital.

When an injectable drug is needed, one may choose from aqueous epinephrine, Sus-Phrine, or terbutaline. In general, terbutaline has a more specific beta agonist but loses a degree of its specificity when given by injection. Studies comparing equal doses of epinephrine and terbutaline showed similar increase in heart rate; however, it has been our experience that terbutaline provides more bronchodilation for a given increase in heart rate than does epinephrine and is tolerated better.

Repeated examination of the patient is the best way to assess his response to therapy. Peak expiratory flow measurement provides an objective measure of the patient's response to the bronchodilator medication. In addition, the response of the patient's PEFR to a bronchodilator allows the physician to predict more accurately whether the patient is likely to require admission.

The patient may have a good response to the above measures with clearing of wheezing and significant increase of PEFR. However, beta-2 agents act only to reduce bronchoconstriction and have no significant acute effect on airway edema, which complicates wheezing attacks of more than a few hours' duration. Pulmonary function abnormalities may persist for weeks after the episode of acute asthma. Thus, after release from the office or emergency room, the patient should continue a beta-2 agent and/or theophylline for at least one to two weeks after an acute episode. If the child has an inadequate response to therapy in the emergency room, he has status asthmaticus and should be admitted to the hospital.

Allergic Rhinitis

Howard Eigen, M.D.

As the chief point of entry to the respiratory tract, the nasal passages are exposed to a wide range of allergens, irritants, and infectious agents. The nasal turbinates function to increase the surface area of the nasal mucosa, to add moisture to the inspired air, and to filter foreign material. Normal nasal secretions are carried posteriorly by the cilia and swallowed automatically. The symptoms of allergic rhinitis are chiefly caused by histamine release from sensitized mast cells when an IgE-mediated reaction occurs. Reflex nasal engorgement may also play a role.

It is often difficult to establish whether the etiology of rhinitis is infectious or noninfectious. Parents often complain that a child has a "cold" (coryza) or has repeated "colds," although the absence of associated constitutional symptoms, e.g., fever, malaise, myalgia, or runny nose, makes an infection unlikely. Compared with allergic rhinitis, infectious rhinitis is more often associated with a cough, especially in the daytime. Regardless of the etiology, the nasal drainage may appear purulent owing to the presence of eosinophils in allergic and neutrophils in infectious rhinitis. A child with a constantly runny nose without constitutional symptoms is likely to have noninfectious rhinitis, i.e., allergic rhinitis, perennial vasomotor rhinitis, or nonallergic rhinitis.

Allergic rhinitis, with congestion of the mucous membranes induced by allergens and mediated by IgE antibodies, is typically characterized by periodic (seasonal) or continuous sneezing, watery rhinorrhea, itching, and nasal obstruction. Vasomotor rhinitis is due to an over-responsiveness of nasal tissues to change in such physical factors as temperature, noxious odors, and, occasionally, position of the head. These patients usually do not have a history of specific allergic disease. Nasal obstruction is a more significant portion of the symptom complex than rhinorrhea. Because it is not IgE-mediated, immunotherapy is not useful. Unfortunately, drug therapy rarely provides symptomatic relief. Nonallergic rhinitis simulates allergic rhinitis in that the nasal mucous membranes are often pale and eosinophilia is present; however, this disorder is not associated with a specific immunological characterization. Although immunotherapy is not recommended in these patients, the symptoms often respond to steroids or antihistamines.

ETIOLOGY

Allergic rhinitis occurs in atopic children who are exposed to specific, usually inhalant, allergens to which they have been sensitized. Seasonal symptoms are usually related to airborne pollens: tree pollens in the spring, grasses in early summer, and weeds in late summer and early fall. Perennial symptoms are more likely if the child is also sensitized to molds and house dust. Molds are present as inhalant antigens for the entire summer, whereas house dust, presumably the house dust mite, spread through the heating system, is a source of antigen during the winter. Although a seasonal pattern may be superimposed on a perennial problem, there is insufficient time between seasons for the nasal mucosa to recover fully; therefore, the child suffers year-round rhinitis, exacerbated when seasonal allergens are prevalent.

PHYSICAL EXAMINATION

Children with allergic rhinitis often have behaviors that attempt to relieve itching or to clear nasal secretions. The allergic salute, in which the patient pushes his nose upward with the palm of his hand to relieve airway obstruction and itching, is a common habit. The frequent use of the allergic salute to relieve symptoms induces a transverse nasal crease across the bridge of the nose of children with persistent symptoms. Nose wrinkling or twitching and mouth wrinkling are other attempts to relieve nasal itching. Allergic shiners, characterized by a dark discoloration of the lower orbitopalpebral groove, are often associated with edema of the same area leading to bags under the eyes. Swelling of the nasal mucous membranes interferes with venous drainage of the suborbital venous arcades, leading to venous stasis and discoloration of the lower orbital skin. The conjunctivae are often injected, and Dennie's lines may be seen radiating from the inner corner of the eye along the lower orbitopalpebral groove. Examination of the nose often reveals swollen, light-blue turbinates covered by clear mucus. In children with perennial symptoms, this bluish color is lost and the nasal mucosa becomes red and swollen. The mucosa of the nasal floor may heap up, giving rise to the illusion of another turbinate along the floor of the nose (the "fourth turbinate" sign). Hypertrophic lymphoid follicles on the posterior pharynx (cobblestoning) and geographic tongue may also be noted. The classic allergic gape, the result of constant mouth breathing, may be a prominent facial feature.

EVALUATION

With a clinical picture of seasonal symptoms of rhinorrhea, congestion, and nasal itching, especially with a positive family history, the diagnosis of allergic rhinitis can be made clinically. When symptoms are not classic or seasonal, laboratory studies may be necessary.

Seventy to 80 per cent of patients with allergic rhinitis have nasal eosinophilia. Positive reactions may be demonstrated to specific antigens given intradermally or by scratch test. Although radioallergosorbent immunoassay (RAST) will identify antigen-specific IgE antibodies in the serum, it is more expensive and, by some reports, less sensitive than skin testing. Total IgE serum concentrations of less than 20 I.U./ml makes allergy highly unlikely. Many patients have both asthma and rhinitis. Hay fever sufferers have a higher than normal incidence of bronchial reactivity even if they have not wheezed. Nasal polyps are uncommon in allergic rhinitis.

TREATMENT

Unfortunately, it is rare for a child with allergic rhinitis to be sensitive to a single antigen, such as cat dander, the source of which can be removed from his environment. Most are sensitive to multiple inhaled allergens, including those, such as pollens, that cannot be avoided. House dust precautions and the use of electronic precipitators or special high-efficiency filters reduce the allergen load but are unlikely, in themselves, to relieve the symptoms.

A logical first therapeutic step is to prescribe an antihistamine preparation that inhibits H_1 receptors. Oral antihistamines are well absorbed and begin to act within 15 to 30 minutes. A list of the major classes of antihistamines and their dosage is included in Table 63–7. Side effects, especially in young children, include excitation and irritability. Oversedation may occur in older children, as may excessively dry mouth or inspissated secretions. Combination products are not necessary for the treatment of allergic rhinitis, but they may, at times, provide more relief than an antihistamine alone. In addition to an antihistamine, many preparations include an alpha-adrenergic sympathomimetic drug that shrinks nasal mucosal membranes by causing constriction of arterioles in the nasal plexus. Some decongestants, such as ephedrine and pseudoephedrine, also cause stimulation of beta receptors, leading in time to vasodilation and rebound congestion. Although phenylpropanolamine has direct and indirect alpha effects, it does not have as much rebound potential. Other products contain methoscopolamine, whose atropine-like effect aids in further drying of secretions. Hyperactivity is the most common side effect of decongestants in children.

Over time larger doses of antihistamines used

Table 63–7. ANTIHISTAMINE CLASSIFICATIONS

Class (Nonproprietary Name)	Trade Name	Dosage	
		Adult	*Child*
Ethanolamines			
Diphenhydramine hydrochloride	Benadryl	25-50 mg 3-4×/d*	5 mg/kg/day 3-4 divided doses
Alkylamines			
Triprolidine hydrochloride	Actidil	2.5 mg 2-3 ×/d	< 2 yr—0.6 mg 2-3×/d > 2 yr—1.25 mg 2-3×/d
Chlorpheniramine maleate	Chlor-Trimeton;	4 mg 3-4×/d	0.4 mg/kg/day 3-4 divided doses
	CTM (delayed action); Histadur; Rhinihist	8-12 mg 2×/d	
Brompheniramine maleate	Dimetane	4 mg 3-4×/d	0.4 mg/kg/day 3-4 divided doses
	Dimetane (delayed action) Extentabs	12 mg 2×/d	
Piperazines			
Hydroxyzine	Atarax; Vistaril	25-100 mg 3-4×/d	2 mg/kg/day 4 divided doses
Phenothiazines			
Promethazine hydrochloride	Phenergan	12.5 mg 2-3×/d	1 mg/kg/24 hr
Trimeprazine tartrate	Temaril	2.5 mg 4×/d	3 yr only—2.5 mg 3×/d 6 mo-3 yr—2.5 mg 3×/d
Azatadine maleate	Optimine	1-2 mg 2×/d	No recommendation
Clemastine fumarate	Tavist	2.68 mg 2×/d	No recommendation

*×/d = times daily

alone or combined with a decongestant may be required to achieve the desired effect. This may be avoided by changing to an antihistamine from a different chemical class when symptoms reappear. Some clinicians recommend that antihistamines be routinely rotated on a 2 to 4 week schedule, taking care that the change is not between two brand names with essentially the same formulation. In chronically symptomatic children, giving the antihistamine and decongestant separately rather than as a fixed combination permits rotation of the antihistamine without changing the decongestant as well as a more precise adjustment of dosage.

The use of antihistamines in asthmatic children is not contraindicated as once thought. Relief of nasal symptoms may result in less mouth breathing and postnasal drip, both of which may exacerbate asthma through stimulation of upper airway receptors.

When specific allergens can be identified by skin testing, immunotherapy may be appropriate for children with severe allergic rhinitis. Careful skin testing to corroborate a history of seasonal symptoms provides a basis on which to prepare an extract. Pollen-induced allergic rhinitis is more amenable than that from dust and animal dander. Usually, it is necessary to prescribe an antihistamine for symptomatic relief during the early phase of immunotherapy.

Sodium cromolyn (Nasalcrom), used as a 4 per cent solution by nasal instillation, either as a spray or as drops, is also effective in controlling allergic rhinitis. Preschool children rarely tolerate nasal spray, and cromolyn requires consistent use in order to maintain its effectiveness. Glucocorticoids, especially beclomethasone, can be used by nasal spray to treat allergic rhinitis. Although not tolerated by preschool children, these agents may be effective in the older child with severe allergic rhinitis. Systemic steroids for allergic rhinitis are contraindicated. Vasoconstricting nasal sprays should not be used in the treatment of chronic rhinitis because of their rebound effect. Rhinitis medicamentosa or chronic rebound congestion can occur with overuse of such nose drops. If they are to be employed for short periods of time, it is helpful to use them unilaterally so as to leave one nostril free of rebound. The use of vasoactive sprays should be limited to five days.

REFERENCES

Aas, K.: Hyposensitization in housedust allergy asthma. Acta Paediatr. Scand., *60*:264, 1971.

Bell, T., and Bigley, J.: Sustained release theophylline therapy for chronic childhood asthma. Pediatrics, *62*:352, 1978.

Ben-Zvi, Z., Lam, C., Hollman, J., et al.: An evaluation of the initial treatment of acute asthma. Pediatrics, *70*:348, 1982.

Commey, J. O., and Levison, H.: Physical signs in childhood asthma. Pediatrics, *58*:537, 1976.

Corrao, W. M., Braman, S. S., and Irwin, R. S.: Chronic cough as the sole presenting manifestation of bronchial asthma. N. Engl. J. Med., *300*:634, 1979.

Eigen, H., Laughlin, J. J., and Homrighausen, J.: Recurrent pneumonia in children and its relationship to bronchial hyperreactivity. Pediatrics, *70*:698, 1982.

Gurwitz, D., Mindorff, C., and Levison, H.: Increased incidence of bronchial reactivity in children with a history of bronchiolitis. J. Pediatr., *98*:551, 1981.

Minor, T. E., Dick, E. C., DeMeo, A. N., et al.: Viruses as precipitants of asthmatic attacks in children. J.A.M.A., *227*:292, 1974.

Norman, P. S.: An overview of immunotherapy: Implications for the future. J. Allergy Clin. Immunol., *65*:87, 1980.

Permutt S: Physiologic changes in the acute asthmatic attack. *In* Austen, K. F., and Lichtenstein, L. M. (Eds.): Asthma. New York, Academic Press, 1972.

Rooney, J. C., and Williams, H. E.: The relationship between proved viral bronchiolitis and subsequent wheezing. J. Pediatr., *79*:744, 1971.

Snyder, R. D., Collipp, P. J., and Greene, J. S.: Growth and ultimate height of children with asthma. Clin. Pediatr., *6*:389, 1967.

Tabachnik, E., Scott, P., Correia, J., et al.: Sustained-release theophylline: A significant advance in the treatment of childhood asthma. J. Pediatr., *100*:489, 1982.

Turner-Warwick, M.: On observing patterns of air flow obstruction in chronic asthma. Br. J. Dis. Chest, *71*:73, 1977.

64

DIABETES MELLITUS

William B. Weil, Jr., M.D., Michael L. Netzloff, M.D., Patricia J. Salisbury, R.N., M.S.N., Robert J. Shaffer, M.A., and Bruce E. Wilson, M.D.

Definition and Frequency

The term *diabetes mellitus* describes a group of conditions characterized by carbohydrate intolerance with hyperglycemia and glycosuria. Formerly, the major divisions of diabetes mellitus were "juvenile onset type" and "adult onset type." These terms have been replaced by Types I and II or the terms "insulin dependent diabetes mellitus" (IDDM) and "noninsulin dependent diabetes mellitus" (NIDDM), respectively, since, while each predominates in its age group as signified by the old terms, there is some overlap.

The hallmark of Type I or insulin dependent diabetes is inadequate insulin production, either absolute or relative to the glucose present. The incidence of insulin dependent diabetes approximates 1 in 600 school age children and is less than that in preschool children. Despite the frequency of IDDM, its etiology remains unclear.

Etiology

Data would seem to indicate either that IDDM is a process requiring a multifactorial sequence for clinical expression or that several different disease processes may all result in the symptom complex we now term insulin dependent diabetes mellitus. Genetically, an increased risk (two- to fourfold) has been seen with HLA haplotypes B8, Dw3, and Dw4. Other genetic patterns not related to the HLA locus have been suggested, but clear documentation of any given modes of inheritance has not been established. Virological studies have implicated several viruses which attack the pancreas during the course of other clinical diseases. In at least one case, successful transplant of a virus located in the islet cells of a boy with diabetes resulted in the development of diabetes in several laboratory mice. The association of IDDM with several known autoimmune processes, such as Hashimoto's thyroiditis and

Addison's disease, as well as the presence of islet cell antibodies and the recent reports associating IDDM with juvenile rheumatoid arthritis, have suggested an autoimmune etiology.

Natural History

In a majority of individuals with IDDM, there is a common pattern to their clinical course. At present, most children are identified by the presence of glucose in their urine after presenting to their primary care provider with a history involving the classic triad of polyuria, polydipsia, and polyphagia. Typically, children appear to undergo a gradual onset of glucose intolerance with increasing symptoms. Eventually there is a relatively rapid change to ketoacidosis unless treatment has been undertaken.

When started on insulin, the children usually show an initial requirement of approximately 0.75 to 1.25 units per kilogram per day. In a period of a few weeks, this requirement will decrease rapidly to less than 0.5 u/kg/day, even reaching zero in some patients. The ensuing period, usually referred to as the "honeymoon period," may last from several weeks to many months, with six months being the modal period. During this stage, hypoglycemic reactions and significant hyperglycemia are uncommon, as the child's own pancreas is producing insulin in response to appropriate stimuli, but in an inadequate amount.

After this relatively stable period, there is a gradual rise in the daily insulin requirement. Some months after the end of the honeymoon period, the amount of insulin required will approximate 1 u/kg/day. Gradual increases in the total daily dose are thereafter dictated by the child's rate of growth, until early adolescence when there may be another increase in insulin, to as high as 1.5 units/kg/day. In late adolescence, the dosage again stabilizes as the growth velocity falls. This final dosage (again about 1 u/kg/day) varies little through the transition to adulthood.

The major problem for most individuals with diabetes is the risk of complications. These complications can be divided into (1) acute, (2) subacute, and (3) chronic. The acute complications of ketoacidosis and hypoglycemia are those that the primary care provider sees most frequently. Diabetic ketoacidosis (DKA) is the result of a relative lack of insulin activity either because too little was given or because the metabolic need increased rapidly.

Hypoglycemia is the result of a relative excess of insulin activity because of overdosage or reduced need, secondary to increased physical activity or decreased food intake. Its onset is usually acute and often correlates with the time of peak insulin activity. The degree of hypoglycemia is variable, ranging from mild sympathomimetic symptoms to coma with seizures. In cases where oral carbohydrate is not tolerated and there is no venous access, intramuscular glucagon (1 mg) can be utilized for treatment.

The primary subacute complication of IDDM is lipodystrophy of the areas where injections are given. Repeated injection into the same area results in sequestering of insulin in the tissues with resultant hypertrophy, hypoesthesia, and poor insulin absorption. Control of glucose metabolism is often erratic as a consequence. Lipodystrophy may also result from poor injection site rotation. Although time and avoiding the areas as injection sites will resolve lipodystrophy, the process may take one to two years. Lipodystrophy has also been treated by injection of the highly purified insulins directly into the atrophied areas. This has not been highly successful in resolving the process. Currently, children with significant lipodystrophy are placed on the more highly purified insulins (e.g., pork insulin) and the nonlipodystrophic sites are utilized.

It is the chronic complications that the patients and their parents often find the most anxiety provoking. These include peripheral neuropathy, renal disease, and retinopathy. It is important to realize that these are manifestations of microvascular disease. Large vessel disease (e.g., atherosclerosis) is not associated with IDDM in the early decades of life. The course of the chronic complications can be highly varied and we recommend referral to the appropriate subspecialist (nephrologist, ophthalmologist, etc.) with the primary care provider continuing to coordinate the various aspects of the patient's management.

The association between all or any of the long-term complications of IDDM and either the wide fluctuations of blood glucose levels characteristic of IDDM, or an underlying unknown defect associated with the insulin deficiency itself, is controversial. There is evidence to support a primary role for metabolic derangements in the development of microvascular complications, as well as data to support a primary role for genetic factors. Most likely, the microvascular disease, as with insulin dependent diabetes in general, represents a heterogeneous group of disorders, evolving from multifactorial etiologies. It is important to note that not all patients develop long-term complications. Studies have shown that up to 20 per cent of patients have escaped microvascular disease after 25- to 40-year follow-ups.

Philosophy of Care

A management plan for the child with diabetes mellitus is determined by that which we know, based upon substantiated data, and that which we believe, based to a large extent on hypothesis, inference, ambiguous data, and personal values. Because there is more information that we are unsure about than what is established fact, it is helpful to consider first the personal aspects of care and thus establish a value-based framework into which the agreed-upon data can be placed.

Currently, care for a child with diabetes typically begins in an office, clinic, or emergency room and is quickly moved to a hospital setting. Instances in which the initial hospitalization is avoided are increasing and could become the dominant approach in the foreseeable future. As children developing diabetes are more often being recognized prior to the development of ketoacidosis, the major reason for hospital care in most situations is to provide time to orient the child and family to the illness and to the technical aspects of treatment. If one is fortunate enought to have the time and resources to accomplish such orientation in an ambulatory setting, the only child that should require hospitalization would be the one with DKA. The plan presented in this chapter anticipates reduced inpatient care by recommending a minimum of educational tasks to be carried out in the hospital: enough to get the child home and able to be given insulin, to have urine tested, and to have rudimentary understanding of the interaction between insulin, food, exercise, and emotional stress. The remaining educational tasks can then be accomplished in an ambulatory setting. It is recognized that if an ambulatory educational program is not feasible, a more prolonged hospital stay will be required to accomplish the instructional program.

The extent to which one utilizes the hospital in the initial care falls in the realm of personal beliefs, as we have no data on the efficacy of long hospital stays, brief hospital stays, or no hospitalization on the long-term outcome of the disease process. Therefore, our use of a brief hospital period is based on value judgments regarding the negative impact of inpatient experiences on the child and family when contrasted with the positive impact of reducing anxiety by establishing the treatment program in a controlled hospital environment. A family that is experienced in caring for a child with diabetes will have a lesser need for hospital care of a second child with diabetes than will a family with little medical knowledge and high levels of anxiety. It is also appropriate to recognize that there are economic and other social factors involved in the decision regarding hospital admission.

One major ideological controversy that has dominated the management of insulin dependent diabetes mellitus for several decades involves the degree of control of blood sugar that one attempts to obtain. In general, most physicians would prefer total normalization of blood sugar if this were reasonably possible. As will be described later, it may be possible to approach this goal quite closely in a few selected patients by using multiple injections of regular insulin or with an "open loop" pump system. In the future such an achievement may be obtainable in more patients with the use of "closed loop" insulin pumps or transplanted islet cells. However, currently one must still weigh the emotional cost of increasingly rigorous measures to improve blood sugar control against the potential benefits that might accrue from such measures in both short- and long-term physical health. The problem can be stated functionally: if it is not possible to obtain completely normal blood sugars, how useful is it to increase the number of insulin injections, obtain more frequent measures of urinary and blood glucose, prescribe more restrictive diets, and suggest greater regularity of exercise and other life events with the hope that these will improve the child's general health, decrease the prevalence of complications, and delay the onset of those complications which do occur?

A further question is which of the above measures will be most effective in achieving the desired outcome and which will be counterproductive because they generate negative behaviors in the patient and/or the family. If one prescribes procedures that the patient and the family find excessively onerous, one may find less compliance than if one were to adopt a more moderate approach. An example of this situation is in the use of carefully calculated and prescribed diets. In our experience, many children will experience less stable blood sugars on a prescribed diet than on one that is self-selected from a somewhat limited food list. This response pattern may occur for several reasons: the family may be unable to maintain the restricted regimen with the result that the child will experience increasingly frequent dietary excesses. Since emotional tension, operating through insulin counter-regulatory hormones, may be the most important determinant of glucose homeostasis, the conflict between the child and family generated around the diet may increase to the point that the emotional state of the child creates wider fluctuations in glucose levels than would occur with a more moderate dietary plan. Additionally, the child's daily energy requirements may vary widely, and if the daily food intake is relatively fixed, the child may experience alternating episodes of hypo- and hyperglycemia.

In summary, it should be recognized that management of the child with diabetes involves both personal value judgments of the physician and family and the application of established biochemical, physiological, and behavioral data. The extent of hospitalization, the type of diet plan, the measures used to assess glucose metabolism, the selection of insulin mixtures, and the frequency of daily injections are issues that reflect this dualism in development of a management plan.

INSULIN

Insulin is the most important part of the management of the child with IDDM. The products currently produced are vastly different from the first available in the 1920s. Three basic types of insulin are now produced. Short acting insulins peak approximately 2 hours after injection and have a duration of 4 to 6 hours. Intermediate acting insulins peak in approximately 8 hours and last 16 to 32 hours. Long acting insulins peak in approximately 18 hours and last up to 48 hours. The risk of night-time hypoglycemia is severe when long acting insulin is taken in the morning, and therefore such insulin is seldom used in children. These three types of insulin are sold under a variety of brand names (see Table 64–1).

Table 64–1. INSULIN TYPES

Short Acting	Intermediate Acting	Long Acting
Regular (B/P, B, P)	Lente (B/P, B, P)	PZI (B/P)
SemiLente (B/P)	NPH (B/P, B, P)	Ultralente (B/P)
Actrapid (P)	Lentard (B/P)	Ultratard (B)
	Monotard (P)	

B/P = Beef-pork combination
B = Pure beef
P = Pure pork

Until 1973 all insulins came in two concentrations, U-40 and U-80. Because this led to many measurement errors, a third concentration, U-100, was introduced to replace U-40 and U-80. The pharmacist may dilute U-100 insulin into other concentrations for the patient who is taking extremely small amounts of insulin. U-10 insulin works well with infants and children taking less than five units per day.

The method used to produce U-100 insulin resulted in a product that was significantly purer than the older insulins. Several European companies further refined the technique for removing proinsulin and insulin-like substances from their products to produce an insulin that is 99.99 per cent pure, so-called monocomponent insulin. In 1979 Eli Lilly began marketing a product to replace their U-100 insulins. This insulin, marketed as Improved Single Peak insulin, is more purified than the previous U-100 insulin but less purified than monocomponent insulin. At the same time, monocomponent insulin was approved for sale in the United States. Lilly, Novo, and Nordisk now market monocomponent insulins in the United States.

The majority of insulin produced is a combination of beef and pork insulin. Although pork insulin is closer to human insulin structurally, not enough pigs are slaughtered to produce pure pork insulin exclusively. Pure beef insulin is also produced for those individuals who are allergic to pork or who will not use pork insulin for religious reasons. Currently all pure pork or pure beef insulins from Lilly are monocomponent. All insulins produced in Europe are monocomponent; however, some are pure pork, some pure beef, and some beef-pork mixture (see Table 64–1).

Monocomponent insulins are used primarily for individuals with lipodystrophy unrelated to injection technique. It may also be of some use to the individual with local cutaneous reactions to insulin injections. The cost of monocomponent insulin makes it less desirable for general use.

The insulins currently available are stable at room temperature and do not need to be refrigerated. Insulin may be inactivated if allowed to freeze or reach extremely high temperatures such as in a closed car.

A variety of sites may be used in any age individual: posterior aspect of the arms; the deltoid region; abdomen; the upper outer quadrant of the buttocks; the anterior, lateral, and posterior thigh; the calf; and the upper back.

Most newly diagnosed patients are discharged from the hospital on a mixture of regular and lente insulins in a ratio of 1 u regular to 3 u lente with a total dose of 0.75 to 1.25 kg/day. Lente has the advantage over NPH of staying suspended longer. If NPH is not adequately mixed each time it is used, it becomes more and more concentrated as the bottle is emptied. Patients may also encounter problems if alcohol from a wet alcohol swab is allowed to pool on the top of the insulin bottle. Small amounts of alcohol may mix with and denature the insulin.

When using two injections of insulin a day, the total dose will be about the same as on one injection per day. The schedule is begun using a ratio of approximately 4 units of lente with 2 units of regular before breakfast and 2 units of lente and 1 of regular before supper.

EXAMPLE

A 12-year-old girl, weighing 40 kg, with diabetes for four years, is on a single injection of 30 units of lente and 10 units of regular before breakfast. She is having occasional reactions in the mid-afternoon, but her urine is 5 per cent glucose in the morning. On two injections per day, she would take 16 units of lente and 8 units of regular before breakfast and 8 units of lente and 4 units of regular before supper (total = 36 units). This is slightly less than her previous dosage but may be sufficient because of better distribution. However, a 24-hour urine glucose divided into three 8-hour collections would be helpful in determining if she were having excessive glucosuria. If a 24-hour urine contained more than 25 grams of glucose (100 kCal or 5 per cent of her estimated caloric intake), then the insulin that should be increased would be based on the distribution of glucosuria in the three 8-hour specimens.

URINE TESTING

Urine testing remains the most frequently used method of assessing diabetes control. The day-to-day test results are used to reflect trends in control, i.e., generally high tests or generally low tests. Test-to-test fluctuations may be the result of fluctuations in blood glucose but may also reflect changes in hydration and urine concentration. Test results may also be influenced by other medications being taken (Table 64–2).

A variety of different products are available for testing urinary glucose and ketones. Because of inconsistencies between products when reporting results by pluses, all products for testing glucose are now reported in percentages. The American Diabetes Association recommends the 2-Drop Clinitest Method for testing glucose because of its ability to pick up levels of glucose as high as 5 per cent or above. Its major disadvantage is that it requires a certain amount of time and equipment to perform the test, making compliance more difficult. Another product frequently used is Keto-Diastix. Although this is a simple dipstick method, it has several disadvantages. The Keto-Diastix's highest reading is 2 per cent or above, which does not allow for differentiation among 2, 3, and 5 per cent. It is also a poor choice for the ketosis-prone child, as the presence of ketones depresses the glucose reaction, leading to falsely low readings. Both Acetest tablets and Ketostix are available for testing urinary ketone levels. At the time of diagnosis both the child and his family are taught urine testing using the 2-Drop Clinitest Method and Acetest tablets.

While in the hospital the child may be asked to check second-voided specimens four times a day. However, at home a first-voided specimen twice a day (before breakfast and before supper) will generally give adequate information. The first-voided specimen gives a better indication of control over a longer period of time, whereas the second-voided specimen more closely reflects the blood sugar at the time of collection.

Table 64–2. EFFECTS OF VARIOUS AGENTS ON URINE TESTS IN DIABETES

	Testing Material			
	Ketodiastix		*Clinitest*	*Acetest*
Substances	*Test for Glucose*	*Test for Ketones*	*Tablets*	*Tablets*
Cephalosporins	0	0	False pos.	0
Nalidixic acid	0	0	False pos.	0
Probenecid	0	0	False pos.	0
L-Dopa	False neg.	False pos.	0	False pos.
Ascorbic acid	Falsely low	0	False pos.	0
Aspirin	0	0	0	False pos.
Bromsulfophthalein	0	False pos.	0	False pos.
Urinary ketones	Falsely low	True pos.	0	True pos.

0 = No effect

Since a child is unlikely to have random ketonuria, ketones are not tested routinely. If the child's urine glucose is 5 per cent or above or if the child is feeling ill, ketones are checked. Most children over the age of six years are able to test their own urine reliably.

After the period of initial adjustment to diabetes, education concerning urine testing continues. If the child or family has had exposure to other individuals with diabetes, they may want further information on other testing methods such as Ketodiastix or Testape. Families are often taught the 1-Drop Clinitest Method at this time. If the child's urinary glucose is 5 per cent or above, the urine may be diluted further in order to establish glucose levels of 6 to 10 per cent or above. One drop of urine, 10 drops of water, and 1 Clinitest tablet are placed together. The resulting color is compared with the 2-Drop Method chart and the percentages are doubled. If the 1-drop test reading is less than 6 per cent, then the original 2-drop test is considered more accurate, with the true reading being approximately 5 per cent.

Since so many variables affect individual day-to-day random urine and blood tests, the 24-hour urine test is considered a more accurate assessment of basic control. The family is taught to collect the specimen at home, check the glucose level, and measure the volume. Simple arithmetic results in the amount of glucose spilled in 24 hours. Volume in milliliters (or cups × 240) × percentage of glucose (expressed in decimal form) = grams of glucose/ 24 hours. The test may be divided into two 12-hour segments or three 8-hour segments in order to locate the time of greatest glucose spill. It is important to emphasize to the child and family to make the day of collection as normal a day as possible. Using this method the goal is to keep the glucosuria less than 5 per cent of the total caloric intake for the day. Most children who are spilling more than 5 per cent of their calories become symptomatic with polyuria, polydipsia, and so on. The 24-hour urine provides a relatively simple and inexpensive test to assess diabetes control.

EXAMPLE

A 6-year-old girl estimated to be consuming about 1600 calories has a 24-hour urine volume of 1200 ml with 3 per cent glucose.

1200 × 0.03 = 36 gm glucose

36 gm glucose × 4 cal/gm = 144 calories

5 per cent of 1600 calorie intake = 80 calories

Therefore, this child has excessive glucosuria and needs either more insulin or a better distribution of the insulin she is taking provided she is not eating excessively or is otherwise ill.

Diet

Since the preinsulin era, the dietary intake of the person with diabetes has been considered a major element in the management plan. Even with the advent of crystalline insulin, diet has remained the foundation of treatment, and increasing the carbohydrate value of the diet is accompanied by increasing the insulin administered. This construct of the role of food in diabetes requires a stable intake of energy, a constant proportioning of food between each meal and snack, and a constant portion of the daily calories derived from fat, protein, and carbohydrates.

To provide some variety in the foods of such a diet and to influence compliance positively, the exchange list system was developed jointly by the American Diabetes Association and the American Dietetic Association. There has been general acceptance of this diet system in the care of the adult with diabetes, but even with the adult patient, the use of a prescribed diet has recently been questioned. Because the physical activity of children is highly variable day to day and as a result, caloric expenditure is altered, it does not seem appropriate to try to maintain a child on a diet that is constant from day to day. If caloric intake varies with expenditure, the result will be more stable blood sugar values, less tendency for the child to "steal" food, and less anxiety in the family about the child eating when he/she isn't hungry.

Therefore, we have adopted a self-prescribed diet that has the following characteristics:

1. Total food intake depends on the child's appetite.
2. Simple carbohydrates (sweets) are discouraged in favor of starch and fructose-containing foods.
3. Three meals a day with two snacks: (a) a predominantly carbohydrate snack in mid-afternoon, and (b) a predominantly protein-fat snack at bedtime.
4. No added salt and the use of polyunsaturated fats are encouraged.
5. The composition of diets (analyzed from diet diaries) indicates that on the average, about 50 per cent of the calories come from carbohydrate, 15 to 20 per cent from protein, and 30 to 35 per cent from fat.

It is our judgment that the use of such "self-prescribed" diets in children usually results in more stable management, fewer hypoglycemic reactions, less emotional tension in the home (itself a stabilizing factor), and more appropriate growth in weight and stature.

SICK DAY ROUTINE

The majority of children with intercurrent illness or mild to moderate ketoacidosis can be managed at home through frequent phone contacts, regular insulin every 4 to 6 hours, and copious oral fluids. By dividing the total daily units of insulin normally taken into proportions of 1/3, 1/4, 1/4, and 1/6 taken as regular insulin before breakfast, before lunch, before supper, and at bedtime, respectively, the child is switched to a four shot per day routine. When calculating the total units normally taken, both morning and evening doses of insulin must be included if the patient is on two injections per day.

The family is instructed to call before the normal morning dose of insulin is given if the child is showing signs of illness or is hyperglycemic and ketotic. One third of the total daily units is given as regular insulin and the family is asked to collect a second-voided specimen before lunch. The noon dose of insulin is adjusted based on the noon urine results. Normally children will drop the ketone level first and then the glucose level will fall. If there is no change in the glucose and ketones or if they are rising, then the noon dose is increased. The dose may be raised by 25 to 100 per cent depending on a variety of subtle signs. A parent's description of signs of dehydration, or Kussmaul breathing, weight loss, abdominal pain, vomiting, and headache are all taken into consideration for decision making. At times the level of anxiety in the parent's or child's voice may influence the decision on dosage. Previous experience with this individual gives the best information for selection of a dosage.

Occasionally a child will drop the glucose level but will maintain the ketone level. In this case, the insulin dose may be maintained or increased and more oral fluids containing calories are provided. The routine is repeated before supper and bedtime. If at any time the urine tests become negative for both glucose and ketones, then that dose of insulin is withheld.

Twenty-four hours of this routine is usually sufficient to bring the child back under control and improve the status of the intercurrent illness. Since the child is not being given any intermediate acting insulin and frequently the bedtime dose of regular insulin is withheld, the child may awaken with higher urinary glucose than usual the next morning. The family should be warned of this and instructed to give a small amount of extra regular insulin with the normal morning dose.

Maintaining hydration during the sick day is most important, particularly with the child who is hyperglycemic and having an osmotic diuresis. Caloric requirements can be achieved through the intake of carbohydrate-containing fluids such as regular soda pop, e.g., colas or ginger ale, and juices. These are alternated with noncaloric fluids such as water, iced tea, and diet soda pop to achieve a balance of fluids, calories, and electrolytes. We have found that Gatorade makes an excellent fluid replacement, as it contains appropriate electrolytes, is relatively low in sugar, and is well tolerated by the child who is nauseated. Other substances well tolerated by children include Jell-O, popsicles, ice cream, and sherbet. Like the insulin dose on sick days, the caloric intake can be adjusted to deal with hypoglycemia.

The sick day routine using four shots of regular insulin is the safest method to use, as the dose can be adjusted as the condition of the child changes. If the child has already taken an intermediate acting insulin and refuses to eat or begins to vomit, profound hypoglycemia with or without seizures may result. This is particularly true in the younger child, and close supervision is required. In the older child or adolescent who is not prone to vomit and will cooperate with drinking, a modification in the sick day routine may be made. The normal dose of intermediate acting insulin having been given, the dose of short acting insulin is increased by 10 to 20 per cent of the total daily units. Again the child is evaluated using second-voided urine specimens before lunch, before supper, and at bedtime, and regular insulin is given as needed. Caution must be used with the noon dose, as this insulin will peak at approximately the same time as the morning intermediate acting insulin. Likewise there is a risk of hypoglycemia with the bedtime dose, particularly if the child is not eating well.

DRINKING, DRUGS, AND SEX

Adolescents often wonder what effect their diabetes will have on their relationships with their peers. Frank discussion with the adolescent of the problems of drinking, drugs, and sex may relieve some anxiety and prevent some problems with diabetes control.

Although we discourage the use of alcoholic beverages, individuals with diabetes can drink them if changes are made in their insulin routine. The extra calories consumed through alcohol must be balanced with extra insulin in order to prevent hyperglycemia. However, the individual must be warned that when alcohol is first consumed it inhibits gluconeogenesis, which may then result in a hypoglycemic reaction. This may be especially profound if the adolescent has skipped a meal in an attempt to balance his intake of extra calories. We advise the individual who wants to drink not to skip meals but rather take an extra dose of regular insulin before going out. A dose of 10 to 20 per cent of the total daily units is sufficient for a moderate intake of alcohol. It is important to discuss the amount of alcohol consumption in concrete terms, as the adolescent's view of moderation may be quite different. This insulin dose will usually handle 2 to 3 12-oz beers, 2 to 3 oz of hard liquor, or 2 to 3 6-oz glasses of wine. The individual is encouraged to choose drinks with the fewest calories such as light beers, white wine, or hard liquor with diet soda pop as mixers. Having something to eat when first beginning drinking will prevent hypoglycemia. The individual is also instructed to check a second-voided urine specimen before going to bed and to take an additional 5 to 10 per cent of the total daily units as regular insulin if hyperglycemic or ketotic at that time. This routine has worked well with the majority of adolescents and young adults who choose to drink. Those who have had difficulty have drunk to excess with resulting vomiting necessitating switching to a sick day routine.

Most adolescents are not aware that marijuana use may mimic or disguise hypoglycemia. Whether the individual has diabetes or not, marijuana use creates a sensation of hunger or the so-called munchies. The individual with diabetes may regard this as hypoglycemia and consume excess calories. If already hypoglycemic, the problem may not be recognized and severe symptoms may result. The effect is cumulative if combined with alcohol, as is often the case. Adolescents are cautioned not to engage in marijuana use when alone. Their peers should also be informed that if the individual with diabetes loses consciousness while using marijuana, emergency care should be sought.

Many adolescents with diabetes wonder whether they should have children of their own. They can be counseled that the chance of their children developing diabetes is only slightly greater than for the general population. The next question is often what effect the diabetes will have on the pregnancy. For the male with diabetes there is no apparent effect of diabetes on the offspring. However, the adolescent male must be cautioned that he is as fertile as any other adolescent and appropriate contraceptive measures must be employed. There appears to be an increased risk for abortion and a variety of birth defects in the infant of the diabetic mother. Recent data would point to hyperglycemia during the period of organogenesis as a contributing factor. The adolescent female must be aware of this relationship and the need for strict control before and during a pregnancy. Because of this relationship contraception for the sexually active adolescent is essential.

It has been our finding that these subjects first need to be discussed briefly with 11- and 12-year-olds. The subject needs to be handled delicately so that the activities are not condoned but rather the child is given an option for further information, when or if he chooses to become involved. The subject is again discussed with the older adolescent with further details being given.

EMOTIONAL CONSIDERATIONS

Children and adolescents with IDDM present physicians with stimulating and complex management problems. Yet the technical difficulties of the regimen may appear simple in comparison with the psychosocial difficulties. Nevertheless, with patience and insight on the physician's part, those children and families who are the most frustrating and time-consuming can ultimately gain the most from professional services, as well as providing the physician with greater understanding of general illness-related behaviors.

Diabetes in children is a particularly good model of chronic disease processes for several reasons: frequent contact with the physician over many years is required; the treatment is complex and potentially dangerous, yet generally occurs in the home; the success of transmission and execution of this complex regimen may affect the long-term outcome; the disease and treatment may induce or exacerbate psychological problems in the child and family and, in turn, may alter the disease course.

From a psychological viewpoint, the period of diagnosis is a crucial time for all parties involved in the treatment. The physician's and staff's attitudes and actions can leave a lasting impression on the child and parents. Parents usually experience a number of overlapping feelings, including disbelief, shock, anger (directed at the physician, the staff, themselves, each other, the disease, or even the child), guilt, and grief. This list is not inclusive and there is no absolute order or sequence. The initial adjustment period may be brief, protracted, or never fully completed. Young parents, a single parent, or parents with few children may be at greater risk for problems during this stage than will older, more experienced parents in a stable marital relationship.

During the period of long-term management, school age children frequently focus on food deprivations, injection pain, and disgust with urine testing. Adolescents commonly experience feelings of separateness from their peers, of being different and "out of it." Many males will compensate through sports. Females are more prone to experiment with wide alterations in food intake in keeping with the propensity of adolescent girls to be concerned about obesity.

For some families, the burden of chronic disease is particularly destabilizing. In such cases there is usually a preceding history of marital discord. This may be open and aggressive or covert, frequently hidden, or contained by one of the couple's long working hours, different interests, and/or a general absence of communication between spouses. Those patterns may be exacerbated by the increased demands of a medical regimen. The father may become increasingly inaccessible; the mother may feel increasingly burdened and resentful. They may disagree on diet and other aspects of treatment and argue about heredity (guilt), and the quality of the marriage will further deteriorate. Often, fathers will be enduring a silent state of desperation, with strong feelings of guilt, fear, anger, and displacement, but lacking the skills or a safe forum to express them. Nevertheless, patients will perceive many of these problems and their emotional stress may lead to increasing management difficulties including "emotional" ketoacidosis, or more or less deliberate attempts to sabotage the treatment and thereby draw the parents' attention away from their fighting and back to themselves via illness.

Most physicians cannot devote the time required to serve as marriage counselors even when their patient's health is at risk. In serious cases of family difficulty, a tactful referral to a social worker, clinical psychologist, or psychiatrist is in order. Any reference to fault, blame, or mental illness should be avoided; rather, one should express the ideas that chronic illness is a stressful situation for any family to experience, and the perspective of an objective, trained specialist can help many parents to communicate their feelings safely and to cope more effectively with the situation.

Even in more typical families, it is important for the physician or other provider to meet and involve both parents and possibly other members of the family. For example, the mother's burden and father's alienation can be lessened if he is encouraged to give injections on weekends or whenever he has the time. Of course, the situation can be reversed when the mother is fully employed outside the home.

There are other nodal points in the course of the illness and the child's development when problems frequently may occur. The patient's adolescence may give the physician as many headaches as it does their parents; one must not forget the stress endured by the patients themselves. A familial perspective reveals two concurrent processes: the child's ambivalent striving for independence and identity versus security and safety, and the parents' desire to keep and control their children (and their own youth), yet a yearning for their own freedom from the worries of caring for children. Thus, patterns of extreme behaviors on both parties' parts are sometimes seen: children will demand autonomy, particularly around their regimen, but may behave so cavalierly as to invite parental interference, while parents may promise independence and responsibility, yet become more nagging and repressive. Naturally, diabetes treatment is a perfect issue over which parents and children will struggle.

The physician's role can be eased if he/she recalls the developmental context of adolescent difficulties; i.e., it is a normal part of coming of age in our culture. Frequently, continued reliance on honest discussion and respectful listening can ameliorate problems during adolescence. In practice, this means eliciting statements of feelings, values, and goals from all parties, including the physician, and attempting to negotiate for common ground.

Typically, reference to ambivalent feelings and behavioral contradictions will occur readily enough. The medical team may wish to employ "behavioral contracts" between parent and child or physician and patient, in which each side alters behavior to achieve a goal, e.g., mother: no nagging about urine tests; child: six tests per week. Clearly, the contracts must be fair and flexible and permit saving "face" for all concerned. The general trend throughout adolescence will be toward greater independence on the patients' part. By the time the adolescent is preparing to leave home, the patient is usually seen alone during visits. This is also a period in which discussion about self-care, family and career planning, and other maturity-related issues may be frankly addressed by the physician.

Finally, some attention must be addressed to long-term complications. While they are rarely seen in the pediatric age range, they are a grave concern to patients, family, and physician. At some point, the medical consultants are obliged to discuss the possible occurrence of later problems. These discussions should not aim at regimen adherence through fear, nor should they be white-washed and vague. Rather a calm, factual approach, leavened with concern, is generally the best received.

In summary, there are several important themes. First is the importance of simple listening. Time spent discussing the patient's concerns will help to build the trust necessary for a solid relationship in the future. Second, attention must be paid to the developmental nature of the patient, parent, physician, and disease course. Different periods require different approaches. Finally, there are a number of challenging and changing roles required of the physician or health care team. At times, technical medicine in the form of emergency treatment, aspects of regimen, and so on, are paramount; at others, the role of social worker or psychologist will become important. Under ideal circumstances, with maturing patients and interested physicians, a partnership between both can evolve.

MANAGEMENT GOALS AND ASSESSMENT

Accurate assessment of the patients' status is critical for achieving good management. There are a number of techniques available for this, utilizing both urine and blood testing. Urine testing is described in detail elsewhere in this chapter. Generally the spot urine tests are utilized to help in day-to-day management and to reflect changes caused by growth, changes in activity, changes in diet, or changes related to stress—either physical or emotional. A divided 24-hour specimen provides more information in terms of the actual amount of glucosuria and its timing. Utilizing both techniques, one can more accurately regulate the total insulin dose, the number of shots administered, and the ratio of short to intermediate acting insulin in each shot.

Blood testing is considerably more controversial. There are two basic tests currently in use for ambulatory care. Determinations of glycosylated hemoglobin (Hgb A_{1C}) have been recommended as a method evaluating control, integrating the times of hyperglycemia over a four- to six-week period. Unfortunately, it has recently been found that there are two fractions to Hgb A_{1C}. One is a stable fraction that does indeed provide an evaluation over several weeks. The second is a labile fraction that represents only the status of several hours prior to specimen collection. These can be separated by a dialysis procedure, but the majority of commercial laboratories are not currently doing this, thus casting some doubt on the usefulness of the results.

Home monitoring of blood glucose has been recommended as a more accurate replacement for the currently utilized urine glucose determinations. Indeed, this may be true for the post-adolescent patient for whom exercise, diet, and other variables have settled into a routine that results in a comparatively stable level of blood sugar. Unfortunately, for the majority of patients in the pediatric age range, the blood sugar is highly variable, with wide swings occuring during the day. The single spot sample, either blood or urine, fails to provide any information as to where the level is heading. Thus we feel that for routine monitoring, first-voided urines provide more data. Further considerations of frequent blood glucose measurements must include the risk of osteomyelitis and permanent disfiguration from multiple capillary samples, as have been documented in infants requiring repeated capillary samplings. The use of multiple daily blood glucose determinations needs further examination before being recommended for general use. Single blood glucose determinations can be useful in situations when one either has confusing data from urine testing or is at the extremes of either negative sugar in the urine or 10 per cent spillage, to determine the patient's exact status prior to administration of some kind of therapy.

Even with the currently available methods of assessment, it is common for a patient to be chronically receiving too much or too little insulin. Unfortunately, it is relatively easy for efforts aimed at achieving optimum control to result in over-insulinization with periods of hypoglycemia and rebound hyperglycemia (often referred to as the Somogyi phenomenon). These patients often report excessive weight gain or periods of symptoms such as ravenous hunger, headaches, or shakiness suggestive of reactions, and yet have a history of pronounced glucosuria sometimes with ketonuria, prompting the physician to increase the insulin dose. It is important to realize that rebound hyperglycemia follows very quickly after an episode of rapid fall in glucose and that ketones can be produced during the period of hypoglycemia. Thus, it becomes very important to consider the patient's over-all symptoms, as well as urine and serum test data, when adjusting insulin doses.

The routine care for all patients with diabetes should include regular screening for signs of complications of diabetes and for indications of associated diseases. Palpation of the thyroid gland and symptom review for Hashimoto's thyroiditis, possibly with periodic screening for antithyroid and antimicrosomal antibodies, should begin during the initial phase of the child's management. Also, examination of injection sites for early lipodystrophy should be a part of each examination. As the child's course progresses, and usually by five to seven years after diagnosis, microvascular complications should be considered. At this time, funduscopic examinations, peripheral neurological examinations, and occasional urine screens for proteinuria should be added to each patient's regimen.

OPEN AND CLOSED LOOP INSULIN DELIVERY SYSTEMS

In the normal person, a functional pancreas responds to blood glucose levels with varying amounts of released insulin, thus regulating the blood glucose within relatively narrow limits. The patient with IDDM lacks endogenous insulin and thus has no such sensitive feedback system.

In an attempt to duplicate the normal process, an "open loop" insulin pump has recently been introduced. This delivers insulin subcutaneously at programmed basal rates with preprandial pulse dose increments. "Closed loop" systems monitor the current blood sugar and adjust the dose of infused insulin on this basis, thus duplicating the pancreas as an "artificial pancreas." The latter is not yet available and awaits the development of a portable glucose monitor.

As another technique for correcting the insulinopenia of IDDM, pancreas or β cell transplants have been tried in experimental animals. This work is progressing slowly because of the problem of immunological rejection.

Until now, control of glycemia at physiological levels has been impossible. However, recent studies suggest that use of the open loop insulin delivery system may allow adequate control of glycemia as well as control many of the other associated metabolic abnormalities. Whether this apparently improved metabolic control will decrease the pathology associated with IDDM remains to be seen.

The initial use of the insulin pump is not simply a matter of strapping the instrument on the belt and inserting the needle subcutaneously. Patient selection and establishing the infused insulin dose are extremely important. Prior to its use on an outpatient basis, the patient must be admitted to a hospital or clinical research setting for a period of two to five days. The basal infusion dose ranges from 12½ to 15 mU per kilogram per hour. The total basal dose is then subtracted from the patient's usual total daily dose on conventional treatment and the remainder is given as four pulse doses, 15 to 30 minutes before meals. The usual distribution of insulin is 30 to 35 per cent before breakfast, 25 per cent before lunch, 25 per cent before dinner, and 15 to 20 per cent before the evening snack. The basal infusion rate and preprandial pulse doses are altered based on the previous day's blood glucose concentrations, which are brought as close to normal as possible. Cooperation of the patient and family is necessary, since home blood glucose monitoring with the Dextrometer or other such instrument is essential to judicious management of the patient on the insulin infusion. Initial monitoring of preprandial pre-insulin infusion blood glucose levels would appear essential to the safe management of the protocol. It should be emphasized that this discussion concerns the battery-operated insulin infusion pumps and not the recently advertised mechanical models, which are no more than a syringe connected to tubing.

Finally, the recent reports of hypoglycemia and other complications and/or sudden deaths in patients using the insulin infusion pumps raise the questions of whether this therapy can be continuously, safely, and effectively applied to a large number of individuals.

In addition to therapies such as the open loop system with frequent monitoring, a regimen of regular insulin injections four times a day also appears to restore the metabolic state of the patient with IDDM close to normal. A multicenter study using these techniques is in progress to establish the relationship between control of hyperglycemia and specific complications of diabetes.

REFERENCES

Abraira, C. M., de Bartola, R. D., and Myscofski, J. W.: Comparison of unmeasured versus exchange diabetic diets in lean adults. Body weight and feeding patterns in a 2-year prospective pilot study. Am. J. Clin. Nutr., *33*:1064–1070, 1980.

Bright, G. M., Blizzard, R. M., Kaiser, D. L., and Clarke, W. L.: Organ-specific autoantibodies in children with common endocrine diseases. Pediatrics, *100*:8–14, 1982.

Cahill, G. F., and McDevitt, H. O.: Insulin-dependent diabetes mellitus: The initial lesion. N. Engl. J. Med., *304*:1454–1465, 1981.

CDC: Deaths among patients using continuous subcutaneous insulin infusion pumps—United States. MMWR, 31 (No. 7):80–82, 87, 1982.

Champsaur, H. F., Bottazzo, G.-F., Bertrams, J., Assan, R., and Bach, C.: Virologic, immunologic, and genetic factors in insulin-dependent diabetes mellitus. Pediatrics, *100*(1):15–20, 1982.

Chase, H. P., and Jackson, G. G.: Stress and sugar control in children with insulin-dependent diabetes mellitus. Pediatrics, *98*(6):1011–1013, 1981.

Daneman, D., Wolfson, D. H., Becker, D. J., and Drash, A. L.: Factors affecting glycosylated hemoglobin values in children with insulin-dependent diabetes. Pediatrics, *99*(6):847–853, 1981.

Dorchy, H., Mozin, M.-J., and Loeb, H.: Unmeasured diet versus exchange diet in diabetes. Am. J. Clin. Nutr., *34*:964–965, 1981.

Langdon, D. R., James, F. D., and Sperling, M. A.: Comparison of single- and split-dose insulin regimens with 24-hour monitoring. Pediatrics, *99*(6):854–861, 1981.

MacGillivray, M. H., Bruck, E., and Voorhess, M. L.: Acute diabetic ketoacidosis in children: Role of the stress hormones. Pediatr. Res., *15*:99–106, 1981.

Rizza, R. A., Gerich, J. E., Haymond, M. W., et al.: Control of blood sugar in insulin dependent diabetes: Comparison of an artificial endocrine pancreas, continuous insulin infusion, and intensified conventional insulin therapy. N. Engl. J. Med., *303*:313–318, 1980.

Rosenbloom, A. L., Kohrman, A., and Sperling, M.: Classification and diagnosis of diabetes mellitus in children and adolescents. Pediatrics, *99*(2):320–323, 1981.

Rudolf, M. C., Genel, M., Tamborlane, W. V., Jr., and Dwyer, J. M.: Juvenile rheumatoid arthritis in children with diabetes mellitus. Pediatrics, *99*(4):510–524, 1981.

Sherwin, R. S., Tamorlane, W. V., Genel, M., and Felig, P.: Treatment of juvenile onset diabetes by subcutaneous infusion of insulin with a portable pump. Diabetes Care, *3*:301–308, 1980.

Teuscher, A.: The place of the "monocomponent" insulins in the therapy of diabetes mellitus. Schweiz. Med. Wochenschr., *105*:485–494, 1975.

White, N. H., Waltman, S. R., Krupin, T., and Santiago, J. V.: Reversal of neuropathic and gastrointestinal complications related to diabetes mellitus in adolescents with improved metabolic control. Pediatrics, *99*(1):41–45, 1981.

65

OBESITY

Gilbert B. Forbes, M.D.

Strictly speaking, obesity (*obedere, obesus*—to devour) is a condition manifested by an increased amount of body fat. Its importance stems from the fact that it is the commonest form of "nutritional" disorder in Western society today and from the reluctant admission by modern medicine that treatment is relatively ineffectual. Since methods for determining body fat content (densitometry, body water, or potassium content [Forbes, 1962]) are too cumbersome for routine use, body weight is the commonly accepted criterion. Yet by any criterion the definition is an arbitrary one. Use of the 90th percentile, for instance, means that 10 per cent of the population is judged to be overweight. Some use the term "per cent overweight" or body mass index (weight/height^2); others prefer to measure the thickness of the skin plus subcutaneous tissue, as estimated by special pinch calipers. The recent compilation of normative data on weight for height should be helpful (NAS data, 1975). From the practical standpoint, however, excessive obesity can be recognized at a glance.

Man ranks among the fatter of mammals: the neonate is 14 per cent fat; at age 18 years the average boy contains about 12 per cent and the girl about 25 per cent fat (Forbes, 1962, 1972). The changes in body fat with age are reflected in the data on triceps skinfold thickness shown in Figure 65–1.

EPIDEMIOLOGY AND PATHOGENESIS

Body weight can increase only in the face of a positive energy balance. Except for those rare instances in which fat accumulation is accompanied by a decline in lean, the onset of obesity can be traced to excess food, reduced physical activity, or both. Food intake may decline

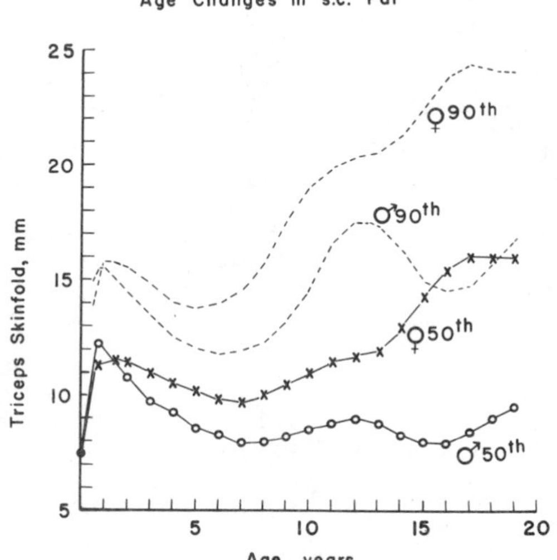

Figure 65–1. Median and 90th percentile values for triceps skinfold thickness. (Redrawn from Tanner, J. M., and Whitehouse, R. H.: Arch. Dis. Child., *50*:142–145, 1975.)

somewhat once body weight has been stabilized at a high level, since the maintenance of excess weight requires fewer calories than its production.

The obese patient is a prime example of the role of denial in the causation of illness (Forbes, 1967). Caloric intakes solicited by routine questioning are often underestimated.* Direct observation (Waxman and Stunkard, 1980; Stunkard and Kaplan, 1977) testifies to the excessive intake and the rapid eating pattern of the obese. An easy way to document this is to offer an 1800 calorie diet for a few days; the comparison with the child's previous diet will be obvious. Food preferences, "junk foods," and carbohydrates are blamed without reason. The parent is hopeful that some endocrine or metabolic disorder is at fault, a vain hope that has been shared by the profession in its vigorous, unrelenting, and thus far futile search for such a cause.

It has been shown that gastrointestinal absorption is normal in obese patients, that caloric distribution of the food consumed is normal, that basal metabolic rate is normal or slightly increased when referred to height, and that patients lose weight in a predictable manner under controlled dietary conditions. There is no proof that they use food in a more efficient manner. Some do exhibit relative insulin resistance, a blunted plasma growth hormone response to provocative stimuli, and increased adrenocorticoid excretion, but these are secondary phenomena, not primary; indeed, they can be induced by deliberate overfeeding of normal subjects.

Many obese patients exhibit a diurnal variation in appetite: a poor breakfast, or none at all, a modest lunch, and then an increasing craving for food as night comes on (Stunkard et al., 1955). This craving is manifest by a poor tolerance for meal delay and by the rapidity with which food is consumed.

Most of the excess weight is fat. The lean body mass is either normal or modestly increased to constitute 10 to 30 per cent of the excess weight (Forbes, 1964; Forbes and Welle, 1982). Generally speaking, obese children are a little taller than normal, bone age is slightly advanced, and sexual maturation, at least in girls, occurs a bit earlier; hemoglobin levels are slightly higher (Garn and Clark, 1975). Longitudinal data show that the acceleration in stature occurs either coincident with or shortly after the excessive weight gain, never before (Forbes, 1977). These findings speak strongly against thyroid, pituitary, or adrenal malfunction as causative factors in obesity. Children with early-onset obesity have an increase in the total number of adipocytes (Hirsch and Knittle, 1970). Overnutrition thus speeds up growth and maturation, just as undernutrition slows it.

Familial factors are of great importance. The majority of obese children have at least one obese parent. Eating patterns do vary among families, and some mothers stress food intake more than others. Garn and Clark (1975) even found an interspouse relationship for both fatness and leanness. Studies of twins and of adopted children also reveal the presence of a genetic factor in obesity (Foch and McClearn, 1980). Among animals, relative body fatness is species-dependent, and strains of mice are known in which obesity is inherited according to Mendelian laws (Mayer, 1963). While the importance of genetics cannot be denied, the relative contribution of environment and heredity in human obesity is still under debate.

The incidence of obesity is inversely related to social class; this fact alone should provide a clue to the curious investigator. Girls are more frequently affected than boys. In certain patients, precipitating factors can be identified: an enforced period of bed rest; a part-time restaurant job; a situational frustration (domestic upheaval, removal to a new location and

*The child may limit his food intake in anticipation of his visit to the doctor, and hence the dietary history may not be representative. An eight-year-old patient of mine observed on *ad libitum* diet in hospital took only 2000 calories daily for a full two weeks, after which his intake gradually rose to 4000 calories.

hence a new school, etc.); the taking of a full-time job by mother, which may be perceived as neglect. I have been impressed by the frequency with which the onset has followed tonsillectomy. A chart of previous heights and weights is helpful in dating the onset.

The role of decreased physical activity is a clear one. Casual observation confirms the slower walk and the more deliberate movements of the obese child and the lack of ability for sustained physical exertion. More weight is gained in winter than in summer, long hours are spent at television, and competitive sports are rarely engaged in. Exercise does require energy, and it is often forgotten that such a simple procedure as walking consumes 300 calories per hour.

Certain phenomena indigenous to modern culture conspire to augment food intake and decrease physical activity. We in America, and throughout Western society, produce an abundance of food, and it is food of high biological quality, widely available, and attractively advertised. Such a surfeit is without parallel in human history and hence represents a new environmental challenge. School lunch programs are widespread. Nutritionists advocate generous allowances of most nutrients in their zeal to see to it that no one is underfed. Our forebears were obliged to walk to school; our children are obliged to ride. The modern child partakes of our adult sedentary ways: immobilized by television, discouraged from walking or cycling by heavy traffic and a paucity of sidewalks, and dependent on the automobile for transportation, his energy expenditure is small indeed.

Normal individuals must possess some finely integrated mechanism(s) for balancing food intake and caloric output, for body weight (in the nongrowing person) varies no more than 1 or 2 per cent over long periods of time. This balance is obviously disturbed in obesity, and since adipose tissue is the only organ capable of great changes in size, fat accumulates as a result of what can only be construed as relative hyperphagia. In discussing this phenomenon, Hamburger (1957) distinguishes between *hunger* and *appetite*: the former is an unconditioned, innate response to the physiological need for food, whereas appetite is a learned psychological pattern involving pleasurable anticipation, a mechanism for dealing with emotional rather than nutritional needs. It is appetite which is at fault in obesity.

The onset of obesity may be associated with situational factors. There are other children for whom eating has become a compulsion, the so-called "developmental" obesity. In my experience, these children tend to be immature, passively dependent, easily upset, petulant, demanding, and fearful of their role in life. Some are obviously depressed, one manifestation of which is the breakfast time anorexia. As Bruch (1957) so aptly put it: "Whether we like it or not . . . we must learn to recognize that for many people overeating and being fat is a balancing factor in their adjustment to life. Ineffective as it is, it represents the best form of adaptation that such people have been able to make . . . without the comfort of eating, life may become so threatening and lacking in any satisfaction there is danger of serious mental illness if reducing is enforced." Later this perceptive student of obesity commented that excessive feeding may have been perceived as cementing the child-mother relationship, and that for the older child a large body size may confer a sense of self-importance (Bruch, 1973, 1975). Such children often have been treated as precious possessions from their earliest years by frustrated, and often obese, parents whose only response to their children's needs was to stuff them with food.

These considerations go far in explaining some of the cardinal features of obesity, namely the vain hope that help can come without dietary restriction, the tendency to invest "reducing" pills and "fad" diets with magic properties, the very high rate of treatment failure, and the marked proclivity for childhood obesity to continue into adult life.

Mayer (1963) has reviewed the various types of experimental and genetic obesities in animals. These include obesities following lesions of the ventromedian nucleus of the hypothalamus and those due to ACTH-secreting tumors. Some are associated with a decrease in lean weight, and hence differ in this respect from the usual form of human obesity. In man, obesity is known to occur in Cushing's syndrome, in some patients with insulinomas, in hypopituitarism, and in the Lawrence-Moon-Biedl syndrome. It is regularly seen in those given large doses of adrenocortical hormones over long periods of time. Yet all of these together explain only a small fraction of the total.

An interesting though rare type of obesity is that known as the Prader-Willi syndrome. It is characterized by muscle hypotonia and failure to thrive in infancy, delayed psychomotor development, hypogenitalism, latent diabetes, and, when obesity begins, compulsive eating.

DIAGNOSIS

The clinical picture is usually sufficient. The increase in subcutaneous fat is usually generalized; a "buffalo hump" is common, as are colored striae over the thighs and breasts. The striae of Cushing's syndrome can be distinguished from these because they are usually wide (0.5 cm or more) and purplish-red in color, and the overlying skin is thin. Mild dyspnea is frequent, and the blood pressure often shows a moderate elevation by the cuff method. Genu valgum is occasionally seen, and intertrigo is common. In examining the genitalia, the pubic fat pad should be vigorously compressed if the true size of the penis is to be appreciated. On rare occasions pubic hair appears early, a manifestation of the secondary hyperadrenocorticism also seen in some obese adults.

The two most important measurements to make are *stature* and *bone age*; if these are normal or above, and particularly if there has been no tendency for height growth to decline, the "endogenous" factors noted above are most unlikely to be present.

The principal condition to be excluded is the "stocky" child whose increased weight is due largely to his large body frame. Such children have good muscle development and firm subcutaneous tissue turgor and are apt to be tall and to have inherited the body build of their parents.

On rare occasions the increased work of breathing leads to alveolar hypoventilation and CO_2 narcosis, the so-called pickwickian syndrome.

PREVENTION

The tendency for childhood obesity to persist into the adult years is well known. Recent evidence suggests that overweight babies are more likely to become obese adults than are thin babies (Charney et al., 1976). Thus it is possible to identify at an early age those who are at risk: those born to obese parents and those who gain weight rapidly during infancy, as well as those whose mothers use food as a means of controlling behavior.

Reasonable, although as yet unproven, preventive measures include the following: breast feeding ("nursing is a useful way both to restore energy balance in the mother and to prevent obesity in the baby" [Mann, 1974])—after all, the supply of breast milk is limited; delay in introduction of solid foods; counseling of mothers to give food only in response to hunger, not as a pacifier; a reorientation of family life toward low calorie foods and toward the ritualization of total meal-time behavior; and the promotion of physical exercise. Incidentally, the high solute-to-calorie ratio of skim milk makes this an inappropriate food for the young infant.

MANAGEMENT*

Here I must admit a feeling of pretentiousness, for I have had so little personal success. But I am not alone, for despite the usual, and often gratifying, initial response to treatment, the reported long-term success rate is dismally poor in children (Stunkard and McLaren-Hume, 1959).

The only means by which weight can be lost is for energy expenditure to exceed intake. Either activity must increase or food intake decrease; the laws of thermodynamics still hold.

For the adolescent a diet of fewer than 1400 to 1600 calories can rarely be tolerated. Attention should be paid to protein, vitamin, and iron content. There is no real advantage to special caloric distribution, such as fad diets are wont to offer, or to unusual spacing of meals. Many need to be reminded of proper techniques for preparing meals: frying adds significant calories, canned fruits may contain sugar, and so forth.

The child with "situational" obesity deserves an understanding of his problem, reassurance, and support, as well as emphasis on the potentially satisfying aspects of his life, together with help in dealing with the particular problem.

Appetite-suppressant drugs and thyroid preparations are of little help.

Behavior modification is currently gaining in popularity, but here, too, the long-term results are still in doubt. A review of the few reports by authors who have followed their patients for at least a year shows that on average only 7 per cent of initial weight is lost, and as is the case with dietary therapy the dropout rate is high (Foreyt et al., 1981). Details of the technique can be found in Stunkard's book (1980).

Fasting leads to rapid weight loss, but this technique has obvious limitations. Large numbers of obese adults, and some adolescents,

*A clear distinction must be made between the subject of this chapter, the obese child, and the more common problem of the moderately overweight adult. The latter may benefit from an approach which combines rational motivation (the health hazard) with certain embellishments, such as placebo (drugs), variety (fad diets), and peer pressure (lay groups).

have now been subjected to one of several surgical procedures—intestinal by-pass, gastric by-pass, gastroplasty, biliary-pancreatic by-pass (Faloon et al., 1977; Joffe, 1981). Many lose significant amounts of weight (40 kg or more), and some report a gratifying improvement in general well-being. However, the complication rate is rather high and involves serious abnormalities of liver, bone, joints, and kidney in addition to GI tract, so careful postoperative follow-up is mandatory. Generally speaking, these operations have been restricted to those with morbid obesity who are judged capable of tolerating the procedure.

Mention should be made of the so-called protein-sparing modified fast, which is a 300 to 800 calorie diet consisting principally of protein. Initial weight loss is fairly rapid, and the proportion of the loss estimated to be lean tissue is less than that observed during a true fast. However, some lean is lost, and the diet is not without life threatening hazards (Lantigua et al., 1980).

The "developmental" type of obesity is a most difficult problem. While some patients may prove to be candidates for low calorie diets or for surgery, both Hamburger (1957) and Bruch (1957) have cautioned against enforced weight loss in these patients, for some will then develop more serious emotional disturbances. Attempts to improve physical activity are rarely successful, appetite suppressants have only a temporary effect, and formula diets may be resented. This is the "hard core" group whose life adjustment centers on the process of eating, and who are literally caught in the dualistic trap of hyperphagia and inactivity. Psychiatric referral may be necessary. One wonders whether diet therapy should even be attempted, for Hamburger (1957) reminds us that "Despite a decreased life expectancy, obesity relating to addiction to food may be a healthier adaptation than addiction to alcohol or other drugs, or a serious depression."

It must be remembered that fat is a high caloric substance, and even under the most ideal circumstances the rate of weight loss will be distressingly slow. For example, studies of fasting adults show that although they lose weight rapidly at first, the average daily loss over long periods is only 500 to 800 grams.

One can only conclude that obesity, although it may be a solace to the patient, is the bane of the modern physician. The present, often sophisticated conceptualizations of this condition have not led to a satisfactory treatment for this "relatively incurable disorder" (Mann, 1974). It cries out for a new approach.

REFERENCES

Bray, G. A. (Ed.): Obesity in Perspective. Washington, D.C., U.S. Government Printing Office, DHEW Pub. # (NIH) 75–708, 1975.

Bruch, H.: Psychiatric aspects of obesity. Metabolism, *6*:461, 1957.

Bruch, H.: Eating Disorders: Obesity, Anorexia Nervosa and the Person Within. New York, Basic Books, 1973.

Bruch, H.: The importance of overweight. *In* Collip, P. J. (Ed.): Childhood Obesity. Acton, MA, Pub. Sciences Group, 1975.

Charney, E., Chamblee, H., McBride, M., Lyon, B., and Pratt, R.: The childhood antecedents of adult obesity: Do chubby infants become obese adults? N. Engl. J. Med., *295*:6, 1976.

Faloon, W. W. (chairman): Conference on jejunoileostomy for obesity. Am. J. Clin. Nutr., *30*:1, 1977.

Foch, T. T., and MacClearn, G. E.: Genetics, body weight, and obesity. *In* Stunkard, A. J. (Ed.): Obesity. Philadelphia, W. B. Saunders Co., 1980, pp. 48–71.

Forbes, G. B.: Methods for determining composition of the human body. Pediatrics, *29*:477, 1962.

Forbes, G. B.: Lean body mass and fat in obese children. Pediatrics, *34*:308, 1964.

Forbes, G. B.: The great denial. Nutr. Rev., *25*:353, 1967.

Forbes, G. B.: Growth of the lean mass in man. Growth, *36*:325, 1972.

Forbes, G. B.: Nutrition and growth. J. Pediatr., *91*:40, 1977.

Forbes, G. B., and Welle, S. L.: Lean body mass in obesity. Int. J. Obesity, in press.

Foreyt, J. P., Goodrich, G. K., and Gotto, A. M.: Limitations of behavioral treatment of obesity: Review and analysis. J. Behav. Med., *4*:159, 1981.

Garn, S. M., and Clark, D. C.: Nutrition, growth, development and maturation: Findings from the ten-state nutrition survey of 1968–1970. Pediatrics, *56*:306, 1975.

Hamburger, W. W.: Psychological aspects of obesity. Bull. N.Y. Acad. Med., *33*:771, 1957.

Hirsch, J., and Knittle, J. L.: The cellularity of obese and non-obese human adipose tissue. Fed. Proc., *29*:1516, 1970.

Joffe, S. N.: Surgical management of morbid obesity. Gut, *22*:242, 1981.

Lantigua, R. A., Amatruda, J. M., Biddle, T. L., Forbes, G. B., and Lockwood, D. H.: Cardiac arrhythmias associated with a liquid protein diet for the treatment of obesity. N. Engl. J. Med., *303*:735, 1980.

Mann, G. V.: The influence of obesity on health. N. Engl. J. Med., *291*:178, 226, 1974.

Mayer, J.: Obesity. Ann. Rev. Med., *14*:111, 1963.

National Academy of Science: Data from Recommended Reference Population, Dept. HEW, Center for Disease Control, Atlanta, 1975.

Stunkard, A. J. (ed.): Obesity. Philadelphia, W. B. Saunders Co., 1980.

Stunkard, A. J., Grace, W. J., and Wolff, H. G.: The night-eating syndrome: Pattern of food intake among certain obese patients. Am. J. Med., *19*:78, 1955.

Stunkard, A. J., and Kaplan, D.: Eating in public places: A review of reports of the direct observation of eating behavior. Int. J. Obesity, *1*:89, 1977.

Stunkard, A. J., and McLaren-Hume, M.: The results of treatment for obesity. Arch. Intern. Med., *103*:79, 1959.

Tanner, J. M., and Whitehouse, R. H.: Revised standards for triceps and subscapular skinfolds in British children. Arch. Dis. Child., *50*:142, 1975.

Waxman, M., and Stunkard, A. J.: Caloric intake and expenditure of obese children. J. Pediatr., *96*:187, 1980.

66

RECURRENT INFECTIONS

Martin B. Kleiman, M.D.

A common parental complaint is that a child appears to be having more frequent or more severe infections than what is perceived as "normal." This complaint deserves careful attention. The past several decades have seen an enormous increase in our understanding of host immune function and the recognition of abnormalities of those important mechanisms which predispose patients to frequent, unusual, and/or severe infections; however, *the incidence of the recognized immune dysfunctions is very low* and, therefore, the decision to begin a complex laboratory investigation must be a carefully reasoned one. This chapter will present an approach designed to enable the physician to establish whether his patient's complaint of recurrent infections strongly suggests (1) an abnormality of immune function; (2) a condition or abnormality that may predispose to localized infection in the absence of general immune dysfunction; (3) that the symptoms are adequately explained by environmental and host factors and are within the range of normal; or (4) a low parental threshold for the perception of illness or other misconceptions concerning health and disease. These last two categories are features of pseudofever of unknown origin (pseudo-FUO) (Kleiman, 1982).

NATURE OF THE INFECTIONS

A careful, accurate description of the parent's perception of the child's symptoms is essential and should include the following information:

1. Onset: At what age did recurrent infection begin?
2. System involvement and location: Are the infections stereotyped or varied in their pattern? Is a single site (e.g., middle ear, lung, throat) affected? Is the site of involvement constant, e.g., pneumonia always in the right middle lobe?
3. Type: Are infections due to viruses, fungi, or bacteria, or are all types seen? Do they "appear" to respond to antibacterial therapy?
4. Frequency and severity: Frequency is defined in terms of the length of the interval between two clinically apparent infections. It is important to distinguish a recrudescence of the original infection after the cessation of antibiotics, e.g., inadequately treated sinusitis, from recurrence. Is there periodicity, seasonal effects, and so on?

Children vary greatly in their response to infections. Severity may be judged by the degree and duration of fever, the extent of prostration and diminished activity, weight loss, time spent in bed, out of school, or in the hospital, and the intensity of the local manifestations of the inflammatory process.

Documentation of complaints with hospital records, laboratory values, radiographs, culture results, and so on, is important for adequate evaluation.

FACTORS AFFECTING SUSCEPTIBILITY TO INFECTION AND THE PARENTAL COMPLAINTS

Parental Expectations

It is important to estimate the parental threshold for anxiety. Few adults appreciate the number of viruses (numbering several hundred) and bacteria (nearly 100 different types of pneumococci and beta hemolytic streptococci alone) to which children are exposed and by which they may become infected. Most normal children experience approximately 100 infections by the time they are 10 years old—an average of about one infection every five or six weeks. In most normal children, only a small number of these infections are severe enough to be clinically apparent. Parents differ markedly in the degree of equanimity with which they can tolerate these frequent but usually mild departures from good health and healthy behavior in their child.

Environmental Factors

The environment has an extremely important role in the frequency and intensity of exposure to infection. The young child's social environment is usually limited to home, school, day care facility, or outdoor and indoor play areas. Factors that are important in the transmission of infections are crowding in the home, particularly in sleeping quarters, and the size and sibling order of the family. School age siblings often acquire infections in the community and transmit them into the home. In recent years, as more women have entered the work force, daycare centers and babysitting groups have become more important in the transmission of infection, especially in children younger than two years. These settings are ideal for disease transmission, since children are usually in the infant and toddler age groups, often in diapers, and many children may be enrolled. A careful history will often associate change in the frequency of infection with a change of daycare or babysitting arrangements.

The drying effect of indoor heating, irritating fumes of chemical irritants, or the circulation of airborne microbes and allergens by forced air heating or air conditioning systems may all act to compromise the natural protective role of the mucociliary transport of the respiratory tract and either mimic or aggravate symptoms of respiratory infection.

Host Factors

The susceptibility and symptoms of the host may be influenced by genetic or environmental factors. Heredity influences the response to infection in a number of ways, many of which are poorly understood. A striking similarity to the child's complaint may often be elicited in a parent (e.g., recurrent croup, bronchitis, tonsillitis, or otitis media) and the fact that the parent outgrew this pattern of illness is reassuring.

Cystic fibrosis is a common hereditary disease in which there are repeated episodes of respiratory infection. Suspicion may be raised by the family history. A sweat test is required to exclude this condition.

Allergic reactions of the respiratory tract may mimic or predispose to infection. The allergic response itself may be triggered by infection, so that inquiry concerning allergic tendencies in the child and family and examination for physical or laboratory evidence of allergy as well as infection should be considered.

Congenital anatomical abnormalities or those acquired from trauma, foreign bodies, or previous illness may affect the functional integrity of the respiratory, gastrointestinal, or urinary tracts and lead to recurrent infections, the principal characteristic of which is recurrence in the same site.

Finally, since development of the multiple cellular, humoral, and biochemical components of the immunological defense system is under genetic control, we have come to recognize a variety of immunodeficiency syndromes, many of which are hereditary. Some arise from congenital malformations, as of the thymus, or from a variety of noxious events occurring during infancy or childhood, for example, protein-calorie malnutrition, radiation injury, certain virus infections, drug reactions, and the use of immunosuppressive agents for the treatment of neoplastic, collagen-vascular, and immunological disorders.

CLINICAL CHARACTERISTICS OF THE IMMUNODEFICIENCY SYNDROMES

Immunodeficiency predisposes to infections that are diverse both in the sites affected and in the nature of the infecting agents. Infections are more frequent and more severe and may persist longer than in normal children. Although infections in immunodeficient children are often caused by the same common pathogenic microorganisms that cause infection in normal children, clinical manifestations tend to be quantitatively different. Therefore, the physicians' suspicion of immunodeficiency disease should be aroused by (1) infection due to an unusual organism not normally pathogenic; (2) recurrence of an infection to which the child should have become immune by virtue of prior infection or immunization; or (3) an unusually persistent, severe, or progressive course of a common, usually mild infection (thrush, vaccinia, and so forth).

The immunological system consists of cellular and humoral portions. Phagocytic cells engulf microorganisms and process their antigens. Lymphoid cells are responsible for the specificity of recognition, cellular and humoral immunity, and immunological memory. Lymphocytes are divided into a T cell or thymus-dependent system, which mediates delayed hypersensitivity and immunity to most viruses, fungi, and mycobacteria, and a B cell system, from which antibody-secreting plasma cells are derived. Humoral factors include the lymphokines and antibodies derived from antigen-stimulated T and B cells, respectively. The complement system is a series of circulating plasma proteins which, when activated, release mediators of inflammation and amplify the other systems. Phagocytosis is essential for the removal and final destruction of invading pyogenic bacteria. It is then not surprising that quantitative or functional abnormalities of components of the immunological apparatus give rise to differing clinical pictures (Table 66–1).

Acquired and secondary deficiencies of the host defenses are quite common. In fact, the frequency of the acquired immunodeficiencies far exceeds that of primary immunodeficiency syndromes. Conditions associated with secondary immunodeficiency include malnutrition, severe diarrhea and protein-losing enteropathy, extensive burns, lymphoreticular malignancy, immunosuppressive therapy, uncontrolled diabetes mellitus, chronic renal failure, and diseases with persistent replicating antigens (infectious or malignant).

DEFICIENCIES OF THE PHAGOCYTIC SYSTEM

Quantitative deficiency of neutrophils (neutropenia or agranulocytosis), which may be hereditary but usually is due to drugs, hypersplenism, or bone marrow failure, deprives the body of its front-line defense against pyogenic organisms. Neutropenia may be cyclic in occurrence and result in a regular periodicity of infection.

The most common qualitative defect of polymorphonuclear leukocyte function, in which phagocytosis occurs normally but the ingested organisms are not killed, is the functional abnormality seen in chronic granulomatous disease. In this condition, the findings include fever, which may be suppressed but not eradicated by antimicrobial therapy, hypergammaglobulinemia, and enlargement of the reticuloendothelial organs due to granuloma and microabscess formation. The NBT (nitroblue tetrazolium) test or bactericidal tests serve to identify patients with this inborn error of leukocyte metabolism.

Splenic dysfunction, due to hereditary or congenital absence of the spleen or to splenectomy, predisposes to overwhelming sepsis and meningitis, especially in the child younger than five years of age. The spleen is the principal organ for removal of microorganisms from the blood of nonimmune animals. Functional asplenia due to autosplenectomy is probably one of several factors responsible for the severe pyogenic infections in children with sickle cell disease. The diagnosis of anatomical or functional asplenia may be suspected by the presence of Howell-Jolly bodies in the peripheral blood smear and confirmed with radionuclide scan.

T CELL DEFICIENCIES

Pure functional T cell deficiency seems to occur in only one rare, congenital immunodeficiency disease—the pharyngeal pouch or DiGeorge syndrome. Partial or complete absence of parathyroids results in neonatal tetany and subsequent hypoparathyroidism. There is also a variable tendency to acquire recurrent viral, fungal, and bacterial infections. Persistent thrush and malformations of the facies, ears, and great vessels are common. T cell function gradually improves in some children; an implant of fetal thymus restores T cell function very rapidly.

The most serious T cell deficiency occurs as a major feature of severe combined immune deficiency, a hereditary abnormality with either X-linked or autosomal inheritance, in which T cell and B cells are absent. Patients have a rudimentary epithelial thymus, lymphopenia, lymph nodes consisting of stroma and macrophages only, chronic pulmonary infection, chronic diarrhea, candidiasis, wasting, and an extraordinary susceptibility to infections of all kinds. This disease, formerly always fatal in the first year or two of life, may now be cured by bone marrow transplantation from a properly matched donor or by immunopotent cells from fetal liver.

Partial T cell deficiency develops in ataxia-telangiectasia, somewhat later than the primary clinical manifestations which occur in childhood, and account for the name of the disorder. cell deficiency may also be a part of several other rare syndromes.

T cell deficiency should be suspected if there is (1) persistent or recurrent thrush (candidiasis) despite antifungal treatment; (2) absence of delayed skin test reactivity to Candida antigen (after a year of age, when most children react positively); or (3) failure of blood lymphocytes to respond to stimulation with certain mitogens.

B CELL DEFICIENCIES

The antibody deficiency syndromes (hypogammaglobulinemia, agammaglobulinemia) serves as a general name for deficiency of the humoral factors especially important for the

Table 66–1. MAJOR IMMUNODEFICIENCY SYNDROMES

Syndrome	Unusual Infection	Signs and Symptoms	Screening Tests
Neutropenia	Staphylococcal; gram-negative bacterial	Mouth ulcers (cyclic)	WBC and differential
Chronic granulomatous disease	Chronic recurrent infection with staphylococci and gram-negative bacteria	Hyperplasia of reticuloendothelial system	NBT test, bactericidal test of leukocytes
Absence of the spleen	Overwhelming sepsis, pyogenic infection	Howell-Jolly bodies	Radionuclide scan for spleen
T cell deficiency Pharyngeal pouch (DiGeorge syndrome)	All types (thrush)	Neonatal tetany facies; malformation of great vessels	Serum PO_4 and a Ca, delayed hypersensitivity (Candida skin test), poor response of lymphs to PHA
Severe combined immune deficiency	All types (thrush)	Onset early (2-3 mo) wasting, runting, chronic pneumonitis	Lymphopenia, hypogammaglobulinemia, absent thymus, absent PHA response
B cell deficiency Transient hypogammaglobulinemia	Pyogenic	Both sexes; onset at 2 to 6 mo; recurrent fever, bronchitis with wheezing; normal tonsils and adenoids	Low IgG for age with low IgA, IgM
X-linked agammaglobulinemia	Recurrent pyogenic infection	Boys only: onset up to 3 yr., effusion large joint; absent or tiny tonsils or adenoids	Very low IgG ($<$ 100 mg/dl) with low or high IgM Delayed hypersensitivity normal, positive Schick after diphtheria immunization
Common variable	Pyoderma, tonsillitis, otitis media, sinusitis, pneumonia	Both sexes, any age; sprue-like syndrome common, lymph nodes small or large	Low IgG, variable IgA, IgM; delayed hypersensitivity variable
Wiskott-Aldrich syndrome	Skin infections, otitis media, pneumonia	Boys only: eczema, thrombocytopenia	IgM low, isohemagglutinins absent
Ataxia-telangiectasia	Sinopulmonary infection (late)	Both sexes, ataxia in infancy; telangiectasia 5 to 6 yr; sinusitis and bronchitis in adolescence	IgA absent (80%), delayed hypersensitivity diminished
Complement deficiency	Pyogenic infections	Sepsis; signs of autoimmune disease	C3, C4, CH_{50}

Table 66–2. MEAN IMMUNOGLOBULIN SERUM LEVELS (mg/dl) IN HEALTHY INDIVIDUALS AT VARIOUS AGES*

Age	IgM	IgA	IgG	Range: *Lowest IgG*	Range: *Highest IgG*
Newborn	11	2	1030	645	1244
1 to 3 months	30	21	430	272	762
4 to 6 months	43	28	427	206	1125
7 to 12 months	54	37	661	279	1533
13 to 24 months	58	50	762	258	1393
25 to 36 months	61	71	892	419	1274
3 to 5 years	56	93	929	569	1597
6 to 8 years	65	124	923	559	1492
9 to 11 years	79	131	1124	779	1456
12 to 16 years	59	148	946	726	1058
Adults	99	200	1158	569	1919

*From figures in Stiehm, E. R., and Fudenberg, H. H.: Serum levels of immune globulins in health and disease. A survey. Pediatrics, *37*:715, 1966, a study based on 296 normal children seen in well child clinic of University of California, San Francisco, and 30 normal adults. Small size of sample may affect variability, particularly in older age groups. Method = radial diffusion with precision within 10 per cent. Range of values given for IgG to show extent of variation.

phagocytosis of pyogenic bacteria. The clinical expression of these disorders is recurrent, severe pyogenic infections due to *Staphylococcus aureus*, pneumococci, *Hemophilus influenzae*, meningococci and, to a lesser extent, beta hemolytic streptococci and other organisms. Infections usually affect the skin, bones, joints, tonsils, paranasal sinuses, middle ears, bronchi, lungs, and leptomeninges. Infected individuals respond normally to antimicrobial therapy; however, recurrences of the same infection are common.

The basic deficiency in most cases is either (1) absence or marked reduction in the number of B cells or (2) a qualitative defect that prevents antigen-stimulated cells from transforming to plasma cells or the release of specific antibody by plasma cells. In any case, the result is antibody deficiency. This syndrome may occur in infancy as transient hypogammaglobulinemia due to a delay in maturation of B cell function; in males in early childhood as X-linked agammaglobulinemia; or in either sex at any time of life in the common variable or acquired forms of hypogammaglobulinemia. Partial or selective deficiency of one of the major immunoglobulin classes (IgG, IgM, or IgA) or of one of the subclasses of IgG may occur, in which case the range of infections may be narrower.

Recognition of these deficiencies depends upon accurate measurement of immunoglobulin in relation to age (Table 66–2) and previous immunological experience. Prompt and vigorous antimicrobial treatment of bacterial infections and regular injections of prophylactic gamma globulin in sufficient doses to maintain an adequate serum concentration of IgG can maintain agammaglobulinemic patients in good health for many years.

COMPLEMENT DEFICIENCIES

Several disorders have been described in which major components of the complement system are either absent or function suboptimally. Patients with absence of C3 or C5, dysfunction of C5, or absence of C3b inactivator have frequent pyogenic infections. Recurrent gonococcal and meningococcal infections have been associated with abnormalities of some of the late complement components. Often, patients with complement deficiencies present with autoimmune disorders such as systemic lupus erythematosus, arthritis, glomerulonephritis, or angioedema.

PHYSICAL SIGNS SUGGESTIVE OF IMMUNODEFICIENCY

Features of the physical examination that suggest recognized immunodeficiency syndromes include generalized lymphadenopathy (chronic granulomatous disease), absent or reduced lymphoid tissue (antibody, polymorph, and complement deficiencies), ataxia, telangiectasia, alopecia, intractable eczema (Wiskott-Aldrich and Job-Buckley syndromes), petechiae (Wiskott-Aldrich syndrome), partial albinism

(Chediak-Higashi syndrome), hyperelastic skin associated with joint laxity, and short-limbed dwarfism. Children with abnormalities of cell-mediated immunity often fail to thrive.

Clinical Characteristics of the Immunodeficiency Syndromes

1. Infection due to an unusual organism, not normally pathogenic.
2. Recurrence of a specific infection to which the child should have become immune by virtue of prior infection or immunization.
3. Unusually persistent, severe, or progressive course of common, usually mild infection (thrush, vaccinia, and so on).

THE DIAGNOSTIC CROSSROADS—IMMUNODEFICIENCY SYNDROME OR PSEUDO-FUO

The physician must now decide whether the information collected from the interview, medical records, and physical examination is suggestive enough of an immunodeficiency disorder to warrant further laboratory pursuit. The experience of most primary physicians as well as subspecialists asked to evaluate children with recurrent infections has been that the minority are found to have an identifiable immunodeficiency syndrome. Similarly, it is the exception that a child is found to have any identifiable biomedical cause for the recurrent fevers.

Pseudo–Fever of Unknown Origin

The majority of patients referred for evaluation of recurrent or persistent fever are found to have, singly or in combination, mild self-limited illnesses, behavioral problems, parents with misconceptions concerning health and disease, or families under stress. This syndrome has been termed pseudo-FUO (Kleiman, 1982) and is an identifiable clinical disorder that may be quickly and accurately diagnosed and effectively managed. Table 66–3 summarizes those features most frequently recognized in children with recurrent infection who are found to have pseudo-FUO.

The evaluation summarized thus far will provide sufficient information with which to identify this syndrome. If the data collected suggest that the problem is pseudo-FUO, laboratory tests should not be obtained, since this serves to augment doubt in the parents. There is also a risk that the physician may overinterpret values at the extremes of normal or be made uncertain by occasional false-positive values. Although it may be quicker and less demanding to order a series of tests which may be interpreted as normal or abnormal than to deal directly with the problems of frightened parents and child, such an approach does not cure the patient.

Table 66–3. CHARACTERISTICS OF THE CHILD WITH PSEUDO-FUO

1. Absence of documented, persistent fever.
2. Lack of objective, abnormal physical findings.
3. Previous history of significant or near fatal illness.
4. Parental fear of malignancy or crippling disease.
5. Frequent environmental exposure to illness.
6. Absence of persistent weight loss.
7. Normal ESR and platelet count.
8. Large number of missed school days due to subjective morning complaints.
9. Discordance of fever and pulse rate.
10. Family member with exposure to a medically related area.
11. Majority have, singly or in sequence, mild self-limited diseases, behavioral problems, parents with misconceptions concerning health and disease, or families under stress.

The most frequent finding in pseudo-FUO is the striking contrast between the well-nourished and healthy child and the many subjective symptoms offered in the interview. A careful history frequently leads to recollection of an initial illness often associated with physical, behavioral, or subjective symptoms, usually of some severity, e.g., tiredness, weight loss, irritability, or headache. The accompanying fever may well have persisted longer than that usually associated with a self-limited illness, and abnormal physical findings, radiographic changes, and/or mild laboratory abnormalities may also have been present. Occasionally there is the kind of overestimation of the seriousness of the initial illness that one sees in the "vulnerable child syndrome" (Green and Solnit, 1964), a disorder in which the parents secretly believe, following the recovery of their child from an earlier serious illness, that the child will die prematurely. The ensuing history usually reveals that the objective signs of the initial illness have improved, as manifested by weight gain, disappearance of fever, return to more normal levels of activity, and improvement of radiographic and laboratory abnormalities. Despite the improvement, continued parental concern may be reflected in a lowered threshold for recognition of symptoms. A cycle of frequent temperature measurement is initiated and mild, even trivial subjective symptoms become foci for concern, especially in association with normal diurnal peaks of body temperature or periodic simple febrile illnesses. By this time the child, sensing parental and often grandparental concern and responding to frequent queries as to "how he feels," begins to believe that he is, indeed, sick and he behaves accordingly. Once analyzed in this fashion, the initial complaint of recurrent fever resolves into a series of etiologically unrelated episodes misperceived by the parents, sometimes the older child, and, occasionally, the physician as recurrent illnesses superimposed on a chronic disorder.

OFFICE EVALUATION OF SUSPECTED IMMUNODEFICIENCY

Table 66–4 summarizes a group of laboratory tests that may be selected to screen a patient in whom there is strong suspicion of an immunodeficiency syndrome. If these tests are all normal and an immunodeficiency syndrome is still strongly suspected, the child is best referred to a clinical immunologist for evaluation. The immunodeficiency disorders require long-term, consistent medical supervision. Some of these patients, even those with severe combined immune deficiency, are now curable if treated early; others may be maintained in good health for many years.

Table 66–4. SCREENING TESTS FOR SUSPECTED IMMUNODEFICIENCY

Type of Immunodeficiency	Tests
B cell deficiency	1. Quantitative immunoglobulins (IgG, IgA, IgM). Age-related normal values crucial. 2. Isohemagglutinin titers (anti-A, anti-B). 3. Schick test or serum for tetanus and diphtheria antibody titers.
T cell deficiency	1. CBC and platelet count, sedimentation rate, absolute lymphocyte count. 2. Skin tests to ubiquitious antigens (Candida, SKSD, trichophyton).
Phagocytic deficiency	1. CBC, absolute neutrophil count. 2. NBT test.
Complement deficiency	1. C3, C4 levels; CH_{50}.

MANAGEMENT

Success in management will depend upon the skill with which the physician sorts out the underlying causes of the child's susceptibility. If history, physical examination, or laboratory tests suggest an immunodeficiency syndrome, then a plan of management should be outlined by a clinical immunologist, who should remain available to the primary physician for consultation and referral.

If history, physical examination and appropriate screening tests exclude a recognized immunodeficiency syndrome, a systematic, long-term plan is no less required.

If it is found that parental misconceptions concerning health and disease may underlie the problem, these misconceptions should be dealt with directly. Emphasis should be placed upon major areas of concern identified during the interview. These should include the absence of signs indicative of malignancy or crippling disease, the explanation for periodic fevers, the likely sources of frequent environmental disease exposures, the negligible likelihood of damage caused by fever itself, and the individual hereditary tendency for some children, different even in siblings, to have fever with simple illnesses.

Environmental control to reduce exposure may be elected. An example would be substituting a babysitting group with only a few children for a large daycare center. One must take special care not to add additional anxiety and guilt to a mother who is forced to work outside the home to support her family. Usually, reassurance that the illnesses will be self-limited and result in no permanent health problems is all that is necessary. It is best, before the fact, to discourage the pursuit of "medical" cures such as fad diets, gamma globulin supplements, vitamins, bacterial vaccines, chronic antimicrobial therapy, and tonsillectomy.

The child's strengths should be emphasized, especially normal growth and development despite the presence of the recurrent fevers. The family and child should leave the consultation confident in a diagnosis of health, not disease.

REFERENCES

Baehner, R. L.: Hematology of infancy and childhood. *In* Nathan, D. G., and Oski, F. A. (Eds.): Disorders of

Leukocyte Function and Development. Philadelphia, W. B. Saunders Co., 1974, pp. 493–519.
Geppert, L. J.: Composition of pediatric practice at a permanent army base in the antibiotic era. Pediatrics, *22*:336, 1958.
Green, M., and Solnit, A. J.: Reactions to the threatened loss of a child: A vulnerable child syndrome. Pediatrics, *34*:53–66, 1964.
Kleiman, M. B.: The complaint of persistent fever: Recognition and management of pseudo fever of unknown origin. Pediatr. Clin. North Am., *29*:201, 1982.
Meyer, R. J., and Haggerty, R. J.: Streptococcal infections in families. Factors altering individual susceptibility. Pediatrics, *29*:539, 1962.
Rosen, F. S.: Primary immunodeficiency. Pediatr. Clin. North Am., *12*:533, 1974.
Rosen, F. S., Alper, C. A., and Janeway, C. A.: The primary immunodeficiencies and the serum complement defects. *In* Nathan, D. G., and Oski, F. A. (Eds.): Disorders of Leukocyte Function and Development. Philadelphia, W. B. Saunders Co., 1974, pp. 529–577.
Stiehm, E. R., and Fudenberg, H. H.: Serum levels of immune globulins in health and disease. A survey. Pediatrics, *37*:715, 1966.

67

CONSTIPATION

Joseph F. Fitzgerald, M.D.

Difficulties with defecation and elimination are common in infants and children. These problems are usually mild and short-lived if proper attention is provided during the acute phase. An alteration in the diet may correct the problem, but, occasionally, stool softeners must be employed. Although chronic constipation most commonly follows an inadequately treated acute episode, in a small percentage of cases it is secondary to a more generalized pathophysiological process. Persisting difficulties with defecation may result in stool-withholding and eventual encopresis (see Chap. 68).

ETIOLOGY

Physiological constipation, a common type in children, usually begins in infancy, especially when the diet is changed from human to cow's milk. The stools become firm, smaller in quantity, and less frequent. Great effort is often necessary to expel stool. The anal irritation that often follows can lead to a pattern of withholding. This may be the major initial event in the development of psychogenic constipation. In the older child, alteration of the bowel pattern for any reason may result in constipation, anal irritation, and a withholding pattern. Psychological factors, diet, and the overuse of enemas or laxatives may be contributory. Parents often relate the development of constipation in older children to a stressful event; however, Levine (1975) found that children who are not constipated undergo similar stresses. Emotional disturbances often disappear with relief of the constipation. There is little doubt, however, that emotional problems contribute to the symptom in some cases.

Although it is rarely the chief complaint, constipation may accompany systemic disorders. A lack of fecal bulk, as in undernutrition, leads to infrequent, small, and firm stools. Dehydrated patients, as well as children with infantile renal acidosis, diabetes insipidus, hypothyroidism, and idiopathic hypercalcemia, pass small, dry stools. Amyotonia congenita, cerebral palsy, infectious polyneuritis, and congenital absence of abdominal musculature interfere with the act of defecation and lead to constipation. Constipation frequently accompanies spinal cord lesions due to a loss of mechanosensory receptors, which results in impaired sensation of rectal fullness and sphincteric dysfunction. Obstructive lesions, including anorectal stenosis, intrinsic and extrinsic tumors, and cicatrizing diseases (e.g., Crohn's disease, necrotizing enterocolitis) are associated with a decreased stool frequency. Redundancy of the rectosigmoid colon, which predisposes to constipation, may accompany chronic illness and malnutrition, or it may rarely be a primary finding in otherwise normal children (dolichocolon of Martinotti).

Loening-Baucke and Younoszai (1982), measuring anal sphincter function, found the internal anal sphincter weaker and less responsive to rectal distention in chronically constipated children compared with nonconstipated children. Their suggestion that internal sphincter dysfunction might be the cause of chronic constipation in some children is difficult to assess at this time.

CLINICAL MANIFESTATIONS

Constipation may be the only symptom, but in chronic cases anorexia, vomiting, failure to thrive, persistent abdominal distention, and excessive flatulence may be reported. Chronic stool retention, evident on rectal examination and on abdominal radiographs, is a common cause of recurrent abdominal pain in children.

Abdominal distention is usually not marked with functional constipation, since gas escapes normally. Fecal masses are often palpated on abdominal examination. Anal disease may be present. Digital rectal examination reveals variable amounts of firm or inspissated stool in the rectal ampulla. Marked abdominal distention raises the possibility of Hirschsprung's disease, especially when the rectum is empty on digital examination; this disorder is highly unlikely when fecal soiling is present. A lax anal sphincter, abnormally flat buttocks (sacral agenesis), or a deep pilonidal dimple with hair tuft (spina bifida occulta) suggests neurological disease.

EVALUATION

A thorough history and physical examination usually precludes the need for additional evaluation; however, anteroposterior and lateral abdominal radiographs are occasionally indicated to help assess the degree of gaseous distention and the amount of stool in the colon. When the possibility of aganglionosis remains, an *unprepared* colon study should be obtained (Franken, 1975). The radiographic diagnosis of congenital aganglionosis (Hirschsprung's disease) depends on the demonstration of a transition from normal-size (aganglionic bowel) to dilated (normally innervated) colon. Detection of the transition zone is more difficult in the prepared colon. Delayed radiographs (24 and 48 hours) may be of value if the initial study is not diagnostic. Additional studies, when necessary, include anorectal manometry (Tobon et al., 1968; Meunier et al., 1976) and rectal biopsy (Campbell and Noblett, 1969).

MANAGEMENT

Dietary corrective measures, useful in cases of simple constipation of short duration, include increasing the intake of fluids and of dietary residue (bran, whole grain cereal, fresh fruits, and vegetables). One to two teaspoonfuls of barley malt extract added to a feeding two to three times daily has been used successfully in infants with unusually firm stools. Stool softeners can be prescribed in older children. Dioctyl sodium sulfosuccinate (5 to 10 mg/kg/24 hours), alone or in combination with other agents, is a safe agent that may be administered for extended periods of time. It is usually ineffective, however, when voluntary stool retention exists.

A bowel training program is instituted in older children. The parents (and older patient) are provided with simple, specific explanations of the gastrocolic reflex, the role of rectosigmoid filling, and the effects of meals on bowel-wall tension and pressure. Davidson et al. (1963) stressed the importance of supporting the feet in order to obtain proper mechanical advantage while passing stool. Mineral oil in a dose of 30 to 75 ml is prescribed twice daily between meals for the patient who is recalcitrant to the above measures. A sweetened beverage or hard candy may be taken simultaneously or immediately afterwards to eliminate the oily sensation. The dosage of oil is tapered slowly and discontinued after four to six months. An occasional patient with a profoundly hypotonic colon benefits from a stimulant laxative that acts primarily on the colon (e.g., senna); however, it is our practice to avoid stimulants except in patients with neurological diseases.

The child with a neurological disorder poses an especially difficult problem. In an effort to increase the amount of fiber in the diet, we often prescribe a bulk-type stool softener such as psyllium hydrophilic mucilloid and empty the rectum before an impaction forms with a daily bisacodyl suppository or saline enema.

Anal fissures often accompany constipation and probably play an important role in the development of a stool-withholding pattern. A fissure near the mucocutaneous junction may not be seen unless the infant is in the knee-chest position, the buttocks are spread widely apart, and a bright light is used. A well-lubricated anoscope or otoscope speculum may be used to visualize lesions not evident on external inspection. They should be treated promptly. Small enemas should be administered to clear impactions and a stool softener, such as dioctyl sodium sulfosuccinate, prescribed to prevent their formation. The mother is instructed to dilate the anal sphincter once or twice daily with a well-lubricated covered finger or glycerine suppository. If this regimen fails, one ounce of mineral or olive oil can be introduced into the rectum with an ear syringe at bedtime. An anesthetic agent, e.g., dibucaine, can be applied to the anal verge prior to defecation.

REFERENCES

Campbell, P. E., and Noblett, H. R.: Experience with rectal suction biopsy in the diagnosis of Hirschsprung's disease. J. Pediatr. Surg., *4*:410, 1969.

Davidson, M., Kugler, M. M., and Bauer, C. H.: Diagnosis and management in children with severe and protracted constipation and obstipation. J. Pediatr., *62*:261, 1963.

Fitzgerald, J. F.: Difficulties with defaecation and elimination in children. Clin. Gastroenterol, *6*:283, 1977.

Franken, E. A., Jr.: Gastrointestinal Radiology in Pediatrics. Hagerstown, MD, Harper and Row, 1975, p. 323.

Levine, M. D.: Children with encopresis: A descriptive analysis. Pediatrics, *56*:412, 1975.

Loening-Baucke, V. A., and Younoszai, M. K.: Abnormal anal sphincter response in chronically constipated children. J. Pediatr., *100*:213, 1982.

Meunier, P., Mollard, P., and Jaubert de Beaujeu, M.: Manometric studies of anorectal disorders in infancy and childhood: An investigation of the physiopathology of continence and defaecation. Br. J. Surg., *63*:402, 1976.

Tobon, F., Reid, N. C. R. W., Talbert, J. L., and Schuster, M. M.: Nonsurgical test for Hirschsprung's disease. N. Engl. J. Med., *278*:188, 1968.

68

ENCOPRESIS

Morris Green, M.D.

Encopresis with functional megacolon secondary to chronic constipation is characterized by repeated fecal soiling owing to the involuntary passage of feces into the underpants of a child over four years of age in the absence of neurological or other anatomical factors. Fecal soiling or smearing of the underclothing with soft, formed, or liquid stool is a consistent finding, usually occurring during the waking hours, most commonly in the late afternoon, but rarely during sleep. Voluminous stools may be passed periodically. Commonly the child is unaware of his odor or of the sensation that he needs to go to the toilet. Colicky abdominal pain may be reported in younger children.

Rectal examination reveals a large rectal vault packed with firm or hard but, occasionally, soft feces. Large amounts of stool may be noted on abdominal palpation. An occasional child will have only rectal retention with a megarectum rather than a megacolon. Abdominal distention is usually minimal. An anal wink reflex is present. In the presence of a characteristic history and physical examination, a barium enema is not indicated. A plain film of the abdomen is helpful, if the physician is uncertain about the amount of fecal retention.

The chronic constipation that regularly precedes the onset of encopresis may be due to painful defecation secondary to an anal fissure, coercive bowel training, fear of the toilet, or voluntary withholding of stools. The accumulation of a fecal mass secondary to chronic constipation causes distention of the rectum and activation of sensory receptors in the rectal wall. Relaxation of the puborectalis muscle and internal sphincter follow reflexly. With succeeding relaxation of the levator ani and shortening of the anal canal, the external sphincter becomes incompetent and allows leakage of feces around the impaction.

MANAGEMENT

When encopresis has been present for months or years, the child and the family come to the doctor ashamed, discouraged, and frustrated. Their resignation needs to be dispelled by the doctor's assurance that this physiological problem is, in fact, common and can, in time, be mastered—although this may take months and recurrences may occur. To achieve this goal, the following steps in management must be meticulously explained and followed. Most children can be treated on an ambulatory basis, but hospitalization may be necessary initially when the fecal impaction is very large, compliance is uncertain, or enemas given by the mother seem psychologically inappropriate.

I. Explanation

Both the parents and the child need an understandable, concrete explanation of why the fecal soiling occurs. This is usually best accomplished by drawing a diagram of the rectosigmoid area, the anal canal, and the sphincters. Referring to the diagram, one may demonstrate how a hollow viscus like the colon will elongate and enlarge proximal to a chronic partial obstruction—the fecal mass—with resultant loss of tone and increase in absorptive surface. Demonstrating the plain film of the abdomen may make the explanation graphic. It may then be shown how removal of the impaction in the rectum will correct the fecal seepage and over time permit the colon to regain normal size and tone.

II. Cleansing out the retained stool
   A. Hypertonic phosphate enemas (adult Fleet enemas) should be repeated two to three times at 12-hour intervals. Usually three enemas are required.
   B. The first series of enemas should be followed by a bisacodyl (Dulcolax) suppository twice a day for one day and then a bisacodyl tablet on the third day.
   C. A plain film of the abdomen may then be obtained to ensure adequate cleansing. If retained stool is still present, the cycle of enemas and suppositories will need to be repeated until all the retained stool is passed.

III. Mineral oil

Once the bowel is cleansed, light, unsweetened mineral oil is prescribed to overcome voluntary stool withholding. This will generally require 30 to 75 ml twice a day between meals. To improve its taste and acceptance, the oil may be refrigerated, mixed in fruit juice or ice cream, or followed by a sweetened beverage or hard candy. Excessive leakage of the mineral oil may follow a recurrence of the fecal retention. After four to six months, when the colon has returned to more normal size and regular bowel habits have been achieved, the mineral oil may be gradually tapered in amount and then discontinued.

IV. Bowel training

The child is to sit on the toilet for 10 minutes twice a day at the same time, preferably after breakfast and dinner. Use of a kitchen timer permits the child to clock himself.

V. Other measures
   A. Excessive milk intake is discouraged.
   B. A high roughage diet is encouraged, including the use of bran cereal or wafers if accepted by the child.

VI. Reinforcement
   A. A calendar should be posted at home and the child asked to check off each time he takes mineral oil or sits on the toilet.
   B. For younger children, a star may be given for each day's compliance with a "surprise" toy for each week's achievement.
   C. The child and family should report to the doctor by phone once a week and, if geographically convenient, be seen once a month.

VII. Relapse
   A. The parent and child should be advised initially that relapses may occur and that they do not mean ultimate failure.
   B. If a relapse occurs, adjustment of the mineral oil dose or a repeat cycle of cleansing enemas is required.
   C. The physician should continue to reinforce his expectation that in time the child will recover normal bowel function.

VII. Counseling

When psychosocial problems are evident, counseling is indicated either by the pediatrician or by another mental health professional.

REFERENCE

Levine, M.D.: Encopresis: Its potentiation, evaluation, and alleviation. Pediatr. Clin. North Am., 29:315, 1982.

69

UNDESCENDED TESTIS

Michael E. Mitchell, M.D.

The term *cryptorchidism* is a general term derived from the Greek root "crypto," which means hidden, and "orchis," or testis. The observation that one or both testes do not reside in the scrotum should bring to mind four different diagnoses: (1) mobile or retractile testis, (2) ectopic testis, (3) true undescended testis, and (4) absent testis.

A mobile or retractile testis is the most common explanation for a nonpalpable scrotal testis. It is also the most frequently missed of the different diagnoses. Because this represents a normal variation in anatomy, diligence and persistence on the part of the physician can avert needless therapeutic intervention. A history of previous scrotal presence of the testis in question should encourage repeat, careful examination before hormonal or surgical therapy. Examination should be performed in warm, quiet surroundings. The patient must be relaxed. Then, with the patient in the supine position, gentle pressure is applied with the examiner's finger tips along the inguinal canal while gently milking the canal contents toward the scrotum. Passive observation with the patient erect may also be effective. Any testis that is, thereby, brought well into the scrotum needs no further intervention.

Ectopia of the testis is felt to result from abnormal attachments of the gubernaculum and subsequent "misdirection" of descent. The testis is normal and is most commonly located in the subcutaneous tissue anterior to the fascia of the inguinal canal. Rarely, ectopic testes are located in the thigh or even on the contralateral side. Unlike the mobile testis, the ectopic testis cannot be manipulated into position and will not reposition with gonadotropin. Testicular ectopia is a surgical condition that, like the true undescended testis, should be treated early.

The true undescended testis remains a topic of considerable discussion and debate as to pathophysiology (i.e., is the testis not down because it is primarily abnormal or does it become abnormal because it is primarily not down?). The ultimate truth is not at hand, and the debate may stem from the fact that there are a variety of different mechanisms for failure of descent ranging from dysgenesis of the testis (as in Klinefelter's syndrome) to hormonal abnormalities (abnormality in the hypothalamic-pituitary gonadal axis) to mechanical problems (as in prune-belly syndrome).

Several findings seem to be consistent. First, most testes descend in the first year of life (Scorer, 1964). Second, undescended testes left untreated are associated with decreased fertility, and the earlier the testis is brought into the scrotum, the greater potential for fertility (Ludwig and Potempa, 1981; Mengel et al., 1981). Histological studies also support this finding (Hedinger, 1979), which is true for unilateral and bilateral pathology. Third, the untreated undescended testis has a much higher potential for tumor degeneration, and early reports seem to show that early treatment reverses this potential (Martin, 1979). Because histological changes occur as early as three years of age, and in view of the above reasons, orchiopexy is now recommended between the ages of one and two years. Gonadotropin (HCG) may be effective in the unilateral case but should always be given in the bilateral nonpalpable testis case to facilitate diagnosis. This may be therapeutic as well.

Unilateral absence of the testis is a diagnosis made at the operating table after inguinal and intraperitoneal exploration. Bilateral anorchia with normal genitalia is a medical diagnosis (Levitt et al., 1978). With HCG stimulation (500 to 1000 IU/day for 3 days), the absence of a significant serum testosterone increase (10 times over base line) in the presence of elevated FSH and LH levels in a prepubertal male should indicate the absence of functioning testicular tissue. Surgical intervention should not be pursued. Testosterone supplementation will be necessary at puberty.

REFERENCES

Hedinger, C. H. R.: Histological data in cryptorchidism: Diagnosis and treatment. Pediatr. Adolesc. Endocrinol., *6*:3, 1979.

Levitt, S. B., Kogan, S. J., Engel, R. M., et al.: The impalpable testis: A rational approach to management. J. Urol., *120*:515, 1978.

Ludwig, G., and Potempa, J.: Der optimale Zeitpunkt der Behandlung des Kryptorchismus. Dtsch. Med. Wochenschr., *100*:618, 1975.

Martin, D. C.: Germinal cell tumors of the testis after orchiopexy. J. Urol., *121*:422, 1979.

Mengel, W., Zimmermann, F. A., and Hecker, W. C.: Timing of repair for undescended testes. *In* Fonkalsrud, E. W., and Mengel, W. (Eds.): The Undescended Testis. Chicago, Year Book Medical Publishers, Inc., 1981, pp. 170–183.

Scorer, C. G.: The descent of the testis. Arch. Dis. Child., *39*:605, 1964.

70

MUSCULOSKELETAL DISORDERS

Congenital, Developmental, and Nontraumatic

G. Paul DeRosa, M.D.

This chapter will stress the physical examination of the musculoskeletal system. Only topics that (1) occur frequently, (2) need prompt orthopaedic referral, or (3) elicit unnecessary parental anxiety will be discussed. Attempts will be made to alert the practitioner to potential pitfalls in diagnosis. Many of the so-called orthopaedic deformities in the neonatal period are merely the result of "intrauterine packing," and as such have excellent prognosis; others are transmitted genetically, so a careful family history and " a look at" mother and father will frequently lead to a diagnosis and, in turn, prognosis for the problem at hand.

EXAMINATION OF THE NEONATE

In the unclad newborn, all four limbs should be moving in a random, purposeless fashion. If the child fails to move an upper extremity, paralysis secondary to brachial plexus palsy (birth trauma) versus pseudo-paralysis of the limb must be considered. The latter may be secondary to fracture of the clavicle or humerus, separation of the upper humeral epiphysis, or neonatal sepsis involving the proximal humerus and adjacent shoulder joint.

The Head, Neck, and Upper Extremities

Place a hand behind the baby's shoulders and gently lift forward. The head gently falls backward, and the neck is easily visualized. The "V" made by the two sternocleidomastoid muscles attaching to the sternum and clavicle is easily seen and palpated. The medial end of the clavicle, the sternum, and the entire anterior shoulder are easily examined in this position. Feel for the crepitus of fracture (later for the healing wad of callus of a neglected clavicular fracture); palpate for the tight band of a contracted sternocleidomastoid muscle or the "tumor" in the sternocleidomastoid muscle that frequently accompanies congenital muscular torticollis. The head should be easily rotated to the right and the left so that the chin touches each shoulder. Lateral inclination of the head so that the ear touches the adjacent shoulder on either side should be easily accomplished. Any resistance to motion, limited motion, or pain on attempted motion should be carefully evaluated by adequate AP and lateral cervical spine films. If one cannot incriminate a contracted sternocleidomastoid muscle for the limited motion, one must inspect the cervical spine for anomalies of failure of segmentation, i.e., the Klippel-Feil syndrome, or generalized "confusion of the cervical spine."

Torticollis has been associated with a higher than normal incidence of congenital dislocation of the hip, so when torticollis is seen, an even closer inspection of the lower extremities is in order. Frequently, children are seen who have (1) a persistence of head molding, (2) a torticollis, (3) long C-shaped scoliosis from occiput to sacrum, and (4) asymmetry of the hip abduction. Best termed the *molded baby syndrome*, the prognosis is usually good for complete resolution *provided* the asymmetrical hip abduction is overcome by stretching of the adducted hip to prevent hip subluxation.

The shoulder and elbow should be put through a passive range of motion. Fracture separation of the upper humeral epiphysis will be manifest by crepitus in the shoulder region. Radiographs will not be helpful until 7 to 10 days after delivery when the healing periosteal new bone formation becomes ossified.

The elbow flexion contraction of the newborn (30 to 45 degrees) may be present up to age six weeks, but full flexion should always be present. Pronation and supination of the forearm (not hand or wrist) should be full in the newborn. If rotation is limited, congenital synostosis of the proximal radius and ulna is the cause. This may be evident on radiographs as a bony bridge but

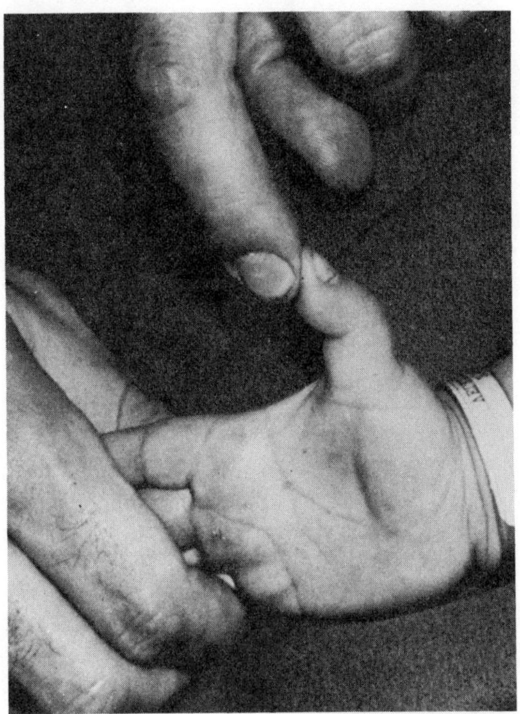

Figure 70–1. The interphalangeal joint of the thumb fails to fully extend. Palpation at the base of the thumb revealed a node on the flexor tendon. Surgical release of the tendon sheath allowed full function.

more than likely will be present as a cartilaginous or fibrous bridge that will ossify later.

The final part of the head and upper limb exam is inspection of the hand. Observe the grasp reflex and note that extension of the fingers elicits flexion of the thumb. Be certain to passively extend the thumb fully! Contracture of the interphalangeal joint may be present, or the deformity may be secondary to a trigger thumb, owing to a discrepancy in size between the flexor tendon and its synovial sheath (Fig. 70–1). Most trigger thumbs resolve spontaneously, but those still present after six months should be surgically released.

The Spinal Column

The child is placed prone on the examining hand, and inspection of the back from occiput to sacrum is accomplished. Each spinous process should be felt in line to be certain that an underlying bony abnormality is not overlooked. While major malformations such as myelomeningocele will readily be apparent, a hairy patch, a pigmented nevus, or a sacral dimple or pit is sometimes only the cutaneous manifestation of an underlying malformation of the vertebral column. This defect, which frequently includes not only the osseous structures but also the spinal cord and nerve roots, is collectively called the *spinal dysraphism syndrome*. If the lower extremities and sphincter function appear normal, then the cutaneous manifestations may simply be recorded. Frequently, however, older children are brought to the pediatrician with the complaint of delayed continence, either bowel or bladder; a loss of continence; or a misshapen foot, either cavus or varus, that was *not* present at birth. These complaints must be considered due to the spinal dysraphism syndrome until proven otherwise.

Children with congenital problems of the lower extremities, foot deformities, and particularly asymmetrical findings such as atrophy or hemihypertrophy should be suspected of having an underlying vertebral anomaly. The young child with a congenital scoliosis usually does not have a neurological problem unless there is associated diastematomyelia, myelodysplasia, or sacral agenesis. Because of the high incidence of associated kidney and bladder problems, routine intravenous pyelogram is a necessity for all children found to have vertebral anomalies.

The Lower Extremities

For this phase of the examination, the child should be placed on his back on a firm examining surface with the hips and knees flexed. One should be careful not to extend the neonate's hip or knee forcibly, as flexion deformities as great as 60 degrees may be present at the hip and up to 45 to 50 degrees at the knee. Full flexion, of course, is always maintained. By placing the feet side by side, with the soles on the table, allowing the hips and knees to flex, one can ascertain the relative height of the knees. If one knee is at a lower level (a positive Galeazzi sign or Allis sign), one can assume that the shortened knee is secondary to either a dislocation of the hip on that side, a congenitally short femur, or both. If the knees are at the same level, one can assume that (1) both hips are reduced and in the sockets, or (2) both hips are dislocated. If the perineum appears unusually wide and there are deep groin creases on both sides, one must suspect that bilateral dislocations of the hip have occurred. After inspection for Galeazzi's sign, each hip should be examined separately to determine hip joint stability, dislocatability, and reducibility.

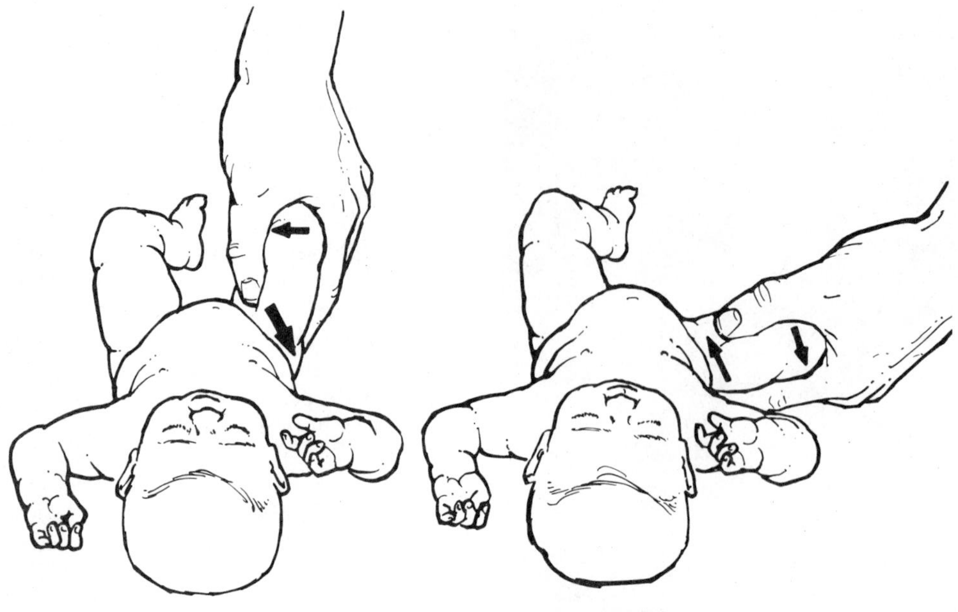

Figure 70–2. Proper method of performing the Provocative maneuver of Barlow and accompanying Ortolani "jerk sign".

The Neonatal Hip Examination

In the newborn, the examiner should be less concerned about range of motion of the hip joint than the stability of the hip itself. Attempting to abduct the infant's hips to the point that the thighs touch the examining table serves only to hurt the infant, cause spasm, and preclude an adequate examination. We must determine the following: (1) Is the hip reduced? (2) Is the hip dislocated? (3) If reduced, is it dislocatable? (4) If dislocated, is it reducible?

The classic Ortolani "jerk sign" of the dislocated hip reducing into the acetabulum should be tested. The flexed hip is abducted gently, the examiner's long finger on the greater trochanter. As abduction is increased, pressure on the trochanter from behind lifts the femoral head back into the socket with a palpable, visible, and sometimes audible "jerk." Unfortunately, the term "click" has been substituted for "jerk" in the pediatric literature. It is the *movement* of the hip and *not* the sound that is the positive finding.

A variation of the Ortolani test has become known as the provocative maneuver of Barlow (Fig. 70–2). The examination is performed by placing the hip in the most unstable position of flexion and slight adduction (the other hand stabilizes the pelvis with the thumb on symphysis and fingers on sacrum). Gentle downward pressure with hand and lateral pressure with the thumb over the adductor region pushes the unstable hip out of the acetabulum. At this point, the Ortolani maneuver of abducting the thigh and lifting on the trochanter with the long finger will reposition the femoral head into the acetabulum with the classic jerk sign of Ortolani. The normal hip *will not* dislocate. The femur may break, but the hip will not dislocate! (The author has treated two cases of fractured femur secondary to overenthusiastic examinations.) It is a gentle test performed upon a *quiet* infant. It does no good to overpower the screaming baby!

The incidence of the positive jerk sign of Ortolani is one to three per 1000 live births, whereas the incidence of a positive provocative maneuver of Barlow may be as high as 15 per 1000 live births. This lends credence to the belief that hip joint laxity is a prime factor in congenital dislocation of the hip.

Probably there is no single cause of congenital dislocation of the hip. Rather, the etiology is multifactorial, with both mechanical and physiological factors combining to produce instability and subsequent dislocation. That 60 per cent of affected children are first-born suggests mechanical causes. Breech presentation also plays a significant role in etiology. Post-delivery environmental factors may also contribute to the development of hip instability and dislocation. In the first months after delivery, the normal physiological position is one of flexion and abduction. Societies in which infants customarily are wrapped onto a cradle board or swaddled to maintain hip extension have an incidence of dislocation 10 times that in populations that do not follow such practices.

TREATMENT

If simple splintage in the reduced position can be accomplished, a near-normal or normal femoral head in the acetabulum will develop in 96 per cent of cases. If the diagnosis is not made and the hip is left dislocated or becomes dislocated in the first several weeks after birth, adaptive changes quickly occur, and the chances of having a normal hip diminish greatly. As the child grows, clinical evidence of the untreated dislocation becomes more obvious (Fig. 70–3). Ortolani sign becomes negative as the child gets older (two to four months). The femoral head becomes trapped outside the acetabulum, and the muscle groups, especially the adductors and the flexors, become shortened about the hip. The adductor tightness is reflected in limited abduction of the thigh. The shortening is then apparent in extra skin folds, deep thigh creases, and the positive Galeazzi sign (unequal height of knees).

Routine x-ray examination in the newborn period to detect typical CDH is *not* reliable. The x-rays may not reveal the dislocation. The usual bony landmarks are not visible, since the infant's pelvis and head and neck of femur are all cartilage at this point in time. The radiolucent cartilage does not allow for accurate measurement of bony landmarks. Therefore, negative findings on radiographs *do not rule out* the presence of dislocation or dislocatable hips. Reliable radiographic signs usually do not become apparent until two to four months following the dislocation. By this time, the characteristic findings of a "shallow acetabulum," a laterally placed femoral neck, and a delay in the ossification of the capital femoral nucleus are all "tip-offs" to the diagnosis. It is stressed that the physical examination in the newborn period is the *only reliable test* for hip joint stability.

Many commercially available splints and harnesses are available today. There is no one best design, and the orthopaedic surgeon should use the one with which he is most comfortable.

Examination of the Knee, Leg, and Foot

An uncommon problem but a *true orthopaedic* emergency is the congenital dislocation or subluxation of the knee (Fig. 70–4). Immediate management within the first few hours after birth can usually result in a satisfactory and nearly normal knee. Delay of as little as 24 hours may render the knee irreducible and require traction and/or surgical procedures. If the leg, ankle, and foot are normal and one can palpate a patella in the area anterior to the knee, reduction should be achieved immediately by gradually flexing the knee with gentle traction on the tibia. The knee is bent as far as possible without force. At this point, an aluminum and foam finger splint with an elastic wrap or tape is applied. This is removed on a twice-daily basis so that further flexion can be accomplished until 90 to 100 degrees of flexion is achieved. In our experience, this has met with good success, provided it is accomplished in the first six hours after birth. In cases that have gone longer than 24 hours, we have had to

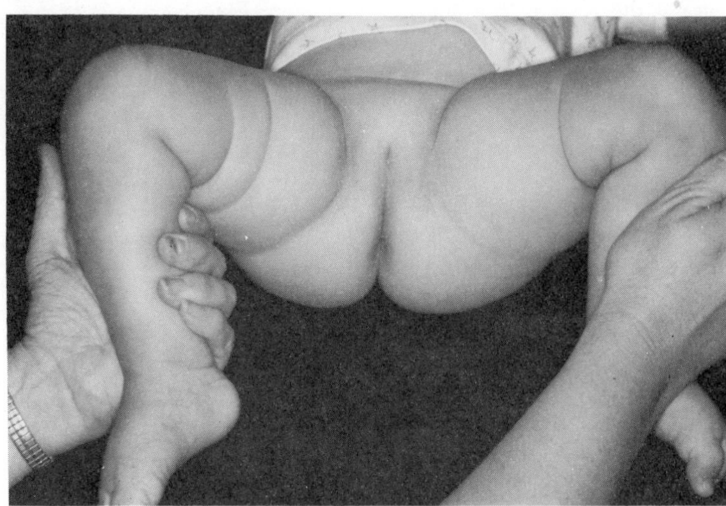

Figure 70–3. Ten month infant with classic signs of hip joint dislocation: deep groin crease, extra skin folds, limited abduction and positive Galeazzi sign.

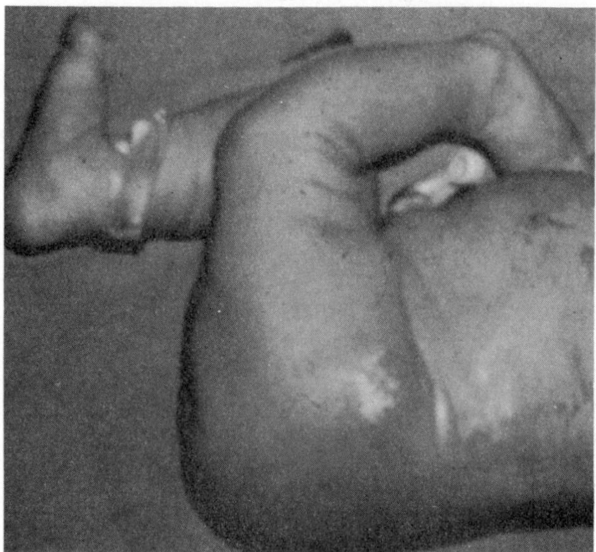

Figure 70–4. Newborn with congenital dislocation of the left knee (genu recurvatum).

resort to distraction pin techniques to reduce the dislocation. Frequently, a dislocation of the hip exists in association with the hyperextended dislocated knee, so once the knee has been flexed and treated, care should be taken that a dislocation of the hip is not overlooked.

It is common for most babies who are packed in utero to have outwardly bowed, medially rotated legs, so-called internal tibial torsion. This is the norm. The child can usually be folded back into the intrauterine position, and one can decide which leg was over the other by the amount of outward curving and medial rotation (Fig. 70–5). Of more importance than the outwardly curved tibia is a sharp, angular anterior or lateral bowing. Anterolateral bowing of the tibia has been classified as benign provided there is a medullary canal visible on radiograph, or "at risk" for fracture if there is a cyst at the apex of the anterolateral bow (Fig. 70–6). Frequently, these children are born with a fracture through the bowed portion of the tibia or suffer fracture within the first year of life. Such fractures fail to unite and become congenital pseudarthroses of the tibia. These pseudarthroses are associated in over 70 per cent of cases with neurofibromatosis. Anterolateral bowing of the tibia with a narrow, sclerotic canal or cystic changes is an orthopaedic emergency. These tibiae should be protected from impending fracture by casts or braces throughout the growth of the child. In contradistinction, posterior or posterior medial bowing at the junction of the middle and lower thirds of the tibia, termed *kyphoscoliosis of the tibia*, usually will spontaneously improve with growth of the child. The only problem is usually a slight leg length inequality of 1 to 1.5 inches at time of skeletal maturity.

Metatarsus adductus, either a supple or rigid

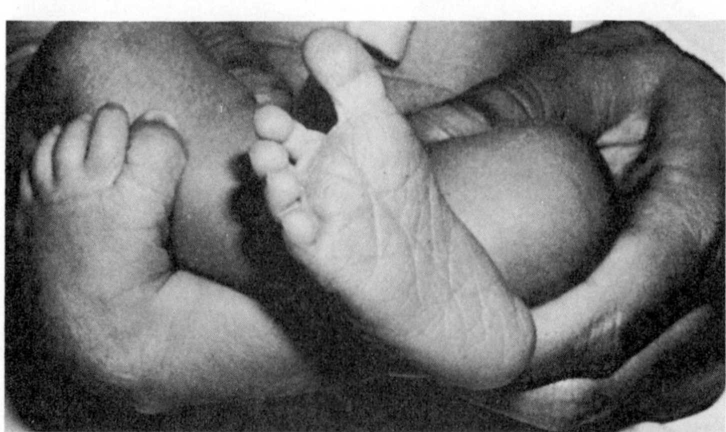

Figure 70–5. Neonate being folded into the in utero position.

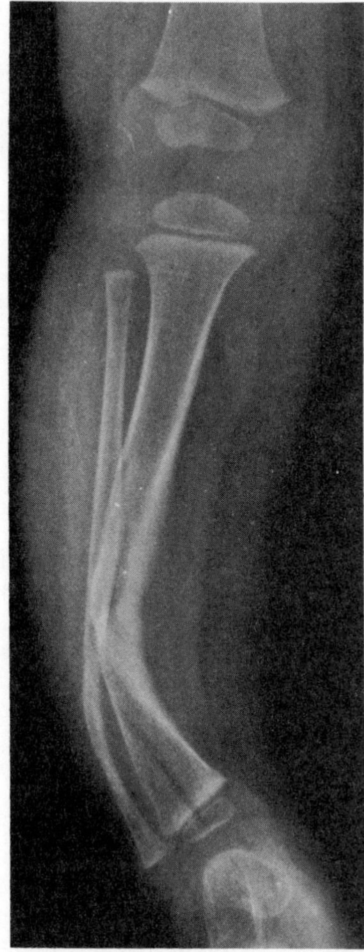

Figure 70–6. Anterior lateral bow of the tibia. No medullary canal is evident. Sclerosis in the area indicates this tibia is "at risk" for fracture.

deformity of the forefoot medially deviated from the midfoot and hindfoot, is a common newborn foot problem. Many of these are simply the result of intrauterine packing and with gentle passive stretching and avoidance of prone sleeping the problem will spontaneously abate. Those that are rigid and do not overcorrect beyond neutral on passive stretching should be vigorously manipulated and placed in serial plaster casts to stretch the contracted parts and allow for a normal fitting of shoes in the future. If the foot is supple and fully overcorrectable beyond neutral, and upon stimulation demonstrates all four motor groups of dorsiflexion, plantarflexion, evertors, and invertors, passive manipulation is all that is usually necessary. If the foot is at all rigid and incapable of being overcorrected, manipulation and serial plaster are mandatory. True clubfoot, that is, congenital talipes equinovarus, is a frequent problem in the newborn (Fig. 70–7). The entire foot is deviated toward the midline with the heel in varus and equinus and the rest of the foot inverted. The goal of treatment is a clinically and radiographically corrected foot that is flexible and fits into conventional shoes. In the newborn, the treatment should begin at once with manipulation of the clubfoot and application of either plaster casts or adhesive strapping. Adhesive strapping is certainly much easier to use in the newborn period, since manipulations (Fig. 70–8) can be carried out at each diaper change by the mother by elongating the medial border of the foot, attempting to reduce the midfoot upon the hindfoot, and pulling the os calcis down out of equinus. If one relies upon plaster casts, these need to be changed at frequent intervals, for the correction does not come from the casts but from the manipulation of the foot. Aggressive, early treatment will lessen the likelihood that surgery will be required, but if a plateau is reached, with no further gains made by the manipulation and application of either plasters or splinting, surgery is indicated. The goal is to have a plantigrade foot, unfettered by plaster casts or splints, at the time the child begins to cruise and bear weight.

Calcaneal valgus foot position is most likely the result of the intrauterine posturing. These children have a higher incidence of dislocation of the ipsilateral hip. Thus, whenever a calca-

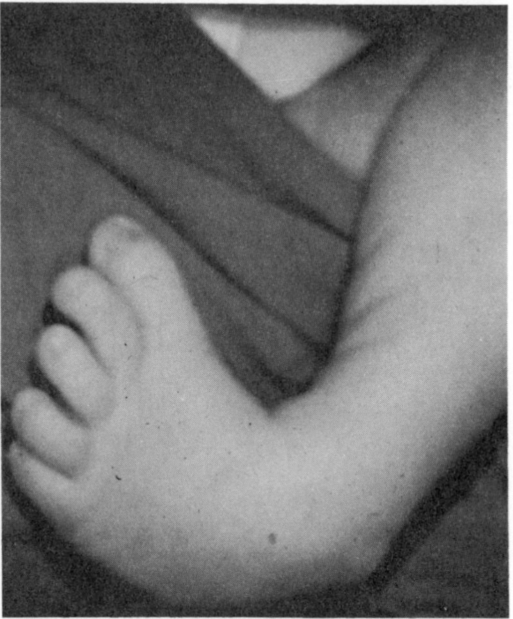

Figure 70–7. Talipes equinovarus, i.e., clubfoot deformity in the newborn. The entire foot deviates toward the midline.

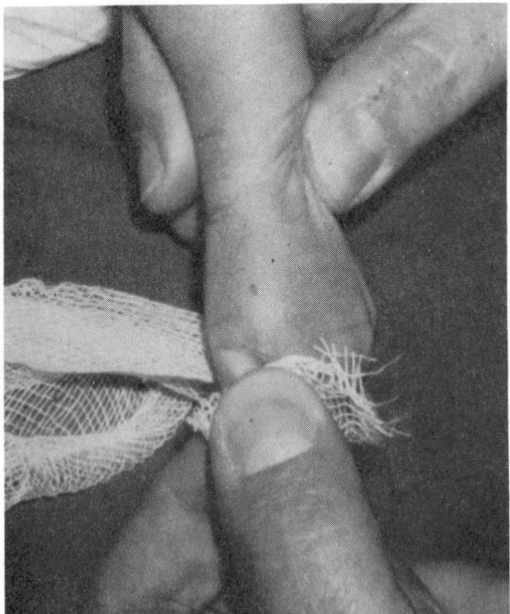

Figure 70–8. Manipulation of clubfoot. Elongation of the medial border of the foot attempted to reduce the midfoot (navicular) upon the hindfoot (talus).

neal valgus foot is seen, careful attention should be paid to the examination of the hips. Generally, passive manipulation, gently stretching out the anterior structures with or without splinting between manipulations, will correct the valgus deformity. On occasion, strapping or plaster may be necessary for more rigid deformities. Care must be taken not to confuse a calcaneal valgus foot with a pes convex valgus or a rocker bottom foot deformity (Fig. 70–9). This is a difficult orthopaedic problem requiring considerable expertise. The talus is in vertical alignment so that the hindfoot and forefoot are both deformed (Fig. 70–10). The posterior structures (capsule and Achilles tendon) are very tight, as well as the anterior structures. Usually the deformity is very rigid, with no motion available at the ankle joint. This birth defect may be associated with arthrogryposis, Turner's syndrome, or other congenital anomalies involving the central nervous system. Orthopaedic surgeons distinguish between idiopathic vertical talus and that with a neurological basis. The great majority of these will come to operative intervention. Early treatment yields a more satisfactory result than allowing the foot to remain uncorrected into the walking years.

ROTATIONAL PROBLEMS OF THE GROWING LOWER EXTREMITIES

As stated before, most babies are packed in utero with their hips and knees flexed and with one tibia overlapping the other, accounting for varying degrees of outwardly curved tibia and medially rotated feet and ankles (see Fig. 70–5). In addition, the feet may wrap about the opposite member and achieve marked adductus or positions that are usually passively correctable. In general, if normal growth and development are allowed to take place, the legs begin to unwind. Longitudinal studies have shown the bimalleolar axis (that is, a line running from the medial malleolus through lateral malleolus) externally rotates during the first several years of life. Many individuals, however, persist in having outwardly bowed, medially rotated tibia and feet, and they are brought to the physician with the complaint of "toeing-in" or tripping while walking. If one takes a good history and observes the child's sitting and sleeping habits, he will find that in a great majority of cases, the child sits with knees flexed, the feet internally rotated, and his bottom resting on his feet. This perpetuates the internal rotation deform-

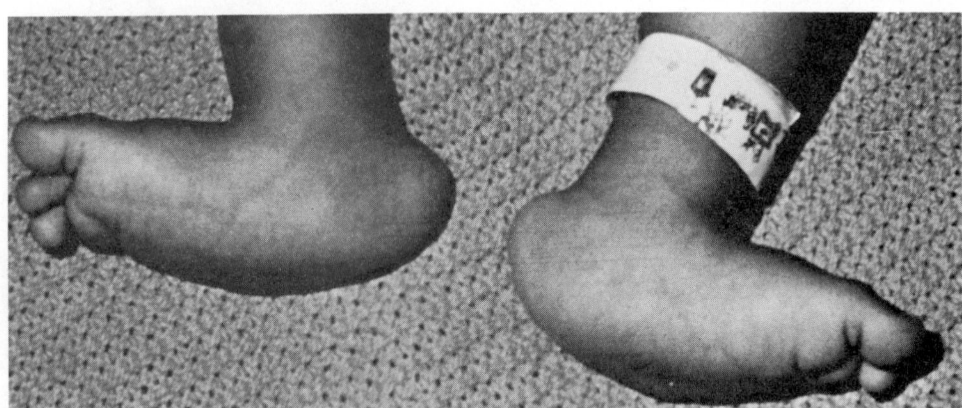

Figure 70–9. Rocker bottom foot. Extremely rigid with motion taking place only in the forefoot.

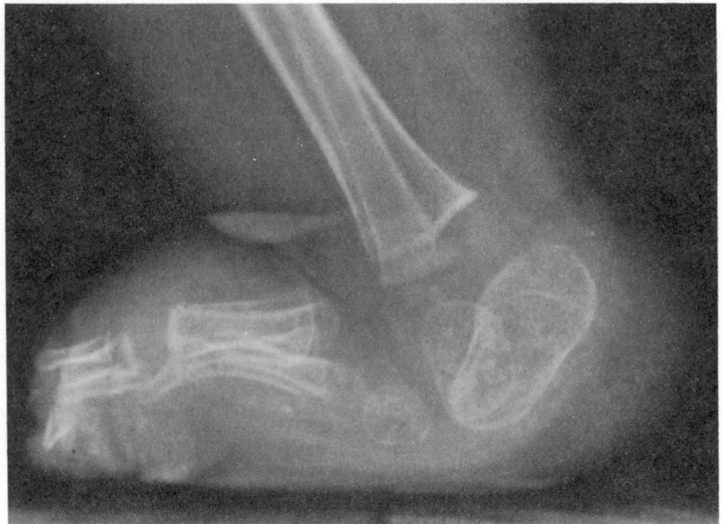

Figure 70–10. Lateral radiograph of congenital vertical talus (rocker bottom foot). The heel is in equinus, the talus pointing directly towards the floor, the midfoot dislocated upon the dorsum of the talus.

ity. Likewise, the child sleeps on his abdomen with his knees tucked up under his chest and his bottom coming down on his internally rotated feet (Fig. 70–11). For this reason, normal growth and development of the normal evolution of external rotation cannot take place, and persistent "internal tibial torsion" or medial rotation is the rule. Treatment consists of altering the child's sleeping and playing habits so that external rotation rather than internal rotation is encouraged.

If the child's habit of sleeping on his abdomen cannot be stopped, a Denis Browne splint or a detachable Fillauer bar applied to the shoes is indicated. This treatment does not correct the deformity but merely allows normal growth and development to take place. Certain guidelines are in order: (1) the width of the bar should be no wider than the width of the hips; an arbitrary rule is that no bar should be wider than six inches; (2) the feet should not be forcibly externally rotated. Only 10 to 15 degrees of external rotation is needed. Extreme rotations or wide bars will have the adverse effect of knee ligament damage, which may be irreparable if allowed to progress. Normally, the time needed for correction is from 6 to 18 months.

Another cause for toeing-in in the ambulatory

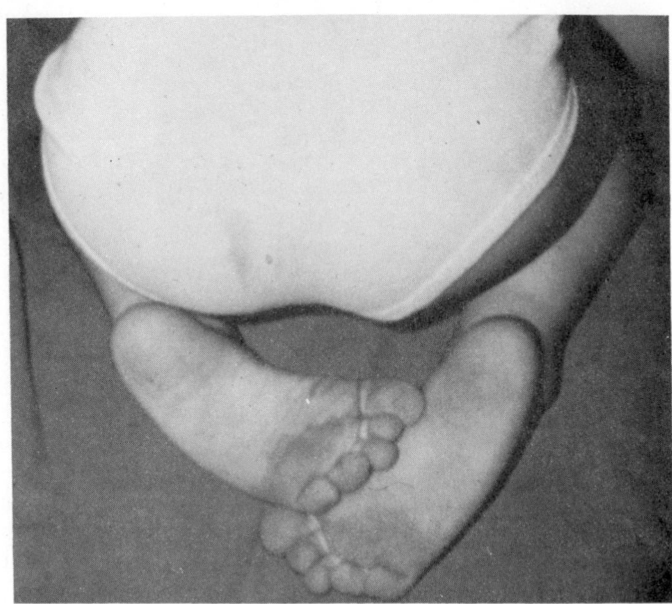

Figure 70–11. Toddler with "toe in" gait assuming his most comfortable sleeping position. The internally rotated feet are being subjected to increased internal forces by the weight of the buttocks.

child is persistent *femoral neck anteversion*. All children are born with the femoral head and neck inclined in a more anterior direction than in the adult. As the child kicks out of the flexion deformity of the neonate and starts a sitting balance to develop a lumbar lordosis rather than the long C infantile curve, the acetabulum assumes a more vertical relationship and the femoral neck usually undergoes a decrease in the anteverted angle. Failure to untwist, so to speak, will lead to excessive amounts of internal rotation of the hip at the expense of external rotation, the hip joint capsule being the restraint that prevents external rotation at the hip. These children classically walk with their kneecaps pointing inward, the so-called "squinting patellae" (Fig. 70–12). When they run, their feet usually whip out to the side, giving the appearance of a clumsy, slow child. This gait is due to muscle contraction of the hip internal rotators seating the femoral head deeply into the socket for stability. The thigh, knee, and, consequently, leg and foot are internally rotated. The knee flexion and extension arc is now "out of line" with the forward progression of the body and consequently less effective. The child is slower, since the normally smooth coordinated mechanics of running are altered. If asked to walk slowly, most of these children can control rotation so that their feet point straight ahead. This requires conscious effort on their part and is, therefore, fatiguing. This is why their gait deteriorates near the end of the day with increased toeing-in. Provided that habits which enhance internal rotation (i.e., sitting in a "W" on the floor and abdominal sleeping) are interrupted early, most toeing-in will "unwind" acceptably by age eight or nine. There are few indications for more aggressive treatment. Shoe prescriptions with wedges or twister cable braces have no place in the treatment of anteversion of the hip or internal rotation of the tibia. What is needed is an adequate explanation of the anatomical reason that the child toes-in. This explanation plus the usually good prognosis for acceptable correction, provided that poor habits are corrected, is sufficient in most cases. In the remainder, especially in those children who have only 0 to 10 degrees of external rotation, osteotomy of the femur may be indicated.

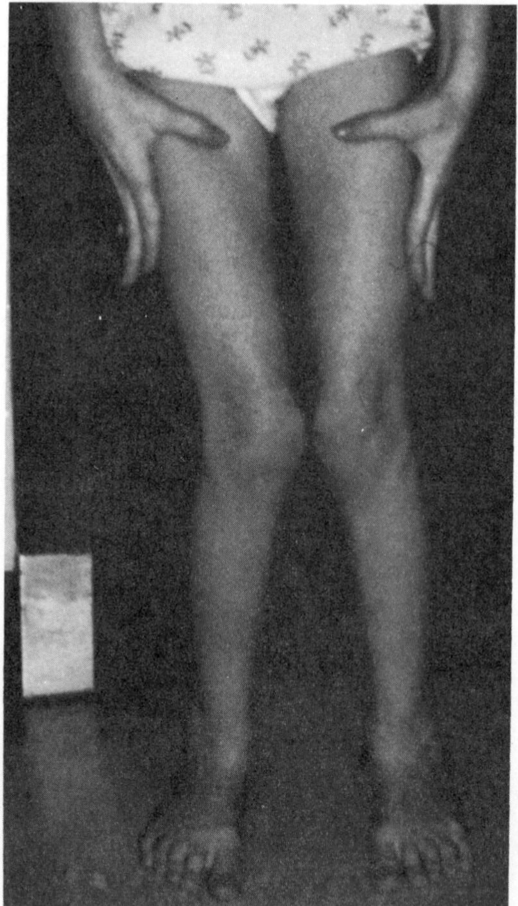

Figure 70–12. Six year old girl with complaint of "toe in" gait. She demonstrates the "squinting patellae" of the excessively anteverted hips.

A word of caution concerning the use of twister cable braces for femoral anteversion must be offered. These devices apply external rotation torque to the foot and ankle. While the child is in the device, he may indeed walk with the foot straight ahead or externally rotated. This external rotation force may have a deleterious effect upon the medial collateral ligament of the knee or the deltoid ligament of the ankle and subtalar joint. For these reasons, the use of twister braces in children who have femoral anteversion as their sole orthopaedic problem is to be condemned.

EXTERNAL ROTATION CONTRACTURE

In contrast to those children who "toe-in," there are those who "toe-out." This posture may be present at birth and diminish as the child begins to walk. There is significant parental anxiety, as the family feels the child is crippled and doing harm to his foot and ankle. The physical findings are just the reverse of the anteverted hip. There is excessive *external rotation* but limited internal rotation at the hip. Radiographs should be made to rule out a dislocation of the hips.

The etiology of toeing-out is an abduction/external rotation contracture of the soft tissues around the hip secondary to intrauterine position. The treatment includes (1) adequate explanation to the family of the anatomical nature of the problem; (2) gentle passive stretching exercises of the external rotators by internally rotating the femurs at each diaper change; and (3) the avoidance of sleeping positions that perpetuate the posture, i.e., the "spread eagle" or frog prone position.

THE "NONCORRECTIVE" CORRECTIVE SHOE

Much ado is made about special or "corrective" shoes in the treatment of common pediatric foot problems. There is no such thing as a corrective shoe! It is a misnomer! Shoes are meant to *protect* the foot, *not* correct it. Shoes protect the foot from sharp objects and cold.

In general, shoes should be flexible and fitted long enough to prevent the toes from being pinched and wide enough so the forefoot is not crowded together. Rigid shoes prevent motion and should be avoided. The sole should be of a nonskid material to prevent the toddler from slipping. The upper should be soft and porous, especially in warm climates. It is best to avoid "fad" shoes or odd-shaped shoes and those with excessive heel height and pointed toes. The shoes should not be expensive.

The altering of shoes with wedges and heels has been a popular mode of treatment for the flexible flat-footed child or the child who toes-in or toes-out. There is no scientific basis for these altered shoe prescriptions, and the practice should be avoided.

If a child presents with a flexible foot that has a normal range of motion and is supported by normal muscles that plantarflex, dorsiflex, evert, and invert the *foot*, then that foot is normal for *that child*! It does not need treatment! It needs to be allowed to grow and develop in normal fashion.

In contrast, the child who presents with a painful and/or rigid foot or one that has an excessively high arch (pes cavus) should be referred for evaluation. Rigid feet may be secondary to tarsal coalition (abnormal bony bridges between the bones); cavus feet may be secondary to neuromuscular disease (peroneal muscular atrophy) or the spinal dysraphism syndrome.

KNOCK-KNEES AND BOWLEGS

There is a varus position of the tibia in the newborn that gradually diminishes in the first two years of life—the so-called physiological bowing. After age two, the tibia swings like a pendulum into a valgus position. This is usually present until age four to eight. About age eight, most children will have the tibiofemoral alignment of the adult. Because of variation in genetic background, these fluctuations of the "tibial pendulum" may take excessive swings and cause parental anxiety. This anxiety may be allayed by documented serial examinations and good quality radiographs revealing no underlying bony abnormality. If bowing persists beyond age two years and if it specifically is confined to the tibia, one must suspect Blount's disease (tibia vara), a disorder that most generally requires surgical correction (Fig. 70–13).

Knock-knee that is physiological and not secondary to underlying disease has an excellent prognosis. Secondary knock-knee is sometimes seen in overweight patients with paralytic conditions, juvenile rheumatoid arthritis, or endocrinopathies and following infection or injuries to the growth plates. The latter usually require surgical correction.

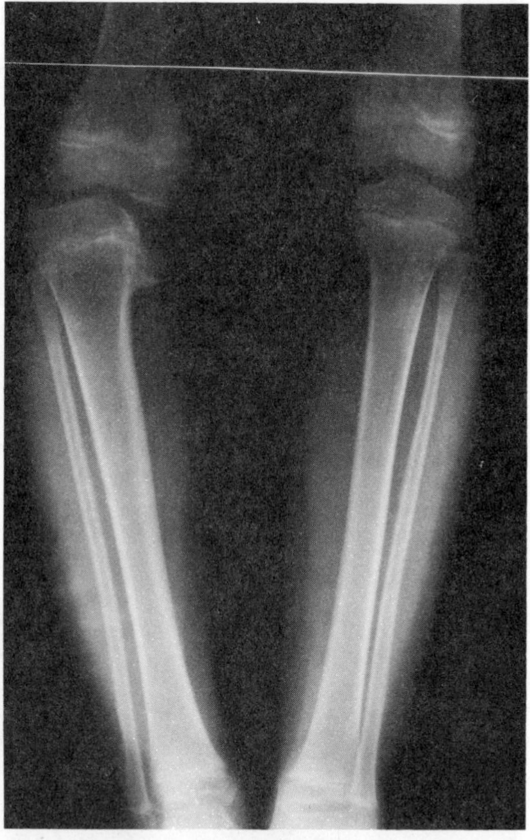

Figure 70–13. Standing AP radiographs of a five year old child with normal tibio-femoral alignment in the child's right and Blount's disease on the child's left leg.

Hip Syndromes of Childhood and Adolescence

The child who limps frightens the family if there is no history of trauma or evident bruising or tenderness. Excluding trauma, the toddler who limps most likely has toxic synovitis of the hip or the irritable hip syndrome. If the child refuses to walk, one must also consider a discitis or disc space infection in the lumbar spine.

In the child from age four to nine years, the limp is most likely associated with either toxic synovitis of the hip or Legg-Calvé-Perthes disease. Toxic synovitis of the hip is better termed *transient synovitis* or *the irritable hip syndrome*, thereby describing the symptoms and duration of the illness rather than its etiology. The cause remains unknown; injury, low grade viral infection, and allergic hypersensitivity have all been incriminated, but no hard evidence supports any cause. The children are not systemically ill at the time of the synovitis. Bed rest until the signs of limited hip motion have abated is sufficient treatment. There may be several bouts of the affliction. It is tempting to consider transient synovitis as a prelude to Perthes disease, but proof of the correlation is lacking. In the case of Perthes disease, the limp predominates over the pain, which may be localized to the thigh or medial side of the knee. When the child is first seen, significant muscle atrophy of the thigh has often occurred. Any limping child requires an accurate assessment of the gait pattern and careful evaluation of the spine by palpation and range of motion examination.

The examination of the hip can easily be accomplished by (1) the simple abduction test and (2) the prone internal rotation test. With the patient lying supine on the examining table, the hips and knees are flexed with feet on the table side by side. The patient is asked to let his knees fall apart, keeping the feet together. The hip that is irritable or inflamed for whatever cause will have a limited range of abduction compared with the opposite noninflamed side (Fig. 70–14). Similarly, when placed in the prone position with the knee flexed 90 degrees, internal rotation is markedly limited on the affected side. In our experience, these two tests are most sensitive for hip joint pathology. Good quality AP and frog lateral x-rays of the pelvis should be made if hip pathology is suspected. Single hip x-rays are not as helpful as the pelvis film, especially for comparison of affected to uninvolved side.

In the age group from 4 to 9, unexplained limp without fever is Legg-Perthes disease until proven otherwise. The treatment is variable depending upon the locale and orthopaedic surgeon, but, in general, one is trying to preserve function by decreasing inflammation of the hip by whatever means necessary and restoring nearly full motion until the lesion has healed. The limping adolescent from age 9 to 17 must be considered to have a slipped epiphysis of the hip until proven otherwise. Many adolescents will be referred to the orthopaedist with thigh or knee pain of varying degree and duration carrying a folder of normal knee x-rays. One must be aware that the pain may

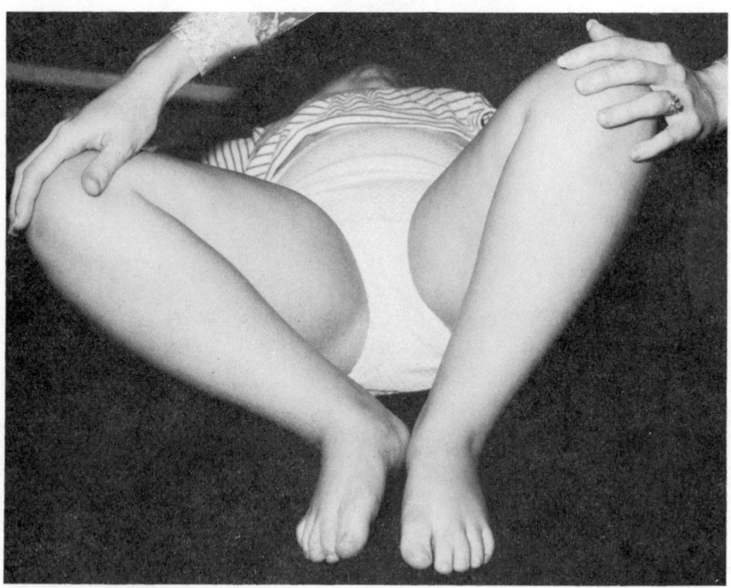

Figure 70–14. Simple abduction test demonstrating limited abduction of the left hip in the flexed position. The child has Perthes disease of the left hip.

be referred to the inner aspect of the thigh and knee and that careful hip evaluation as described above is necessary to rule out hip joint pathology. The treatment for slipped capital femoral epiphysis is (1) make the diagnosis and (2) *prevent further slipping*! This can be accomplished by internal fixation using threaded pins or bone grafting procedures to stimulate epiphyseal plate closure. The sequelae of severe slips and avascular necrosis secondary to severe slips are far too large a price to pay for these young people. It behooves us to pay particular attention to the adolescent who complains of thigh or knee pain.

Osgood-Schlatter's Disease

Knee pain in the active adolescent is usually the result of direct trauma. Many young people complain of knee pain when in actuality the pain is localized to the tibial tubercle. If direct compression upon the tubercle reproduces the pain or accentuates the pain, a diagnosis of Osgood-Schlatter's disease may be made. This usually self-limiting lesion is related to inflammation of the attachment of the infrapatellar tendon into the tibial tubercle and thereby to the proximal tibial growth plate. Good quality anterior and posterior x-rays are needed, not so much to make the diagnosis of Osgood-Schlatter's disease, but to rule out other disorders such as a low grade osteomyelitis or an osteosarcoma that may mimic Osgood-Schlatter's disease. Once these significant problems are ruled out, attention can be given to limiting the child's activities with the advice that the lesion will most likely heal but will take some time. Many children need to be converted from running and jumping sports to swimming in order to give an outlet for their energies. It is stressed again that Osgood-Schlatter's disease is a very common lesion of the adolescent knee and is self-limiting, not requiring treatment other than avoidance of those activities that enhance the pain. Once the pain has abated, direct trauma may play a significant role in aggravating the condition, so it is stressed that knee pads should be worn in order to eliminate some of the second and third episodes of decreased activity.

SCOLIOSIS

School screening programs have encouraged the pediatrician to become more aware of scoliosis and spinal deformities. Why so much fuss about a crooked back? Long-term studies on untreated scoliosis patients have revealed an increased risk of death from cardiopulmonary causes. Almost all adult scoliosis patients have significant back pain. Many are disabled because of symptoms of fatigue and pain. Furthermore, curves in excess of 60 degrees in the thoracic area will continue to progress after skeletal maturity, as will lumbar curves in excess of 40 degrees. Female patients who become pregnant may also experience an increasing curve following delivery of the baby. For these reasons and many others, aggressive treatment of the child with a spinal deformity is justified.

CLASSIFICATION AND ETIOLOGY

The broadest categories of scoliosis are *nonstructural* and *structural* scoliosis. Nonstructural scoliotic curves are extremely flexible and show correction upon side bending of the patient toward the convex side of the curve. In structural scoliosis, the curve fails to correct upon such side bending and is quite rigid.

After a careful history and physical examination, most scoliosis patients presenting to the pediatrician will probably have their condition categorized as "idiopathic"; that is, the true etiology remains obscure. If, however, we look closely at these patients and their families, we find that a great number of the families will give a history of curves in other family members, so-called familial or genetic scoliosis. If a family has one child with a curvature of the spine, then all the children in that family must be examined and observed throughout their growth period for the occurrence of scoliosis. Counseling the parents and the patient is important. Based upon present knowledge, a person who has scoliosis has a one in three chance of having children with scoliosis.

Depending upon the age at the time of recognition of the curve, familial scoliosis is designated as infantile (if less than three years of age at onset), juvenile (three to eight years of age at onset), or adolescent scoliosis. In the United States, the most common form of idiopathic scoliosis is the adolescent onset variety, that is, the child aged 10 to 14 just prior to the last rapid growth spurt. It is in this group of children that school screening is most rewarding. The overall incidence of scoliosis is variously quoted in the orthopaedic literature as being between 4 and 8 per cent of the normal population. Not all of these people need active treatment, because *not all scoliotic curves are progressive*! Only about 2 per cent of the population have progressive spinal curves requiring active treatment. It is of major importance that all children be screened for scoliosis at each examination by the pediatrician. Each routine visit and each preschool and school physical is an opportunity for the physician to examine the spine for malalignment. The examination requires only about 30 seconds, but if properly performed may yield a lifetime of dividends. In the neonatal period, the examination is performed both in the prone position and with the child suspended. In all older children, the examination should be performed in the standing position.

THE EXAMINATION

Observe from the back (Fig. 70–15). Careful attention is given to the following areas: (1) Are the shoulders of unequal height? (2) Is there an obvious curve of the spine or the spinous processes? (3) Is there a prominent scapula? (4) Are there asymmetrical waist creases? (5) Is there a tilt of the pelvis or unequal leg length? (6) Does one arm hang away from the trunk farther than the other? The patient should then bend forward, as if touching his toes, and the spinal alignment should be checked in the "forward bending" position (Fig. 70–16). Both sides of the thorax and trunk should be at the same level in forward bending. If they are not, scoliosis is present. These simple observations can satisfactorily screen out most scoliotic curves. If there is concern that any of the above are present, an x-ray of the spine should be obtained in the standing position. The film should include the vertebral column in its entirety, from occiput to sacrum.

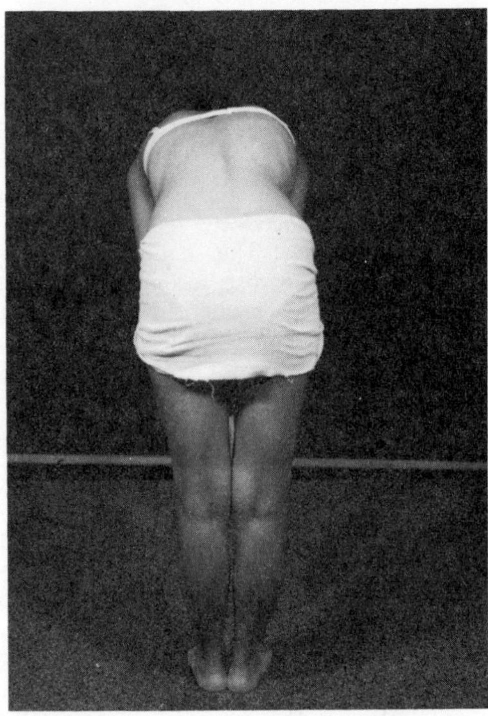

Figure 70–16. Forward bending test demonstrating a right thoracic scoliosis.

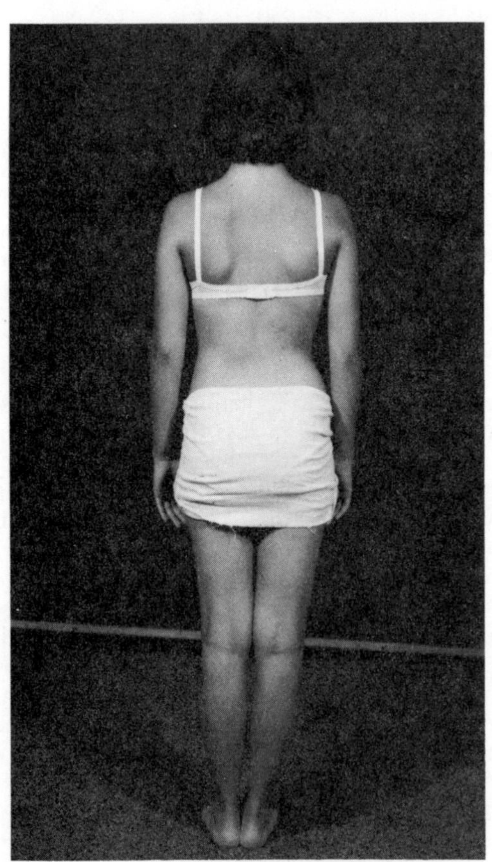

Figure 70–15. See text.

MEASUREMENT OF THE CURVE
(Fig. 70–17)

The severity of the scoliotic curve is determined by careful measurement of the spinal x-ray. Curves may be of any pattern, but the most typical idiopathic adolescent curve is that of a right thoracic curve, that is, the majority of the curvature occurs in the thoracic vertebrae, and it is convex to the patient's right side.

GUIDELINES FOR TREATMENT

The best treatment for scoliosis is early detection and prompt referral to a facility equipped to provide complete scoliosis care. Treatment of children with scoliosis falls into three categories: (1) observation, (2) bracing and exercise programs, and (3) surgery. Although

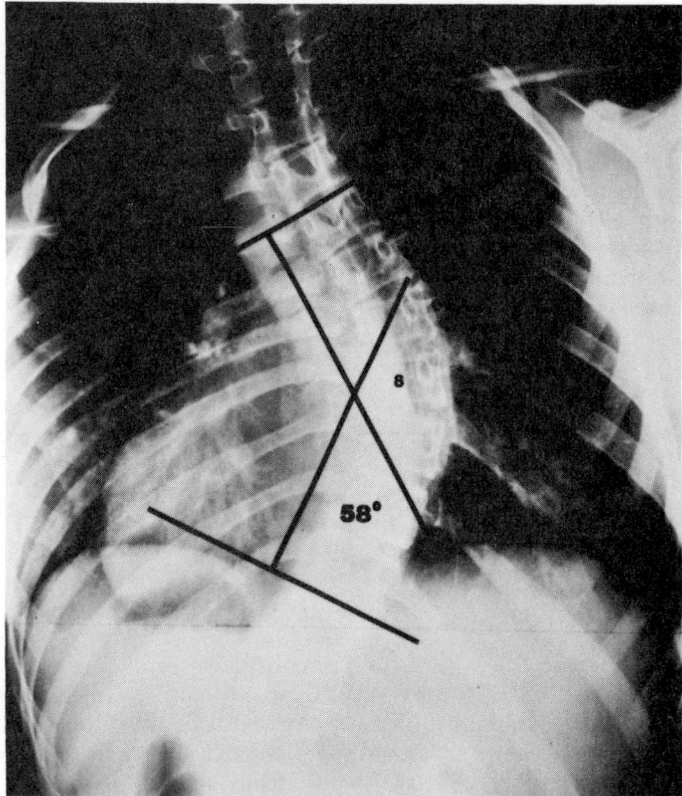

Figure 70–17. Measurement of a right thoracic curve. Top limit of the curve is superior border of T5. Lower limit of the curve is the inferior border of T11. Apex of curve is T8. The angle of intersection of the perpendicular lines to the limit vertebrae borders is the degree of spinal curvature.

treatment must be individualized to each patient, the following general comments may be made. Spinal curvature measuring less than 20 degrees in a skeletally immature patient may be observed at frequent intervals, i.e., every six months with routine repeat x-rays. All subsequent x-rays must be compared with the original film so that true progression is not minimized by observer bias or overlooked due to measurement error. Curves greater than 20 degrees and less than 45 degrees deserve aggressive treatment with a brace program and an active exercise routine. The goal of all therapy in scoliosis is to prevent further deformity. If the curve is found and treatment begun early with rigid adherence to the treatment protocol, the need for spinal surgery for children with idiopathic scoliosis may be obviated.

If brace treatment is indicated, the child must be willing to spend 23 hours each day in her brace and perform exercises as prescribed by the doctor and supervised by the physical therapist. Exercises for scoliosis fall into two categories: (1) general conditioning and spinal flexibility and (2) in-brace exercises to extend the spinal column and isometric exercises to push against and away from the pads of the brace. The use of a mirror is encouraged for the in-brace exercises. The mirror facilitates the visual proprioceptive feedback mechanism; i.e., the child contracts muscles and sees a result from the exercise. Patients and families must be counseled that exercises alone do not cure scoliosis! They make the child look and feel better. They make the child aware of her posture and methods to effect changes in her posture. Exercises keep the spine flexible, enabling the brace to function more effectively.

Brace wearing must be continued until vertebral growth has ceased. This is usually determined by the appearance of the iliac apophysis on the x-ray. Families and patients should understand that growth does not cease at the same age for all patients and that the wearing of the brace must be continued until that individual child has reached skeletal maturity as determined by her x-rays. In children whose curves are greater than 45 or 50 degrees, and in whom spinal growth still remains, brace therapy will not be satisfactory. These larger curves have a greater propensity for progression; hence the need for stabilization of the curve surgically.

ELECTROSPINAL STIMULATION

There are experimental protocols wherein the scoliotic child is treated by electrically stimulating the muscles on the convex side of the curve during sleeping hours. No long-term studies are yet available to compare this mode of treatment with brace therapy; hence it is still experimental. It is hoped that early detection by school screening and aggressive treatment will preclude the need for surgery in these patients.

REFERENCES

Hensinger, R., and Jones, E.: Neonatal Orthopaedics. New York, Grune and Stratton, 1981.

Lloyd-Roberts, G. C.: Orthopaedics of Infancy and Childhood. London, Butterworths, 1971.

Sharrard, W. J. W.: Pediatric Orthopaedics and Fractures. London, Blackwell Scientific Publications, 1979.

71

INFLAMMATORY BOWEL DISEASE

Joseph H. Clark, M.D., and Joseph F. Fitzgerald, M.D.

Ulcerative colitis is an inflammatory disease of the colon which is limited to the mucosa and, to a lesser extent, the adjacent submucosa. Crohn's disease is characterized pathologically by discontinuous and transmural involvement of the bowel wall and by the presence of non-caseating granulomas. Gryboski and Spiro (1978) noted that 20 per cent of pediatric patients with Crohn's disease had diffuse small bowel disease, 20 per cent had only terminal ileal involvement, 50 per cent had ileocolitis, and 10 per cent had isolated colon disease.

The majority of patients with inflammatory bowel disease are older than 10 years at the time of diagnosis (Fig. 71–1). Although both ulcerative colitis and Crohn's disease have been reported in infants, necrotizing enterocolitis and milk-induced colitis can present clinical pictures which may be temporarily indistinguishable from inflammatory bowel disease. There is no appreciable sex difference in either Crohn's disease or ulcerative colitis. Several epidemiological studies have shown that inflammatory bowel disease has a higher incidence among Caucasians, especially those of Jewish heritage.

The etiologies of ulcerative colitis and Crohn's disease are unknown, but it appears likely that an interaction of multiple factors is operative such as genetic influences, the actions

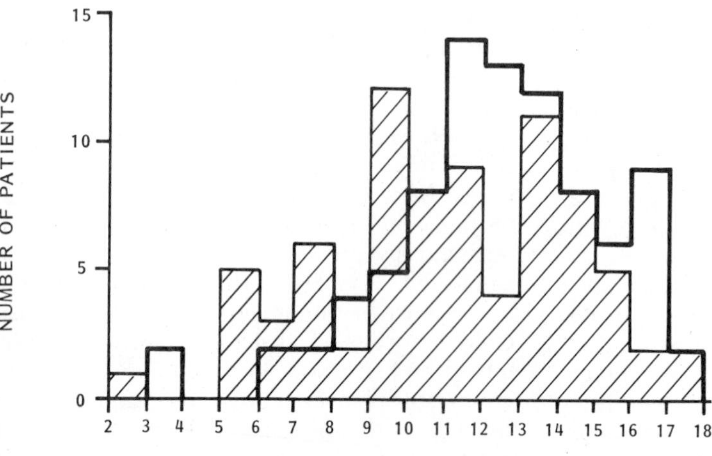

Figure 71–1. Chronological age at the time of diagnosis in 165 patients with inflammatory bowel disease. Diagonally lined areas represent patients with Crohn's disease; bold line represents patients with ulcerative colitis. The majority of patients are diagnosed after nine years of age; Crohn's disease predominates in patients less than eleven years of age with inflammatory bowel disease.

of an external agent or agents, altered immunological and other defense mechanisms, etc. (Kirsner and Shorter, 1982).

CLINICAL MANIFESTATIONS

Diarrhea, abdominal pain, weight loss, anemia, and fever are the cardinal symptoms of inflammatory bowel disease (Table 71–1). Diarrhea, often bloody, is the dominant symptom in ulcerative colitis, whereas abdominal pain predominates in Crohn's disease. Arthritis, the most common extraintestinal manifestation of both diseases, has been more commonly associated with Crohn's disease in our experience.

Erythema nodosum, pyoderma gangrenosum, and other dermatological manifestations are seen in both disorders and correlate with disease activity. Special emphasis needs to be placed on the high incidence of perianal and anal disease in inflammatory bowel disease, especially Crohn's disease involving the colon. The typical Crohn's fissure is a broad-based, midline, indolent lesion with undermined edges. Such lesions should always suggest Crohn's disease, and operative treatment should be avoided until this diagnostic possibility is excluded.

Clubbing of the fingers has been observed in ulcerative colitis and, more commonly, in Crohn's disease. Liver disease can accompany both disorders, although symptomatic lesions such as chronic aggressive hepatitis and pericholangitis are more common with ulcerative colitis in our experience. Urological manifestations accompanying inflammatory bowel disease, primarily Crohn's disease, include hydronephrosis, renal and vesical calculi, and nephrocalcinosis. Occasionally, uveitis and aphthous lesions accompany inflammatory bowel disease.

Growth retardation is a frequent complication of inflammatory bowel disease, especially Crohn's disease. Occasionally, growth failure is the initial clinical manifestation and precedes other symptoms or signs by years. Retardation of linear growth and bone age as well as delayed sexual maturation are observed. The etiology of the growth retardation is probably due to inadequate caloric intake, but malabsorption, gastrointestinal protein loss, chronic inflammation, and corticosteroid therapy play some role. Crohn's disease involving the cecum and ascending colon is more commonly associated with growth failure. Reversal of growth retardation occurs following nutritional restitution either by intravenous hyperalimentation or oral supplementation (Kelts et al., 1979; Kirschner et al., 1981).

Table 71–1. RELATIVE FREQUENCY OF PRESENTING SYMPTOMS AND SIGNS IN PATIENTS WITH ULCERATIVE COLITIS AND CROHN'S DISEASE

	Crohn's Disease	Ulcerative Colitis
Diarrhea	+ + + +	+ + + + +
Hematochezia	+ +	+ + + + +
Abdominal pain	+ + +	+ + + +
Weight loss	+ + + +	+ +
Fever	+ +	+
Growth failure	+ +	+
Oral lesions	+	
Perianal disease	+	
Finger clubbing	+	
Arthritis	+	
Liver disease		+
Abdominal mass	+	

EVALUATION

The diagnosis of inflammatory bowel disease is suggested by a careful history and thorough physical examination. Supportive data are obtained by lower gastrointestinal endoscopy and gastrointestinal radiography. Since the rectosigmoid mucosa is abnormal in 95 per cent of patients with ulcerative colitis and 40 to 50 per cent of those with Crohn's disease, proctosigmoidoscopy is the first step in the evaluation. Anesthesia may be required for the patient less than 10 years of age. This procedure should be performed without prior preparation in order to obtain the maximal amount of information and to avoid artifactual alterations that could result in misinterpretation. Hypertonic enemas can produce mucosal alterations indistinguishable from mild colitis.

The endoscopic features of ulcerative colitis are inflammation, edema, friability (punctate bleeding following minor trauma such as gentle rubbing with a cotton swab), and pinpoint ulceration. Pseudopolyps may be seen. Diffuse mucosal involvement is the rule. The features of Crohn's disease are less specific although deep, broad, serpiginous ulceration, occasionally producing a "cobblestone" appearance, may be seen. More typically, patchy areas of edema and inflammation are noted in the rectosigmoid colon. These abnormal areas are not especially friable. Not uncommonly, a nonspecific picture is seen in Crohn's disease, i.e., patchy areas of mucosal atrophy associated with a prominent submucosal vascular pattern.

The proctoscopic features of ulcerative colitis are similar to those in shigellosis and amebic colitis, although characteristic ulceration is classically seen in the latter. In early infancy, milk-induced colitis and the enterocolitis of Hirschsprung's disease have endoscopic features indistinguishable from ulcerative colitis.

We routinely examine the rectal mucus for pus cells and amebae. Rectal biopsies are useful when the endoscopic features are equivocal. Not uncommonly, the diagnosis of Crohn's disease is established on the basis of a granuloma in the biopsy specimen.

Contrast radiographic studies are obtained after proctosigmoidoscopy. Suspected severe colitis is an exception to this dictum, since a contrast study in such patients could result in toxic dilatation or perforation. In this situation, the study is deferred until the disease is under control. Intestinal preparation is unnecessary for patients with significant diarrhea; others require individualized preparation. It is our practice to examine the entire gastrointestinal tract of all patients suspected of having inflammatory bowel disease. In addition to a radiographic small bowel series, we currently utilize colonoscopy rather than barium enema to determine the extent of colonic involvement.

Laboratory tests performed during the evaluation include a complete blood count, erythrocyte sedimentation rate, platelet count, and protein electrophoresis. The stool is cultured and examined for ova and parasites if the patient has diarrhea. If the patient is anemic, the blood smear is examined and a reticulocyte count is obtained. The serum iron and iron binding capacity are determined. The patient with Crohn's disease may have a complex anemia resulting from iron, folate, and B_{12} deficiencies. The urine of a patient with ileitis should be examined for oxalate crystals. The patient's nutritional status is most readily assessed by measuring the serum proteins and carotene. The leukocyte count is often evaluated in patients with active disease; band forms and eosinophils may be associated with systemic manifestations. Liver function tests (AST, ALT, alkaline phosphatase, and fractionated bilirubin) are obtained to rule out asymptomatic liver disease. An amebiasis hemagglutination titer should be obtained before steroid therapy is initiated.

TREATMENT

The control of active disease is the goal of medical therapy (Table 71–2). Adrenocorticoids are prescribed to suppress the active disease, while other measures are instituted to prevent exacerbation. Prednisone is administered to all patients with active disease at 2 mg/kg/day (maximum of 60 mg) as a single daily dose, or rarely in a divided daily regimen. Positive nitrogen balance is necessary for maximal steroid effect. We have been impressed that adequate intestinal healing does not occur until cushingoid facies are seen. Hospitalization for intravenous hydrocortisone and hyperalimentation may be necessary.

Salicylazosulfapyridine (SASP), an early sul-

Table 71–2. TREATMENT OF INFLAMMATORY BOWEL DISEASE IN THE AMBULATORY SETTING

I. Low-residue, nonirritating, lactose-free diet
II. Mild sedative
   e.g., phenobarbital + belladonna; loperamide
III. Antispasmodic
IV. Anti-inflammatory medications (in order of initiation)
   A. *Ulcerative colitis:*
      1. SASP (50–75 mg/kg/day)
      2. Steroid retention enema (at bed-time)
      3. Prednisone (1–2 mg/kg/day to 60 mg/day)
         Single AM dose —+ response→ Alternate-day therapy
         No ↓ response
         Divided dose (± azathioprine)
   B. *Crohn's disease:*
      1. SASP (50–75 mg/kg/day)—colon involvement
         or
      2. Prednisone (1–2 mg/kg/day to 60 mg/day) as above

fonamide derivative, has been utilized in inflammatory bowel disease for almost 40 years. The active moiety appears to be 5-aminosalicylic acid, although the mechanism of action is incompletely known (Koltz et al., 1980). The dosage is maintained at 50 to 75 mg/kg/day (maximum 4 grams daily) to avoid gastrointestinal side effects. Hemolytic anemia and leukopenia may be observed. While the role of SASP in maintaining a state of remission for ulcerative colitis is clearly documented, the National Cooperative Crohn's Disease Study recently failed to show any advantage for SASP over placebo in adults with quiescent disease (Summers, 1979). SASP is effective in the treatment of active colonic Crohn's disease as well as active ulcerative colitis.

The role of dietary management in the treatment of inflammatory bowel disease is open to debate. Certainly the imposition of an unnecessarily rigid diet on a pediatric patient may have a negative net effect. On the other hand, common sense would suggest that certain foods may impede the healing process. Hence, we initially institute a low-residue, nonirritating diet. Further, in light of the reports of the association of hypolactasia and ulcerative colitis, we eliminate milk from the diet of these patients. We discuss these restrictions honestly with the patient in order to obviate the feelings of guilt which could follow "indiscretions." We assure the patient that it is our intention to relieve the dietary restrictions when we feel that active disease has been suppressed.

Since the gastrointestinal tract is affected by cerebral influences, we usually prescribe a mild sedative such as phenobarbital (1/4 to 1/2 grain) in combination with an anticholinergic to relieve spasm and decrease motility. Hematinics are employed as necessary, and a daily multivitamin is prescribed.

Perianal disease is treated with sitz baths and topical therapy with combination antibiotic-steroid ointment. Metronidazole (20 mg/kg/day) has been shown to be effective for persistent perianal disease in the absence of active bowel disease (Bernstein et al., 1980).

Azathioprine may be added to augment the effectiveness of corticosteroids. Steroid retention enemas and foams have limited usefulness. Ulcerative colitis limited to the rectum without systemic symptoms (ulcerative proctitis) may be treated with a steroid foam agent in addition to SASP. Six of the 171 patients in our series had ulcerative proctitis.

Treatment evaluation is initially performed at 2- to 4-week intervals. Later, the patient can be seen at 6- to 12-week intervals. The treatment program can be altered when all parameters indicate suppression of the active component of the disease. At this point, patients receiving prednisone are placed on either an alternate-day program or a single daily dosage regimen. If suppression is maintained, we decrease the dose by 5 mg every four to six weeks with the hope that we can discontinue the prednisone and maintain the patient on SASP alone. Low-dose SASP is maintained indefinitely. A recrudescence is managed by reinstitution of daily steroid therapy at a higher level. An alternate-day program is not suitable for an occasional patient, and weaning is performed on a single daily dosage regimen exclusively.

The dietary restrictions are gradually relaxed, and the patient is allowed to control his own diet while avoiding foods that produce symptoms.

Proctosigmoidoscopic examination of patients with ulcerative colitis is performed whenever the patient is symptomatic or Hemoccult-positive stool is found. Barium enemas should be performed in all patients with ulcerative colitis after approximately 5 years to determine the presence of colonic narrowing, which may be difficult to appreciate endoscopically. Prophylactic colectomy after 10 years of ulcerative colitis is no longer recommended, since these patients may be followed with yearly colonoscopy to identify dysplastic changes. Colectomy may be performed as part of an endorectal "pull-through" procedure with preservation of the rectal muscle sheath. This allows for only a temporary ileostomy and the preservation of anal continence. Of the 24 patients with ulcerative colitis who required surgery in our series, eight have undergone an endorectal "pull-through" operation.

Radiographic studies of the small bowel are performed on all patients with symptomatic Crohn's disease. Colonoscopy is very useful in the evaluation of Crohn's disease. Surgery is generally avoided in patients with Crohn's disease due to the high rate of recurrence, although the risk of recurrence varies with the disease location. Thirty-three of our patients with Crohn's disease have required surgery for internal fistulae, intestinal obstruction, poor response to medical therapy, and growth failure.

SUMMARY

Inflammatory bowel disease is being recognized with increasing frequency in the pediatric population. The cardinal symptoms of these chronic diseases are diarrhea, abdominal pain, fever, and weight loss. The most difficult patients to diagnose are those whose initial symptoms are only weight loss or fever, since so many other diseases may be responsible. Anemia and perianal disease are frequently seen. Proctosigmoidoscopy, gastrointestinal radiography, and rectal biopsy are the essential diagnostic maneuvers. Treatment is nonspecific and directed at suppression of the active disease and elimination of factors that might contribute to disease activity. The patient with inflammatory bowel disease may present challenging problems to the practitioner. Early consultation with a pediatric gastroenterologist will usually be of benefit.

REFERENCES

1. Bernstein, L. H., Frank, M. S., Brandt, L. J., et al.: Healing of perianal Crohn's disease with metronidazole. Gastroenterology, 79:357, 1980.
2. Crohn, B. B., Ginzburg, L., and Oppenheimer, G. D.: Regional ileitis: A pathologic and clinical entity. J.A.M.A., 99:1323, 1932.
3. Gryboski, J. D., and Spiro, H. M.: Prognosis in children with Crohn's disease. Gastroenterology, *74*:807, 1978.
4. Hamilton, J. F., Bruce, G. A., Abdourhaman, M., and Gall, D. G.: Inflammatory bowel disease in children and adolescents. Adv. Pediatr., *26*:311, 1979.
5. Kelts, D. G., Grand, R. J., Shen, G., et al.: Nutritional basis of growth failure in children and adolescents with Crohn's disease. Gastroenterology, *76*:720, 1979.
6. Kirschner, B. S., Klich, J. R., Kalman, S. S., et al.: Reversal of growth retardation in Crohn's disease with therapy emphasizing oral nutritional restitution. Gastroenterology, *80*:10, 1981.
7. Kirsner, J. B., and Shorter, R. G.: Recent developments in nonspecific inflammatory bowel disease II. N. Engl. J. Med., *306*:837, 1982.
8. Klotz, U., Maier, K., Fischer, C., and Heinkel, K.: Therapeutic efficacy of sulfasalazine and its metabolites in patients with ulcerative colitis and Crohn's disease. N. Engl. J. Med., *303*:1499, 1980.
9. Summers, R. W., Switz, D. M., Sessions, J. T., Jr., et al.: National Cooperative Crohn's Disease Study: Results of drug treatment. Gastroenterology, *77*:847, 1979.
10. Wells, C.: Ulcerative colitis and Crohn's disease. Ann. R. Coll. Surg. Engl., *11*:105, 1952.
11. Werlin, S. L., and Grand, F. J.: Severe colitis in children and adolescents: Diagnosis, course and treatment. Gastroenterology, *73*:828, 1977.

72

JUVENILE RHEUMATOID ARTHRITIS AND DERMATOMYOSITIS

Murray H. Passo, M.D.

JUVENILE RHEUMATOID ARTHRITIS

Juvenile rheumatoid arthritis (JRA) is the most common chronic arthritic condition in children. The incidence of JRA is estimated to be near that of childhood cancer and muscular dystrophy.

Diagnostic Criteria (Table 72–1)

The patient must have objective evidence of arthritis defined as joint swelling or limitation of motion with heat, pain, and/or tenderness. Subjective complaints alone, such as pain or tenderness, represent an arthralgia, not arthritis. Patients with JRA complain of inactivity stiffness in the morning and also after napping or sitting for prolonged periods of time. The arthritis must be persistent for a minimum of six weeks. Other conditions, including traumatic, infectious, neoplastic, hematologic, orthopedic, and metabolic conditions as well as other connective tissue diseases, must be excluded (Brewer et al., 1977).

Clinical Manifestations (Table 72–1)

JRA can be divided into three major subtypes—systemic, polyarticular, and pauciarticular onset, defined by the clinical manifestations during the first six months of the disease. A few children change from one subtype to another in the course of their disease.

Systemic Onset Type

The onset of this subtype is commonly before five years of age, and almost an equal number of boys and girls are affected. A clinical hallmark

Table 72–1. DIAGNOSIS OF JUVENILE RHEUMATOID ARTHRITIS

Diagnostic Criteria
Arthritis—swelling or limitation of motion plus pain, tenderness, or warmth
Chronicity—greater than six weeks
Exclusion of other diseases (see text)
Clinical Subtypes
Systemic Onset
Fever
Rash
Lymphadenopathy
Hepatosplenomegaly
Pericarditis
Seronegative*
Polyarticular—more than five joints
Seronegative—rheumatoid factor −
Seropositive—rheumatoid factor +
Pauciarticular—less than five joints
Early childhood onset—female, ANA +, under five years of age*
Late childhood onset—male, HLA-B27+, over 8 years of age*

*Majority of patients

is the daily or twice-daily fever to 103°F or more, with the temperature spike characteristically occurring in the late afternoon or evening. A wide diurnal variation of temperature between 97 and 105.5°F in a single day is the usual pattern. The characteristic "rheumatoid" rash, present in about 90 per cent of the patients, is a salmon-colored macular or maculopapular eruption present on the trunk, extremities, and occasionally the face, and in areas that have been irritated by underclothing or pressure. Usually nonpruritic, the rash is evanescent, appearing fleetingly in conjunction with the fever. It may be brought out by the so-called Koebner phenomenon performed by gently traumatizing the skin.

The arthritis of systemic onset JRA may lag behind the systemic features by several months to years. Symmetrical polyarthritis including the knees, small joints of the hands and feet, wrists, ankles, and cervical spine is usual, although some children have only a few joints involved. Approximately 25 per cent of these children have significant morbidity, persisting into adulthood, from erosive, deforming arthritis.

In addition to generalized lymphadenopathy, splenomegaly and hepatomegaly occur in approximately half of the patients. Pleuritis, pericarditis, and, occasionally, peritonitis sometimes occur.

The hemogram can be remarkable with anemia in the 6 to 7 gm/dl range, a polymorphonuclear leukocytosis with counts in excess of 20,000, and thrombocytosis with platelet counts in excess of 500,000. The erythrocyte sedimentation rate, elevated in the majority of patients, is a useful parameter with which to follow disease activity. Tests for rheumatoid factors and antinuclear antibodies are almost uniformly negative.

Polyarticular Onset Type

Approximately 40 per cent of the children have the polyarticular onset subtype in which females outnumber the males by 2:1. More than five joints are involved in the first six months of the disease in the absence of severe systemic signs. A symmetrical polyarthritis involving both large and small joints is the outstanding feature of this subtype. Involvement of the temporomandibular joints and cervical spine may cause micrognathia or retrognathia in some patients.

This subtype is further divided into seropositive and seronegative for rheumatoid factors, with the majority of patients being seronegative. In seronegative patients, the arthritis is usually of mild to moderate severity, and subsequent cartilage destruction and severe deformity are uncommon. Approximately 10 per cent of JRA patients, mostly school age or adolescent females, have a positive rheumatoid factor test and their disease closely resembles adulthood rheumatoid arthritis. Rapidly progressive, erosive arthritis lasting into adulthood and causing significant morbidity commonly occurs.

Pauciarticular Onset Type

Approximately 40 per cent of patients have pauciarticular onset defined as involvement limited to four or fewer joints. Most of these patients are not systemically ill, although occasional mild systemic manifestations may occur. There are at least two distinct subgroups, early and late childhood onset.

The early childhood subgroup consists predominantly of females with disease onset before five years of age. Up to 60 per cent have a positive ANA, with titers that tend to be lower than in the systemic lupus erythematosus (SLE) group. Joint involvement is of mild to moderate intensity and often asymmetrical, involving large joints such as knees, ankles, elbows, wrists, and, rarely, small joints of the hands or feet. The sacroiliac joints and the spine are spared. These children are at the highest risk for chronic iridocyclitis, and up to 50 per cent may have eye involvement (Schaller, 1980). It is estimated that up to 75 to 95 per cent of the children who develop iridocyclitis are in the pauciarticular subtype. The activity of the joint disease is independent of the activity of the eye disease.

Since the eye involvement is largely asymptomatic, routine serial slit lamp examinations are recommended. In the high-risk group—ANA positive pauciarticular—patients should be examined every three to four months throughout childhood and adolescence. Patients with a previous bout of iridocyclitis, irrespective of subtype, should be followed at least every three to four months or more often depending on the activity of the eye disease. Polyarticular and systemic onset patients should be followed no less than every six months.

The late childhood subgroup usually consists of school age or adolescent males, with the arthritis affecting predominantly the large, weight bearing joints. Approximately 60 to 80 per cent of these patients are HLA-B27 positive. It is now recognized that some patients of this subgroup subsequently develop sacroiliitis and lumbodorsal spine involvement in early adulthood.

Malignancies, especially leukemia and neuroblastoma, may mimic JRA; however, the involvement tends to be disproportionately painful when compared to the objective physical findings. X-rays may show metaphyseal rarefaction, periosteal reaction, or lytic lesions, findings that would be unusual in early phases of JRA.

Table 72–2. MANAGEMENT OF JUVENILE RHEUMATOID ARTHRITIS

Goals of Treatment
1. Reduction of pain and swelling
2. Normal range of motion and muscle strength
3. Foster psychosocial normalcy
4. Patient understanding of disease and treatment rationale

Management—Multidisciplinary, Comprehensive
- Physician—Pharmacological
  - First line—aspirin, NSAIDs
  - Second line—chrysotherapy, D-penicillamine, antimalarials
- Physical Therapy
  - Evaluation
    - joint assessment
    - functional muscle strength
    - activity level
    - posture
  - Treatment
    - exercises
    - heat
    - joint protection
- Occupational Therapy
  - Evaluation of activities of daily living
  - Splints and adaptive devices
- Social Service
  - Psychosocial and financial counseling
- Orthopedics
  - Bracing recommendations
  - Operative management
    - soft tissue release
    - synovectomy
    - joint replacement
- Ophthalmology
  - Serial slit lamp examination

All members participate in education, motivation, and psychosocial needs.

Parameters for Follow-up
- Duration of stiffness
- Swelling
- Range of motion
- Activity level and school attendance
- Hemoglobin, salicylate level, SGOT, sedimentation rate
- Growth
- Psychosocial adjustment

Management of JRA (Table 72–2)

The management of juvenile rheumatoid arthritis requires a comprehensive multidisciplinary approach with the following goals: (1) reduction of pain and swelling; (2) restoration or maintenance of normal range of motion and muscle strength; (3) psychosocial normalcy; and (4) patient understanding of the disease and its treatment.

Pharmacological Management

The mainstay of pharmacological management remains salicylates. Although the most commonly used salicylate is aspirin, several other salicylate products are available, including sodium salicylate, choline salicylate (Arthropan), salsalate (Disalcid), and magnesium-choline salicylate (Trilisate).

Aspirin is prescribed by dosage per weight in patients less than 26 kg starting with 75–100 mg/kg/day. A simple rule of thumb is to prescribe one baby aspirin (75–81 mg)/kg/day. In patients over 25 kg one can induce toxicity with that mg/kg dosage. In those children, 6 to 12 adult aspirin per day are prescribed depending on the size of the patient. Aspirin is best taken three to four times a day and need *not* be given on a fixed, hourly schedule. Salicylates accumulate and reach a steady state at approximately five to seven days. In the anti-inflammatory range of 20 to 30 mg/dl, the plasma salicylate level will not vary greatly. This permits taking the aspirin at mealtime and bedtime. Late night-time doses can be omitted.

One attempts to reach a level of 20 to 30 mg/dl and to modify the dosage accordingly as the child grows in order to maintain that level. When initiating aspirin therapy, one must not increase the dosage in too large increments, especially after a level of 15 mg/dl has been obtained. A small increment of 10 to 15 per cent may be all that is necessary to generate a level of 20 mg/dl or higher.

Signs of toxicity include tinnitus and hearing loss; CNS changes, either somnolence or hyperactivity; and hyperventilation. In younger children auditory changes are less reliable. Gastrointestinal discomfort may be largely prevented by giving the salicylate product with food or milk at mealtime. Hepatotoxicity, manifest by an elevation of the SGOT and SGPT, is usually asymptomatic, although a few patients experience vomiting, anorexia, and abdominal pain. Serial SGOTs are usually obtained along with the salicylate level during the early months of management. Enzyme elevations tend to be transient and usually return to near-normal or normal within a few weeks. In those patients in whom the enzyme elevation is dose related, a reduction in the dosage may be all that is necessary to reduce the SGOT yet maintain therapeutic anti-inflammatory levels.

Salicylates usually require several weeks to reach maximal efficacy. If they have proved to be nonefficacious after three to six months of therapeutic levels, another nonsteroidal anti-inflammatory drug may be tried. Currently, Tolectin (30 mg/kg/day in three or four doses) and Naprosyn (10 mg/kg/day in two doses) are approved for use in children. Several additional agents are awaiting FDA approval.

Additional pain relief may be provided with concomitant prescription of acetaminophen. The use of narcotic analgesics is discouraged. Superficial heat or ice may provide additional analgesia. Local steroid injections are considered when one or a few joints are particularly bothersome.

Augmentation of therapy beyond first line anti-inflammatory drugs is necessary in some patients with such drugs as gold, antimalarials, and D-penicillamine. These drugs are reserved for patients with progressive disease which has been unresponsive to salicylate or nonsteroidal anti-inflammatory therapy consistently provided for six months or more, plus adjunctive therapy such as physical and occupational therapies. The initiation of these agents should be determined by physicians experienced in their indications and usage.

Steroid therapy is indicated for severe systemic manifestations such as pericarditis and myocarditis. Although articular disease rarely requires steroid therapy, occasionally low-dose steroids are used in unremitting arthritis to permit return to some semblance of normal function.

Physical Therapy and Occupational Therapy

The treatment program is aimed at (1) pain relief, (2) maintaining or improving range of motion and muscle strength, (3) teaching joint protection and improved body mechanics, and (4) education.

Heat therapy is recommended for pain relief and muscle relaxation. Morning stiffness is reduced by a morning bath or shower. Heat should be used for no more than 20 to 30 minutes, as there is little additional benefit from more prolonged therapy. Heat therapy is utilized prior to exercises to relax the periarticular musculature and improve performance. A home paraffin bath can be helpful in reducing hand or foot pain and increasing range of motion. Electric heating pads are rarely recommended because improper usage in some cases has caused local burns.

Cold therapy is preferred by some patients because of its analgesic effects, especially when patients experience marked pain with movement or with reduction of contractures.

A home exercise program is prescribed to maintain or improve range of motion and muscle strength. Stretching exercises are prescribed for contractures. The program is carried out by the patient and/or his parents on a once- or twice-a-day schedule.

After assessing the activities of daily living, an occupational therapist teaches efficient ways to carry out daily functions without adding injury and wasteful effort. Assistive equipment and adaptive devices (elevated toilet seats, bathtub bars, etc.) may be prescribed to improve the patients' ability to care for themselves.

Splinting is usually carried out by the occupational therapist. Night-time splints rest the joint and maintain optimal functional position. Splints are also utilized for correction of contractures and other deformities. The heat malleable plastic splints can be modified as the child grows or as contractures are reduced. Such splints are usually well tolerated even by the very young toddler.

Assessment of Clinical Course

Follow-up requires frequent re-evaluation while the disease is being brought under control. The prognosis in this disease is relatively good, with approximately 50 to 70 per cent of the patients entering adulthood with little or no functional disability. Frequent rechecking for rheumatoid factor and ANA is not necessary except in special circumstances. The hemoglobin can reflect improvement because anemia from chronic inflammation is corrected as the disease is controlled. A declining hemoglobin may reflect clinical deterioration or gastrointestinal blood loss. The erythrocyte sedimentation rate is followed, recognizing that in some patients it is normal during significant bouts of inflammation, whereas in others it is persistently elevated despite clinical improvement.

The child is encouraged to participate in normal activities as tolerated. Most children can attend school, although modifications in the schedule and layout of the classes may be necessary. At least part-time school attendance is important for peer interaction and social adjustment. Homebound tutoring is discouraged unless the child is extremely ill. Participation in physical education is also advised wherever possible. Often the patient is able to carry out his own physical therapy program during physical education class. Contact sports are often inappropriate because of continued joint involvement, but swimming is strongly encouraged.

Table 72–3. DIAGNOSIS AND MANAGEMENT OF DERMATOMYOSITIS

Clinical Manifestations
- Cutaneous
  - heliotropism, violaceous hue
  - face, trunk, extensor surfaces of elbows, knees, knucles
  - cutaneous infarctions
  - edema
- Muscle
  - weakness—proximal greater than distal
  - +/− tender
- Gastrointestinal
  - distention
  - pain
  - hemorrhage
  - perforation
- Pulmonary
  - aspiration pneumonia
  - respiratory insufficiency
  - fibrosis
- Cardiac
  - arrhythmias

Diagnostic Evaluation (referable to myopathy)
- Muscle enzymes—CPK, aldolase, SGOT, SGPT, LDH
- EMG
- muscle biopsy
- pulmonary function tests
- esophagram

Management
- Pharmacologic—steroids, occasionally immunosuppressive agents
- Physical therapy—active and passive range of motion, conditioning
- Supportive pulmonary care
- Psychosocial considerations
- Long-term follow-up essential

Late Complications
- Contractures
- Calcinosis
- Pulmonary fibrosis
- Change to another connective tissue disease

JUVENILE ONSET DERMATOMYOSITIS (JODM)
(Table 72–3)

Dermatomyositis is a chronic inflammatory multisystem disease that is manifested primarily in the skin and muscle. Additional involvement may occur in the pulmonary, cardiac, gastrointestinal, articular, and rarely, renal systems. The onset is commonly between 4 and 10 years of age, with a mean age of approximately 6 years, and females are affected approximately twice as often as males. The clinical onset of the disease may be sudden or insidious, and a prodromal phase including fatigue, irritability, and malaise may antedate the rash and weakness by several weeks or months.

The characteristic rash, which may precede, accompany, or follow the onset of muscle weakness, is observed in the periorbital area, over the malar eminences, chest, extensor surfaces of the elbows, knees, fingers, and medial malleoli. There may be a brawny edema of the subcutaneous tissues. Periungual erythema with capillary nail bed changes is also seen. The facial rash is erythematous, with varying degrees of violaceous hue or heliotropism. Low grade fever is seen in the majority of patients, but 5 to 10 per cent may manifest a 40° F temperature spike, usually associated with fulminating disease. The hallmark of the muscle disease is weakness, which is more prominent in the proximal than the distal musculature; hence, the shoulder and hip girdle and abdominal and neck muscles are weakest. Muscle tenderness may or may not be present.

Laboratory Investigation

The serum muscle enzymes are abnormal in the majority of patients, but they are occasionally normal. The most common abnormality is seen in the creatine phosphokinase and aldolase; however, SGOT, SGPT, and LDH are also abnormal in many patients. The ANA, rheumatoid factor test, and immunoglobulins are abnormal in some patients. Histocompatibility studies indicate an increase in HLA-B8 (Pachman and Cooke, 1980). The electromyogram is positive in the majority of patients. Nerve conduction velocities are normal. The muscle biopsy shows evidence of myositis. The blood count and erythrocyte sedimentation rate, which may be normal, should not be used as indicators of disease or normalcy.

Treatment

The majority of patients require corticosteroid therapy. The usual dosage of prednisone is 2 mg/kg/day divided into three doses. Once response begins with improved stamina and muscle strength and a reduction in the muscle enzymes, the corticosteroids can be changed to a single daily dose and tapered over the course of the next several months. The cutaneous manifestations are not as predictably amenable to steroid therapy, and they may continue to be active despite adequate control of the myositis. Patients who are not controlled with steroid therapy alone may be tried on immunosuppressive agents.

In addition to pharmacological management, extreme care must be taken to prevent deformity. Physical therapy should be instituted with passive range of motion early in the course of the disease to prevent muscle shortening with progressive contractures. Occupational therapy is helpful in making splints to maintain joints in functional positions. Active range of motion and conditioning exercises can be gently instituted as the patient improves.

Course and Prognosis

Many patients recover within two years never to have a relapse again. Conversely, some patients are extremely refractory to treatment and experience a pernicious course of rash, fever, muscle weakness, and eventual death. Overall, however, the prognosis is favorable and restoration of independent function is possible in the majority of cases.

REFERENCES

Ansell, B. M.: Rheumatic Disorders in Childhood. London, Butterworth & Co., Ltd., 1980.

Banker, B. Q., and Banker, M. V.: Dermatomyositis (systemic angiopathy) of childhood. Medicine, *45*(4):261–289, 1966.

Bohan, A., and Peter, J. B.: Polymyositis and dermatomyositis, Part I and Part II. N. Engl. J. Med., *292*:344–347, 403–407, 1975.

Brewer, E. J., Jr., et al.: Current proposed revision of JRA criteria. Arthritis Rheum., *20*(2) Suppl.:195, 1977.

Brewer, E. J., Giannini, E. H., and Person, D. A.: Juvenile Rheumatoid Arthritis, 2nd Ed. Philadelphia, W. B. Saunders Co., 1982.

Hanson, V.: Systemic lupus erythematosus, dermatomyositis, scleroderma, and vasculitides in childhood. *In* Kelley, W. B. (Ed.): Textbook of Rheumatology. Philadelphia, W. B. Saunders Co., pp. 1327–1348, 1981.

Miller, J. J., III (Ed.): Juvenile Rheumatoid Arthritis. Littleton, MA, PSG Publishing Co., Inc., 1979.

Pachman, L. M., and Cooke, N.: Juvenile dermatomyositis: A clinical and immunologic study. J. Pediatr., *96*(2):226–234, 1980.

Petty, R.: Epidemiology of juvenile rheumatoid arthritis. *In* Miller, J. J., III: Juvenile Rheumatoid Arthritis. Littleton, MA, PSG Publishing Co., Inc., 1979, p. 12.

Proceedings of the Conference of the Rheumatic Diseases of Childhood. Arthritis Rheum., *20*(2) Suppl:145–636, 1977.

Schaller, J. G.: Juvenile rheumatoid arthritis. Pediatr. Rev., *2*(6):163–174, 1980.

Smiley, W. K.: The eye in juvenile chronic polyarthritis. Clin. Rheum. Dis., *2*(2):413–428, 1976.

73
HEADACHES

Morris Green, M.D.

The diagnostic possibilities of chronic or recurrent headaches are listed in Table 73–1.

DIAGNOSTIC POSSIBILITIES

Muscle Contraction Headaches

Muscle contraction, presumably secondary to tension, is the most common cause for recurrent or persistent headaches. The complaint may be described as a "tight band around the head," "pressure from the outside," or persistent aching. While such headaches are usually generalized, the discomfort may begin in the muscles of the neck, shoulders, or occiput and migrate anteriorly to the frontal region. Usually there are no prodromal symptoms, but nausea, vomiting, dizziness, or nervousness may occur concurrently.

Table 73–1. CAUSES OF HEADACHE

I. Muscle contraction headache
II. Vascular (migraine) headaches
  A. Classic migraine
  B. Common migraine
  C. Complicated migraine
    1. Hemiplegic or hemisensory migraine
    2. Ophthalmoplegic migraine
    3. Acute confusional states
    4. Basilar migraine
    5. Alice-in-Wonderland syndrome
  D. Cluster headache
III. Combined headache—muscle contraction and vascular
IV. Traction headache
  A. Intracranial tumors; hematoma
  B. Brain abscess
  C. Intracranial malformation
  D. Arteriovenous malformations
  E. Pseudotumor cerebri
  F. Central nervous system leukemia
V. Inflammatory disease of the central nervous system
VI. Post-traumatic headache
VII. Ocular disorders
VIII. Sinusitis
IX. Hypertension
X. Psychogenic
  A. Conversion reactions
  B. Depression
  C. Hypochondriasis

Migraine Headaches

Although migraine headaches in children over seven years of age may be similar to those in adults, more frequently young children present with cyclic vomiting and generalized, severe headaches. Classic migraine hemicranial headaches occur in the retro-orbital, frontal, or temporal regions, usually repeatedly on the same side. Prodromal or concurrent symptoms include photophobia, nausea, vomiting, abdominal pain, pallor, sweating, facial flushing, eyelid edema, and mood changes. Scintillating scotomata, hemianopsia, zigzag lines, blurred vision, or paresthesias are less frequent in children than in adults. Initially unilateral and throbbing or pulsating, the headache usually becomes generalized and constant. While episodes generally last two to three hours, they may persist 48 hours or longer. Children commonly sleep during or after the attack. Migraine and muscle contraction headaches may occur simultaneously. Eighty-five per cent of the parents of children with migraine have a history of headaches, and 70 per cent have classic migraine.

Complicated migraine is accompanied by neurological deficits. Ophthalmoplegic migraine, which involves the oculomotor and, less frequently, the abducens nerve, is rare in early childhood. Twelve to 24 hours after the onset of the headache, eye pain, nausea, and vomiting develop along with sudden, usually unilateral, ptosis, dilatation of the pupil, and reduced mobility of the eye. These findings may persist for days or weeks. Hemiplegic migraine, at times familial, is characterized by neurological deficits, such as aphasia, paresthesias, hemiparesis or hemisensory loss, which may last for hours to days. Headache usually follows on the contralateral side.

Basilar artery migraine may occur from late infancy through adolescence with a sudden onset of transient bilateral blindness, vertigo, ataxia, dysarthria, tinnitus, blurred vision, oculomotor abnormalities, ataxia, loss of consciousness, paresthesias around the mouth and the distal extremities, and cranial nerve deficits. Severe headache—bifrontal, temporal, or occipital—and vomiting follow. Acute confusional states persisting 10 minutes to 24 hours may be the initial or later manifestation of a migraine episode in older children and adolescents. Accompanying symptoms may include agitation, apprehensiveness, and combativeness. The Alice-in-Wonderland syndrome is characterized by olfactory, gustatory, and auditory hallucinations, micropsia, metamorphosia, and other distortions of time and space.

Cluster headaches, characterized by bursts of one to three headaches a day over a period of weeks, are uncommon in children. In addition to severe headaches, the patient may develop unilateral conjunctival injection, rhinorrhea, and lacrimation.

Traction Headaches

Causes for traction headaches include intracranial tumors, hematoma, brain abscess, arteriovenous malformations, pseudotumor cerebri, and central nervous system leukemia. Headache is less commonly a symptom of intracranial tumors in children than in adults and is rarely the presenting symptom. Although headaches due to a brain tumor usually occur in the morning shortly after arising and disappear after a brief time, they may be present at other times, e.g., awakening the child from sleep. They may be precipitated by sudden exacerbations in intracranial pressure caused by coughing, sneezing, straining with a bowel movement, or change in position. Traction headaches are usually described as dull, deep, and intermittent, although occasionally steady. They also may be intense and incapacitating. That a headache may be temporarily relieved by aspirin does not rule out an intracranial mass lesion. Temporary lessening of the headache may also be due to separation of the sutures. Severe and prolonged headaches and those that have changed in character, fail to respond to medication, or are accompanied by a change in personality or vomiting are worrisome.

Rupture of an intracranial aneurysm may be accompanied by excruciating headache, photophobia, meningeal signs, and impaired consciousness. Arteriovenous malformations may produce a sudden headache, obtundation, focal neurological defect, signs of meningeal irritation, and increased intracranial pressure. In addition to severe headache, patients with pseudotumor cerebri may have blurring of vision, diplopia, nausea, vomiting, and bilateral papilledema. The neurological examination and computerized axial tomography are normal. Symptoms may persist for weeks. Central nervous system leukemia causes headaches, irritability, diplopia, polyphagia, and rapid weight gain.

Post-traumatic Headaches

Post-traumatic headaches occurring in children after a severe head injury, especially one leading to unconsciousness, may persist for months or years. The patient may also complain of dizziness, nervousness, heightened sensitivity to noise, inability to concentrate, hyperactivity, sleep disturbance, and difficulty controlling anger. While the child's emotional reaction to the injury may have been unusually severe, the premorbid emotional adjustment and current environmental stresses should be explored. Unsettled litigation related to the accident seems to contribute to persistence of the symptoms in some cases. The differential diagnosis includes a chronic subdural hematoma.

Ocular Disorders and Sinusitis

Headache may be caused by eyestrain secondary to uncorrected refractive errors, astigmatism, muscle imbalance, or impaired convergence. Other ocular symptoms may include burning, tearing, conjunctival hyperemia, blurring, and dizziness. Since photophobia and conjunctival injection may accompany severe headache of any cause, they do not necessarily indicate the presence of eye disease. Sinusitis or inflammation and engorgement of the nasal turbinates are infrequent causes of chronic headache in children.

Hypertension

Chronic hypertension is an unusual cause of chronic headache in children. Acute hypertensive encephalopathy like that associated with acute glomerulonephritis is manifested by severe headache, nausea, vomiting, confusion, seizures, and transient focal neurological findings.

Psychogenic Headaches

Identification with a relative or other important person or a conversion reaction are other possible mechanisms for psychogenic headaches. Constant, dull headaches, lasting for days, are almost always psychogenic, most frequently due to depression. Severe and frequent headaches are a common feature in patients with psychogenic purpura (autoerythrocyte sensitization, Gardner-Diamond syndrome).

THE DIAGNOSTIC APPROACH

The Interview

The pediatric interview is the most helpful tool in understanding the cause of headaches. Both migraine and muscle contraction headaches may be precipitated by stress, e.g., arguments between the child and someone close to him. They may also be associated with disappointment, rejection, intense excitement, anxiety, and fear of failure as in school examinations, auditions, recitals, or contests. Patients with migraine headaches report numerous precipitating factors including excessive noise, confusion, illness, foods (cheese, chocolate, or citrus fruits), alcohol, menstruation, oral contraceptives, extreme exertion, emotional stress, fasting, loss of sleep, prolonged sleep, and lengthy viewing of television or movies.

Children with either muscle contraction or migraine headaches and, at times, their families may have difficulty with feelings of aggression, anger, or resentment, especially toward significant persons. Unaware of a relationship between headaches and feelings, they are unlikely to volunteer this association. Since these feelings are often unconscious, the child may deny their presence. Although muscle contraction or migraine headaches may be precipitated by events that immediately evoke anger, the child who is chronically inhibited from its direct expression by strong parental disapproval, personal discomfort, or guilt may carry a burden of intense resentment. It is appropriate to ask the child what kinds of things make him mad, how he deals with his anger, and how he would like to manage it. Similar information should be obtained from the parents. The presence of anxiety and depression in the child should also be explored.

The Physical Examination

The physical and neurological examination should include careful funduscopy, testing of visual fields, and screening for visual acuity, ability to converge, and phorias. Re-evaluation is indicated periodically, especially in the first four to six months after onset of the headache.

Procedures

Since it is unusual for headaches to be the only manifestation of a seizure disorder, an electroencephalogram is rarely helpful. Computerized tomography is indicated if an intracranial structural mass lesion is suspected. Since the vast majority of headaches in children are due to muscle contraction or migraine, it is rarely necessary to carry out laboratory procedures such as CT scan, EEG, or skull roentgenograms. A good history, negative physical examination, and a therapeutic trial reliably make the diagnosis most of the time.

TREATMENT

Children and their parents are often greatly relieved to learn that their concerns about the possibility of a brain tumor or "increased pressure" are needless. The reassurance of a meticulous physical examination and the physician's clarification of the etiology of the headache may, in itself, lead to a diminution of the complaint. Prevention and treatment of migraine and muscle contraction headaches are facilitated by attention to the child's daily schedule. This may include the suggestion that the child consider a less strenuous day, reducing the number of his extracurricular activities; avoiding excessive fatigue, excitement, or television viewing; and adopting a regular time for sleep and meals. The physician's periodic reinforcement may be required to support such changes. Although the child may not elect to reduce his schedule, his understanding of the relation between such stress and headaches help him accept this discomfort as an unpleasant side effect of being a perceptive and intensely involved person.

Drug Therapy

Drug therapy is difficult to evaluate because headache is subjective, emotional factors play a prominent contributory role, and responses to pain, discomfort, and medication are highly individual.

Aspirin and acetaminophen provide highly effective symptomatic relief. The dosage of both aspirin and acetaminophen is 5 to 8 mg/kg/dose, every 4 hours as necessary. Propoxyphene hydrochloride is sometimes used as a substitute for aspirin. Codeine, although highly effective in the treatment of severe headaches, is rarely indicated in children. Phenobarbital or other mild sedatives may be used with aspirin for a limited time as an adjunct in the management of severe muscle contraction headaches. Phenytoin or phenobarbital (3 to 5 mg/kg) has been used in anticonvulsant doses for the prophylaxis of migraine headaches.

Diazepam may be used in a dose of 2 to 5 mg, depending on the age of the child, for symptomatic relief of an unusually severe muscle contraction headache. Amitriptyline in a dosage of 1 to 2 mg/kg may be useful with muscle contraction, migraine, or combined headaches, especially in the depressed teenager. Fifty mg is generally the starting dose in adolescents. The dose may be gradually increased over several weeks to a total of 200 mg a day in divided doses.

If aspirin or similar mild analgesics alone or with a sedative do not relieve migraine headaches, Fiorinal may be taken at the onset of the headache and again in one hour. Depending upon the age of the child, the initial dose is one to two tablets with another tablet an hour later as needed. Midrin in a dosage of two capsules at the onset of a headache and another capsule one hour later as needed may be used as an alternate drug. In adolescents whose classic migraine pain does not respond to these analgesic agents, the combination of ergotamine tartrate and caffeine may be tried. The patient should take one or two tablets of a preparation such as Cafergot during the prodromal phase or at the first sign of a headache. If symptomatic relief is not obtained, the dose may be repeated every 30 minutes for four times. The total dosage, once determined, can be taken initially. If nausea and vomiting are prominent prodromal symptoms, a rectal suppository or sublingual preparation may be used. Ergotamines should not be used in the treatment of complicated migraine or for prepubertal children.

Migraine prophylactic medication may be considered in children who have more than four or five headaches a month. In controlled studies, cyproheptadine hydrochloride (Periactin) in a dosage of 0.3 mg/kg/day in three divided doses has been thought to reduce the number and severity of migraine episodes. Propranolol, a highly useful drug for the prophylaxis of migraine headaches whether of the common, classic, or complex form, may be used in all age groups and is the agent of choice for the older adolescent. In children under 12 years of age the dose is 5 to 10 mg t.i.d.; over that age, the dose is 10 to 20 mg t.i.d. A higher dose may be used, but not over 30 to 40 mg q.i.d. Propranolol is contraindicated in patients with asthma, other pulmonary disorders, and cardiovascular disease. Clonidine has also been used for migraine prophylaxis.

Biofeedback training and relaxation therapy are recently explored techniques for the treatment of chronic muscle contraction and migraine headaches in children.

REFERENCES

Honig, P. J., and Charney, E. B.: Children with brain tumor headaches. Am. J. Dis. Child., *136*:121, 1982.

Prensky, A. L.: Headaches. *In* Gellis, S. S., and Kagen, B. M. (Eds.): Current Pediatric Therapy 10. Philadelphia, W. B. Saunders Co., 1982, p. 73.

Shinnar, S., and D'Souza, B.: Migraine in children and adolescents. Pediatr. Rev., 3:257, 1982.

Thompson, J. A.: Diagnosis and treatment of headache in the pediatric patient. Curr. Probl. Pediatr. *10*:5, 1980.

74

CHRONIC FATIGUE

Morris Green, M.D.

Chronic fatigue, lassitude, or "lack of energy" is occasionally reported in older children and adolescents. Table 74–1 is an etiological classification of fatigue. Depression is probably the most common cause of the child's awakening tired and needing to rest frequently during the day. Masked school phobia should also be considered in older children who complain of chronic fatigue. A comprehensive pediatric interview and physical examination, supplemented by laboratory examinations considered clinically indicated (mono spot test, SGOT, BUN, serum creatine, CBC, T_3, T_4, sedimentation rate, and chest x-ray) will usually permit a diagnosis to be readily established. The management of many of the etiological disorders is discussed in other chapters.

Table 74–1. ETIOLOGICAL CLASSIFICATION OF FATIGUE

I. Emotional	IV. Endocrine
A. Depression	A. Cushing's disease
B. Masked school phobia	B. Addison's disease
C. Grief	C. Hypo- and hyperthyroidism
D. Hyperventilation syndrome	D. Primary hyperaldosteronism
II. Infectious	V. Allergic
A. Infectious mononucleosis	VI. Sleep Disorders
B. Hepatitis	VIII. Cardiac
C. Tuberculosis	IX. Miscellaneous
D. Histoplasmosis	A. Sarcoidosis
E. Chronic infections	B. Myasthenia gravis
III. Hematology/Oncology	C. End-stage renal disease
A. Anemia	D. Chronic pulmonary disease
B. Leukemia; lymphoma	

75

PEDIATRIC DERMATOLOGY

Sidney Hurwitz, M.D.

It has been estimated that 20 to 30 per cent of children and adolescents seen by pediatricians and family practitioners present problems related directly or indirectly to the skin. This chapter is designed to provide physicians with information that will enable them to deal effectively with common skin problems in the pediatric age group (Hurwitz, 1981a).

IMPETIGO

There are two basic forms of impetigo: (1) a thick-crusted variety which is primarily streptococcal in origin and (2) a bullous form which is associated with phage group II staphylococci (Fig. 75–1). Lesions due to streptococci frequently affect the lower extremities, appear in

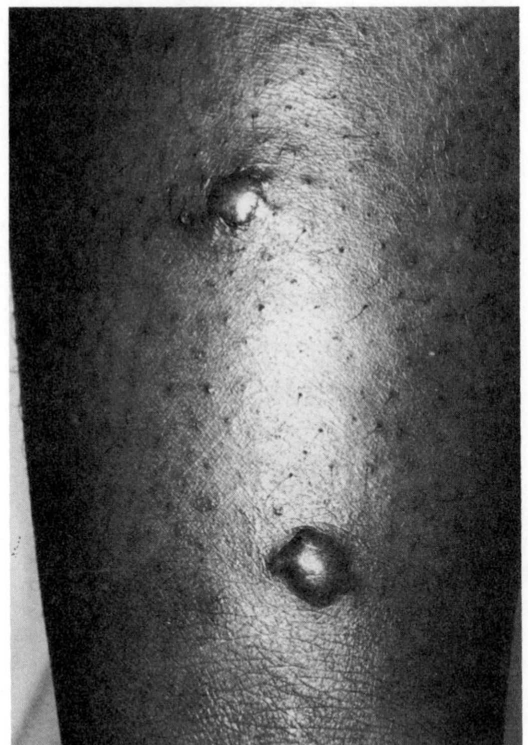

Figure 75–1. Bullous impetigo. Characteristic of group II staphylococcal infection. (This and all other illustrations in this chapter are from Hurwitz, S.: Clinical Pediatric Dermatology. Philadelphia, W. B. Saunders Company, 1981.)

hot summer months, and often consist of punched-out ulcers on the legs with superimposed crusts. Trauma and insect bites contribute to the pathogenesis, and fever and lymphadenopathy are frequent early features of this disorder. Lesions of staphylococcal impetigo generally affect the face, trunk, and extremities, do not appear to have a seasonal predilection, and consist of superficial blisters that rupture and leave a scalded appearance (Table 75–1).

In older children, simple uncomplicated impetigo frequently responds to gentle washing of lesions, removal of crusts, and drainage of blisters and pustules, thus helping prevent local spread and reaccumulation of crusts. If crusts are firmly adherent, warm soaks or compresses are useful. Topical antibiotics are frequently highly effective in treatment of early superficial pyoderma due to *Staphylococcus aureus*. In cutaneous infections due to beta-hemolytic streptococcus or persistent staphylococcal infection, however, systemic antibiotics produce swifter response and fewer failures.

Children with streptococcal impetigo are best treated with systemic antibiotics, but owing to changing patterns and increasing resistance to penicillin, penicillin G is generally not recommended for the treatment of *Staphylococcus aureus* infection. Such individuals are best treated with erythromycin for a period of 7 to 10 days. For those acutely ill or with severe forms of bullous impetigo, however, dicloxacillin should be administered. Although the risk of developing glomerulonephritis following skin infection with a nephritogenic strain of streptococci is high (12 to 28 per cent), systemic antibiotics may eliminate cutaneous streptococci but do not prevent glomerulonephritis due to streptococcal impetigo.

STAPHYLOCOCCAL SCALDED SKIN SYNDROME

Staphylococcal scalded skin syndrome (SSSS) is a distinctive dermatitis caused by an exfoliative toxin termed "exfoliatin," generally elaborated by coagulase-positive group II staphylococci, usually but not necessarily phage type 55 or 71, occasionally group I, type 52 (Melish and Glasgow, 1971). This disorder is characterized by three phases: erythematous, exfoliative, and desquamative. It often begins with a prodromal period, malaise, fever, irritability, and generalized erythema with a fine, stippled sandpaper appearance and exquisite tenderness of the skin.

The exfoliative phase is heralded by exudation and crusting around the mouth and sometimes the orbits, and separation of crusts surrounding the mouth, producing radial fissures which give this disorder its characteristic appearance (Fig. 75–2). The upper layer of the epidermis may become wrinkled or may become removed by a light stroking (often peeling off like a wet tissue paper—Nikolsky's sign).

Table 75–1. CLINICAL FEATURES OF STREPTOCOCCAL AND STAPHYLOCOCCAL IMPETIGO

	Streptococcal	Staphylococcal
Invasion Sites	Traumatized skin (particularly lower extremities)	Face, trunk, extremities
Seasonal	Frequently in hot, humid months	No seasonal predilection
Characteristics	Vesicles, ulcers, and crusts	Bullae and "scalded skin"

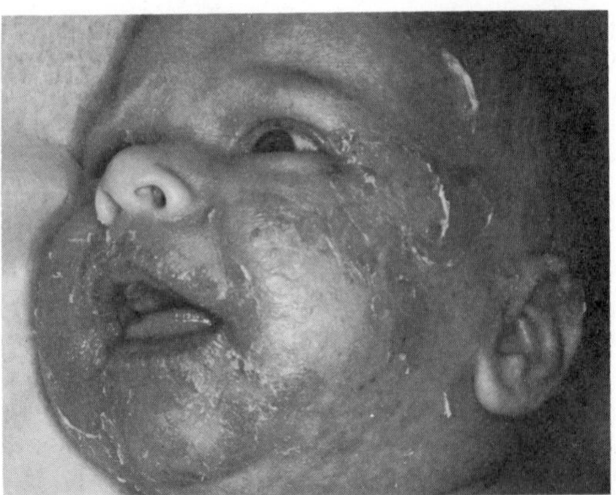

Figure 75–2. Staphylococcal scalded skin syndrome due to group II phage-type 71 staphylococcus.

Shortly thereafter the patient develops flaccid bullae and eventual exfoliation of the skin.

The diagnosis of staphylococcal scalded skin syndrome can be verified by isolation of coagulase-positive *Staphylococcus aureus* from pyogenic foci on the skin, conjunctivae, ala nasi, and nasopharynx and in stools and occasionally blood. The organism is not recovered from blisters or areas of exfoliation.

Treatment requires prompt initiation of antistaphylococcal therapy to eradicate the focus of infection and eliminate further toxin production. Topical antibiotics are ineffective. Since most staphylococcal antibiotics are resistant to erythromycin, penicillinase-resistant antistaphylococcal agents such as dicloxacillin are preferred.

DIAPER DERMATITIS

Diaper dermatitis (diaper rash) is perhaps the most common cutaneous disorder of infancy and childhood. Seen most frequently in infants and children less than two years of age, diaper dermatoses usually begin between the first and second months of life and, if not properly controlled, may recur at intervals until the child no longer wears diapers. Diaper dermatitis is not a specific diagnosis but refers to a group of disorders initiated by a combination of factors, the most significant being prolonged contact with or irritation by the urine and feces, maceration by wet diapers and impervious diaper coverings, and, in a high percentage of cases, secondary infection with *Candida albicans* (Table 75–2) (Leyden et al., 1977).

Table 75–2. DIAPER DERMATITIS

1. A symptom complex
2. Etiology (a combination of factors)
   a. Prolonged contact or irritation by urine and feces
   b. Maceration due to wet diapers and impervious diaper coverings
   c. High incidence of secondary infection with *Candida albicans*
3. May be the first sign of a more severe or systemic disorder

The management of diaper dermatitis is directed at keeping the area clean and dry and limiting irritation and maceration by the avoidance of occlusive diaper coverings. Frequent diaper changes, especially at night, thorough cleansing, and the judicious use of topical therapy may be sufficient to keep the patient free from this disorder. Severe and secondarily infected dermatitis should be treated systemically with appropriate antibiotics. Candidal infection is characterized by a beefy red color, a sharp marginated edge, and pinpoint pustulovesicular satellite lesions (Fig. 75–3). Candidal infections require topical application of an antimonilial agent, preferably miconazole (Monistat-Derm) or clotrimazole (Lotrimin or Mycelex). Low-potency topical corticosteroids applied lightly in a thin film are effective in inflammatory or contact dermatitis and will hasten recovery of damaged skin. For recurrent diaper dermatitis, preparations such as 1:2:3 ointment (a combination of Burow's solution 10.0, Aquaphor 20.0, and zinc oxide, q.s. ad 60.0) are particularly helpful (Hurwitz, 1981a).

ATOPIC DERMATITIS

Atopic dermatitis, one of the most common disorders of infancy and childhood, is a hereditary condition characterized by a chronic, pruritic, eczematoid eruption in an individual with a personal or familial tendency toward atopic disease such as asthma or allergic rhinitis (Hurwitz, 1981b). The disorder can be divided into three phases, based upon the age of the patient and the distribution of lesions: infantile atopic dermatitis, atopic dermatitis of childhood, and atopic dermatitis of the adolescent and adult.

Infantile atopic dermatitis usually begins between two and six months of age on the cheeks, forehead, or scalp and then extends to the trunk or extremities in scattered, often symmetrical patches (Fig. 75–4). Although scaling and crusting of the scalp may suggest seborrheic dermatitis, the severe itching, a history of atopy,

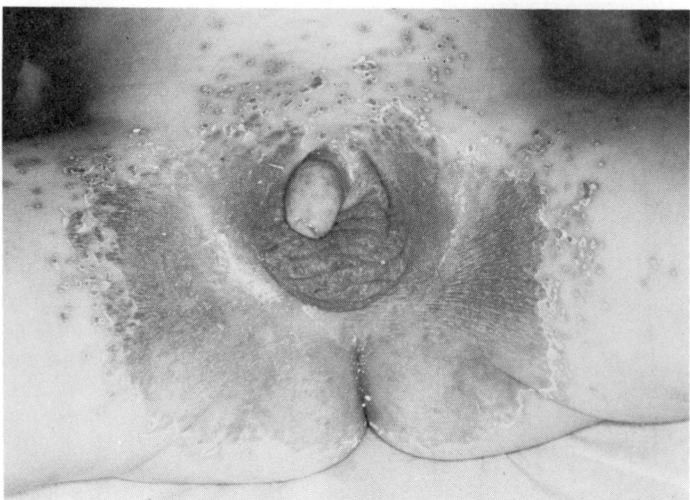

Figure 75–3. Candidal (monilial) diaper dermatitis with sharp margination and pustulovesicular satellite lesions.

and the character and distribution of lesions help differentiate the two disorders.

The childhood phase usually occurs from 4 to 10 years of age. Affected individuals are less likely to have exudative and crusted lesions and have a greater tendency toward chronicity and lichenification. The classic areas of involvement in this group are the wrists, ankles, antecubital and popliteal regions, and feet. Remission generally occurs before the age of 10 or 12, but the disorder may merge into the succeeding adolescent and adult phase.

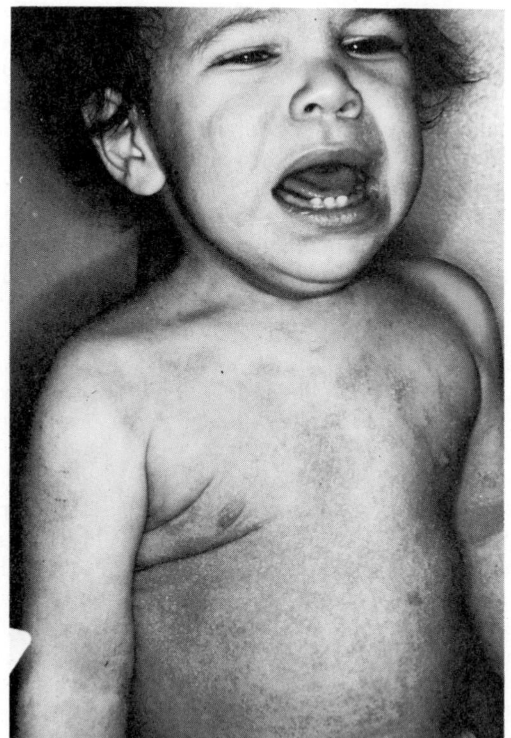

Figure 75–4. Atopic dermatitis. Characteristic facies and generalized eczematous eruption.

The adolescent and adult stage of atopic dermatitis begins at or around 12 years of age and frequently persists into the early twenties or later. Predominant areas of involvement include the flexor folds, face and neck, upper arms and back, and dorsal aspect of the feet, hands, fingers, and toes. The eruption in this age group is frequently characterized by dry and thick lesions, confluent papules, and the formation of large lichenified plaques. Weeping, crusting, and exudation may occur, usually the result of superimposed external irritation or infection.

The diagnosis of atopic dermatitis is based upon the aggregate of signs, symptoms, stigmata (atopic pleats, dryness and itching of the skin, keratosis pilaris, increased palmar markings, and lichenification), course, and associated familial findings.

The disease is characterized by severe spasmodic itching and its consequences. Clinically, it is recognized as a pruritic erythematous papular and vesicular eruption with edema, serous discharge, and crusting. Sites of predilection frequently are helpful. In chronic forms of atopic dermatitis, scaling, lichenification (Fig. 75–5), hyperpigmentation, thickening, and fissuring are characteristic (Hurwitz, 1981b).

Secondary infection is the most common complication seen in atopic dermatitis. At times associated with group A beta-hemolytic streptococci and, even more frequently, staphylococcal organisms, the skin of patients with atopic dermatitis appears to be inherently favorable for *Staphylococcus aureus* colonization. Postin-

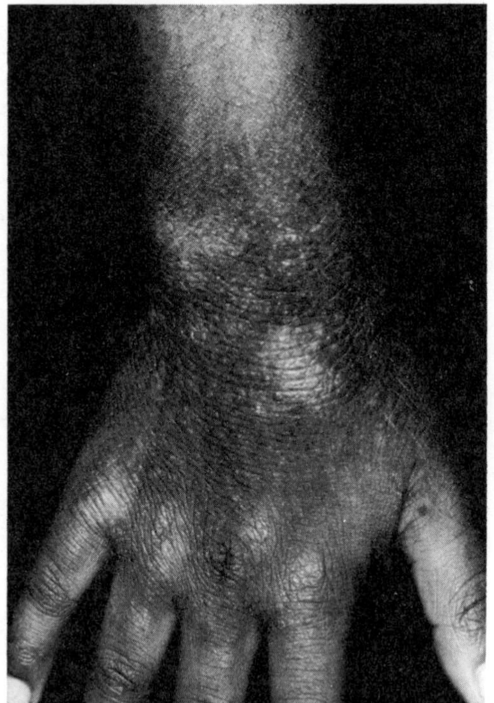

Figure 75–5. Lichenification. A hyperpigmented thickened leathery reaction to persistent rubbing and scratching in a patient with chronic atopic dermatitis.

flammatory hypopigmentation may be noted following involution of eczematous lesions. Since this defect is primarily epidermal, post-inflammatory hypopigmentation generally improves with time without a need for active therapy. Kaposi's varicelliform eruption caused by *Herpes virus hominis* is characterized by umbilication of vesicles.

The treatment of atopic dermatitis depends on the management of dry and itching skin. Patients should be instructed to limit bathing and to use lubricants to help moisten and rehydrate the skin. A mild soap such as Dove or Neutrogena may be used. For individuals who prefer to bathe more frequently, an alternate program may be utilized. In this regimen (the wet method) the patient may soak in a tepid or lukewarm bath for a period of 20 minutes or more. While the child is wet, preferably while still in the water, a thin coating of petrolatum is applied liberally to the skin.

Cetaphil lotion may be used instead of soap and water as a cleansing and lubricating agent for individuals with dry skin. This hydrophilic lotion may be applied liberally and rubbed gently over the skin once or twice a day (without water) until a light foaming occurs. Following removal by light wiping with a soft cotton cloth or cleansing tissue, a protective lubricating film remains.

Although benefit from dietary restrictions may be interpreted with skepticism, many physicians advocate the elimination of specific foods in the management of atopic dermatitis especially in the first year or two of life. In such instances specific foods may produce an urticarial reaction that may initiate pruritus and scratching, resulting in exacerbations of atopic dermatitis. For such individuals potential allergenic foods may be eliminated until the disorder is controlled.

As the child grows older, food reactivity frequently diminishes. It should be noted, however, that food allergies are not a cause but may act as triggering factors. Effective therapy, therefore, requires a careful history, observation of ingestants that might trigger exacerbations, particularly during the first year or two of life, a temporary elimination of suspected food allergens, and, of primary consideration, judicious management of the dry and itching skin characteristic of this disorder.

Skin tests and hyposensitization are of little value and are rarely necessary in the management of children with atopic dermatitis. Topical steroid preparations, however, are extremely effective but they must be carefully selected. This involves the correct strength and proper formulation for the particular eruption (Table 75–3). Considering the wide use of topical corticosteroids, there have been relatively few reports of adverse reaction due to their absorption. When applied over large areas of dermatitic skin, or when used under occlusion, the possibility of systemic absorption must, however, be considered. This is particularly true for infants and small children where suppression of the pituitary-adrenal axis and growth retardation have been documented. Other potential side effects of topical corticosteroids, particularly when used under occlusion or for long periods of time, include cutaneous atrophy, steroid rosacea, striae, telangiectasia, and perioral dermatitis.

Potent topical steroids, when used judiciously, may be used in small areas for short periods of time with relatively little risk of absorption. Once the disorder is under control, however, it is advisable to taper the therapy to a moderately potent topical corticosteroid and, as the disorder continues to improve, to one of the less potent hydrocortisone formulations. This gradual reduction of topical steroid potency over a period of weeks is advisable in an effort to avoid a rebound phenomenon that tends to

Table 75–3. ORDER OF POTENCY OF TOPICAL STEROIDS (from most to least potent)

I.	Diprosone ointment 0.05% Florone ointment 0.05% Halog cream 0.1% Lidex cream 0.05% Lidex ointment 0.05% Topicort ointment 0.25% Topsyn gel 0.05%
II.	Aristocort cream 0.5% Diprosone cream 0.05% Florone cream 0.05% Flurobate gel 0.025% (Benisone gel) Topicort cream 0.25% Valisone lotion 0.1% Valisone ointment 0.1%
III.	Aristocort ointment 0.1% Cordran ointment 0.05% Kenalog ointment 0.1% Synalar cream (HP) 0.2% Synalar ointment 0.025%
IV.	Cloderm cream 0.1% Cordran cream 0.05% Kenalog cream 0.1% Kenalog lotion 0.025% Synalar cream 0.025% Valisone cream 0.1% Westcort cream 0.2%
V.	Tridesilon cream 0.05% Locorten cream 0.03%
VI.	Topicals with hydrocortisone, Alphaderm, dexamethasone, Flumethalone, prednisolone, methyl prednisolone

Updated from Hurwitz (1981a) and Stoughton (1976).

occur when topical steroids are too rapidly discontinued. Following the gradual reduction of topical corticosteroids, the disorder frequently can be controlled with a regimen of limited baths, frequent lubrication, and antipruritics (as needed) in an effort to minimize the dryness and itchiness inherent in this disorder (Hurwitz, 1981a).

Open wet dressings (Table 75–4) and appropriate antibiotics are frequently important in the treatment of secondary infection. Systemic steroids, however, should be reserved only for those few, extremely severe cases that cannot be controlled by other means.

Table 75–4. OPEN WET DRESSINGS

Action

1. Soothing, cooling, and antipruritic
2. Removal of crusts and debris
3. Astringent and antibacterial effect
4. Hydration

Technique

1. Handkerchief, diaper, or strip of bed sheeting
2. Tepid or room temperature
3. Moderately wet (not dripping)
4. Remoisten at intervals

From Hurwitz (1981b).

Pityriasis Alba

Pityriasis alba is a common cutaneous disorder characterized by discrete asymptomatic hypopigmented patches on the face, neck, upper trunk, and proximal extremities of children and young adults (Fig. 75–6). Individual lesions vary from one to several centimeters in diameter and have sharply delineated margins and a fine branny scale.

The cause is unknown, but the disorder appears to represent a nonspecific dermatitis (possibly a mild form of atopic dermatitis). Most cases appear following sun exposure and result from a disturbance in pigmentation of the affected areas. Topical hydrocortisone formulations and lubrication followed by sun exposure appear to diminish the dry skin and fine scaling, allowing repigmentation of involved areas, generally within a period of several weeks (Hurwitz, 1981a).

SEBORRHEIC DERMATITIS

Seborrheic dermatitis is a term used to refer to an erythematous, scaly or crusting eruption

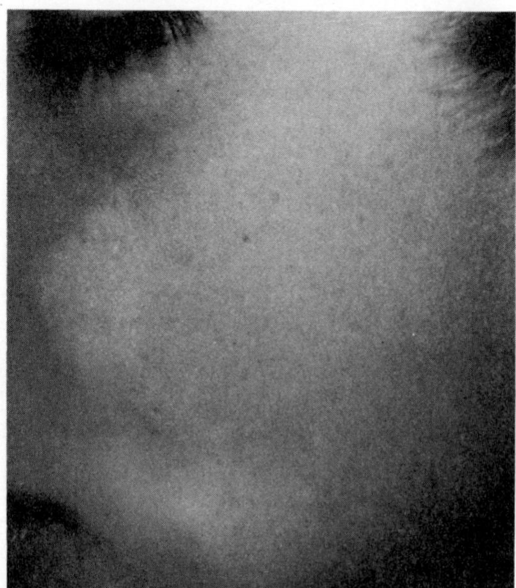

Figure 75–6. Pityriasis alba. Circumscribed scaly hypopigmented lesions on the cheek.

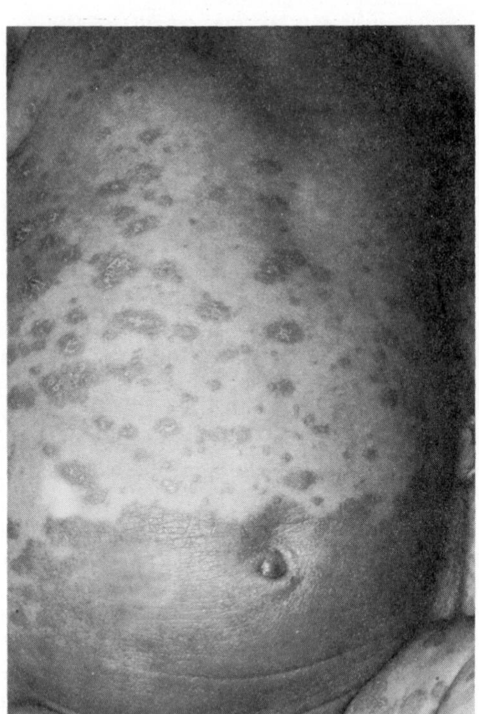

Figure 75–7. Seborrheic dermatitis. Greasy well-marginated scaly eruption on trunk and diaper area.

that occurs primarily in the so-called seborrheic areas, namely the scalp, face, and postauricular, presternal, and intertriginous areas (Fig. 75–7). The specific etiology of this disorder remains unknown. Although it may continue throughout life, it is most commonly seen in infancy between the second and tenth weeks of life, usually clears spontaneously by 8 to 12 months of age, and generally does not recur until the onset of puberty.

The therapy of seborrheic dermatitis depends on the nature, severity, and location of the disorder. The scalp should be treated with antiseborrheic shampoos. If the scales are thick and adherent, removal can be facilitated by the use of slightly warm mineral oil or petrolatum. In stubborn or persistent cases, wrapping the scalp with a warm damp towel before shampooing may assist in removal of thick scales and crusts, or the use of "P&S" liquid (Baker/Cummins) may be helpful.

Mothers should be instructed that when the scalp is shampooed, gentle scrubbing of the scalp is safe and often necessary in order to facilitate removal of thick adherent scales. For stubborn or persistent lesions, a topical corticosteroid lotion, such as 1 per cent hydrocortisone or 0.01 per cent Synalar or Fluonid solution, alone or in combination with 3 to 5 per cent sulfur precipitate or salicylic acid, or both, is frequently effective. These formulations may be applied two or three times a day.

NUMMULAR ECZEMA

Nummular eczema is a cutaneous eruption characterized by discoid or coin-shaped plaques of eczema. Lesions are composed of minute papules and vesicles which enlarge by peripheral extension to form discrete, round or oval, erythematous, often lichenified and hyperpigmented plaques varying in size from one to several centimeters in diameter (Fig. 75–8). They usually occur on the extensor surfaces of the hands, arms, and legs, as single or multiple lesions on dry or asteatotic skin. The specific etiology is unknown. It seems to appear in a cold or dry environment and is aggravated by excessive bathing and local irritants such as wool or harsh or drying soaps.

Effective therapy depends upon limited baths, frequent lubrication, and potent topical steroids, preferably in an ointment base or under occlusion (assuming, of course, that associated secondary infection is controlled).

CONTACT DERMATITIS

Contact dermatitis may be defined as an eczematous eruption produced either by local exposure to a primary irritating substance or by an acquired allergic response to a sensitizing substance. When the dermatitis is due to a nonallergic reaction of the skin, it is termed an *irritant contact dermatitis;* when it is a mani-

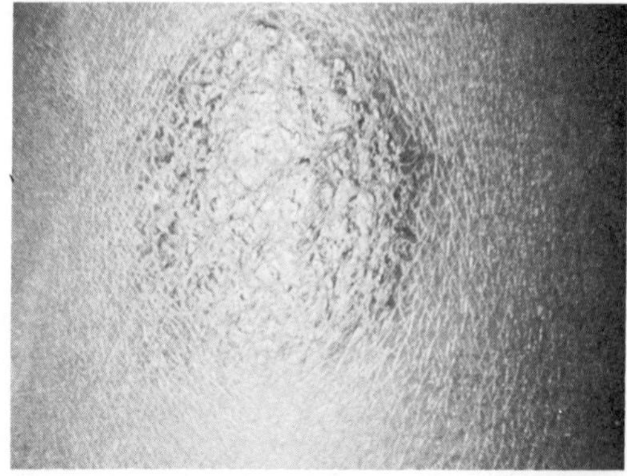

Figure 75–8. Nummular eczema. A well-circumscribed papulovesicular coinshaped lesion on the pretibial area of a patient with ichthyosis vulgaris.

festation of delayed hypersensitivity to a contact allergen, it is termed *allergic contact dermatitis*.

Primary irritant dermatitis may be produced by harsh soaps, bleaches, detergents, solvents, acids, alkalis, fiber glass particles, baby oils, bubble baths, certain foods, saliva, talcum powder, urine, feces, and intestinal secretions.

The diagnosis of allergic contact dermatitis is made on the appearance and distribution of skin lesions, aided, when possible, by a history of contact with an appropriate allergen. Acute eczematous lesions are characterized by an intense erythema accompanied by edema, papules, vesicles (sometimes bullae), oozing, and a sharp line of demarcation between the involved and normal skin. Chronic lesions are characterized by lichenification, fissuring, scaling, and little or no vesiculation.

The management of irritant and contact dermatitis is aided by topical corticosteroids. They are helpful in suppressing the pruritic manifestations and give temporary relief. In severe and incapacitating cases of poison ivy, oak, or sumac (Rhus) dermatitis, short-term systemic corticosteroid treatment may be indicated. Systemic steroid therapy may be initiated with dosages in the range of 20 to 30 mg of prednisone or its equivalent per day, with gradually tapering dosages over a period of two to three weeks. Premature termination of systemic steroid therapy may result in rapid rebound, with return of the dermatitis to its original intensity. The use of injectable steroids, however, should be discouraged, since the dosage can be neither modified nor terminated in the event of adverse reaction or need for change in therapy. Of further consideration in this respect is the fact that atrophy may at times occur as a sequela of intramuscular steroid therapy.

Desensitization to the oleoresin of poison ivy by the systemic administration of Rhus antigen is frequently disappointing and often produces undesirable side effects. It is probably best reserved for extremely sensitive patients who cannot avoid repeated exposure to the antigen.

PSORIASIS

Psoriasis is a common inherited disorder characterized by erythematous scaly papules or plaques with a predisposition for the elbows, knees, extensor surfaces of the limbs, genitalia, and lumbosacral area (Table 75–5).

Classic lesions of psoriasis consist of round, erythematous, well-marginated patches with a full, rich, red hue covered by a characteristic grayish or silvery-white scale (Fig. 75–9). Lesions almost invariably begin as small, reddish, pinpoint to pinhead-sized papules surmounted by fine scales. These papules coalesce and form patches or plaques that measure from 1 to 3 centimeters or more in diameter.

Table 75–5. PSORIASIS

1. Autosomal dominant with incomplete penetrance
2. Round, erythematous, well-marginated patches or plaques with rich red hue and mica-like scale
3. Bilaterally symmetrical pattern with predilection for scalp, elbows, knees, lumbosacral, and anogenital regions
4. Bleeding points on removal of scale (Auspitz's sign)
5. Nail changes
   a. In 25 to 50%
   b. Pitting, discoloration, crumbling of nail plate
   c. Subungual keratosis
   d. Onycholysis (separation of nail from nail bed)

The hallmark of psoriasis is the silvery micaceous (mica-like) scale that is generally attached at the center rather than the periphery of lesions. Removal of this scale results in fine punctate bleeding points (Auspitz's sign). The Koebner phenomenon, a special feature seen in psoriasis as well as in certain other skin

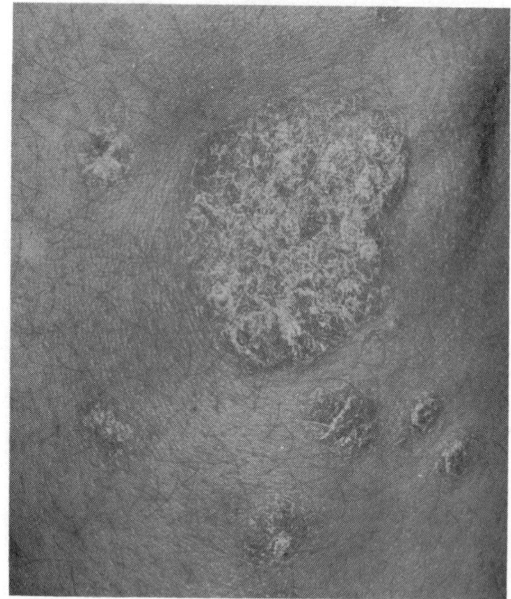

Figure 75–9. Psoriasis. Well-marginated papulosquamous lesions with mica-like scale.

disorders (verrucae, Rhus dermatitis, lichen planus), is the occurrence of patches of psoriasis that develop as a reaction to nonspecific injury. In addition to its clinical value as a diagnostic sign, this phenomenon is frequently seen as a precipitous cause of psoriasis and should be emphasized to all patients afflicted with this disorder.

The Koebner phenomenon is particularly significant in childhood psoriasis when drop-like (guttate) lesions appear suddenly over a large part of the body surface. Two-thirds of patients with guttate psoriasis give a history of an upper respiratory infection, generally but not necessarily streptococcal in origin, one to three weeks before the onset of an acute flare of the disorder. Lesions are round or oval in configuration and generally occur in a symmetrical distribution over the trunk and proximal aspects of the extremities (occasionally the face, scalp, ears, and distal aspects of the extremities) (Fig. 75–10).

The nails appear to be affected in 25 to 50 per cent of patients with psoriasis. Pitting is probably the best known and most characteristic nail change. Generally seen as small irregularly spaced depressions measuring less than 1 millimeter in diameter, larger depressions or punched-out areas of the nail plate may also be noted. Other psoriatic nail changes include discoloration, subungual hyperkeratosis, crumbling and grooving of the nail plate, and onycholysis (separation of the nail plate from the nail bed).

Topical corticosteroids are often the mainstay of local therapy for psoriasis. Although high-potency topical cortisteroids such as Halog and Florone cream or ointment applied two or three times a day are helpful in short-term management of severe recalcitrant lesions, most patients respond well to moderate- or low-potency steroid formulations. Tars still remain a highly effective therapeutic modality. Cosmetically acceptable preparations are now available for baths and as creams or lotions, and formulations of tar in a gel base (Estar gel and Psorigel) are safe, effective, and cosmetically acceptable. These may be used twice a day alone or, when necessary, in combination with topical corticosteroids. One may apply the tar, rub it in gently, and then apply the topical corticosteroid and rub it in right over it.

Most psoriatic patients are benefitted by exposure to sunlight and are frequently better during the summer months. Advantage should be taken of this in planning the activities of the psoriatic child. Appropriate precautions, however, must be exercised, since overexposure may result in sunburn or exacerbation of the disorder.

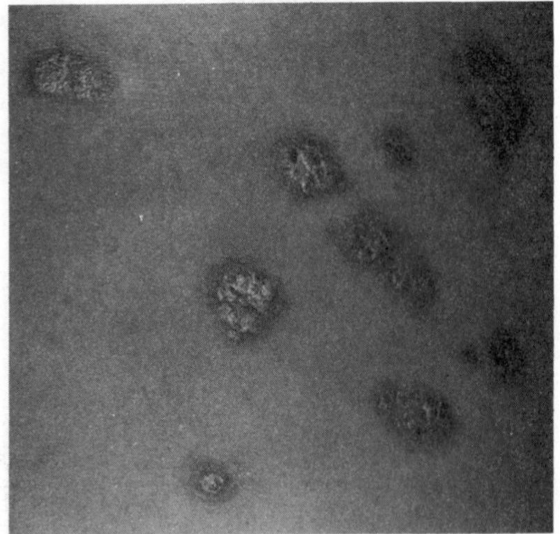

Figure 75–10. Guttate (droplike) psoriasis frequently occurs as a sequela of an upper respiratory infection (generally, but not necessarily, streptococcal in origin).

PITYRIASIS ROSEA

Pityriasis rosea is an acute, benign, self-limiting disorder with a peak incidence in adolescents and young adults. The eruption follows a distinctive pattern, and 70 to 80 per cent of cases start with a single isolated lesion, the so-called herald patch. It may occur anywhere on the body, most commonly the trunk, upper arms, neck, and eyes. This initial lesion is seen as a sharply defined oval area of scaly dermatitis (2 to 5 cm in diameter) with a flat, pink or brown center and a red, finely scaled, and slightly elevated border.

After an interval of 5 to 10 days a secondary generalized eruption appears in crops, generally sparing the face. These clinically distinctive lesions resemble the herald patch in morphology but are smaller and generally more ovoid in configuration. On the thorax the long axis of individual lesions runs parallel to the lines of skin cleavage in what has been described as a "Christmas-tree" pattern (Fig. 75–11). Typical of these secondary lesions is a fine scaly edge with a characteristic cigarette paper–like "collarette" scale. Occasionally, particularly in young children, lesions may be papular, vesicular, pustular, urticarial, or even purpuric in nature, particularly during the early stages of the eruption. Less commonly, some patients may show an inverse distribution of lesions on

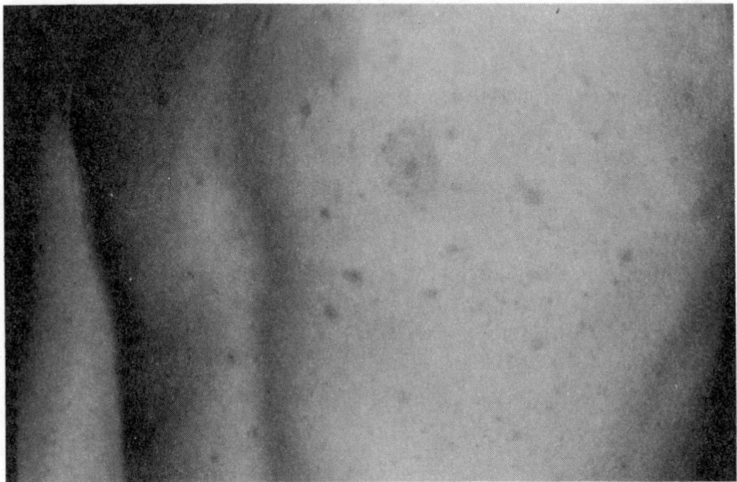

Figure 75–11. Pityriasis rosea. Christmas-tree pattern in lines of cleavage.

the face, wrists, and extremities, which may or may not spread centrally to include the trunk.

Most patients require no treatment beyond reassurance. Healing generally begins after a period of 2 to 4 weeks, and is usually complete by 6 to 12 weeks. Pruritus usually responds to topical antipruritic lotions and mild topical corticosteroid formulations. Exposure to ultraviolet light or sunshine generally tends to hasten resolution of lesions.

ICHTHYOSIS

Ichthyosis refers to a group of hereditary conditions characterized by dryness and scaling. These disorders have been divided into four major classes: (1) ichthyosis vulgaris (autosomal dominant); (2) sex-linked ichthyosis (X-linked recessive); (3) lamellar ichthyosis (autosomal recessive); and (4) epidermolytic hyperkeratosis (autosomal dominant).

Ichthyosis vulgaris is the mildest and most common form of ichthyosis (its incidence has been estimated as 1 in 250 to 1000 persons). The disorder is usually noticed after the first three months of life. Scales are most prominent on the extensor surfaces of the extremities, particularly in cold and dry weather. Scales on the pretibial and lateral aspect of the lower leg are large and platelike, resembling fish scales. The flexural areas are spared. In other areas small, white, branlike scales may be seen. Scaling of the forehead and cheeks, common during children, generally diminishes and clears with age.

The management of all types of dry skin consists of retardation of water loss, rehydration and softening of the stratum corneum, and alleviation of scaliness. Ichthyosis vulgaris and X-linked ichthyosis can be managed well by topical application of emollients and the use of keratolytic agents to facilitate removal of scales from the skin surface. Urea, in concentrations of 10 to 25 per cent, available as Carmol-10, Aquacare/HP, or Ultramide lotion, has a softening and moisturizing effect on the stratum corneum, and propylene glycol (40 to 60 per cent in water) applied overnight under plastic occlusion hydrates the skin and causes desquamation of scales. Alpha hydroxy acid preparations such as lactic acid (Lacticare lotion) are also beneficial.

EPIDERMOLYSIS BULLOSA

The term *epidermolysis bullosa* refers to a group of inherited disorders characterized by bullous lesions that develop spontaneously or as a result of varying degrees of friction or trauma. The absence or presence of permanent scarring allows this disorder to be divided into two major groups: those that result in complete healing without scarring and those that inevitably produce scars.

The treatment of epidermolysis bullosa is palliative, with avoidance of trauma and control of secondary infection. Oral phenytoin recently has been suggested for the treatment of dystrophic forms of this disorder (Eisenberg et al., 1978). Dosages of 2.5 to 5.0 mg/kg of body weight per day, to a maximum dose of 300 mg per day (a dosage high enough to obtain serum levels of 5 to 12 μg per milliliter), have proven to be helpful in the treatment of some individuals.

PIGMENTED MOLES AND NEVI

The incidence of nevocellular nevi in newborn infants is slightly more than one per cent (Jacobs and Walton, 1976). This incidence increases throughout infancy and adulthood, reaching a peak at puberty and adolescence. The size and pigmentation of lesions also increase at puberty, during pregnancy, or following systemic estrogen or corticosteroid therapy. Described on the basis of the location of the nevus cells, they may be designated as junctional (Fig. 75–12), intradermal (Fig. 75–13), or compound lesions (Fig. 75–14). Junctional nevi have nevus cells confined to the dermoepidermal junction, intradermal nevi have these nests in the dermis alone, and compound nevi have nevus cells in both locations (Table 75–6).

Junctional nevi are generally hairless, light to dark brown or brownish black macules. Ranging in size from 1 mm to 1 cm in diameter, their surface is smooth and flat, and skin furrows are preserved. Although most lesions are round, elliptical, or oval and show a relatively uniform pigmentation, some may be slightly irregular in configuration and color. *Compound nevi* may be present at birth but are more common in older children and adults. They tend to be more elevated and vary from a slightly raised plaque to a lesion of a somewhat papillomatous nature. They are flesh-colored to brown, may have a smooth or warty surface, and, particularly when seen on the face, may contain dark coarse hairs. In late childhood and adolescence, compound nevi frequently tend to increase in thickness and depth of pigmentation. It is at this stage that many children are brought to a physician for evaluation. *Intradermal nevi* are usually dome-shaped, attached by a broad base or pedunculated, and range in size from a few millimeters to a centimeter or more in diameter. Often clinically indistinguishable from compound nevi, they vary in color from nonpigmented lesions to those of varying shades of brown to black.

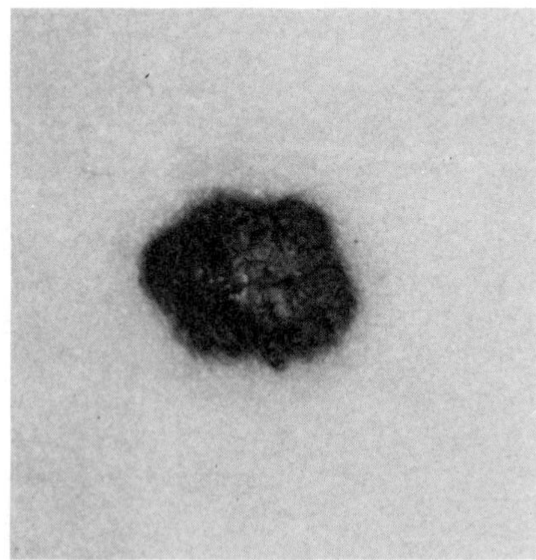

Figure 75–13. Intradermal nevus. A dome-shaped, slightly elevated, irregularly pigmented nodular lesion.

The management of pigmented nevi is usually related to their cosmetic appearance or the fear of malignant change. The majority of lesions require no treatment. With careful clinical evaluation, the patient frequently can be reassured as to their benign nature. In the past, many authors advocated routine excision of pigmented lesions in certain anatomical locations (palms, soles, and genitalia), owing to the belief that the likelihood of malignant transformation was greater in these areas. It now appears that prophylactic removal of all pigmented lesions

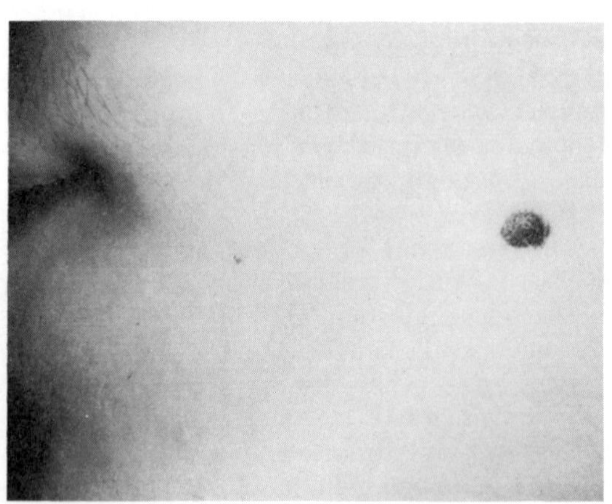

Figure 75–12. Junctional nevus. In contrast to a malignant melanoma, the skin surface is generally smooth and flat, and skin furrows are preserved.

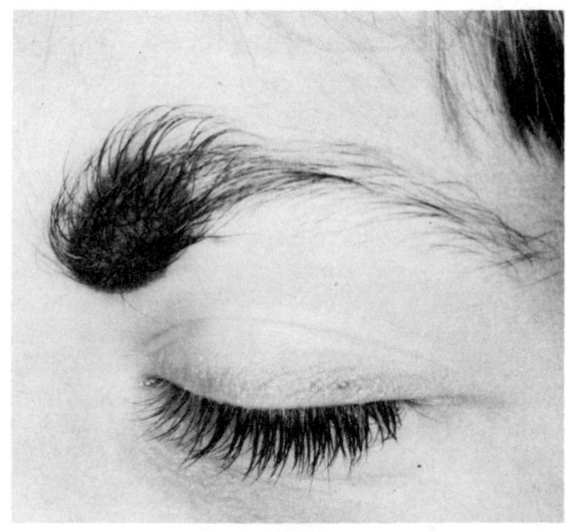

Figure 75–14. Compound nevus. Compund nevi tend to be more elevated, have a smooth or papillomatous surface, and, particularly when seen on the face, may contain coarse hairs.

Table 75–6. CHARACTERISTICS OF PIGMENTED MOLES AND NEVI

	Location	Characteristics
Junctional nevi	Nevus cells confined to dermoepidermal junction	Generally hairless; light to dark brown or brownish black; 1 mm to 1 cm in diameter with a smooth flat surface
Intradermal nevi	Nevus cells located in the dermis	Usually dome-shaped; may be pedunculated or attached by a broad base; size varies from a few mm to 1 cm or more; color varies from non-pigmented to shades of brown or black
Compound nevi	Nevus cells located both at dermoepidermal junction and in dermis	Slightly raised flesh-colored to brown; slightly raised plaques to papillomatous lesions; surface smooth or warty; dark hairs may be present

in these areas is neither warranted nor feasible. Removal of lesions in areas of trauma is probably more a matter of convenience than a bona fide prophylactic measure. Biopsy for diagnosis is recommended in pigmented lesions with (1) any change in color, especially the appearance of shades of red, pink, gray, white, or blue or the spread of pigment from the lesion into the surrounding skin, (2) irregularity of the border, (3) irregularity in pigmentary pattern, (4) pigmented satellite lesions, and (5) and symptoms such as pain or itching. Any suspicious lesion should be totally excised, whenever possible, and subjected to histopathological examination.

VASCULAR NEVI

Congenital vascular malformations occur in a high percentage of newborn infants. In a study of over 1000 infants seen in the first 48 hours of life, strawberry hemangiomas appeared in 2.6 per cent, port-wine stains (nevus flammeus) in 0.3 per cent, and salmon patches in 40 per cent.

Strawberry hemangiomas may be present at birth but generally develop in the first few postnatal weeks. They initially appear as small, well-demarcated telangiectatic macules or papules, as clusters of closely packed pinhead lesions, or as bright punctuate stippled or fine thread-like telangiectases surrounded by an area of localized pallor. During the first five weeks of life these lesions become vascularized and grow to present the strawberry type lesion, a raised bright or purplish red lobulated tumor with well-defined borders (Fig. 75–15).

At least 90 per cent of strawberry and cavernous hemangiomata undergo complete or partial resolution. Accordingly, fewer than 10 per cent of hemangiomas, whether they are strawberry, cavernous, or mixed, constitute any cosmetic handicap. Because of the tendency for most hemangiomas to regress completely, or almost completely, over 98 per cent of cases require no therapy. The final result in untreated lesions is generally far superior to that obtained from most forms of therapeutic intervention. Management generally consists of observation; avoidance, whenever possible, of active therapy; and reassurance to the parents. Hemangiomas that require intervention are those that by their size and growth compromise vital structures such as the eyes, nares, auditory canals, pharynx, or larynx; those that have an alarming rate of growth; large, usually cavernous lesions that have an associated thrombocytopenia (Kasabach-Merrit syndrome); or lesions that by their size or location are particularly susceptible to trauma, hemorrhage, or secondary infection.

When intervention is required, intralesional injection of sterile triamcinolone acetonide suspension may result in involution, or a course of

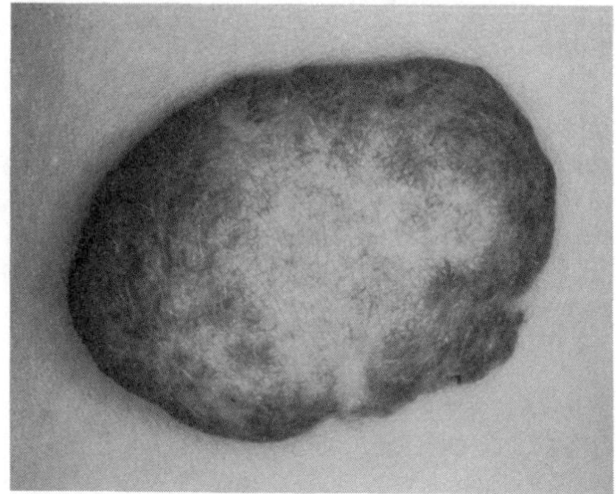

Figure 75–15. Strawberry hemangioma with focal areas of involution.

oral prednisone may be used in a dosage of 2 to 4 mg/kg per day (or its equivalent) for four weeks, followed by alternate-day therapy using the same or doubled dosage for a period of four to six weeks, with gradual tapering of the dosage as the condition warrants. In cases where recrudescence of the hemangioma occurs following reduction of dosage, a second course of therapy may be necessary (Fost and Esterly, 1968).

Salmon patches appear as flat, dull-pink macular lesions (often with telangiectasia) on the nape of the neck, glabella, forehead, upper eyelids, and the nasolabial regions. No treatment is necessary, since 95 per cent of salmon patches (with the exception of those of the nuchal region) generally fade during the first year of life.

Port-wine stains (nevus flammeus) are generally present at birth and usually do not grow out of relation to the growth of the child. They show little tendency toward involution, and treatment heretofore has generally been unsatisfactory. Use of Covermark, a tinted opaque waterproof cream (manufactured by Lydia O'Leary, New York City), can do much to alleviate the cosmetic appearance. Of recent interest are encourgaging studies on the use of argon laser beam therapy. At present, argon therapy is not recommended for children under nine years of age. The darker port-wine lesions with more pronounced vascularity are most responsive to therapy.

Cavernous hemangiomas represent basically the same pathological process as strawberry nevi but are composed of larger mature vascular elements. They are present at birth, grow in proportion to the growth of the individual, and are generally seen as bluish-red masses with less distinct borders. Occasionally a combination of strawberry and cavernous hemangioma may occur. Cavernous-type hemangiomas generally tend to soften and, although little change occurs in their surface area, usually demonstrate a gradual decrease in thickness or volume during the second or third year of life. Cavernous hemangiomas have a lesser growth rate than strawberry hemangiomas and 90 per cent improve by the time the child is nine years of age. Regression of cavernous lesions often is not as complete but generally results in a satisfactory cosmetic appearance.

WARTS AND MOLLUSCUM CONTAGIOSUM

Warts are common viral disorders of the skin. Their incubation period varies from one to six months. Although their course is totally unpredictable, the duration of lesions varies from a few months to five years or more, with 25 per cent disappearing spontaneously within three to six months and 65 per cent disappearing spontaneously within a period of two years.

There is no single effective treatment for warts. They are unpredictable, occasionally highly resistant to therapy, and have a recurrence rate that varies from 5 to 10 per cent no matter what the therapeutic approach. Whether or not warts should be treated depends entirely upon the patient's or parents' desires. Those that are painful, spreading, enlarging, subject to trauma, or cosmetically objectionable should be treated.

Whatever method the physician may select, he should be guided by conservatism if excessive trauma and scarring are to be avoided. The simplest topical agents are keratolytic preparations containing lactic acid, salicylic acid, and flexible collodion. The power of suggestion ("charming of warts") is simple and nontraumatic and in susceptible individuals may cure warts within a few days, leaving no trace of the previous lesions. How this works is unknown; however, it may explain the multiple spontaneous cures attributed to various inert preparations. Cantharidin, a potent blistering agent, available as Cantharone (Seres Laboratories), is easy to use and frequently effective, particularly in the management of periungual and plantar warts. The disadvantage to the use of this agent, however, is the fact that occasionally a ring of satellite warts may develop at the periphery of the blister. Cryosurgery with liquid nitrogen, although at times somewhat uncomfortable, is frequently a highly effective therapeutic approach to the treatment of individuals with multiple warts. Podophyllum resin, often used in the treatment of moist warts (condylomata acuminata), in concentrations of 20 to 25 per cent in tincture of benzoin, acts as a cytotoxic agent, arresting epidermal mitoses with cellular disruption of the hypoplastic tissue. This preparation must be applied carefully only to lesions, with avoidance of adjacent tissues, and must be washed off with soap and water within a period of four to six hours. Electrodesiccation and curettage may be utilized for individual large warts. This procedure must be used with extreme caution in order to reduce potential scarring.

Molluscum contagiosum is a condition characterized by firm, solid, and flesh-colored papules with a waxy or pearly-gray semitranslucent quality and a centrally located dimpled umbilication and pulpy curd-like core that can be expressed with a comedo extractor or a small sterile needle. Lesions consist of epidermal cells infected with a DNA virus of the pox virus group.

Treatment generally depends on minor destructive techniques and should produce as little scarring or discomfort as possible. A sharp spoon curette can be drawn quickly across a lesion without anesthesia. The small amount of bleeding can be managed by applying pressure, or by the use of styptics such as 25 per cent aluminum chloride solution or a ferric subsulfate solution (Monsel's solution). A light application of liquid nitrogen or brief applications of cantharidin or a combination of cantharidin, podophyllum, and salicylic acid (Verrusol or Cantharone Plus) applied for short periods of time (up to two hours) frequently results in the formation of a blister, and after two or three treatments will often result in destruction of lesions. Since the disease is transmissible by autoinoculation, no matter which method of therapy is utilized, care must be taken to make sure that all lesions are destroyed. Other as-yet-inapparent lesions may appear at previously infected sites.

PEDICULOSIS

Human lice are small, six-legged, wingless insects with translucent, grayish-white bodies that become red when engorged with blood. They spend their entire life as ectoparasites, living on man, dependent on the blood they extract from their victims. The varieties of pediculi that attack man include *Pediculus humanus corporis* (the body louse), *Pediculus humanus capitis* (the head louse), and *Pthirus pubis* (the crab louse). Each variety has a predilection for certain parts of the body and rarely migrates to other regions.

Pediculosis Corporis. The body louse generally lives in clothing or bedding and lays eggs on the seams of clothing. Its nits attach firmly to items of clothing and hatch owing to body warmth when the clothing is worn by the human host. The parasite is rarely observed on the skin; it obtains its nourishment by clinging to the patient's clothing and piercing the skin with its proboscis. The primary lesion is a small pinpoint red macule, papule, or urticarial wheal, with a characteristic hemorrhagic central punctum. Owing to the intense pruritus associated with this disorder, primary lesions are frequently obliterated by scratching and, therefore, are seldom seen. Diagnosis is established by a generalized pruritus, parallel scratch marks, fleeting wheals, secondary eczematization, bacterial infection, bloody crusts, and in cases of long duration, postinflammatory hyperpigmentation. The diagnosis can be confirmed by the finding of lice or nits in the seams of clothing.

Pediculosis Capitis. Pediculosis capitis is the most common form of louse infestation. Nits are chiefly found in the hairs above the ears and in the occipital region, usually one-quarter inch or so from the scalp. Nits present away from the scalp and along the shafts or tips of long hairs signify long-standing infection or residual nits from previously treated infestation. Itching is the principal symptom, and infestation is frequently complicated by bacterial infection (impetigo of the scalp, furunculosis, or postoccipital lymphadenopathy) or dermatitis of the posterior neck and upper shoulders (particularly in girls or women with long hair). It is important not to mistake epidermal scales or hair casts as pediculosis capitis or nits.

Pediculosis Pubis. Pediculosis pubis is generally seen in the hairs of the pubic region, but may also involve the eyelashes, beard, mustache, and axillary and other body hairs. Itching may be initial symptom, but in persistent cases eczematization or secondary infection (folliculitis) may occur. A heavy infestation may be accompanied by bluish or slate-colored macules, 0.5 to 1.0 cm in diameter (maculae ceruleae), that do not blanch upon pressure with a glass slide.

Pediculosis Palpebrarum. In children *Pthirus pubis* (occasionally *Pediculus humanus capitis* or *corporis*) may locate in the eyelashes or eyebrows. When the eyelids are involved it usually is related to infestation in an adult, often the mother. In this disorder the nits must be differentiated from the scaling seen in blepharitis associated with seborrheic dermatitis.

One per cent gamma benzene hexachloride (lindane) or synergized pyrethrins (Rid, A-200 Pyrinate) are effective in the treatment of pediculosis capitis and pediculosis pubis. Pediculosis capitis is treated by 1 per cent lindane (Kwell or Scabene) as a shampoo or lotion or by Rid or A-200 Pyrinate. When lindane shampoo is used, the patient's scalp should be thoroughly shampooed for four minutes with one tablespoon or less of the preparation. If the lotion is used, it may be applied to the scalp, left on overnight, and then washed out carefully. A second treatment may be repeated after one week if viable eggs persist. Other children in the family should be examined, and those with evidence of infestation should be treated. Since nits are attached only to the hair shaft, removal may be facilitated by the use of a fine-tooth comb or tweezers, or by soaking the hair with white vinegar or a 3 to 5 per cent acetic acid solution.

In pediculosis pubis, a thin layer of lindane lotion or synergized pyrethrins is applied to the infested and adjacent hairy areas, with particular attention to the pubic mons and perianal region. The lindane lotion is left on for 12 hours, then washed off thoroughly, with reapplication in one week if viable eggs persist. Synergized pyrethrins are left on for 10 minutes and washed off. Sexual contacts should be treated simultaneously, but other household members need not be treated. At the conclusion of therapy, treated individuals should change their underclothing, pajamas, sheets, and pillowcases. These articles should be washed by machine, automatically dried or laundered, ironed, or boiled in order to destroy the remaining ova or parasites.

In pediculosis corporis the body louse ordinarily inhabits only the clothing. Therapy mainly consists of hygiene and frequent showering or bathing, with frequent changing of underclothes and bedding. Underclothes and bedding should be laundered with hot water or boiled. Drycleaning destroys lice in clothing that cannot be laundered. All likely contacts (members of the household and close contacts in institutions) should be examined and treated if there is evidence of infestation.

Pediculosis of the eyelashes may be treated by petrolatum or yellow mercuric oxide applied thickly to the eyelashes twice daily for eight days, followed by mechanical removal of remaining nits. Physostigmine ophthalmic preparations (Eserine) are also effective if applied topically to the eyelid margin (twice daily for 24 to 48 hours). Because of the parasympathetic effect of physostigmine, miosis should be watched for as a possible side effect.

SCABIES

Scabies is a contagious disorder caused by an itch mite, *Sarcoptes scabiei.* Scabies typically presents as a distinctive clinical syndrome of pruritic papules, vesicles, pustules, and linear burrows (Fig. 75–16). Most patients, however, do not present this clear a picture, but rather a mixture of primary lesions, intermingled with or obliterated by excoriation, eczematization, crusting, or secondary infection. The severe itching that accompanies this disorder takes approximately four to six weeks to develop and is thought to be related to sensitization. Until the sensitization occurs, the disorder usually is unrecognized.

In adults and older children, lesions tend to involve the webs of fingers, the axillae, the flexures of the arms and wrists, the belt line, and the areas around the nipples, genitals, and lower buttocks. In infants and young children the distribution is altered and includes the palms, soles, head, neck, and face. Bullous lesions are uncommon, but vesicles are often found in infants and young children, owing to the predisposition for blister formation in this age group (Hurwitz, 1979).

A high percentage of children who develop scabies have been found to develop persistent reddish-brown infiltrated nodules, particularly

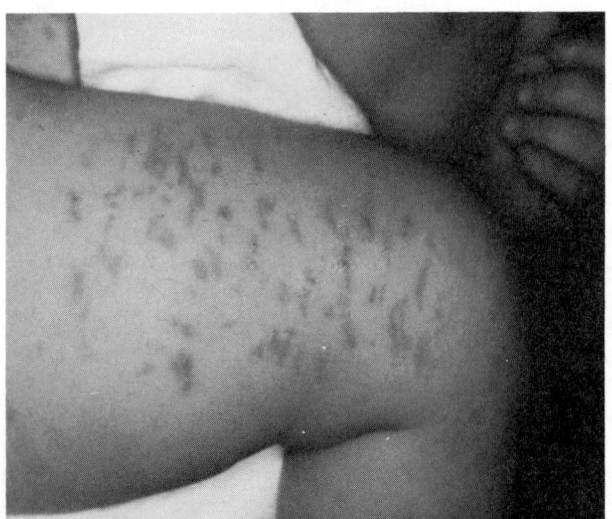

Figure 75–16. Papulovesicular lesions of scabies in a 2½-year-old child.

on the covered parts of the body (the axillae, shoulders, groin, buttocks, and genital area). These lesions, which often persist for months despite adequate therapy, do not indicate persistent infestation.

Eczematous changes due to scratching and rubbing of involved areas or to topical therapeutic agents are common complications of scabies in infants and children. They are frequently aggravated by excessive bathing, overzealous attempts at hygiene, and associated dryness and pruritus. Secondary infection, seen as pustulation, bullous impetigo, severe crusting, or ecthyma, is also a common complication in young children.

The diagnosis of scabies is made by the history of itching, a characteristic distribution of lesions, the recognition of primary lesions, particularly the pathognomonic burrow when present, and the presence of disease among the patient's family or associates. In infants and children, the diagnosis is often overlooked because of the lower index of suspicion and atypical distribution that includes the head, neck, palms, and soles, and obliteration of demonstrable primary lesions as a result of vigorous hygienic measures, excoriation, crusting, eczematization, and secondary infection.

Confirmation of the diagnosis can be made by the microscopic examination of scrapings of suspicious lesions, with demonstration of the adult mite, ova, larva, or fecal matter. The best lesions for microscopic examination are fresh papules or identifiable burrows, ideally those where potential organisms or ova have not been scratched or excoriated. A drop of mineral oil on the suspected lesion frequently allows easier scraping of the lesion and a more definitive identification of the pathogenic organism.

The therapy of scabies consists of topical application of 1.0 per cent gamma benzene hexachloride (Kwell or Scabene), 10 per cent crotamiton (Eurax), 6 to 10 per cent precipitate of sulfur in petrolatum, or a suspension of benzyl benzoate in a 12.5 to 25 per cent concentration (Table 75–7).

Gamma benzene hexachloride, probably the most widely used and most effective, has recently come under scrutiny because of possible central nervous system toxicity associated with inappropriate use. Following the prescribed time of application, generally 8 to 12 hours, the preparation should be washed off thoroughly. A second application may be required one week later to destroy recently hatched larvae not eliminated by the initial treatment, but there is no justification for repeated treatment at frequent intervals. This practice may result in toxicity due to abnormally high blood levels of this potentially toxic agent. For infants, where possible toxic effects become more acute owing to a relatively greater skin surface and possible higher blood level accumulations, 6 per cent sulfur precipitate in petrolatum appears to be safe, effective, and well tolerated. The preparation can be applied nightly for three nights, and if evidence of infestation persists, this regimen may be repeated in one week. As an added precaution, in order to limit overtreatment on the part of patients and their families, only required amounts of the gamma benzene hexachloride should be prescribed, and prescription refills should be strictly limited.

It should be noted that symptoms and signs may not clear for weeks, since the hypersensitivity state does not cease immediately after the eradication of the infection. The patient and his family should be alerted to this possibility so that they will know what to expect and not be tempted to continue excessive therapy. The scabies mite is unable to live for more than five minutes in temperatures above 120° F (50° C) or when away from its human host for two days or more. Thus, if personal clothing and bedclothing of treated individuals are changed, stored, or laundered in a washing machine or dryer, reinfestation can usually be prevented.

Systemic antipruritics, topical antipruritic lotions, and only low-potency hydrocortisone preparations may be appropriate for the management of persistent pruritus and secondary eczematization associated with scabietic infestation. Although current evidence suggests that adequate treatment may fail to reduce the incidence of nephritis following secondary cutaneous streptococcal disease, it seems reasonable to treat all scabies infestations complicated by streptococcal infection with appropriate systemic antibiotics (Hurwitz, 1979, 1981a).

Table 75–7. TREATMENT OF SCABIES

1. 1.0% gamma benzene hexachloride (Kwell, Scabene)
2. 10% crotamiton (Eurax)
3. 6 to 10% sulfur in petrolatum
4. 12.5 to 25% benzyl benzoate
5. Antipruritics (systemic and topical)
6. Appropriate antibiotics when necessary

SUPERFICIAL FUNGAL INFECTIONS

Fungal infections that affect man may be superficial, deep, or systemic. The superficial infections are those that are limited to the epidermis, hair, nails, and mucous membranes. Deep fungal infections are those in which organisms affect other organs of the body or invade the skin through direct extension or hematogenous spread.

There are three common types of superficial fungus infection: the dermatophytoses, tinea versicolor, and candidiasis (moniliasis). The dermatophytes, a group of related fungi that live in soil, on animals, and on humans, digest keratin and invade the skin, hair, and nails to produce a diversity of clinical lesions. They are termed tinea, dermatophytosis, or, because of the annular appearance of the lesions, ringworm. Depending upon the involved site, the infection may be termed tinea capitis, tinea corporis, tinea pedis, tinea cruris, or onychomycosis (tinea of the nails).

Tinea Capitis

Tinea capitis, the most common dermatophytosis of childhood, is a fungal infection of the scalp characterized by scaling and patchy alopecia. Primary lesions are characterized by broken-off hairs, scaling, and partial alopecia (Fig. 75–17). The infected areas are round, oval, or sometimes irregular. There may be coalescence of lesions, with formation of gyrate patterns. Any dermatophyte causing tinea capitis may also produce a sharply demarcated boggy granulomatous swelling called a kerion. This inflammatory lesion, which represents an exaggerated host response, does not necessarily represent persistent dermatophyte infection.

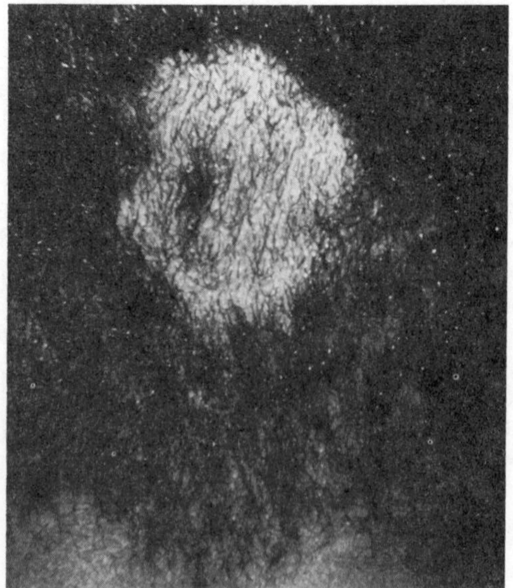

Figure 75–17. Tinea capitis. Broken hairs and scaling in a sharply circumscribed area of alopecia.

Diagnosis of tinea capitis is aided by Wood's light examination, demonstration of the fungus by potassium hydroxide wet-mount preparations of loose hairs removed from suspected areas, and fungal culture. It must be emphasized, however, that a high percentage of hairs, those infected with *Trichophyton tonsurans* (rapidly becoming the most common form of tinea capitis in the United States), do not fluoresce.

Topical antifungal agents do not reach the hair follicle and are ineffective in the treatment of tinea capitis. Oral griseofulvin (10 to 20 mg/kg per day) of the microcrystalline form for periods of six to eight weeks or more, is generally effective against all forms of tinea capitis. If a kerion is present, a combination of prednisone and griseofulvin generally will ensure rapid clearing and help keep atrophy and permanent hair loss to a minimum.

Tinea Corporis

Superficial tinea infections of the nonhairy skin are termed tinea corporis. This disorder is characterized by one or more annular, sharply circumscribed scaly patches with a clear center and scaly vesicular, papular, or pustular border (Fig. 75–18). When multiple lesions are present, they may join together, thus giving rise to bizarre polycyclic configurations. Most patients with tinea corporis respond to topical applications of clotrimazole (Lotrimin or Myclelex),

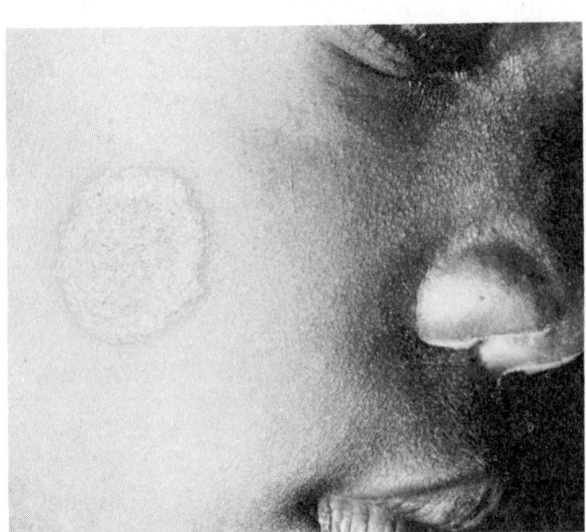

Figure 75–18. Tinea corporis (ringworm) with a circinate papulovesicular border.

haloprogin (Halotex), miconazole (Monistat-Derm), or tolnaftate (Tinactin) gently rubbed onto the affected skin morning and evening. Clearing and relief of pruritus are seen within the first 7 to 10 days after the initiation of therapy. Treatment, however, should be continued for a minimum of two or three weeks after the affected area is clinically clear and fungal cultures are no longer positive. In unusually severe, extensive, or resistant disease, a course of therapy with systemic griseofulvin may be required.

It must be remembered that dermatophytes and Monilia (Candida) are not synonymous and although nystatin is effective against monilial infection, it is ineffective for the treatment of dermatophyte infection. Clotrimazole, haloprogin, and miconazole, however, are effective in the topical therapy of both dermatophytes and monilia.

Tinea Cruris

Tinea cruris ("jock itch") is an extremely common superficial fungus infection of the groin and upper thighs. It is more symptomatic in hot, humid weather and is most frequently noted in obese individuals or persons engaged in vigorous physical activity, those who experience chafing, and those who wear tight-fitting clothing such as athletic supporters, jockey shorts, wet bathing suits, panty hose, or tight-fitting slacks. The eruption is sharply marginated, is usually but not invariably bilaterally symmetrical and involves the intertriginous folds near the scrotum, the upper inner thighs, and occasionally the perianal regions, buttocks, and abdomen. The scrotum and labia are usually spared or only mildly involved unless the eruption is caused by *Candida albicans*, overtreatment, or an associated neurodermatitis. The margins are abrupt and frequently half-moon shaped, and the skin in the involved area is erythematous and scaly.

Treatment consists of topical therapy with clotrimazole, haloprogin, miconazole, or tolnaftate preparations gently rubbed into the affected area and surrounding skin twice daily for a period of three to four weeks, reduction of excessive chafing and irritation by the use of loose-fitting cotton underclothing, and reduction of friction and perspiration by the use of a bland absorbent powder. For dermatophyte-induced lesions that are resistant or recur frequently, oral griseofulvin is indicated for a period of four or five weeks.

Tinea Pedis

Tinea pedis (athlete's foot) is an unusual dermatophyte infection in young children. More common in adolescents and adults, it is the most prevalent ringworm infection seen in adults. Although children are not completely immune, most instances of "athlete's foot" in individuals below the age of puberty usually represent misdiagnosed examples of foot eczema, shoe dermatitis, or other dermatoses.

The disorder may present clinically as an intertriginous inflammation, a vesiculopustular eruption, or a chronic scaling disorder with or without hyperkeratosis. Of these, interdigital lesions are the most common expression of the disorder and appear as fissuring, maceration, and interdigital scaling, generally in the web between the fourth and fifth toes, accompanied by maceration and peeling of the surrounding skin. Contrary to the eruptions seen in foot eczema, the dorsal aspect of the toes and feet generally remain clear.

Tinea pedis frequently is difficult to control because of the moist and warm environment of the feet. Efforts to keep the feet dry are helpful and topical antifungal agents such as clotrimazole, haloprogin, miconazole, and tolnaftate are generally effective.

Candidal (Monilial) Infections of the Skin

Candidiasis (moniliasis) is an acute or chronic infection of the skin, mucous membranes, and occasionally the internal organs, caused by yeast-like fungi of the *Candida* species. Oral candidiasis (thrush) is a painful inflammation of the tongue, soft and hard palates, and buccal and gingival mucosae characterized by whitish-gray, often confluent, friable, cheesy, pseudomembranous patches or plaques on a markedly reddened mucosa. Lesions often respond to careful removal of the curd-like lesions after each feeding by a cotton applicator dipped into a mixture of one-quarter teaspoon of baking soda and one or two drops of liquid detergent mixed in a glass of warm water or to careful removal of lesions by a cotton applicator dipped into a nystatin suspension (Mycostatin Oral Suspension or Nilstat Oral Suspension). Persistent or recurrent lesions may be treated by administration of oral nystatin (Mycostatin or Nilstat Oral Suspension).

Cutaneous candidiasis is generally characterized by a vivid beefy red color with a raised, sharply marginated edge with white scales at the border of lesions and pinpoint pustulovesicular satellite lesions. The treatment of superficial infections of the skin caused by *Candida albicans* consists of topical antimonilial agents such as topical clotrimazole, miconazole, haloprogin, or nystatin. Although Mycolog cream or ointment is also effective, many authorities avoid these preparations because of the presence of a potent corticosteroid (triamcinolone) and possible hypersensitivity to the neomycin, gramicidin, paraben, or ethylenediamine contained in Mycolog. It should be noted that ethylenediamine and parabens are contained in the cream but not in the ointment formulations of this preparation.

Ketoconazole (Nizoral), released in the United States in August, 1981, is an orally absorbed broad-spectrum antifungal agent for the treatment of resistant or recurrent dermatophytoses, tinea versicolor, candiasis (particularly chronic mucocutaneous candidiasis), paracoccidioidomycosis, and to a lesser degree, chromomycosis, blastomycosis, histoplasmosis, and coccidioidomycosis. Although relatively free of severe side effects, it should be noted that hepatic toxicity has been associated with its use. It is suggested, therefore, that until further information is available, this drug should be reserved for severe systemic or incapacitating fungal disorders unresponsive to other or less toxic agents and that liver function studies be evaluated before and at regular intervals during the use of this agent.

Tinea Unguium (Onychomycosis)

Onychomycosis is a chronic fungal infection of the fingernails or toenails caused by *Trichophyton rubrum*, *Trichophyton mentagrophytes*, and *Epidermophyton floccosum* (the dermatophytes that usually affect the hands and feet), and, at times, *Candida albicans*. Although rarely seen in children, the disorder generally occurs in association with tinea infection of the hands or feet, but it may occur as a primary infection or in association with other dermatophytoses. It must be differentiated from psoriasis of the nails, dystrophy secondary to eczema or chronic paronychia, trauma, tetracycline-induced photo-onycholysis, pachyonychia congenita, lichen planus, nail-patella syndrome, and other nail dystrophies.

Despite recent advances in antifungal therapy, topical agents are rarely effective, and oral administration of griseofulvin or ketoconazole (for periods of 6 months for fingernails or 12 to 18 months for toenails) is frequently required. It should be noted that even with long-term systemic therapy, recurrences are frequent.

AUTOSENSITIZATION DERMATITIS ("Id" Reactions)

Autosensitization, frequently referred to as an "id" reaction, is a term used to describe a disorder created by sensitization of the body by circulating antibody or by delayed hypersensitivity to constituents of its own tissues. This disorder is characterized by an acute papulovesicular eruption on the forearms, the flexor aspects of the upper arms, the hands, the extensor aspects of the upper arms and thighs, and, less commonly, the face and trunk. The disorder, nearly always preceded by an exacerbation of a pre-existing dermatitis, infection, rubbing, or inappropriate therapy, should be differentiated from hyperhidrosis, which often affects the hands and feet and appears as a result of excessive production of perspiration, and dyshidrosis (pompholyx), a term applied to a condition of recurring vesiculation of the palms and soles in which hyperhidrosis and retention of sweat precedes the eruption.

Treatment of autosensitization dermatitis consists of proper control of the primary disorder, open wet compresses, antihistamines, and topical corticosteroid preparations such as Florone, Kenalog, or Synalar. Although seldom indicated, a two- to three-week course of systemic corticosteroids may, at times, be necessary in cases that are unresponsive to more conversative therapy.

The treatment of pompholyx (dyshidrosis) frequently is aided by the use of a 20 per cent topical aluminum chloride (available as Drysol–Person, & Covey), open wet compresses, and topical corticosteroid creams.

ACNE VULGARIS

Acne vulgaris, a disorder of the pilosebaceous apparatus, is the most common skin disorder of the second and third decades of life. Acne, which usually begins one or two years prior to the onset of puberty as a result of androgenic stimulation of the sebaceous gland, is attributable to an abnormal keratinization process that results in obstruction of the pilosebaceous unit. Recent controlled studies refute the value of dietary restrictions imposed upon acne patients and, contrary to previous opinions, the disorder has nothing to do with cleanliness or hygiene.

Whereas various drying and exfoliating agents may cause drying and peeling, remove oils from the surface of the skin, and suppress individual lesions to a limited degree, they fail in the effective prevention of new lesions and may impede the proper utilization of effective topical agents currently available for the treatment of acne vulgaris.

As a result of obstruction of the pilosebaceous follicles two types of comedones are formed—open comedones (blackheads) and closed comedones (whiteheads). Recent evidence suggests that it is the closed comedo that is responsible for the problems seen in acne. These lesions are small and skin-colored, lie just beneath the skin surface, and have microscopic openings that keep their contents from escaping. As the sebaceous glands continue to form keratin and sebum, the follicular wall ruptures, expelling sebum into the surrounding dermis, thus initiating the inflammatory process that is seen clinically as papules, pustules, cysts, or nodules. Free fatty acids, the result of hydrolysis of triglycerides within the pilosebaceous follicles, are believed to play an important role in comedogenesis and the formation of inflammatory lesions.

Success of the acne therapy depends upon (1) prevention of follicular hyperkeratosis one eighth of an inch beneath the epidermal surface, (2) reduction of *Propionibacterium acnes* and free fatty acids, and (3) elimination of comedones and papules, pustules, cysts, and nodules that result therefrom. Today, this goal can be achieved by proper selection of available medications, coupled with the cooperation of the patient, and the knowledge, continued interest, and enthusiasm of the physician and his staff.

Of the available topical agents, benzoyl peroxide, vitamin A acid (tretinoin, Retin-A), and topical antibiotics appear to be the most effective topical agents. Benzoyl peroxide is currently available in lotion form or the more potent gel formulation (Benzac W, Benzagel, Desquam-X, Panoxyl, or Persa-Gel), in 5 and 10 per cent concentrations. These formulations cause fine desquamation, help reduce the level of free fatty acids, are bactericidal for *P. acnes*, and decrease inflammation of acne lesions. A relatively low incidence of irritant or allergic contact dermatitis (up to 1 to 2.5 per cent) suggests a degree of caution in their use. A test for possible allergic contact dermatitis, perhaps by an open patch test on the volar aspect of the patient's wrist, prior to the initiation of therapy, appears to be a sensible precautionary measure.

Tretinoin (Retin-A) has several beneficial effects on the skin of patients with acne vulgaris. When applied topically, it stimulates dehiscence of horny cells, resulting in a thinning of the horny layer, an increased cell turnover, a decreased comedo formation, and a sloughing and expulsion of existent comedones from their sebaceous follicles; reduces inflammatory lesions arising from comedones; and enhances transepidermal penetration of benzoyl peroxide or topical antibiotics. Because of its known capacity to cause severe irritation and peeling, topical vitamin A therapy should be initiated conservatively and used sparingly in an effort to prevent irritation associated with the overuse of this agent. If prolonged sun exposure is anticipated, patients may be cautioned to use a sun-protective formulation such as SunDown, Pre-Sun, Pabagel, or Eclipse. Although success in the management of acne vulgaris can be achieved by the use of vitamin A acid or benzoyl peroxide alone, the therapeutic effect is substantially increased by the use of the two agents in combination.

Systemic antibiotic therapy suppresses *P. acnes*, causing a reduction in a concentration of free fatty acids, the primary irritant of sebum. Today the use of systemic antibiotics can be decreased and often eliminated by the use of benzoyl peroxide, tretinoin, or topical antibiotics (Cleocin-T, Staticin, Ery-Derm, A/T/S, Meclan, or Topicycline) alone or in combination (Hurwitz, 1981a). When systemic antibiotics are considered necessary, tetracycline, the antibiotic most frequently prescribed, is effective, inexpensive, and relatively free of side effects. Side effects seen in association with tetracycline include pseudotumor cerebri, gastrointestinal irritation, vaginal moniliasis in female patients, esophageal ulcerations, bullous eruptions around the fingernails and on the hands and, on rare occasions, photo-onycholysis. The incidence of photoreactivity to oral tetracycline is unknown but appears to be extremely low, except for demethylchlortetracycline (Declomycin), in which photosensitivity appears to develop in about 20 per cent of cases.

Oral erythromycin, clindamycin, and minocycline are also beneficial when inflammatory and pustular lesions fail to respond to oral tetracycline. Of these three, erythromycin is the least expensive and has the fewest complications. Long-term systemic use of clindamycin is not recommended owing to the possibility of induced pseudomembranous ulcerative colitis. Minocycline appears to have merit in those patients who are unresponsive to tetracycline or erythromycin therapy. Caution must be exercised, however, since this tetracycline derivative may cause pigmentation and appears to have an affinity for the central nervous system, with a resulting high incidence of headaches and dizziness.

A new oral retinoid (13-*cis*-retinoic acid, Accutane) appears to be highly effective for those individuals with severe pustulocystic acne who are unresponsive to other effective therapy, including systemic antibiotics. This product has multiple side effects and should not be utilized for routine cases of acne vulgaris. Side effects include cheilitis, facial dermatitis, xerosis, conjunctivitis, rhinitis sicca, epistaxis, skin fragility, pruritus, headache, alopecia, appetite changes, and temporary elevation of serum triglycerides and liver enzymes. Because of possible teratogenic effects, Accutane should not be given to patients anticipating possible pregnancy while under therapy with this agent.

VITILIGO

Although chiefly of cosmetic significance, disorders of pigmentation are among the most conspicuous and, at times, among the most cosmetically and psychologically annoying and persistent of cutaneous disorders. Vitiligo, seen in at least 1 to 2 per cent of the population, appears to be an autosomal dominant trait of variable penetrance and in about half of the patients it begins prior to the age of 20 years.

Lesions appear as partially or completely depigmented ivory-white areas. They frequently have an oval or linear contour and vary in size from a few millimeters to large, occasionally segmental areas or almost total depigmentation of the body. Ordinarily, the diagnosis is not difficult, especially when there is symmetrical hypopigmentation about the eyes, nostrils, mouth, nipples, umbilicus, or genitals. Other sites of predilection include exposed areas such as the dorsal surfaces of the hands, the face, the neck, body folds, and areas over bony prominences such as the elbows, knees, knuckles, and shins.

The course of vitiligo is variable. Extension of lesions frequently tends to occur when the patient undergoes severe stress of either emotional or physical nature. Although there is no satisfactory treatment of vitiligo, repigmentation can occasionally be accomplished by the oral administration of psoralen compounds (Trisoralen or Oxsoralen) followed by gradual exposure to sunlight or long-wave ultraviolet light. When treatment is unsatisfactory, lesions can be hidden by the use of cosmetic makeups or aniline dye stains such as Neo-Dyoderm or Vita-Dye.

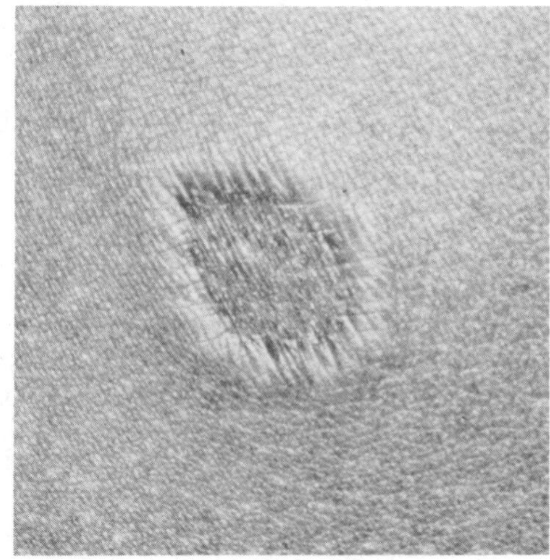

Figure 75–19. Granuloma annulare. Flesh-colored papulonodular lesions in an annular configuration.

GRANULOMA ANNULARE

Granuloma annulare is a relatively common cutaneous disorder characterized by papules or nodules that are grouped in a ringlike or circinate distribution (Fig. 75–19). Although the disorder may occur on any part of the body, it usually begins on the lateral or dorsal surfaces of the hands or feet. The cause of this lesion is unknown.

Lesions of granuloma annulare usually disappear spontaneously, often within a period of several months to years. Since it has been suggested that patients with granuloma annulare may be predisposed to diabetes mellitus, it is reasonable that all such patients be investigated for this possibility. Topical corticosteroids, corticosteroids under occlusion, and intralesional steroids are beneficial in hastening resolution of lesions, but because of the risk of dermal complications with such therapy, reassurance of eventual spontaneous resolution may be all that is necessary.

Occlusion of topical corticosteroids involves covering of treated areas with a polyethylene film such as Saran-wrap or the use of a steroid-impregnated polyethylene film available as Cordran tape. This mode of therapy appears to enhance the penetration of corticosteroids and is particularly effective for short periods of time (8 to 12 hours a day, generally at night, on successive days). Occlusive techniques, however, are contraindicated for prolonged periods of time or in acutely infected or intertriginous areas. When used excessively or improperly, such techniques may result in local infection, miliaria, folliculitis and, with prolonged use, atrophy or striae.

Intralesional steroid therapy involves the injection of 0.1 to 0.3 ml of triamcinolene acetonide in a concentration of 2.5 to 10.0 mg/ml. Caution must be exercised, however, with this form of therapy, since atrophy of the skin may occur when the injection is high in the dermis or when the amount or concentration of the steroid is excessive. This form of therapy, therefore, is probably best managed by a dermatologist who has experience with the proper use of intralesional steroid therapy.

URTICARIA PIGMENTOSA

Cutaneous lesions generally appear as multiple reddish-brown (occasionally yellowish-brown) hyperpigmented macules, papules, or nodular lesions that urticate when traumatized (Fig. 75–20). They may occur anywhere on the body but generally tend to involve the trunk, often in a symmetrical fashion. Individual lesions are usually round or oval, vary in size from 1 millimeter to several centimeters in diameter, and generally are larger in children than in adults.

When seen in children, urticaria pigmentosa has an excellent prognosis. In about one half of the cases in which the disorder has its onset in infancy or early childhood, the lesions disappear by adolescence or early adult life. Although generalized flushing may occur when large amounts of histamine are liberated, the pruritus associated with this disorder is usually mild and intermittent. Urticaria and pruritus may be induced by inadvertent or deliberate rubbing of lesions; exercise; hot baths; the ingestion of spicy foods, cheese, or alcohol; and vigorous rubbing after bathing or showering. Patients should also avoid histamine-releasing drugs such as aspirin, codeine, opiates, procaine, and polymyxin B, and antihistaminic agents such as hydroxyzine should be kept available.

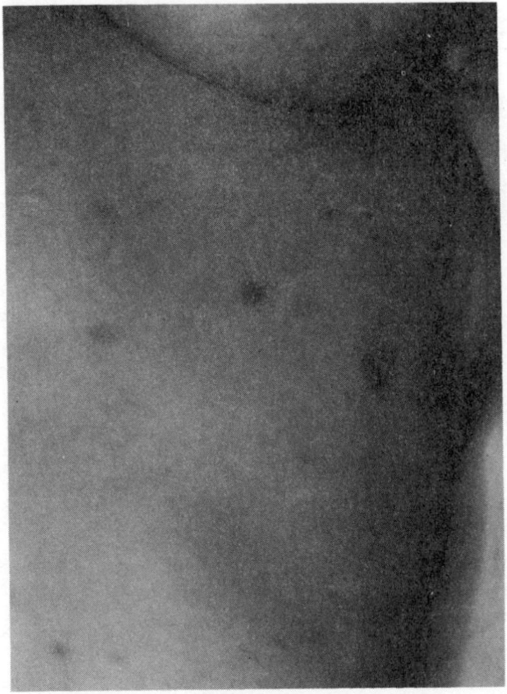

Figure 75–20. Multiple hyperpigmented macules and papules (urticaria pigmentosa) on the chest and abdomen of a young infant.

URTICARIA

Urticaria, a systemic disease with cutaneous manifestations, is characterized by the appearance of transient well-circumscribed wheals that are evident as erythematous, intensely pruritic elevated swellings of the skin or mucous membranes. The exact etiology in a particular patient is often difficult to identify, since it may be associated with hypersensitivity to a multitude of agents such as foods, drugs, infections, serum injections, insect bites, inhalant or contact allergens, and psychogenic factors. Typical lesions have a white palpable center of edema with a variable halo of erythema. They vary in size from pinpoint papules to large lesions several centimeters in diameter. Central clearing, peripheral extension, and coalescence of individual lesions result in a clinical picture of oval, annular, or bizarre serpiginous configurations.

Effective treatment is dependent upon identification of the etiological factor and its elimination whenever possible. Symptomatic treatment consists of antihistamines, of which hydroxyzine (Atarax or Vistaril) appears to be the most effective and the drug of choice. The subcutaneous administration of epinephrine is often effective and particularly beneficial in patients with angioedema and acute or severe urticaria. Although frequently effective in patients with severe or persistent urticaria, because of the side effects, systemic steroids should be reserved for those patients who are unresponsive to other modes of therapy.

ERYTHEMA NODOSUM

Erythema nodosum represents a delayed hypersensitivity syndrome characterized by red tender nodular lesions, usually on the tibial surface of the legs. In children streptococcal and other respiratory infections and primary tuberculosis are the most common causes. Noninfectious disorders that cause erythema nodosum include ulcerative colitis, regional ileitis, and reactions to various drugs, particularly sulfonamides, phenytoin, and contraceptive pills.

The disorder is characterized by symmetrical lesions, which vary in size from 1 to 5 cm in diameter, and occur usually on the pretibial areas, occasionally on the knees, ankles, thighs, extensor aspects of the arms, the face, and the neck. Initially, they appear as bright to deep-red, warm and tender, oval, slightly elevated nodules. After a few days they develop a brownish-red or purplish bruiselike appearance. The eruption usually lasts three to six weeks but may recede earlier if the patient remains in bed. Recrudescences may occur over a period of weeks to months, but attacks are seldom recurrent and arthralgias may precede, coincide with, or follow the eruption in as many as 90 per cent of the cases.

The treatment of erythema nodosum is directed at the cause of the disorder. Bed rest, with elevation of the patient's legs, helps reduce pain and edema. When pain, inflammation, or arthralgia is prominent, salicylates may be helpful. Intralesional corticosteroids frequently cause rapid involution of individual lesions, and oral corticosteroids may be beneficial in persistent or recurrent eruptions.

ERYTHEMA MULTIFORME AND STEVENS-JOHNSON DISEASE

Another systemic disorder highlighted by cutaneous manifestations is erythema multiforme, a distinctive acute hypersensitivity syndrome, again with any number of etiologies: hypersensitivity to viral, bacterial, protozoal, fungal, or *Mycoplasma pneumoniae* infections; sensitivity to food or drugs; immunizations; or connective tissue disorders. Whereas drug reactions and malignancies are important causative factors in older individuals, infectious diseases are the most common cause of erythema multiforme in children (particularly the virus of herpes simplex), with a history of cold sores preceding the development of other lesions by 3 to 14 days.

The clinical spectrum of erythema multiforme ranges from a localized eruption of the skin and mucous membranes to a severe multisystem disorder (Table 75–8). The disease occurs at any age, with the most severe forms occurring in children and young adults. The eruption is symmetrical and may occur on any part of the body, with a predilection for the palms and soles, backs of the hands and feet, and extensor surfaces of the arms and legs. As the disorder progresses, the lesions often extend to the trunk, face, and neck. Oral lesions may occur alone or in conjunction with cutaneous lesions. Seen in 25 per cent of cases, they first appear as bullae with swelling and crusting of the lips and development of erosions of the buccal mucosa, gums, and tongue.

Table 75–8. ERYTHEMA MULTIFORME AND STEVENS-JOHNSON DISEASE

1. A distinctive acute hypersensitivity syndrome
   a. Viral, bacterial, protozoal, fungal, or *M. pneumoniae* infection
   b. Food, drugs, or immunizations
   c. Connective tissue disorders
2. Macular, urticarial, and vesiculobullous (the predominant lesions are dull red to dusky flat macules or sharply marginated wheals)
3. Target lesions (the hallmark of the disorder)
4. A symmetrical eruption with predilection for the palms, soles, extensor surfaces of arms and legs, and backs of hands and feet
5. As the disorder progresses lesions often extend to the trunk, face, and neck
6. Oral lesions seen in 25% of patients

The term *erythema multiforme* should not be applied indiscriminately to any polymorphic eruption. The disorder is a specific hypersensitivity syndrome with a distinctive clinical pattern, the hallmark of which is an erythematous ring (the so-called iris or target lesion) (Fig. 75–21). Although a single type of lesion might

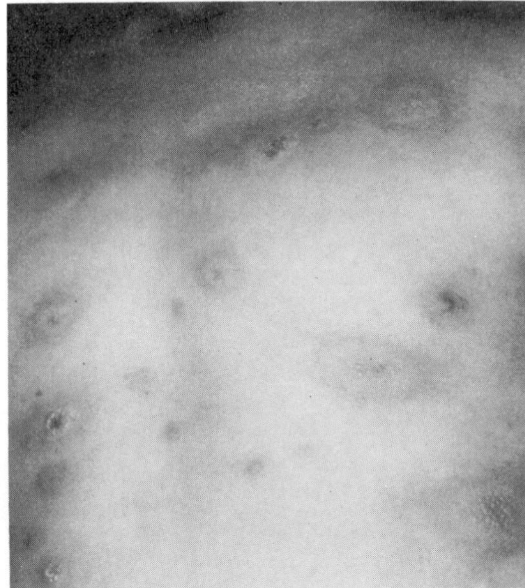

Figure 75–21. Erythema multiforme. Target lesions and marginated wheals with central vesicles.

predominate during a particular attack, the basic lesions are macular, urticarial, and vesiculobullous. The evolution and resolution of individual lesions lasts about a week, but the eruption may continue to appear in crops for as long as two or three weeks, thus contributing to the multiform appearance of the eruption.

Severe forms of bullous erythema multiforme with mucocutaneous involvement have been labeled Stevens-Johnson disease (Fig. 75–22). This disorder is an extremely severe form of bullous erythema multiforme, with high fever, pronounced constitutional symptoms, and widespread bullae, which involve the mucous membranes, conjunctivae, and anogenital areas.

The management of erythema multiforme and Stevens-Johnson syndrome depends upon the clinical status of the patient. A thorough search for and elimination of the underlying cause is imperative. If a drug is suspected, it should be discontinued. Mild cases may subside spontaneously or occasionally respond to antihistamines. Severe oropharyngeal involvement often necessitates frequent mouthwashes, local application of elixir of Benadryl, or topical use of Xylocaine Viscous as an anesthetic. When ocular involvement is present, ophthalmologic consultation should be obtained, the eyes should be cleansed frequently with separation of the eyelids, and topical antibacterial agents should be utilized to prevent secondary infection. Although their use is controversial, many authors feel that steroids in high dosages are indicated in cases with severe skin or mucous membrane involvement, or when there is evidence of appreciable systemic toxicity. Recent studies, however, suggest that the use of systemic corticosteroids in Stevens-Johnson syndrome may actually increase morbidity and cause prolongation of hospital stay (Rasmussen, 1976).

HENOCH-SCHÖNLEIN PURPURA

Henoch-Schönlein (anaphylactoid) purpura appears to represent a diffuse vasculitis caused by hypersensitivity to a variety of etiological factors. Bacterial or viral infections appear to be the most frequently implicated precipitating cause; drugs, food, insect bites, and chemical toxins also have been suggested as possible etiological factors.

Mainly a disease of children and young adults (particularly those between 3 and 10 years of age), the disorder is characterized by a distinctive rash (erythematous papules followed by purpura), abdominal pain, and joint symptoms. Renal disease occurs frequently, but other organ involvement is relatively less common.

Skin lesions consist of small hemorrhagic macules, papules, and/or urticarial lesions, which appear in a symmetrical distribution over the buttocks (Fig. 75–23) and the extensor surfaces of the extremities (particularly the elbows and knees). The disorder usually consists of a single episode, which may last for several days to several weeks. In some cases, however, recurrent attacks may occur at intervals for weeks or months.

Individual lesions occur in crops, tend to fade after about five days, and eventually are replaced by areas of brownish pigmentation, purpura, or ecchymoses. New crops of lesions

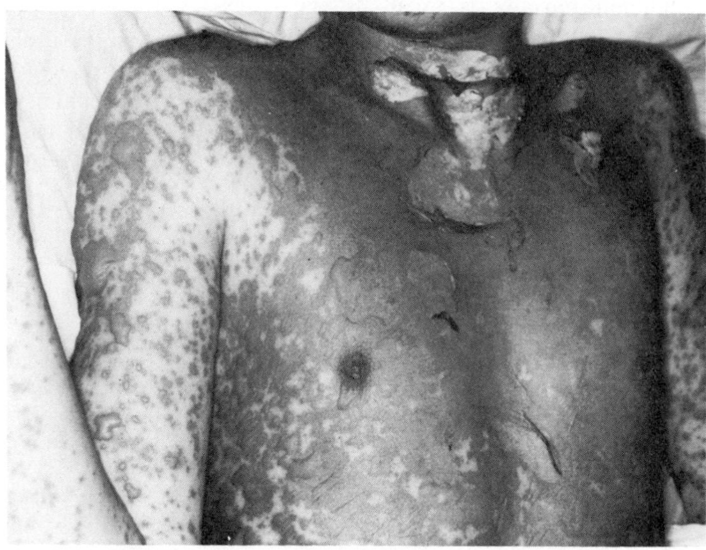

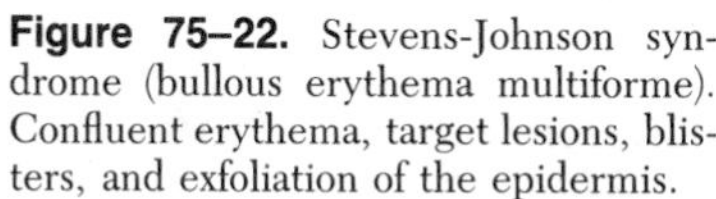

Figure 75–22. Stevens-Johnson syndrome (bullous erythema multiforme). Confluent erythema, target lesions, blisters, and exfoliation of the epidermis.

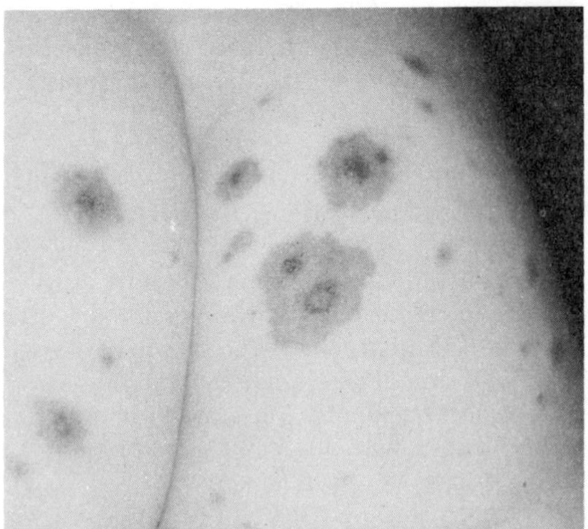

Figure 75–23. Henoch-Schönlein purpura (anaphylactoid purpura). Hemorrhagic macules, papules, and urticarial lesions in a symmetrical distribution over the buttocks of a young child.

frequently occur over the fading lesions of a previous episode, thus giving a polymorphous appearance to the disorder. The presence of palpable purpura will usually clarify the true nature of the disorder. This characteristic finding, created by edema and extravasation of erythrocytes, gives individual lesions their diagnostic palpable and purpuric appearance. When the diagnosis remains in doubt, histopathological examination of a cutaneous punch biopsy generally helps clarify the nature of the eruption. The degree of systemic involvement may vary, with arthritic or gastrointestinal symptoms reportedly seen in as many as two thirds of affected children.

The prognosis for most patients with Henoch-Schönlein purpura is excellent. There is no specific therapy. Throat cultures and appropriate antibiotics are indicated if a specific respiratory illness is suspected and identified. There is little evidence that systemic corticosteroids influence the prognosis of Henoch-Schönlein purpura. Since they may suppress the acute manifestations, they may be justified for short periods in severe cases, particularly those with significant gastrointestinal complications.

KAWASAKI DISEASE

Kawasaki disease (mucocutaneous lymph node syndrome) is a disorder of unknown etiology affecting infants and young children. The disorder has been reported worldwide (Fig. 75–24) (Kawasaki et al., 1974).

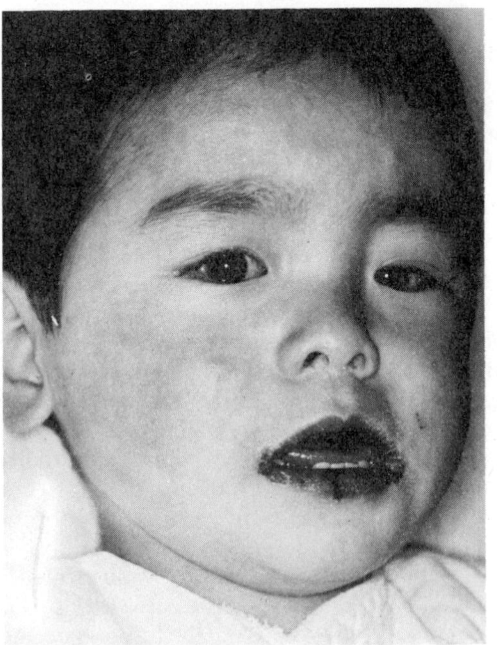

Figure 75–24. Kawasaki disease (mucocutaneous lymph node syndrome). Characteristic facies with maculopapular morbilliform rash, congestion of the bulbar conjunctivae, and hemorrhagic crusting and erosion of the lips. (Courtesy of Dr. Tomisaku Kawasaki.)

Patients with Kawasaki disease exhibit a unique spectrum of six clinical findings that are distinctive and diagnostically helpful: (1) fever lasting more than five days; (2) bilateral conjunctival injection; (3) dry, red, and fissured lips; strawberry tongue; and redness of the oropharynx; (4) erythematous rash; (5) indurative edema of the hands and feet, followed by desquamation of the fingertips; and (6) nonpurulent cervical lymphadenopathy. The diagnosis, based upon the exclusion of other clinically similar diseases, is considered to be established by the presence of fever and four of the five remaining criteria (Table 75–9).

Although occasional cases of Kawasaki disease may be seen in adults and children over 10 years of age, most patients (85 per cent) are under 5 years of age and 50 per cent are under

Table 75–9. DIAGNOSTIC CRITERIA OF KAWASAKI DISEASE

A. Fever lasting more than five days
B. Four of the five remaining criteria:
   1. Conjunctival injection
   2. Oral cavity changes
   3. Exanthem
   4. Changes in the extremities
   5. Lymphadenopathy

2½ years of age. Associated features include cardiac manifestations, central nervous system involvement (extreme irritability, lethargy, and aseptic meningitis), pyuria, rheumatic complications (arthritis and arthralgia), and gastrointestinal manifestations. The prognosis is good in most cases, with improvement usually beginning about the fourteenth day of illness. ECG abnormalities, however, have been found in 70 to 90 per cent of children with this disorder; 27 per cent of patients have shown abnormalities in coronary angiography one to six months after the onset of the disease; and 1 to 2 per cent of the patients, generally young infants with this disorder, may suffer sudden death due to coronary occlusion, myocarditis, inflammation of the A-V conduction system, and rupture of aneurysms. Most deaths, when they occur, appear between the twentieth and fortieth day of the disease. Polycythemia between the fifteenth and twenty-first days of the illness is characteristic and often helpful in diagnosis.

The cutaneous eruption, seen in 92 per cent of the cases, generally begins at the third to fifth day of the illness, simultaneous with or soon after the onset of fever. The polymorphous eruption begins on the extremities as red macules and generally evolves into pruritic urticaria-like plaques. Maculopapular, morbilliform, or urticarial eruptions are frequently seen and in less than 5 per cent of cases scarlatinal or erythema multiforme–like eruptions may be noted.

Generally 14 to 20 days after the onset of fever, a highly characteristic pattern of desquamation begins. Seen in 94 per cent of the patients, it lasts approximately one week. The desquamation generally begins at the tips of the fingers and toes and the junctions of the nails and skin (just beneath the nails) and, over a period of 10 days, gradually progresses to include the fingers, toes, and areas of the palms and soles (Fig. 75–25).

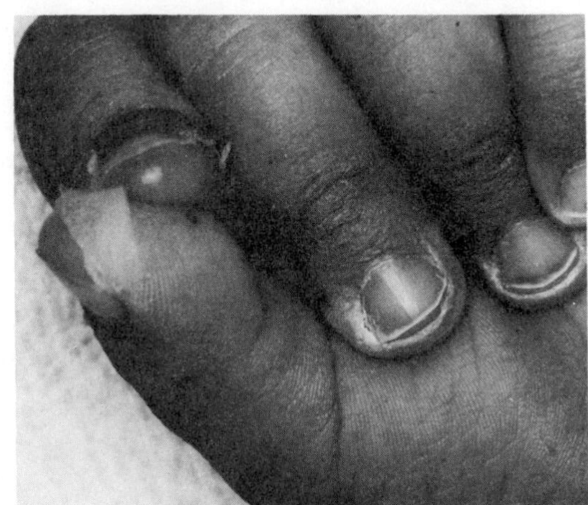

Figure 75–25. Desquamation of the fingers in a patient with Kawasaki disease. (Courtesy of Dr. Tomisaku Kawasaki.)

To date there is no effective or definitive treatment for this disease or its catastrophic sequelae. The most important problem in the management of patients appears to be the ability to detect and prevent coronary aneurysm and myocardial infarction. Present treatment is supportive and generally consists of aspirin, in dosages of 80 to 100 mg/kg/day. Once the patient has become afebrile and there is no evidence of arthritis or arthralgia, the dosage of aspirin may be reduced 20 to 30 mg/kg/day. In patients without complications, aspirin should be continued until the sedimentation rate has become normal. This usually occurs approximately 6 to 10 weeks after the onset of illness. Although systemic corticosteroids have been suggested for the treatment of Kawasaki disease, a recent study suggests that corticosteroids are contraindicated, since there appears to be a higher incidence of coronary aneurysms in patients so treated (Kato et al., 1979).

TOXIC SHOCK SYNDROME

Toxic shock syndrome, first described in 1978, is a recently recognized disorder associated with a staphylococcal infection. It appears to have an incidence of 3 to 6 per 100,000 menstruating females and has a mortality of 8 to 10 per cent. Seen in children, adolescents, and individuals of both sexes, 95 per cent of cases have been seen in females. The youngest case reported to date is that of an 18-month-old male, but most cases appear between the ages of 12 and 52 years of age, with a peak incidence between the ages of 15 and 19 years.

The disorder is characterized by a scarlatinal rash, fever greater than 102°F, desquamation of the palms and soles (one to two weeks later), postural hypotension, and three or more of the following seven associated findings: (1) gastrointestinal (vomiting and diarrhea), (2) muscular (severe myalgia, abdominal tenderness, and elevated CPK), (3) mucous membrane involvement (hyperemia of vaginal, buccal, and conjunctival membranes), (4) hepatitis with elevated bilirubin, (5) hematological changes (particularly thrombocytopenia less than 100,000), (6) central nervous system (disorientation or alterations in consciousness), and (7) renal (renal insufficiency with elevated BUN or creatinine levels).

The diagnosis can be confirmed by the presence of postural hypertension, thrombocytopenia, and culture of *Staphylococcus aureus* from the vagina, throat, nares, conjunctivae, or stools. Treatment consists of removal of tampons, when present; the use of intravenous fluids; vaginal douches with povidone-iodine when vaginal cultures are positive; and beta-lactimase–resistant antistaphylococcal drugs (dicloxacillin, oxacillin, or cephalosporin).

REFERENCES

Eisenberg, M., Stevens, L. H., and Schofield, P. J.: Epidermolysis bullosa: New therapeutic approaches. Aust. J. Dermatol., *19*:1–7, 1978.

Fost, N. C., and Esterly, N. B.: Successful treatment of juvenile hemangiomas with prednisone. J. Pediatr., 72:351–357, 1968.

Hurwitz, S.: Scabies in childhood. Pediatr. Rev., *1*:91–94, 1979.

Hurwitz, S.: Clinical Pediatric Dermatology. Philadelphia, W. B. Saunders Co., 1981a.

Hurwitz, S.: Eczematous eruptions in childhood. Pediatr. Rev., *3*:23–30, 1981b.

Jacobs, A. H., and Walton, R. G.: The incidence of birthmarks in the neonate. Pediatrics, *58*:218–222, 1976.

Kato, H., Koike, S., and Yokoyama, T.: Kawasaki disease. Effect of treatment of coronary involvement. Pediatrics, *63*:175–179, 1979.

Kawasaki, T., Kosaki, F., Okawa, S., et al.: A new infantile acute febrile mucocutaneous lymph node syndrome (MLNS) prevailing in Japan. Pediatrics, *54*:271–278, 1974.

Leyden, J. J., Katz, S., Stewart, R., et al.: Urinary ammonia and ammonia-producing organisms in infants with and without diaper dermatitis. Arch. Dermatol., *13*:1678–1680, 1977.

Melish, M. E., and Glasgow, L. A.: Staphylococcal scalded skin syndrome: The expanded clinical syndrome. J. Pediatr., *78*:958–967, 1971.

Rasmussen, J. E.: Erythema multiforme in children: Response to therapy with systemic corticosteroids. Br. J. Dermatol., *95*:181–186, 1976.

Stoughton, R. B.: A perspective on topical corticosteroid therapy. *In* Farber, E. M., and Cox, A. J. (Eds.): Psoriasis: Proceedings of the Second International Symposium. New York, Yorke Medical Books, 1976, p. 224.

76

BLOOD DISORDERS: ANEMIA AND HEMORRHAGE

Robert L. Baehner, M.D.

A diagnosis of anemia in children requires an appreciation of the normal variations between red cell mass, plasma volume, and age. Table 76–1 documents these changes with age. The causes of anemia can be broadly divided into those due to decreased production of red cells or synthesis of hemoglobin and those due to increased loss or destruction of red cells from the circulation. Most anemias can be diagnosed by relevant historical information, the physical examination, and a careful inspection of a properly prepared peripheral blood smear stained with Wright's stain.

HISTORY

The infant with true anemia at two or three months of age (Hgb less than 9.0 gm/dl) was probably anemic at birth. Newborn infants become anemic from bleeding at birth, exchange transfusions with adult blood which provides less red cell mass, fetal-maternal transfusion, or fetal-fetal transfusion associated with twin births. The most common congenital hemolytic anemia is hereditary spherocytosis, an autosomal dominant disorder of variable severity. Thirty per cent of these patients have parents and families without the disease, suggesting a spontaneous mutation. The more rarely occurring congenital red cell enzymopathies are either autosomal recessive (pyruvate kinase deficiency) or X-linked (G6PD deficiency).

Anemia after six months of age is most often due to iron deficiency. A properly obtained dietary history usually reveals excessive milk intake. This is best estimated by accounting for the number of bottles of milk consumed per night as well as throughout the day. Often the iron-deficient child is fretful and irritable, demanding two or more bottles of milk at night. Most iron-deficient infants consume more than one quart of milk per day, limiting iron intake to less than 1 mg. Excessive milk intake often occurs because of problems in maternal-infant interaction. Although some blood loss in the

Table 76–1. NORMAL BLOOD VALUES IN INFANTS AND CHILDREN

	Cord blood	Day 1	2 weeks	6 weeks	12 weeks	1 year	4 years	8 to 12 years
Hemoglobin (gm/dl)	16–18	19.0 ± 2.8	17.3 ± 2.0	12.0 ± 1.5	11.3 ± 0.9	11.6 ± 0.8	12.6 ± 0.8	13.1 ± 1.2
Hematocrit (%)	53–58	61 ± 7	54 ± 8	36 ± 5	33 ± 3	35 ± 3	37 ± 3	41 ± 3
Red Cells ($\times 10^6/mm^3$)	5.25	5.14 ± 0.7	4.80 ± 0.8	3.40 ± 0.4	3.70 ± 0.3	4.60 ± 0.4	4.70 ± 0.4	4.90 ± 0.5
MCV (u^3)	115	119 ± 9	112 ± 19	105 ± 12	88 ± 8	77 ± 6	80 ± 6	81 ± 7
MCHC (%)	32	32 ± 2	32 ± 3	34 ± 2	35 ± 2	33 ± 2	34 ± 2	34 ± 2
Reticulocyte (%)	3.7	3.2 ± 1.4	0.8 ± 0.6	1.2 ± 0.7	0.7 ± 0.3	0.9 ± 0.5	0.9 ± 0.5	1.1 ± 0.6

Modified from E. C. Albritton: Standard Values in Blood, Philadelphia, W. B. Saunders Co., 1952, p. 38, and Matoth et al.: Acta Paediat. Scand., *60*:317, 1971.

stool occurs in most cases of iron-deficiency anemia, a history of melena is unusual.

After age five, iron deficiency due to dietary reasons is rare. Once the iron-deficient state is identified in the older child, a history and search for gastrointestinal blood loss from chronic epistaxis, peptic ulcer with or without Meckel's diverticulum, duplication of the bowel, or vascular malformations should be made. The menstruating teenager may become iron deficient. Fad diets are also a rare, but occasional, cause of iron deficiency in this age group.

The toddler living in an older home in an urban area may develop lead poisoning by eating plaster, paint chips, and other debris high in lead content. Lead poisoning produces a hypochromic microcytic anemia. This anemia is usually also associated with iron deficiency.

The ethnic background of the anemic patient may be of importance. Thalassemic syndromes due to depression of the gene controlling alpha or beta globin chain synthesis of hemoglobin produce serious, life-threatening hemolytic anemia in the homozygous state and can be confused with mild iron deficiency anemia in the heterozygous form. Thalassemia of the beta globin gene is frequent among individuals immigrating from the Mediterranean Sea area. Depression of alpha globin chain synthesis is most commonly seen in individuals of Chinese ancestry. The incidence of the sickle hemoglobin gene in the American black population is between 8 and 13 per cent, and approximately 0.4 per cent have homozygous sickle cell anemia. Red cell glucose 6-phosphatase dehydrogenase (G6PD) deficiency is X-linked, occurring in approximately 10 per cent of black males. In contrast to Causasian G6PD, seen most often in Italians and Greeks with a chronic hemolytic anemia, G6PD deficiency in black males produces sudden hemolysis on exposure to sulfonamides, nitrofurans, aspirin in large doses, acetophenetidin, and antimalarials.

Chronic diseases such as rheumatoid arthritis, chronic renal disease, cystic fibrosis, regional enteritis, chronic granulomatous disease, and other inflammatory conditions may produce so-called secondary anemias.

SIGNS AND SYMPTOMS

The cardinal sign of anemia is pallor. The fair-haired, light-skinned child is often mistakenly thought to be anemic. If the anemia is gradual in onset, symptoms of easy fatiguability, irritability, decreased play tolerance, and lethargy may be subtle. More severe anemias cause lightheadedness or dizziness and if associated with high output heart failure, produce dyspnea, headache, and chest discomfort. Sudden blood loss or hemolysis may produce shocklike symptoms including anxiety, restlessness, increased thirst, palpitations, nausea, vomiting, and convulsions. After trauma, sudden blood loss into the intestinal tract, abdominal viscus, or retroperitoneal space may not be apparent early when peripheral vasoconstriction and tachycardia predominate. Anemia is noted only a day or two after blood volume has been restored. Pallor associated with the acute onset of a febrile illness often is due to an acquired autoimmune hemolytic anemia.

PHYSICAL EXAMINATION

The anemic patient has pallor of the buccal mucosa, conjunctivae, and nail beds. Although the skin folds of the hands may be white, this finding is difficult to assess in children. Systolic precordial murmurs are present in most moderate and severe anemic states. Hepatosplenomegaly may or may not be noted. The sclerae are usually icteric in hemolytic anemias. Circulating dipyroles produce a gray cast to the skin in hemoglobinopathies such as thalassemia or hemolysis due to an unstable hemoglobin. Purpura and petechiae, or skin and mucous membrane infection, suggest associated depression of platelets and white cell count.

LABORATORY STUDIES

Anemias can be classified based on red cell size, the relative concentration of hemoglobin in the cells, and the presence or absence of polychromasia on the peripheral blood smear. For office practice, the microhematocrit is a valuable and convenient method for determining anemia. A thin blood smear with red cells adjacent but not abutting each other, properly stained with Wright's stain, provides valuable information regarding red cell size, shape, and hemoglobin pigment content. Electronic particle counters are becoming more available in commercial laboratories and office practices to permit rapid calculation of red cell indices. The MCH refers to the mean amount of hemoglobin per red cell (normal equals 28 to 32 micromicrograms/dl). The more informative values are the mean corpuscular volume (MCV), expressing the average red cell volume or size from the hematocrit over the red blood count (normal is 82 to 92 cubic microns), and the mean corpuscular hemoglobin concentration (MCHC), expressing the percentage of hemoglobin over the hematocrit (normal MCHC is 32 to 35 per cent).

Certain practical points for proper collection of blood from finger sticks or heel sticks should be kept in mind. The heel or finger stick must provide free flow of blood. The first drop of blood should be wiped away before collection is made into the microhematocrit tube or the pipette for hemoglobin determination. Cold extremities should be prewarmed to ensure a free flow of blood. The finger or heel should not be squeezed, since extravasated tissue fluid will falsely lower the hematocrit or hemoglobin value.

The most common microcytic hypochromic anemia is iron deficiency. Other causes of microcytic hypochromic anemia include lead poisoning associated with prominent basophilic stippling of red cells on blood smear, the thalassemic syndromes, and occasionally secondary anemias. The FEP test (free erythrocyte porphyrins) is an accurate simple micro method to screen for lead poisoning. Homozygous beta thalassemia produces marked variation in red cell size, targeted red cells, and many nucleated red cells on the blood smear. Target cells are also prominent in sickle cell and hemoglobin C diseases and liver disease and following splenectomy. Beta thalassemia minor produces a very hypochromic microcytic blood smear which the inexperienced observer often confuses with iron deficiency; however, the hypochromia is so profound that if the anemia were due to iron deficiency, the hemoglobin would be less than 5 gm/dl rather than between 8 and 1000 gm/dl, as is the case in thalassemia minor.

The anemia of chronic inflammation or infection, which may be either microcytic-hypochromic or normocytic-normochromic, results from sequestration of iron in the reticuloendothelial system, with less iron available for hemoglobin synthesis by developing red cells in the bone marrow. Serum iron levels are decreased in both conditions; the binding protein for iron, transferrin, is reduced in the anemia of chronic infection or inflammation but is increased in iron deficiency. In iron deficiency anemia the saturation of transferrin is generally less than 10 per cent but is greater than 30 per cent in the anemia of chronic infection or inflammation.

Hemolytic anemias or anemias responding to hematinic therapy are associated with polychromatic red cells on smear correlating with the reticulocytosis. Serum haptoglobin is low, and indirect bilirubin is greater than 1 per cent with chronic hemolysis. Fixed sickle forms are usually present in the blood smear of patients with sickle cell disease, but not those with sickle cell trait. A positive sickle cell screening test does not imply that the patient has sickle cell disease, but simply the presence of sickle hemoglobin. Proof for sickle cell disease must reside in the hemoglobin electrophoresis, which reveals a slightly higher concentration of hemoglobin A than hemoglobin S in the trait and an absence of adult hemoglobin in homozygous sickle cell disease.

The presence of many microspherocytes on the blood smear usually indicates that a patient has congenital spherocytosis, although acquired hemolytic anemia and sequestration anemia due to splenomegaly may also produce spherocytes. The Coulter counter can be used to screen for spherocytosis, since the MCHC is uniquely greater than 35 per cent, and for thalassemia minor where the MCV and MCH are very low (MCV 60 μm^3; MCH 22 nng). A positive direct Coomb's test is found in most cases of acquired hemolytic anemia. Associated viral illness such as infectious mononucleosis due to Epstein-Barr virus, cytomegalovirus infection, and cold agglutinin mycoplasmin pneumonia are diagnostic considerations.

Anemia with normal sized or slightly macrocytic red cells without polychromasia suggests decreased production of red cells in the bone marrow. The reticulocyte count is usually less than 1 per cent. Congenital hypoplastic anemia first described by Diamond and Blackfan is a rare disorder noted in infants generally less than one year of age. Transient erythroblastopenia of childhood, which occasionally follows an upper respiratory infection and subsides in two to eight weeks without specific therapy, may occur in infants and children between one month and six years of age. When the blood smear also reveals diminished platelets and white cells or abnormal white cells, leukemia, lymphoma, or severe aplastic anemia must be ruled out with a bone marrow aspiration or biopsy. True megaloblastic anemias due to folic acid or vitamin B_{12} deficiency are rare. Folate stores in the liver can be depleted in the chronically ill infant or child. Diseases of the small bowel and anticonvulsant therapy produce folate deficiency, whereas surgical resection of the terminal ileum removes the site of vitamin B_{12} absorption.

MANAGEMENT

Iron-Deficiency Anemia

The common mild nutritional iron-deficiency states with a hematocrit ranging between 28 and 32 per cent usually respond to altering the dietary habits of the child, encouraging solid table foods and reducing the milk intake to less than 16 ounces per day. In more severe cases, ferrous sulfate, 6 mg/kg/day of elemental iron, should be administered two or three times daily. Placing the medication on the back of the tongue may minimize the nonpermanent staining of the teeth that may occur. Ferrous sulfate is the drug of choice, since other polysaccharide iron capsules and chewable iron preparations are not well absorbed, even though they produce less gastrointestinal irritation. Generally, the hemoglobin rises a gram per week after ferrous sulfate treatment is initiated. Treatment should be continued for three months after the hemoglobin returns to normal to replace iron stores.

The most common cause for failure to respond to oral iron is lack of compliance. Inspection of the remaining volume of ferrous sulfate medication and of the stools to verify the black color induced by ferrous sulfate confirms compliance. Rarely, intramuscular iron dextran is required because of gastrointestinal intolerance or to ensure that the infant receives the iron. Multiagent hematinics should be discouraged, since they tend to confuse the correct diagnosis. In the hypoproteinemic variety of iron deficiency, it may be necessary to substitute a soy bean or meat base protein for cow's milk, since intestinal losses of proteins and blood are often accentuated by cow's milk protein.

Hemolytic Anemias

Patients with hemolytic anemias are susceptible to aplastic crises when the bone marrow erythron stops producing red cells. Children with sickle cell anemia are more vulnerable to overwhelming pneumococcal meningitis or septicemia. It is advisable that penicillin be available at home to be started at the earliest sign or symptom of serious infection. Some physicians advocate using prophylactic penicillin daily for the first few years of life in patients with sickle cell disease. These patients should receive pneumococcal polysaccharide vaccine if they are over two years of age. Aplastic crises must be treated with transfusion of packed red blood cells in the amount of 10 ml/kg. The frequently occurring painful crises in sickle cell disease are usually treated with analgesics (Codeine and Demerol), and hydration, 3000 ml/M^2/day. If the patient is vomiting, intravenous hydration may be required. At the present time, there is no safe and convenient method for preventing sickling crisis.

SCREENING FOR A BLEEDING DISORDER

When called upon to evaluate the potential seriousness of bruises of the extremities or recurrent epistaxis, the pediatrician must decide when to initiate further diagnostic studies. Elective surgical procedures as well as certain dental procedures may require a preoperative office evaluation to rule out the possibility of underlying coagulation disorders.

Most bleeding disorders can be diagnosed by careful attention in the history to past bleeding episodes and excessive bleeding in the family. Although the male infant with Factor VIII or Factor IX deficiency may escape without serious bleeding at circumcision, the majority of severe hemophiliacs with less than 1 per cent Factor VIII or Factor IX experience bleeding at this time. The family history is negative in 50 per cent of severe cases. On the other hand, those with moderate to mild hemophilia (with factor levels greater than 1 per cent) usually do not bleed from circumcision. Almost all of them have a positive family history. (Hemophilia is discussed in Chapter 77.) Factor VIII and Factor IX deficiency are transmitted as X-linked diseases so that an historical inquiry for similar bleeding episodes in maternal uncles and cousins is required. An in-depth family history with a diagram of a family tree is helpful to account for all family members. Often parents wish to recount this analysis after consultation with other family members.

Apparent abnormalities of coagulation often stem from improper collection and processing of blood samples. The physician should become acquainted with correct methodology and the competence of the coagulation laboratory where these evaluations are performed. Blood for testing is collected by clean venipuncture, thereby reducing chances for contamination from tissue juices that can activate coagulation factors. The samples should be placed in a volume of 3.8 per cent acid-citrate-dextrose (ACD) to provide a final volume of 9 parts whole blood and 1 part ACD. The collection tube is then filled to its proper height and the blood is placed on ice immediately for prothrombin time (PT) and partial thromboplastin time (PTT) determinations. The estimation of platelet number and morphology on peripheral blood smear is made from clean finger stick or heel stick rather than anticoagulated whole blood. Except for the first seven days of the newborn period when vitamin K–dependent factors have not reached normal adult levels (Factor II, VII, IX, and X), there are no major differences between coagulation values obtained from infants, children, or adults.

Only a few tests are really necessary to screen for bleeding disorders. All cases of severe, moderate, and mild Factor VIII and Factor IX deficiencies will have prolonged PTT. The prothrombin time (PT) tests for extrinsic pathway factors include disorders of Factor V, Factor VII, prothrombin (Factor II), and Factor X. Fibrinogen levels can now be assayed quickly and accurately. Thus, all coagulation factors except Factor XIII, fibrin stabilizing factor, deficiency of which is a very rare disorder, are identified with the PTT, PT, and fibrinogen.

Patients with von Willebrand's disease generally have depressed levels of Factor VIII, but they may not be low enough to prolong the PTT. In those cases, a Factor VIII assay is required. In addition, these patients have abnormalities of platelet function due to a deficiency of von Willebrand's factor, a plasma factor affecting platelet adhesiveness and generally also prolonging the Ivy bleeding time. A prolonged bleeding time is characteristic of either thrombocytopenia or abnormal platelet function as observed in von Willebrand's disease, thrombopathy, thrombasthenia, or the effect of aspirin in preventing platelet aggregation due to the blocked secondary release of platelet adenosine diphosphate.

A properly prepared blood smear will give some indication of decreased platelet numbers as well as permit evaluation of platelet morphology. Examination of the sequence of whole blood clot formation, retraction, and lysis also provides useful information. This gives some estimation of the total amount of fibrinogen available for the fibrin clot as well as platelets for contraction. Thus, with this group of simple tests, PT, PTT, fibrinogen, blood smear for platelet numbers and morphology, Ivy bleeding time, and an observation of the clot formation contraction, retraction, and lysis, the physician in an office practice is capable of diagnosing greater than 95 per cent of all hereditary and acquired pediatric disorders of coagulation.

REFERENCE

Nathan, D. G., and Oski, F. A. (eds.): Hematology of Infancy and Childhood, 2nd Ed. Philadelphia, W. B. Saunders Co., 1981.

77

CURRENT CARE FOR HEMOPHILIA

Margaret W. Hilgartner, M.D.

DEMOGRAPHY

Hemophilia A (classic hemophilia) is characterized by a deficiency of the Factor VIII clotting activity in the presence of a nonfunctioning Factor VIII protein. Hemophilia B is characterized by a deficiency of the Factor IX clotting activity in the presence of a nonfunctioning Factor IX protein or complete absence of the protein. The two have similar clinical presentation and can be distinguished only in the laboratory. The incidence of hemophilia in the U.S. is 1/10,000 males for Factor VIII deficiency and 0.25/10,000 males for Factor IX deficiency. It is usually a sex-linked recessive inheritance; however, a large proportion of new cases are due to a high mutation rate, with 25 per cent of new cases without a family history of hemophilia. Prevalence appears to be increasing and may be expected to do so, since the gene is no longer lethal and more hemophiliacs are reproducing (Miller, 1982).

PRESENTATION

Severe hemophilia in those patients with less than 1 per cent of the missing clotting factor is characterized by frequent "spontaneous" painful bleeding episodes. Bleeding may occur at circumcision but usually does not begin until the toddler begins to walk. Bleeding occurs most often into joints—ankles, knees, hips, and elbows—and, if unabated, leads to progressive arthropathy, joint destruction, and crippling.

Patients with moderate disease with up to 5 per cent of the clotting factor may bleed with trauma and then continue to bleed spontaneously into a "target joint," i.e., one joint that seems to have problems more frequently than another; however, the episodes are usually less frequent than those in the patient with severe disease (Aronstan et al., 1979). Patients with mild disease of 10 to 40 per cent bleed only with severe trauma such as surgery, including dental surgery. The frequency and pattern of bleeding vary with each patient and throughout the year in any given patient; for example, some patients may bleed weekly while others bleed monthly with or without trauma. It is this variability that contributes to the difficulties in coping with the disease (Hilgartner, 1979).

Bleeding may occur anywhere in the body, into body cavities, into or around any organ as well as in the joints. It may be controlled with pressure if minor or superficial but usually requires factor replacement for control.

PATTERNS OF CARE

Bleeding episodes can be controlled with replacement of the deficient clotting factor which is obtained from normal human plasma. One ml of fresh normal plasma contains one unit of each of the clotting factors. Factor VIII is found in the cryoprecipitate of fresh frozen plasma and can be resuspended for infusion or further purified, concentrated, and lyophilized. Factor IX can be fractionated with Factors II, VII, and X, concentrated, and lyophilized. The patient deficient in functioning Factor VIII and IX can have his plasma factor level corrected with an intravenous infusion of one of the products as long as necessary for adequate healing. Type and length of therapy are dependent on the magnitude and site of bleeding. For example, a simple bleed into the muscle requires one small infusion which may be given on an outpatient basis, a bleed into a joint requires a larger dose, and abdominal or central nervous system bleeding episodes require hospitalization and 7 to 10 days of daily high dose therapy.

Concentrates are the preferred product for treatment of bleeding episodes for most patients, particularly those on home care programs, because of their ease of storage and administration and their stability. The majority of patients are treated on demand or episodic basis; i.e., they are treated for each bleeding episode as it occurs. Episodic care may be given in a hospital or other ambulatory setting in early childhood when cryoprecipitate or fresh frozen plasma for Factor IX deficiency is used or with concentrate of Factor VIII or IX on the home care program. A very small per cent of the population (4.5 per cent in the NHLI 1972 study) are treated routinely every two to three days on a prophylactic program to maintain a plasma level of greater than 10 per cent clotting factor and to prevent "spontaneous bleeding." A transfusion of 25 to 30 units per kilo every three days may achieve this plasma level. A large number of patients may have short-term prophylaxis for six to eight weeks to allow healing of a damaged joint or persistent synovitis and then return to episodic care. Dosage of product varies with type of hemophilia, the product used, and the severity of the bleeding episode, and the rapidity of treatment following the onset of bleeding; i.e., 10 to 15 units per kilo of concentrate will suffice for a muscle bleed, while 40 to 50 units per kilo are necessary for a serious CNS, retropharyngeal, or retroperitoneal bleed.

HOME CARE

Current treatment of the older child and the adolescent with hemophilia has transformed the hemophiliac from an in-hospital patient to a more independent ambulatory person capable of receiving diagnostic and therapeutic programs in an out-patient facility, at home, or at work. "Self-therapy," frequently called home care, has substantially altered the life style and productivity of these patients. Patient or family members are taught the philosophy of early treatment, the rationale of replacement therapy, and the mechanics of intravenous therapy (Hilgartner and Sergis, 1977). This shift of responsibility of early treatment to the patient or family is possible only when they are willing and able to accept the responsibility. Elaborate medical support and back-up systems must, of course, be available. Children as young as two years of age may be enrolled in such a program if the child and family are able to accept such a role. Those entered in a home care program must have periodic examination, including medical, orthopedic, psychosocial, and dental evaluations, along with laboratory evaluations of liver and renal function, response to transfused factor, and the development of an inhibitor to the replacement product.

COMPREHENSIVE CARE

Since the current care of the hemophiliac extends beyond crisis intervention of bleeding episodes and management of orthopedic complications, care is best given by a comprehensive team. The multidisciplinary approach supported by the HHS Regional Hemophilia Diagnostic and Treatment Centers requires centralization of treatment with regular clinical visits for evaluation and formulation of an individual treatment plan that incorporates medical, dental, psychosocial, vocational, and financial aspects of patient care. The patient and/or the center staff may elect to have the episodic care for bleeding given at the center or through the child's regular physician. If the latter is chosen, copies of the treatment plan are sent to this physician as well as to the patient to make them aware of the current status of the patient and the plans for the interval until the next visit. It is recognized that the skills and facilities of the primary care physician may be well developed for the treatment of many bleeding episodes but that the more severe bleeding episodes and surgical procedures should be treated in the centers where expertise, additional facilities, and paramedical help are available. Communication between the center staff and the general physician is therefore essential so that each may do his part for optimal patient care.

Hemophilia adversely affects the lives of patients in a variety of ways. Most children with this disorder have had a bleeding episode requiring transfusion by the age of four. As they grow, they must cope with the knowledge that they may have a serious, possibly lethal bleeding episode at any time. The stress of bleeding, pain, and immobilization with family separations beginning early in life tend to affect the psychosocial development of the child. These fears, coupled with the overprotectiveness of a family, particularly the mother, can lead to the hemophiliac's becoming either a passive, inactive, and isolated individual whose self-image is very poor or, conversely, a daredevil who rebels against an oversolicitous mother by becoming a defiant overactive boy. Those boys who can adapt and use the experience gained through normal activities of growth and development to understand their disease and the limitations that it may impose usually develop a good masculine identification and a strong sense of self-worth (Handford and Stricler, 1982).

The relationship with the hemophilia team is used for ongoing education and counseling. These services assure that even prior to the birth of a hemophiliac, supportive help is available to reduce the anxiety and problems in parent-infant relationships. Parents can also be counseled long before the onset of the usual need for transfusions about the day-to-day care and precautions required for the infant, toddler, and preschooler. For example, knowledgeable mothers may wish to pad the clothing of infants as they begin to crawl. In our institution a group of parents with children under six years of age meet monthly with the social worker for self-help sessions to reduce anxiety levels and foster normal patterns of parenting for the patient and for his well sibling(s). They also learn that siblings may be neglected and that the problem of the carrier sisters must be recognized early. Very early indications of overprotection or underprotection can be detected and dealt with in such programs.

Other types of intervention have been used for the older child and young adult to decrease stress, anxiety, and fears. Self-hypnosis has been used by LaBaw and others for a number of years with a documented decrease in infusion product (Handford and Stricler, 1982; Varni et al., 1982). Varni believes that a learned system of biofeedback is just as useful (Varni et al., 1982). Whatever mechanism is used, efforts to decrease anxiety appears helpful in assisting the patient to cope with his illness.

The comprehensive team may assist with the development of alternate physical education programs that give the patient appropriate age-related exercise and make him feel part of a program, without the risk of contact sports.

References

Agle, D. P., and Mattsson, A.: Psychiatric factors in hemophilia: Methods of parental adaptation. Bibl. Haematol. *34*:89, 1970.

Aronstan, A., Rainsford, J. G., and Pairter, M. I.: Patterns of bleeding in adolescents with severe hemophilia A. Br. Med. J. *1*:469, 1979.

Gill, F. M., Shapiro, S. J., Palascak, J., Hulton, M. B., Whitehurst, D. A., Poole, W. K., and the Hemophilia Study Group. The natural history of factor VIII inhibitors in patients with hemophilia A. A national cooperative study I. Characteristics of the population, 1980. (Submitted for publication.)

Handford, H. A., and Stricler, E. M.: Psychosocial pro-

gram. *In* Hilgartner, M. W. (Ed.): Hemophilia in the Child and the Adult. New York, Masson Publishing, 1982.
Hilgartner, M. W.: Managing the child with hemophilia. Pediatr. Ann., 8(6):383–403, 1979.
Hilgartner, M. W., and Sergis, E.: Current therapy for hemophiliacs: Home Care and therapeutic complications. Mt. Siani J. Med., *44*:316–331, 1977.
LaBaw, W. L.: Autohypnosis in hemophilia. Haematologia (Budapest) 9(1–2):103–110, 1975.
Miller, C. H.: Genetics in hemophilia and von Willebrand's disease. *In* Hilgartner, M. W., (Ed.): Hemophilia in the Child and the Adult. New York, Masson Publishing, 1982.
Salk, L., Hilgartner, M. W., and Granill, B.: The psychosocial impact of hemophilia on the patient and his family. Soc. Sci. Med. *6*:491–505, 1972.
Varni, J. W., Katz, E. F., and Dash, I.: Behavioral and neurochemical aspects of pediatric pain. *In* Russo, D. C., and Varni, J. W. (Eds.): Behavioral Pediatrics: Research and Practice. Plenum Publishing Corporation, 1982, pp. 177–224.

78
SHORT STATURE

James Wright, M.D.

The growth, multiplication, and differentiation of function of body structures is dependent not only on genetically determined enzymes but also upon supplies of nutrients for protoplasmic synthesis and energy metabolism. Assimilation and transportation of these nutrients to a cellular environment compatible with optimum protein synthesis is necessary for an increase in either cell size or cell number, one or both of which are essential for growth. These same factors, needed for normal growth, are operative from formation of the zygote to full maturity.

The most widely accepted definition of short stature is height that is three or more standard deviations below the mean for age and sex. A rate of growth consistently below that to be expected at the child's developmental age is indicative of the need for evaluation, regardless of position of height on the growth curve. Bone age determination is the usual method of assessing developmental age during infancy and childhood. A dwarf has been broadly defined as an individual who is conspicuously smaller than his peers.

HISTORY AND PHYSICAL EXAMINATION

In the history, evaluation of the child with short stature requires special emphasis on all available prior measurements, beginning with birth weight and length. Social data are of particular importance. The family history should include not only any known case of short stature, but also adult heights and the growth and development patterns of relatives. In the physical examination it is especially important to look for evidence of systemic disease, disproportion of skeletal segments, and status of sexual development.

GROWTH CHARTS

The most commonly used growth charts demonstrate height attainment by plotting height versus age. Percentiles or standard deviations are used to show the wide range of measurements observed in a normal population. The ninety-seventh and third percentiles are approximately equal to two standard deviations above and below the mean. While a plotted measurement on such a chart may indicate short stature, multiple points constituting a growth curve indicate height velocity and the presence or absence of growth failure. The height age of a child corresponds to the age at which his height equals the fiftieth percentile.

BONE AGE

Prior to full maturity, the duration of growth may be predicted by the level of physical maturation. Before the onset of adolescent sexual development, determination of the bone age is used as an index of physical maturation. The Greulich and Pyle atlas of roentgenograms of hand and wrist offers the best standardized method for evaluating skeletal maturation. Roentgenograms of the hemiskeleton for a study of total number of epiphyseal centers offer an alternative method in infants and young children or when clinical impressions are at variance with bone age determined from only the hand and wrist, but it must be remembered that the standard error of the method is fairly large.

LABORATORY STUDIES

The extent of laboratory studies indicated in children with growth failure is determined by the age of the child and by historical data. If there is a history of poor nutrition or interactional problems between the parents and child, a period of observation on an adequate diet may obviate the need for further studies. When the cause of growth failure is not clear, laboratory studies indicated are a complete blood count and urinalysis, including urinary pH. Analysis of the blood should include pH or bicarbonate content, serum cholesterol, sodium, potassium, chloride, blood urea nitrogen or creatinine, calcium, inorganic phosphate, alkaline phosphatase, and total proteins. It is useful to determine the serum T_4 by a radioimmunoassay. X-rays of the hand and wrist for level of skeletal maturation are required. If there is evidence for a central nervous system lesion, or if there is a strong suggestion of hypopituitarism, roentgenograms of the skull should be obtained. In phenotypic females with short stature in whom there is no other obvious diagnosis and in whom stigmata of Turner's syndrome are present, karyotype analysis is indicated prior to further evaluation of endocrine function. The staining of buccal smear to determine presence or absence of Barr bodies should be done only in laboratories with a high volume of such tests and with expert and experienced technical personnel.

ETIOLOGY AND DIAGNOSIS OF SHORT STATURE

Primordial dwarfism, a term traditionally used to designate a child with short stature who does not have a delay in physical maturation, is a diagnosis that should be limited to those children who have intrauterine growth failure with persistent small size. Characteristically, growth is slow from earliest infancy, although epiphyseal maturation and sexual development usually occur at the expected time or at only a slightly delayed rate. Growth hormone levels are usually normal. Other endocrine function studies have also been normal. There is an increased incidence of mental retardation and other developmental somatic abnormalities.

Table 78–1. ETIOLOGY OF SHORT STATURE

1. Intrauterine growth retardation
2. Chromosomal abnormalities
3. Genetic (familial) short stature
4. Constitutional delay in growth and physical maturation
5. Psychosocial short stature
6. Skeletal dysplasias
7. Disorders of carbohydrate, lipid, and protein metabolism
8. Undernutrition
9. Chronic disease (nonendocrine and nonskeletal)
   a. Diseases of cardiovascular system
   b. Diseases of pulmonary system
   c. Diseases of the gastrointestinal system (bowel and liver)
   c. Diseases of the kidney
   e. Diseases of the central nervous system
10. Endocrine disorders
   a. Hypothyroidism
   b. Growth hormone deficiency
   c. Glucocorticoid excess (endogenous or iatrogenic)
   d. Premature closure of epiphyses in precocious sexual development or virilizing syndromes
   e. Pseudohypoparathyroidism

Primordial dwarfism is seen sporadically without other congenital anomalies in some, and in association with a number of characteristic anomalies in others, e.g., progeria, bird-headed dwarfism, peculiar craniofacial anomalies, and hemiatrophy or hemihypertrophy. Little is gained by trying to segregate each patient into a particular diagnostic category. Intrauterine infection such as congenital rubella, syphilis, toxoplasmosis, or cytomegalic inclusion disease is associated with intrauterine growth failure and multiple congenital anomalies.

The clinical features of congenital hypothyroidism or cretinism are well known. Although failure of longitudinal linear growth with resulting short stature is indeed a feature of congenital hypothyroidism, it is rarely the major or only presenting complaint. When acquired hypothyroidism occurs after the age of two years, growth failure may be the principal, or in some cases, the only complaint. Detailed history, however, may elicit such subtle signs and symptoms of hypothyroidism as decreased activity, cold intolerance, increased hours of sleep, a tendency to gain weight, and constipation. Physical signs may include cool and dry skin with sallow complexion, puffiness of the face (especially around the eyes), and coarse, brittle hair. The most characteristic growth pattern in acquired hypothyroidism is an almost complete cessation of longitudinal linear growth.

T_4 by radioimmunoassay is the only chemical determination which must be done initially for the indication of thyroid function. Should the T_4 be low, determination of TSH (thyroid stimulating hormone) should be carried out to determine whether the hypothyroidism is primary or secondary to hypothalamic-pituitary dysfunctions. Most cases are primary.

Hypopituitary dwarfism may be sporadic or familial, organic or idiopathic. Idiopathic hypopituitarism may be most frequently a result of hypothalamic dysfunction rather than a primary defect of pituitary function. Although suprasellar tumors are the principal cause, organic hypopituitarism may be seen in destructive or invasive lesions of the brain, e.g., histiocytosis or Hand-Schüller-Christian disease, which affect releasing homones from the hypothalamus. Patients with organic hypopituitarism usually present for medical attention because of neurological or visual abnormalities, whereas patients with idiopathic hypopituitarism usually present with growth failure or spontaneous symptomatic hypoglycemia. It is necessary to demonstrate failure of response to at least two of the standardized provocative tests for growth hormone release in order to establish a definitive diagnosis of growth hormone deficiency. Pituitary growth hormone does not directly stimulate skeletal growth, but rather the production of somatomedins, which, in turn, stimulate longitudinal linear growth. Failure of somatomedin production in the presence of normal or elevated levels of pituitary growth hormone may be a cause of short stature. Radioimmunoassay of somatomedin C, a serum protein that is growth-promoting and growth hormone–dependent, may prove to be a useful screening test for growth hormone deficiency. Evaluation of thyroid and adrenal function is indicated in a child with deficiency of pituitary growth hormone. Tests for gonadal function are indicated in the teen-age patient.

Psychosocial dwarfism is the term currently used for the short stature observed in children from an emotionally deprived environment. Many patients with psychosocial short stature also have evidence of transient hypopituitarism with growth homone and corticotropin deficiencies. Associated behavioral aberrations may include polyphagia associated with eating garbage and frequent vomiting; polydypsia to the extent of drinking from unusual sources such as toilet bowls; and disoriented sleep patterns associated with night wandering during which foraging for food occurs. Frequently there are other behavioral manifestations such as "flat" personality, withdrawing, and nondiscriminating attachment to parents or strangers. There is an associated retarded bone age and, in adolescents, delayed sexual maturation. Growth rate usually shows a marked increase upon removal of the child from the environment in which the child is living to a more health-promoting setting.

Constitutional delayed growth and physical maturation are observed more commonly in males than in females; however, parental concern for height in males is more evident than for females and contributes to the marked predominance of males reported from most clinics. There is a family history of similar growth and development patterns in approximately 40 per cent of the children seen in the author's clinic. These patients do not have any known endocrine dysfunction, and the cause of the condition which is associated with slow attainment of adult height is unknown. Typically, these children are normal in size at birth and throughout infancy. They fall away from the normal growth curve during the preschool and, perhaps, early school years and then demonstrate a normal growth rate without any "catch-up." During childhood the height of affected children tends to be equivalent to about the fiftieth percentile for the children of the same sex who are two to four years younger. Bone age is characteristically comparably delayed, i.e., by two to four years. Endocrine function studies are normal. A child who has retarded height age, comparably retarded bone age, a history of normal size at birth, and no abnormal endocrine function studies usually has constitutional delayed growth and physical maturation. Because of delay in physical maturation, they usually catch up through a prolonged period of growth prior to closure of the epiphyses.

A diagnosis of Turner's syndrome is always considered in phenotypic females with short stature. This syndrome is associated with short stature, absence or partial failure of sexual development, and some abnormality in sex chromosomes. Associated somatic abnormalities may include micrognathia, peaked palate, webbed neck, lymphedema of the extremities (in infancy), increased carrying angle of the arms, shortened fourth and/or fifth metacarpals, coarctation of the aorta, and renal anomalies such as double collecting system and horseshoe kidney. Moderate pubic hair growth at the usual age of adolescent sexual development is common; however, breast development is absent except in XO/XX mosaics in whom there may be slight development. Sterility is the rule. Short stature is always found, but the degree is variable and there is a genetic component involved in ultimate height. A missing sex chromosome resulting in sex chromosome complement of XO is the most common abnormality in karyotyping. Mosaicism such as XO/XX and XO/XY is also associated with Turner's syndrome, as are abnormalities of an X chromosome observed in XXqi karyotype.

Other systemic disorders may be characterized by growth failure, but this is rarely the principal or only complaint. Severe mental retardation is frequently accompanied by short stature. Children with congenital heart disease or chronic pulmonary disease may be shorter than their healthy peers. Malabsorption which leads to nutritional deficiencies is probably the leading cause of growth failure associated with gastrointestinal disease, although anorexia may be a contributing factor. Retardation of growth may occur in patients with inflammatory bowel disease even in the absence of specific gastrointestinal symptoms. The exact etiology of the growth impairment in children with chronic renal disease remains unknown; however, chronic metabolic acidosis is recognized as a deterrent to normal growth. The diagnosis of children whose short stature is due to osteochondrodystrophies and other skeletal disorders is usually suggested by physical appearance (i.e., disproportion of body segments) and is confirmed by skeletal roentgenograms.

TREATMENT OF SHORT STATURE

There is no effective treatment for primordial dwarfism.

Treatment of both primary and secondary hypothyroidism is replacement with either dessicated thyroid, synthetic T_4, or synthetic preparations that are mixtures of T_4 and T_3. Replacement dosage should be approximately 100 mg of dessicated thyroid per square meter of body surface or the equivalent in one of the other preparations. Growth response to treatment usually consists of "catch-up" growth rate followed by appropriate growth rate for a level of physical development with continued treatment.

Treatment of hypopituitarism involves replacement with the missing hormones from the target glands, i.e., thyroid hormones if thyroid function is deficient, glucocorticoid if adrenocortical function is deficient, sexual steroidal hormones if gonadal function is deficient, and growth hormone. Supplies of human growth hormone are still not adequate to treat all patients with hypopituitarism beginning at the time of diagnosis. The dosage of thyroid replacement is identical to that used in primary hypothyroidism. The amount of glucocorticoid replacement is based on 15 mg of hydrocortisone per square meter of body surface per day. Dosage of sexual steroidal replacement is variable. The amount of human growth hormone used is about 0.1 unit per kilogram body weight three times weekly.

Treatment for psychosocial dwarfism obviously involves alteration of the environment in which the child is functioning, either by transfer to a better one or by major intervention to improve the home in which the child lives.

No treatment is necessary to attain appropriate sexual maturation and genetically determined adult height in constitutional delayed growth in adolescents. After the age of 15, when continued short stature and sexual infantilism are associated with significant psychological problems, a short course of testosterone may be considered for these patients. A long-acting (depot) form of testosterone, 100 mg given intramuscularly every four weeks, may be used for four months. Such treatment should be undertaken with the goals of producing a fairly prompt, noticeable increase in growth rate as well as secondary sexual development, and of attaining a level of maturation of the hypothalamic-pituitary-gonadal axis which will allow the patient to continue his normal sexual development when treatment is discontinued. Treatment should also be undertaken only after assuring the patient that he is not abnormal, that sexual maturation and growth spurt will eventually occur without treatment, and that treatment merely brings about these changes sooner.

Usual management of the short stature of Turner's syndrome involves the use of anabolic steroids for approximately two to three years prior to the initiation of estrogen replacement therapy. Oxandrolone, in a dosage of 0.1 to 0.25 mg/kg body weight per day in one or two doses, is used in the author's clinic. The anabolic steroid is then continued together with the estrogen replacement for approximately another year or until there is fusion of epiphyseal centers evident on x-ray. Treatment with estrogen therapy is then continued. Long-term use of estrogen should always be in conjunction with progesterone. Initial treatment with estrogen utilizes ethinyl estradiol 5 to 10 micrograms or conjugated estrogens (Premarin) 0.3 mg daily on the first 21 days of each calendar month. After six months, dosage of estrogen is increased to 10 to 20 micrograms of ethinyl estradiol or 0.625 mg of conjugated estrogen. Medroxyprogesterone acetate (Provera) 10 mg per day on the 17th through the 21st day of each calendar month is added at the time of the increased dosage of estrogen.

REFERENCES

Beck, G. J., and van den Berg, B. J.: The relationship of the rate of intrauterine growth of low-birth-weight infants to later growth. J. Pediatr., *86*:504, 1975.

Fitzhardinge, P. M., and Steven, E. M.: The small-for-date infant. I. Later growth patterns. Pediatrics, *49*:671, 1972.

Frasier, S. D., and Rallison, M. D.: Growth retardation and emotional deprivation: Relative resistance to treatment with human growth hormone. J. Pediatr., *80*:603, 1972.

Frasier, S. D., Aceto, T., Jr., and Hayles, A. B.: Collaborative study of the effects of human growth hormone deficiency. V. Treatment with growth hormone administered once a week. J. Clin. Endocrinol. Metab., *47*:686, 1978.

Hopwood, M. J., and Becker, D. J.: Psychosocial dwarfism: Detection, evaluation, and management. Child Abuse Neglect, *3*:439, 1979.

Johanson, A. J., Brasel, J. A., and Blizzard, R. M.: Growth in patients with gonadal dysgenesis receiving fluoxymesterone. J. Pediatr., *75*:1015, 1969.

Leonard, M. F., Rhymes, J. P., and Solnit, A. J.: Failure to thrive in infants. Am. J. Dis. Child., *111*:600, 1966.

Lippe, B. M.: Primary ovarian failure. *In* Kaplan, S. A. (Ed.): Clinical Pediatric and Adolescent Endocrinology. Philadelphia, W. B. Saunders Co., 1982.

McDonough, P. G.: Gonadal dysgenesis and its variants. Pediatr. Clin. North Am., *19*:631, 1972.

Pollitt, E., and Eichler, A.: Behavioral disturbances among failure-to-thrive children. Am. J. Dis. Child., *130*:24, 1976.

Powell, G. F., Brasel, J. A., and Blizzard, R. M.: Emotional deprivation and growth retardation simulating idiopathic hypopituitarism. I. Clinical evaluation of the syndrome. N. Engl. J. Med., *276*:1271, 1967.

Powell, G. F., et al.: Emotional deprivation and growth retardation simulating idiopathic hypopituitarism. II. Endocrinologic evaluation of the syndrome. N. Engl. J. Med., *276*:1279, 1967.

Prader, A.: Delayed adolescence. Clin. Endocrinol. Metab., *4*:143, 1975.

Silver, H. K., and Finkelstein, M.: Deprivation dwarfism. J. Pediatr., *70*:317, 1967.

Sobel, E. H.: Abnormal growth patterns in infancy and adolescence. *In* Gardner, L. I. (Ed.): Endocrine and Genetic Diseases of Childhood and Adolescence. Philadelphia, W. B. Saunders Co., 1975.

Soyka, L. F., et al.: Effectiveness of long-term human growth hormone therapy for short stature in children with growth hormone deficiency. J. Clin. Endocrinol., *30*:1, 1970.

Van Wyke, J. J., and Underwood, L. E.: Relation between growth hormone and somatomedin. Annu. Rev. Med., *26*:427, 1975.

Warkany, J., Monroe, B. B., and Sutherland, B. S.: Intrauterine growth retardation. Am. J. Dis. Child., *102*:249, 1961.

79

MUSCULOSKELETAL ACHES AND LIMB PAIN

Murray H. Passo, M.D.

The evaluation of musculoskeletal aches and limb pain is a common problem for the primary care physician. The majority of children who have recurrent limb pain have no demonstrable organic lesion. Reports indicate that up to 15 per cent of school age children have occasional limb pain and that 4.5 per cent of children experience pain severe enough to cause interruption of normal acitivities for longer than three months.

Table 79–1 lists the anatomical structures and the pathological processes involved in the etiology of the pain. Usually a combination of anatomical structures is involved in a single disease process. A crossmatch of these anatomical structures with the pathological processes permits the development of a long list of different disease processes that need to be considered as the cause of the pain (Zohn and Mennell, 1976).

A description of the pain can also be helpful in determining the anatomical and pathophysiological processes that are involved. The profile of pain as described by Engel (1970) includes six dimensions listed in Table 79–2. Pain can be referred from proximal or distal structures, as is the case with hip pain referred to the medial knee. Previous experience with pain as

Table 79–1. EVALUATION OF LIMB PAIN BY CROSSMATCHING ANATOMICAL STRUCTURES WITH PATHOLOGICAL PROCESSES*

Anatomical Structure	Pathology
Bone	Trauma
Hyaline cartilage	Infection
Synovium and joint capsule	Noninfectious inflammation
Ligaments	Metabolic disorder
Muscles and tendons	Neoplasia
Intra-articular meniscus	Congenital anomalies
Bursa	Psychological disorder
Nerve	Idiopathic disorder
Vascular structures	

*Modified from Zohn, D. A., and Mennel, J. M.: Musculoskeletal pain: Diagnosis and Physical Treatment. Boston, Little, Brown and Co., 1976, p. 17.

well as the current emotional status of the patient may influence the intensity of the pain. Knowledge of the intensity of the pain can be helpful when it correlates with objective physical findings or, occasionally, when it is disproportionate but corroborated by other historical or clinical information. The frequency, duration, and variability of episodes is important in analyzing recurrent or intermittent bouts of pain. Additionally, the pattern of involvement is helpful, e.g., migratory, additive, or episodic. The qualitative aspect of the pain, i.e., throbbing, aching, burning, or tingling, may be difficult for children to describe. It is helpful to know whether the pain has modified sleep or daily activities, including vocational, recreational, and school participation. In addition, the physician should be sensitive to whether the complaint is being used for secondary gain. Is

Table 79–2. PAIN PROFILE—A DESCRIPTION OF PAIN

Aspects to be described:

1. Topographical—location, remember referred pain
2. Quantitative—intensity
3. Temporal—chronology, frequency, duration, variability, pattern of involvement
4. Qualitative—characterization, description—throbbing, aching, burning, etc.
5. Associated physiological aspects—effects of activity, rest, movement; aggravating or alleviating factors
6. Behavioral and psychological—changes in life's routine because of the pain, secondary gain, conversion mechanism, depression, anxiety

the child depressed or anxious or seemingly unconcerned?

Complaints of swelling, limitation of motion, alterations in locomotion and usual daily activities, stiffness, fatiguability, weakness, and lack of stamina are sought. One must establish whether the complaints are solely subjective or whether objective changes have been observed. Asking for examples is often helpful in determining the significance of the complaint.

Perhaps the most helpful part of the history in identifying an underlying systemic disease is the thorough review of systems. Since this can be readily accomplished during the physical examination, it requires little additional time. Clues from the review of systems can also provide evidence of a functional or psychosomatic disease. Some of these patients may have pain in numerous areas, including headaches, chest pain, and abdominal pain.

Important items to ask about, since they are often not volunteered, are fever, growth, weight loss, rashes, alopecia, mucosal ulcerations, gastrointestinal dysfunction, menstrual changes, dyspnea, Raynaud's phenomenon, recurrent infection, bruising, nervousness, and school attendance.

Recent immunizations, exposure to hepatitis or blood products, and current medications can be helpful in determining the etiology of pain. One needs to review the family medical history and the current status of the family health and social situations. Children often mimic pain that is present in another family member, and they may develop pain in response to family stress.

A thorough physical examination is necessary to evaluate patients for limb pain, including the spine and all four extremities. The focus of pain should be examined by inspection and palpation for swelling, range of motion, symmetry, cutaneous changes, girth, weakness, alterations in active motion, and sensation.

CLINICAL PAIN SYNDROMES

Chapter 72 on juvenile rheumatoid arthritis describes the typical example of inflammatory arthropathy. The features of inflammatory arthritis include inactivity stiffness, principally manifest as immobility in the morning, after naps, and after prolonged periods of sitting. Pain is usually deep aching, occasionally sharp, and diffusely present throughout the joint. The pain and stiffness are aggravated by initial movement but seem to improve with subsequent activity. Pain may not be a significant feature in young children, and difficulty with locomotion may be more obvious. Swelling is almost uniformly present in these joints, although occasionally thickened synovium and limitation of motion are the only features. One will see such findings in any of the connective tissue diseases, including JRA, SLE, dermatomyositis, occasionally scleroderma, mixed connective tissue disease, and some of the vasculitis syndromes.

Migratory arthritis is defined as involvement of a few joints and subsequent involvement of other joints as the previously affected joints improve. Included in the spectrum of migratory arthritis are acute rheumatic fever, arthritis associated with inflammatory bowel disease, occasionally leukemia and *Neisseria* gonococcal and meningococcal arthritis.

These can be distinguished from mechanical disorders such as patellofemoral pain or chondromalacia patella, which cause most patients to complain of knee pain with retropatellar grinding or a catching sensation and occasionally locking or buckling. The pain is aggravated by activity that loads the patellofemoral joint in flexion, e.g., squatting, climbing stairs, standing from a seated position, running, and kneeling. Compressing the patella down on the femoral condyles, as in sitting with the knees flexed for prolonged periods of time, may also aggravate the pain. Many of these patients have had prior patellar trauma or have patellar malalignment.

On physical examination, the usual patient with the patellofemoral pain syndrome has conspicuous patellofemoral crepitus. The patella may be hypermobile. Knee effusion may be present; however, a tense, warm effusion is rarely seen. The pain may be elicited by the patellofemoral compression test. The examiner holds the patella between his thumb and index finger, pushes it downward and distally against the femur, and then asks the patient to contract the quadriceps muscles by tightening this muscle group or by straight leg raising. The medial border of the infrapatellar surface is often tender, as well as the corresponding surface of the underlying femur.

Most of these patients have patellar malalignment. In patients with valgus knee deformities, such as increased femoral anteversion with external tibial torsion, the quadriceps forces pull the patella laterally with extension. On physical examination there is a widened "Q angle" of greater than 20 degrees. The quadriceps (Q) angle is measured by drawing one line from the anterosuperior iliac spine to the center of the patella and a second line from the center of the patella to the tibial tubercle. The normal angle is 15 degrees or less. Also, patella alta (high-riding, often hypermobile patella) may be noted in some patients with this pain syndrome. At the extreme of malalignment some patients have lateral patellar subluxation. Historically, they describe the knee locking or becoming stuck, with relief of the severe pain only after the subluxation is reduced. X-rays are usually not revealing, although they verify patella alta or patellar malformations and exclude other conditions such as avascular necrosis or osteochondritis dissecans. Several views should be obtained, including anteroposterior, lateral, tunnel, and Merchant's views.

The differential diagnosis for patellofemoral pain *must* include a torn medial meniscus. This can be demonstrated by McMurray's test (tibial rotation test), inability or reluctance to squat or duck walk, and loss of knee motion in either full flexion or extension.

Therapy for patellofemoral pain is largely conservative, with only a small percentage of patients requiring surgery. The mainstay of management is quadriceps strengthening exercises, complemented with aspirin and/or other analgesics. Whether high dose aspirin offers significant improvement is controversial.

Neoplastic disease includes local benign tumors and systemic malignant conditions. Osteoid osteoma, a benign tumor usually occurring in the femur or tibia, causes a boring, aching type of pain especially pronounced at nighttime, often awakening the patient, and characteristically relieved by an analgesic dose of aspirin. X-rays are helpful in establishing the diagnosis.

Nonosseous malignant neoplasms in children, chiefly acute leukemias or metastatic neuroblastoma, commonly cause osteoarticular pain that is usually severe and often disproportionate to the objective physical findings. A careful physical examination, however, often demonstrates tenderness in the area of neoplastic infiltration. Frank arthritis has been reported in some patients. X-ray and laboratory investigations generally yield the proper diagnosis. Occasionally, diagnostic features lag behind the pain by weeks or months.

Growing pains represent a common disorder with a classic clinical picture. Typically nonarticular and located in the calves and thighs, behind the knees, and occasionally in the upper extremities, the pain is described as a mild to severe deep aching occurring in the late evening to night-time. In most cases the pain disappears completely by morning. Parents deny seeing objective signs of swelling, erythema, tenderness, or warmth. The pain, which may last from a few minutes to several hours, may occur after excessive bouts of activity in some patients. Growing pains are alleviated by massage, analgesics, warmth, and a tincture of time. The incidence of this complaint ranges from 4.2 to 33.6 per cent (Hawksley, 1938; Naish and Apley, 1951). Importantly, an additional feature of growing pains is that these children often come from "painful families" and may have a life-long history of somatic complaints including headache and abdominal pain.

Infectious diseases of bone and joint are usually very painful and accompanied by conspicuous physical findings. Swelling, marked limitation of active motion, and extreme pain are the hallmarks of septic arthritis. In osteomyelitis local metaphyseal bone tenderness, adjacent joint swelling, moderate to severe pain, and systemic toxicity are often found. Synovial fluid analysis and appropriate cultures are necessary to sort out these infectious processes from other inflammatory and neoplastic conditions.

The child who does not want to be moved may well have discitis or inflammation of the intravertebral disc. This disorder, characterized by moderate to severe pain, is aggravated by movement. Patients often become apathetic and want to be left alone. Although the pain is often referred to the hip area, examination of the hips does not substantiate joint involvement. The spine is flattened and loses its natural curves. X-ray, bone scan, and physical examination help to establish the diagnosis.

Several idiopathic conditions that present as limb pain have been described. Children with juvenile episodic arthritis/arthralgia (JEA) have recurrent bouts characterized by sudden onset of incapacitating pain and/or tenderness that cause the involved joint to be held in flexion (Brewer et al., 1982). Objective findings such as swelling may or may not occur. Involvement is usually self-limited and the duration a few hours up to several weeks. Laboratory and radiographic examinations are negative. Brewer reports that these children are normally active, often very athletic. This benign condition, which does not progress to a chronic arthropathy, is similar to pallindromic rheumatism, an entity long described in adulthood, except that half of those patients develop a chronic rheumatoid condition subsequent to years of recurrent joint afflictions. Additional investigations are necessary in order to explore functional or psychosocial aspects in many of these patients.

Also included in the idiopathic group are reflex neurovascular dystrophy (Bernstein et al., 1978) and the arthromyalgia syndrome (Bernstein, 1981). Well recognized in adults, reflex neurovascular or reflex sympathetic dystrophy rarely occurs in children. The syndrome is characterized by severe limb pain, signs of autonomic dysfunction or vasomotor instability in the involved limb, and swelling with thermal, color, and perspiration changes. Psychogenic factors may contribute to the etiology in many of these children. In the arthromyalgia syndrome, Bernstein describes older children with persistent or recurrent muscular and articular pain in whom there are no objective findings on physical, radiographic, or laboratory examination; evidence for a psychological etiology is also lacking.

With persistent or recurrent limb pain in children unaccompanied by objective findings, psychosocial factors may be the cause. Prolonged school absenteeism, unexplained fatigue, anorexia, multiple somatic complaints, and evidence of depression may be noted in the interview. Many of these children have a history of a definite antecedent organic insult such as trauma or a virus-like syndrome, but the symptoms linger and the patient does not recover. A return to normal daily activities and personal responsibilities is increasingly resisted. Considerable secondary gain is noted as an additional positive finding for a psychological etiology. Once an underlying organic etiology is ruled out on the basis of the history, the physical examination, or other appropriate procedures, the youngster needs to be rehabilitated by rigorous physical therapy and a concomitant attention to the underlying emotional problems. Return to normal daily activities and, in time, extracurricular activities is essential. Reassurance is extremely important in order to gain the confidence and cooperation of the parents and child. In instances when evidence for a psychosocial etiology is lacking, continued clinical observation and follow-up are indicated. A psychosocial diagnosis should not be made only by exclusion.

REFERENCES

Bernstein, B. H., Singsen, B. H., Kent, J. T., et al.: Reflex neurovascular dystrophy in childhood. J. Pediatr., 93:211, 1978.

Bernstein, B. H.: Diagnostic dilemmas: A rheumatologist's perspective (Continued). *In* Arthritis and Childhood, Report of the Eightieth Ross Conference in Pediatric Research. Columbus, Ohio, Ross Laboratories, 1981, p. 8.

Brewer, E. J., Giannini, E. H., and Person, D. A.: Juvenile Rheumatoid Arthritis, 2nd Ed. Philadelphia, W. B. Saunders Co., 1982, pp. 81–82.
Engel, G. L.: Pain. *In* MacBryde, C. M., and Blacklawn, R. S. (Eds.): Signs and Symptoms: Applied Pathologic Physiology and Clinical Interpretation, 5th Ed. Philadelphia, J. B. Lippincott Co., 1970, pp. 44–61.
Hawksley, J. C.: The incidence and significance of "growing pains" in children and adolescents. J. R. Inst. Public Health, *1*:798, 1938.
Naish, J. M., and Apley, J.: "Growing pains": A clinical study of non-arthritic limb pains in children. Arch Dis. Child., *26*:134, 1951.
Zohn, D. A., and Mennell, J. M.: Musculoskeletal Pain: Diagnosis and Physical Treatment. Boston, Little, Brown and Co., 1976, pp. 15–34.

GENERAL REFERENCES

Ansell, B. M.: Rheumatic Disorders in Childhood. London, Butterworth and Co., Ltd., 1980, pp. 1–17.
Apley, J.: Limb pains with no organic disease. Clin. Rheum. Dis., *2*(2):487–491, 1976.
Oster, J.: Growing pain. Danish Med. Bull., *19*(2):72–79, 1972.
Oster, J., and Nielson, A.: Growing pains. A clinical investigation of a school population. Acta Paediatr. Scand., *61*:329, 1972.
Passo, M. H.: Aches and limb pain. Pediatr. Clin. North Am., *29*(1):209–219, 1982.
Polley, H. F., and Hunder, G. G.: Rheumatologic Interviewing and Physical Examination of the Joints, 2nd Ed. Philadelphia, W. B. Saunders Co., 1978, pp. 1–45.

80

MENTAL RETARDATION

Herbert J. Grossman, M.D.

The American Association on Mental Deficiency defines retardation as "significantly subaverage general intellectual functioning resulting in or associated with concurrent impairments in adaptive behavior, and manifested during the developmental period." Significant subaverage performance is defined as an I.Q. of 70 or below on standardized measures of intelligence. The upper limit is to serve only as a guideline and may be extended upward to an I.Q. of 75, especially in school settings, depending on clinical judgment. The Cattell scale and the Kuhlmann-Binet are commonly used tests for infants or severely retarded children. Since a diagnosis of mental retardation cannot be made on the basis of the I.Q. alone, adaptive behavior must also be significantly retarded as reflected in the degree of independence and social responsibility the child has achieved. Adaptive behavior derives from intellectual, affective, motivational, social, and motor abilities. All these factors contribute and are part of a child's total adaptation to his environment. Measured intelligence will generally correlate with the level of adaptive behavior; however, there will be frequent individual discrepancies in levels of performance on the two dimensions, especially in mild retardation. The ultimate determination of the presence or absence of mental retardation still rests to a great extent on clinical judgment.

Levels of mental retardation based on measured intelligence are defined as mild, moderate, severe, and profound (Table 80–1).

The term "mildly retarded" is often used interchangeably with "educable retarded" while "moderate" retardation is equated with "trainable." The term "dependent retarded" is sometimes used for the severely retarded and the "life support level" for the profoundly retarded. Table 80–2 summarizes some of the developmental characteristics, potential for training, and educational, social, and vocational adequacy.

About 25 per cent of children with mental retardation have a syndrome that is recognizable clinically at birth or early in infancy or childhood. Most instances of mental retardation, however, are not identified until school entrance. Developmental appraisal as a part of well baby assessment may permit early detection of developmental retardation. When the degree of retardation is great, such determinations have prognostic significance.

Table 80–1. LEVEL OF RETARDATION INDICATED BY IQ RANGE OBTAINED ON MEASURE OF GENERAL INTELLECTUAL FUNCTIONING

Term	IQ range for level
Mild mental retardation	50–55 to approx. 70
Moderate mental retardation	35–40 to 50–55
Severe mental retardation	20–25 to 35–40
Profound mental retardation	Below 20 or 25

Table 80–2. DEVELOPMENTAL CHARACTERISTICS, POTENTIAL FOR EDUCATION AND TRAINING, AND SOCIAL AND VOCATIONAL ADEQUACY ACCORDING TO THE FOUR LEVELS OF MENTAL RETARDATION*

Level	Preschool Age (0–5) Maturation and development	School Age (6–21) Training and education	Adult (21 and over) Social and vocational adequacy
Profound	Gross retardation; minimal capacity for functioning in sensorimotor areas; needs nursing care.	Obvious delays in all areas of development; shows basic emotional responses; may respond to skillful training in use of legs, hands and jaws; needs close supervision.	May walk, need nursing care, have primitive speech; usually benefits from regular physical activity; incapable of self-maintenance.
Severe	Marked delay in motor development; little or no communication skill; may respond to training in elementary self-help, e.g., self-feeding.	Usually walks barring specific disability; has some understanding of speech and some response; can profit from systematic habit training.	Can conform to daily routines and repetitive activities; needs continuing direction and supervision in protective environment.
Moderate	Noticeable delays in motor development, especially in speech; responds to training in various self-help activities.	Can learn simple communication, elementary health and safety habits and simple manual skills; does not progress in functional reading or arithmetic.	Can perform simple tasks under sheltered conditions; participates in simple recreation; travels alone in familiar places; usually incapable of self-maintenance.
Mild	Often not noticed as retarded by casual observer but is slower to walk, feed self and talk than most children.	Can acquire practical skills and useful reading and arithmetic to a 3rd to 6th grade level with special education; can be guided toward social conformity.	Can usually achieve social and vocational skills adequate to self-maintenance; may need occasional guidance and support when under unusual social or economic stress.

*From The President's Panel on Mental Retardation: Mental Retardation, A National Plan for a National Problem: Chart Book. Washington, D.C., U.S. Department of Health, Education, and Welfare, 1963, p. 15.

DIAGNOSIS

The etiology of mental retardation ranges from the biomedical, usually clinically evident or diagnosable by laboratory and other procedures, to the biopsychosocial. A comprehensive diagnostic examination for the mentally retarded person is an involved process. No one discipline can necessarily provide all the answers; rather, a comprehensive diagnostic evaluation by an interdisciplinary team is indicated, using a variety of skills and techniques.

A specific professional discipline may have a major role in the diagnosis and evaluation of a child's problems at one age and a minor role at another stage. For example, early in the life of a mentally retarded child the pediatrician may have a considerable role in assessing a given problem. Some time after, when the child is ready for a special program of education, the pediatrician assumes a less active role, and the educator has the major responsibility. There must be a constant reassessment of the problem. Sometimes the problems are primarily medical, sometimes they are primarily psychological, sometimes they are primarily educational, and sometimes they are primarily rehabilitative in terms of specific vocational training.

A careful history and physical examination, including a neurological appraisal, are important in assessing the mentally retarded individual. Laboratory studies in the evaluation of mental retardation can be of great value, but they must be used selectively; e.g., skull x-rays and CT scans may be indicated in some cases.

Chromosome studies are not indicated in most retarded children but are to be considered if a patient has multiple anomalies, especially affecting the face, ears, and distal extremities, or is born small for gestational age. Other indications may include a maternal history of repeated miscarriages, dermatoglyphic abnormalities, unusual facies, macro-orchidism, or a clinically recognizable genetic syndrome. Lysosomal storage diseases are suggested by regression or deterioration of motor and intellectual development, hepatosplenomegaly, skeletal dysostosis, cloudy cornea, cherry red macula, retinal degeneration, and similarly affected siblings. An inborn error in amino acid metabolism is suggested by positive screening tests, unusual odors, metabolic acidosis, failure to thrive, seizures, lethargy, vomiting, unusual hair, ataxia, and other neurological symptoms. Cultural-familial factors are a common cause for retardation and for a disparity between a child's actual performance and his innate abilities. Insufficient social and emotional stimulation from the mother or other caregiver may lead to retarded behavior in infants and young children.

MANAGEMENT

The first step in management is to interpret to the parents the results of the diagnostic studies and their meaning. Two basic goals here are the beginning of parent education and the development with the family of a plan of management based on the child's needs and the availability of services to meet those needs.

What the doctor tells the parents about their child and how he tells them and acts toward them and the child at this time may well determine his future role in the management of the child as well as influence the parents' attitudes toward the child. The importance of parent education (not parent counseling or therapy) at this time is paramount. The greatest source of emotional disturbance in parents is uncertainty—not knowing what has happened and wondering what can be done. The physician must attempt to answer their often unspoken questions: "What is mental retardation?" "What will it mean to my child?" "Can it be cured?" "What will he need?" "In what ways is he like other children (rather than unlike other children)?"

The way in which the physician conducts this initial step in management is critical. Parental dissatisfaction at this point often results in further "shopping around" for physicians.

The emotional reactions of the physician affect the manner and content of his advice to the family. Faced with the parents' need for immediate answers, often an insistence that something be done at once, or their seeming inability to understand or accept his findings, the physician, not unlike the parents, may find himself wishing to be rid of the entire problem. The anger or hostility of the parents, provoking a similar feeling in the physician, may cause him to act in a cold, blunt, or uninterested way. The need for objectivity and awareness of one's own emotional reactions is self-evident.

Particularly during the initial interpretation, it is important that both parents be present. This practice not only reduces the chances of misunderstanding but provides clues in the parental relationship that will be valuable in future management. Sometimes this approach also permits an early start toward uniting the parents to meet the continuing stress of having a retarded child.

Information should be presented factually, emphasizing the child's strengths and potentialities along with his handicaps and vulnerabilities. A focus on the child's deficiencies without attention to his assets and potential for development may cause the parents to interpret any sign of progress as evidence that the doctor's evaluation was wrong. To the best of his knowledge and in a gracious and sympathetic manner, the physician must endeavor to give honest, understandable information regarding the diagnosis and prognosis.

Parents should be given an approximate appraisal of the child's probable rate of development. This is necessary in order to adjust their conception of developmental milestones such as sitting, walking, and talking, and to allow them to begin teaching self-care skills such as feeding and toilet training at appropriate times. Advice from the occupational therapist and physical therapist may assist the parents in approaching these problems of daily care. Emphasis is placed on how to help the retarded child develop motor abilities, as well as teaching the child drinking and eating skills, the use of special equipment that may be helpful, and techniques for toilet training and self-dressing. Relatively simple suggestions about everyday care can make the difference between the mother's ability to manage her child and her complete frustration.

A child at any level of retardation can be helped to improve his personal, social, and intellectual behavior through proper instructional programming. Some skills, such as learning bowel and bladder control, are so complex that they must be subdivided into parts and the central skill taught first. Reinforcement by means of a reward, either food or praise, should be given immediately for any accomplishment. Parents must be warned that progress will be slow and not to become discouraged at the need for constant repetition. Mentally retarded persons are at high risk for psychiatric and behavioral disorders of all types. Although there are currently no psychoactive agents that are specific for mental retardation, there are many agents that may make some retarded individuals more amenable to other forms of treatment.

The development of physical activity and fitness in the retarded is beneficial to their general health and can add to their socialization through greater peer acceptance and improvement in their self-concept. This is particularly applicable in the child with associated physical handicaps.

Socialization should be encouraged at all times. The mentally retarded have difficulty in comprehending the demands of social interaction. Parents should be encouraged to explore all areas of social contact for their child. Some retarded children withdraw and spend hours in meaningless repetitive (stereotyped) behavior unless activities are devised that are particularly attractive to the child, e.g., a favorite game, a ride, or a walk in the park. Group play with peers, either spontaneously with neighbor children or within the more structured atmosphere of a nursery school or day care center, is important in teaching the child the social skills of sharing and cooperation. Social interaction can also be enhanced while encouraging and rewarding vocalization.

THE CHANGING ROLE OF SERVICES FOR MENTALLY RETARDED INDIVIDUALS

During the last decade, a vast increase in options for the care and management of mentally retarded individuals has occurred. Certainly a major factor has been mandatory public education for the handicapped under Public Law 94–142. In addition, even for those individuals more substantially impaired, there is an increase of placement options, including family care homes, nursing homes, and convalescent hospitals. The past 10 to 15 years have witnessed a major change in the social policy geared to broader opportunities and a commitment to have individuals live in their own homes or in communities in home-like settings to the fullest extent possible. There have been major efforts across the nation to depopulate state institutions providing care for the mentally retarded. The belief that smaller is better is common; however, within a given type of residential setting, size per se is not related to the quality of care. Sometimes very small family style homes are more restrictive than are larger boarding care settings in the same geographical region. There is no generally accepted array of definitions for community residential programs such as foster homes, group homes, and board and care homes. Staffing patterns vary greatly as well as the quality of care. The location of facilities and community support are also very crucial factors. Urban settings often provide a greater number of specialized services and opportunities for additional activities including recreation greater than those in rural areas. On the other hand, there is no evidence that rural environments are necessarily segregated or isolated or limit the involvement of mentally retarded persons in their local communities. More important is the need for an array of community support and training options.

RESIDENTIAL PLACEMENT

The most difficult decision is that of residential placement. It is a determination that only parents can and should make based on sound advice from competent authorities. The physician should not make the decision for the parents; neither should he remove his sympathetic support and guidance during this agonizing time.

Timing is critical. Premature introduction of the subject may cause either panic or open hostility on the part of the parents. Almost from the beginning of their awareness that their child is retarded, parents will question the possibility of placement in their own minds and raise it with the physician if given the opportunity. Because of the severe emotional stress that such thoughts arouse, and the need to resolve it, parents are apt to infer any mention of institutionalization by the physician as an out-and-out recommendation. On the other hand, after an adequate period in which they have had an opportunity to work through their real need to do everything possible for their child, they may be able to consider placement as one reasonable and practical alternative in their particular situation. Placement immediately following birth of even the most severely damaged child is rarely indicated.

The effects of placement on the parents and other siblings are often unpredictable. Considerable knowledge of the family and its dynamics is necessary for one to guide the parents properly in this decision. Removal of the child from the home may actually cause an exacerbation of the family troubles, while still resulting in benefit to the child. The effects on siblings are also quite varied. The direct relationships between the normal and retarded siblings are less critical than the nature of their relationships with the parents.

The presence of certain problems in the child may raise serious questions about the need for residential placement. In the adolescent or youth with mild retardation, serious problems in social adaptation may force consideration of residential care. The daily care needs of the severely or profoundly retarded, particularly those with major physical handicaps that limit mobility or require constant nursing care, may, with growth, become intolerable for even the ablest parent. Failure to provide for periodic, regular relief, especially for the mother, may result in a residential placement that would otherwise be unnecessary.

THE FAMILY

The ultimate success of management depends upon the physician's ability to coordinate the necessary health services with the child's eductional and social needs. Few communities have all necessary services and, for those families living in more rural areas, finding programs that meet their needs may be next to impossible. The ingenuity of all concerned will be taxed.

First the physician must understand himself, his emotional reactions to the problem, and their effect on the content and manner of his counseling of the family. He may identify too closely with the parents and feel that they have indeed an intolerable burden, thus failing to deal realistically with the problems of long-term management. Sensing the parents' denial and even open hostility, he may react with his own denial and hostility by using this as an excuse for dismissing the problem, either directly or through his manner. The physician must carefully examine his own feelings both toward the child and his family and toward the problems presented, recognizing that these reactions are common. His objectivity then does not permit these feelings to interfere with the management program.

Physicians are familiar with the reactions of most parents to the shock of the initial diagnosis and their disbelief of it, followed by anxiety and anger projected at physicians and other professionals who sometimes do not offer specific treatment. The parents feel guilt, shame, and chronic sorrow as they begin to question why they have produced a retarded child. "Shopping" for the answer may occur. Often the parent who "pesters" the physician most after the initial "novelty shock crisis" is the one who is most likely to make a satisfactory long-term adjustment. The parents' acceptance of their child's retardation is a slow and emotionally painful process. Counseling is best provided in an ongoing relationship focused on care and management. The physician may not always be the most qualified or the one with the best relationship to provide counseling to the parents; however, he is often the only person who is providing ongoing counseling.

The retarded child's development may suffer if the parents' emotional attitudes or family interactions are distorted. His needs for love and acceptance are the same as those of a normal child. Parents must be made aware of the differences in emotional and intellectual development. Overprotection can slow or impair the learning of self-help skills well within the child's potential. Siblings will resent the undue attention the retarded child receives and, as they grow older, may reflect parental feelings of shame or embarrassment. Parents must be encouraged to discuss the child's problem openly and correct any fears or wrong ideas that the other children may have.

GENERAL REFERENCES

American Academy of Pediatrics Policy Statement. The Doman-Delacato Treatment of Neurologically Handicapped Children. Pediatrics, *70*:810–812, 1982.

Beaudet, A. L.: Genetic diagnostic studies for mental retardation. Curr. Prob. Pediatr., *7*:3, 1978.

Gerald, P. S.: X-linked mental retardation and the fragile-X syndrome. Pediatrics, *68*:594, 1981.

Gottlieb, J.: Mainstreaming: Fulfilling the promise? Am. J. Ment. Def., *86*:115–126, 1981.

Grossman, H. J. (Ed.): Classification in Mental Retardation. Washington, D.C., American Association on Mental Deficiency. 1983.

Grossman, H. J., Simmons, J. E., Dyer A. R., and Work, H. H.: The Physician and the Mental Health of the Child. I. Assessing Development and Treating Disorders Within a Family Context. Chicago, American Medical Association, 1979.

Grossman, H. J., and Stubblefield, R. L.: The Physician and the Mental Health of the Child. II. The Psychological Concomitants of Illness. Chicago, American Medical Association, 1980.

Haywood, H. C., and Newbrough, J. R.: Living Environments for Developmentally Disabled Persons. Baltimore, Universtiy Park Press, 1981.

Hersh, S. P., and Simmons, J. E.: The Physician and the Mental Health of the Child. III. Issues and Skills in Relating Primary Medical Care to the Other Human Services. Chicago, American Medical Association, 1981.

Kolodny, E. H., and Cable W. J. L.: Inborn errors of metabolism. Ann. Neurol., *11*:221–232, 1981.

Landesman-Dwyer, S.: Living in the Community. Am. J. Ment. Def., *86*:223–234, 1981.

Macmillan, D. L.: Mental Retardation in School and Society, 2nd Ed. Boston, Little, Brown and Company, 1982.

Moeschier, J. B., Bennett, F. C., and Cromwell, L. D.: Use of the CT scan in the medical evaluation of the mentally retarded child. J. Pediatr., *98*:63–65, 1981.

Smith, D. W., and Simons, E. R.: Rational Diagnostic Evaluation of the Child with Mental Deficiency. Am. J. Disabled Child., *129*:1285–1290, 1975.

Szymanski, S. S., and Tanguay, P. E.: Emotional Disorders of Mentally Retarded Persons. Assessment, Treatment, Consultation. Baltimore, University Park Press. 1980.

REFERENCES OF PARTICULAR VALUE TO PARENTS

Brown, S. L., and Moersch, M. S.: Parents on the Team. Ann Arbor, University of Michigan Press, 1978.

Dickerson, M. U.: In *Our Four Boys: Foster Parenting Retarded Teenagers*. Syracuse, NY, Syracuse University Press, 1978.

Perlman, L., and Scott, K. A.,: Raising The Handicapped Child. Engelwood Cliffs, NJ, Prentice-Hall, 1981.

Perske, R., and Perske, M.: Hope for the Families: New Direction for Parents of Persons with Retardation or Other Developmental Disabilities. Nashville, TN, Abingdon Press, 1981.

Turnbull, A. P., and Turnbull, H. R., III: Parents Speak Out: Growing with a Handicapped Child. Columbus, OH, Charles E. Merrill, 1979.

81

LEARNING PROBLEMS

Peggy C. Ferry, M.D.

The field of learning disorders has expanded rapidly in the past decade. As more infants and children survive previously fatal disorders affecting brain development, the number of survivors with cognitive dysfunction has increased. Landmark federal legislation in 1975 mandated a wealth of special education programs to meet the needs of children with learning problems and other handicaps. Collaboration between the schools and physicians is occurring at a much greater frequency than in the past. Fellowship training programs have been developed for pediatricians wishing to specialize in learning disabilities, and many physicians now devote a substantial portion of their practice to children with these problems. Rather than being a subspecialized area of pediatrics in which only a very few physicians are skilled, evaluating the child with learning problems has become a standard part of pediatric primary care.

As the primary care physician assumes an increasingly broader role in developmental supervision, prevention, and child advocacy, he should identify children in his practice "at risk" for learning problems and be informed about the appropriate steps in evaluation and management.

PREVALENCE

In a survey by the United States Department of Education in 1980, more than 1.45 million children—or 3 per cent of the entire school age population—were identified as learning disabled. Prevalence figures for individual states vary from 0.39 per cent ot 4.9 per cent, illustrating differences in interpretation of the definition, case-finding, and provision of services. McCarthy (1982) has pointed out that the change in definition of mental retardation (IQ < 60) in the early 1970s led to the reclassification of large numbers of children with IQ's in the 70s and 80s as learning disabled, producing somewhat inflated prevalence figures in subsequent years.

DEFINITIONS

The term *learning disorder* implies school performance significantly below the expected academic level for the child's age. A learning disorder is not a single diagnostic entity, but rather comprises a variety of diagnostic categories that are not mutually exclusive. Learning *disabilities* are more precisely defined (see below). Unfortunately, the label *learning disabled* is often applied to any child who fails to learn, for whatever reason. Specific *learning disabilities* include disorders of listening, thinking, talking, reading, writing, spelling, or arithmetic. The definition should be reserved for use as follows:

> Children with learning disabilities mean those children who have a disorder in one or more of the basic psychological processes involved in understanding or in using language, spoken or written, which disorder may manifest itself in imperfect ability to listen, think, speak, read, write, spell, or do mathematic calculations. Such disorders include such conditions such as perceptual handicaps, brain injury, minimal brain dysfunction, dyslexia and developmental aphasia. Such terms do not include children who have learning problems which are primarily the result of visual, hearing, or motor handicaps, of mental retardation, of emotional disturbance, or of environmental, cultural or economic disadvantage. (Public Law 94-142, Education for All Handicapped Children Act of 1975, 94th Congress)

Another definition more recently proposed is:

> Learning disabilities is a generic term that refers to a heterogeneous group of disorders manifested by significant difficulties in the acquisition and use of listening, speaking, reading, writing, reasoning or mathematical abilities. These disorders are intrinsic to the individual and presumed to be due to central nervous system dysfunction. Even though a learning disability may occur concomitantly with other handicapping conditions (e.g., sensory impairment, mental retardation, social and emotional disturbance), or environmental influences (e.g., cultural differences, insufficient/inappropriate instruction, psychogenic factors), it is not the direct result of those conditions and influences (National Joint Committee for Learning Disabilities) (McCarthy, 1982).

NEUROLOGICAL SUBSTRATES

A great deal is still unknown about the ways in which normal children learn to think, understand and use language, read, and apply mathematical concepts. In early studies of learning disabled children, researchers were reluctant to ascribe a neurological basis for the child's difficulties, since there was not other evidence of "brain damage." Often the child was presumed to be "lazy," poorly motivated, or emotionally disturbed. Recently, however, pediatric neuropsychologists have analyzed cognitive and linguistic deficits in children with learning disorders and have shown specific patterns of cerebral dysfunction (Mattis et al., 1975). For example, dyslexic children show patterns that include language disorder, articulatory and graphomotor dyscoordination, and visual-spatial perceptual difficulties. Pediatric neuropsychologists can be expected to contribute much new knowledge to our understanding of learning disabled children in the future.

Heilman et al. (1976) have outlined a neuropsychological classification scheme for the basic components of communication and learning (Fig. 81–1). While not precisely circumscribed, these areas of cerebral localization provide a useful framework in which to consider childhood learning problems. Heilman's scheme can

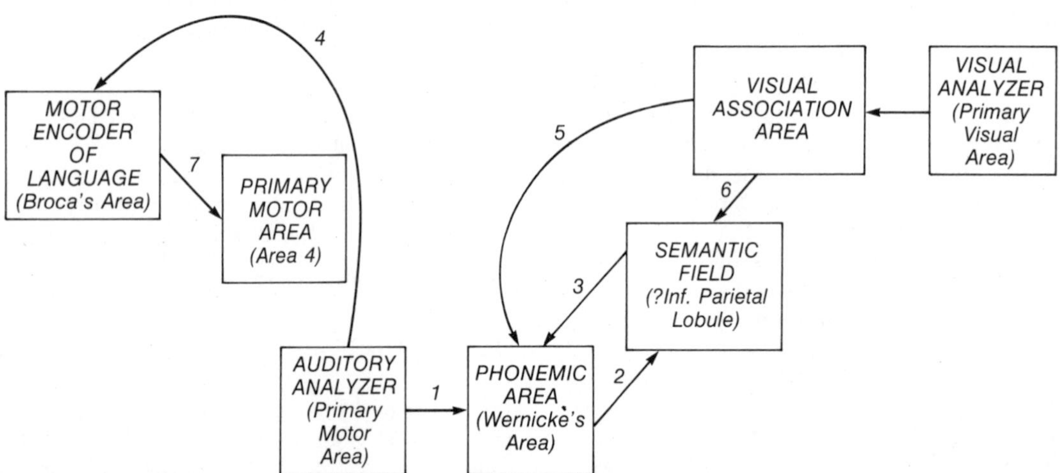

Figure 81–1. Neuropsychologic scheme of basic components of communication and learning in the left cerebral hemisphere. (From Heilman, K. M., Tucker, D. M., and Valenstein, E.: A case of mixed transcortical aphasia with intact naming. Brain, 99:415–426, 1976.)

be superimposed upon the concept of hemispheric specialization, with the left cerebral hemisphere subserving verbal activities and the right hemisphere primarily involved with visual-spatial skills. The seven pathways that process auditory and visual symbols are viewed as connecting neural systems. Lesions in specific areas or pathways produce identifiable clinical neuropsychological syndromes. For example, a child with injury to Pathway 1 would be unable to comprehend spoken language ("word deafness"), but if he had previously learned to read, this skill would remain intact. Similarly, a lesion in Pathway 7 would impair spontaneous speech, naming, and reading aloud, but auditory perception would be unimpaired. These areas of neuropsychological dysfunction correlate with neuropathological changes—for example, a young boy with dyslexia was found to have an area of polymicrogyria and associated cortical dysplasia in the speech region of the left temporal lobe (Galaburda et al., 1979).

Children with learning problems will not uncommonly display evidence of left or right cerebral dysfunction, either on clinical examination or neuropsychological testing. For reasons that are not well understood, but perhaps related to the functional, anatomical, and biochemical asymmetry of the brain, the left cerebral hemisphere, particularly in boys, appears to be especially vulnerable to injury or insult. This observation may account, in part, for the significantly greater percentage of boys than girls with learning problems.

It is not the physician's role to function as an educational diagnostician; however, he should be aware of the types of learning problems that may occur. Just as in a child with a hemiparesis, appropriate knowledge of the area of cerebral injury is useful in planning a therapy program, e.g., encouraging the child to use the hand served by the intact hemisphere. Similarly, the child with a severe expressive language disorder due to left cerebral dysfunction may best be taught by visual means, preferentially using his intact right hemisphere skills.

The pediatrician can also assist parents of learning disabled children with specific cerebral deficits in encouraging the children to use recreational and vocational skills that capitalize on their intact functions; for example, children with left hemisphere lesions and language disorders may be adept at visual-motor skills, artistic activities, drawing, and as later career choices, architecture and engineering.

Much has been written about the behavior problems that may precede, accompany, or follow specific learning disabilities. These problems may also be a reflection of organic brain dysfunction, with or without associated environmental influences. Hyperactivity, the inability or unwillingness to accept parental discipline, a short attention span, and low frustration tolerance may appear to mask an underlying learning disorder. These problems are not synonymous with learning disabilities and should not be equated with them.

Social learning disabilities may play an important role in the child's overall functioning in school and society—for example, the learning disabled child's inability to recognize appropriate facial expressions (from parietal lobe dysfunction) or to "get the point" of stories or jokes (from language disability) may lead to social isolation, poor self-image, and additional behavioral problems.

LEARNING DISORDERS AND DELINQUENCY

The relationship between delinquent behavior and learning disabilities has received increased attention in recent years, as the link between the two problems has become more impressive. A growing body of evidence has shown that youths with learning disabilities are more likely to be found delinquent than those without learning disabilities, although no study has shown that learning disabilities *cause* delinquency. Deficits in concept formation, verbal-symbolic functions, and perceptual organization have been reported in as many as 70 per cent of delinquent boys. Both biological and environmental factors may contribute to antisocial behavior.

A common sequential pattern among learning disabled children is placement in a highly structured program in the elementary school years, followed by very little assistance in secondary school. As the stresses of adolescence appear, the cognitive, social, and emotional difficulties the child had encountered may coalesce, leading to poor self-esteem, depression, and disruptive, aggressive behavior. These problems illustrate the dire need for continuing special education services into secondary and high school levels.

CLINICAL PRECURSORS OF LEARNING DISORDERS

In the past, the majority of children with learning problems had no specific, known med-

Table 81–1. POTENTIAL PRECURSORS OF LEARNING DISORDERS

1. Medical Conditions and Illnesses
   a. Prenatal infections ("TORCH" syndromes, especially CMV)
   b. Low birth weight, perinatal intraventricular hemorrhage
   c. Perinatal asphyxia
   d. Meningitis (especially herpes, bacterial forms)
   e. Cerebral trauma secondary to child abuse or accidental trauma
   f. Juvenile onset diabetes mellitus (especially before age 4 years)
   g. Leukemia (particularly after cranial irradiation and/or intrathecal methotrexate)
   h. Congenital heart disease with infectious or thrombotic complications
2. Surgical Conditions
   a. Open heart surgery (particularly after prolonged cardiopulmonary bypass)
   b. Hydrocephalus
   c. Congenital cerebral malformations (porencephaly, hemiatrophy, particularly if involving the left cerebral hemisphere)

ical illness or developmental brain abnormality that could be identified precisely as the cause for their learning difficulties. In recent years, however, neuropsychological studies of children who have survived a variety of pediatric illnesses or surgery have identified specific learning problems (Table 81–1). A frequent statement by parents of leukemia survivors, for example, is "we thought he was cured of the leukemia but then he started school and couldn't learn." The neurotoxicity of intrathecal methotrexate and CNS irradiation is thought to be responsible for the cognitive deficits in these children (Meadows et al., 1981). It should be stressed that the majority of youngsters recovering from these disorders do *not* have difficulty in school, but as many as one third of survivors of certain pediatric illnesses with CNS involvement may have learning problems. For this reason, it is incumbent upon the practicing pediatrician who is following these youngsters to be on the alert for learning or developmental problems. Office screening and preschool entry referral for psychological assessment may be considered if problems are suspected. In the author's experience, delayed language development in the preschool years is the most useful early predictor of subsequent learning disorders.

ASSESSMENT

The "No Frills," "Mini-Team" Approach

Until recent years, multidisciplinary team evaluation of learning disabled children was common, with a single child often being evaluated by professionals from five or more different professions. While useful in some complex cases, this approach is time consuming, elaborate, expensive, and probably unnecessary for educational planning in most instances. Additionally, constraints of federal funding make such evaluations an unavailable luxury for most school districts in the 1980s. A recent Supreme Court decision that a school district need not supply a sign-language interpreter for a deaf fourth-grader may lead some schools to further reduce services for handicapped children. The decision highlights the financial impossibility of requiring "optimal" education for all youngsters, normal or handicapped.

Experience has shown that a "mini-team" approach, using a physician and psychologist or educational consultant, can provide appropriate planning for most learning disabled children (Tables 81–2 and 81–3). In less than an hour's office time, the pediatrician can obtain pertinent facts about the child's development and school history (the latter to include specific academic information as well as a behavioral history), perform a physical examination, and arrange for vision and auditory screening. Telephone inquiry to schools, either by the physician or by someone trained in his office, can elicit additional information about the child's classroom performance and behavior. Evaluation by appropriate consultants can determine the child's cognitive ability, perceptual strengths and weaknesses, communication ability, academic strengths and weaknesses, and social/emotional adaptation (Culbertson and Ferry, 1982). The physician himself should not administer or interpret psychoeducational tests; rather, he should be aware of the general strengths and limitations of currently available tests and should work collaboratively with his psychological and educational consultants. Appropriate recommendations can then be made for classroom placement. As more and more children with chronic medical conditions and handicaps are being served in the public schools, the physician may contribute to the school's understanding of the child's medical illness, medications, urological and orthopedic devices, and the general contribution of the

Table 81–2. DIAGNOSTIC EVALUATION OF THE CHILD WITH LEARNING PROBLEMS

Step 1	Step 2	Step 3
Initial interview School history Physical examination Vision, hearing screening	School phone call and/or visit Psychological/educational assessment Additional consultation as needed	Meeting with parents, school officials Preparation of I.E.P.

Table 81–3. TAKING A SCHOOL HISTORY

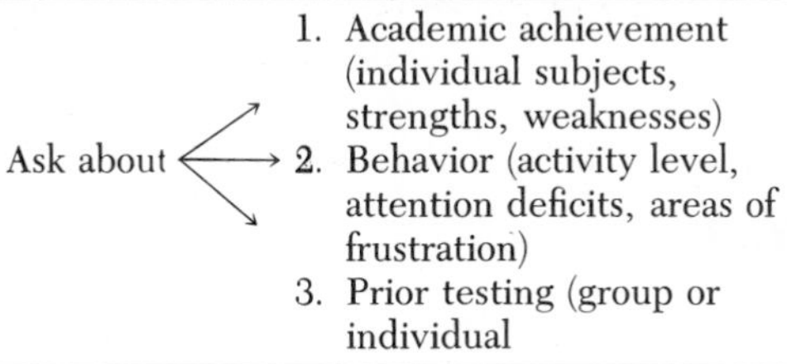

Ask about
1. Academic achievement (individual subjects, strengths, weaknesses)
2. Behavior (activity level, attention deficits, areas of frustration)
3. Prior testing (group or individual

child's underlying medical condition to his well-being in school. School personnel welcome such collaboration.

MANAGEMENT

Passage of Public Law 94-142 (Education for All Handicapped Children Act, 1975), which mandated free appropriate education for children with all types of handicaps (including learning disabilities), was a landmark event for handicapped children. The act was intended primarily as an *educational* one, without full recognition of the inordinate costs involved. However, recent cutbacks in federal spending have curtailed the availability of special programs in the public schools and have limited the scope of this well-intentioned legislation. Problems in the implementation of PL 94-142 have included (1) failure to serve large numbers of children, particularly in the 0 to 3 and 18 to 21 year age group, (2) use of variable placement patterns and an uneven quality of special programs, (3) failure to provide adequate definition of "related services" (physical, occupational, and speech therapy, medical services), (4) creation of a massive new bureaucracy, (5) failure to provide adequate numbers of appropriately trained special education personnel, and (6) failure to appropriate sufficient funds.

Recent recommendations for changes in implementation of PL 94-142 include (1) reducing the federally appropriated dollars for subsequent years, (2) deregulation of the existing statute and removal of the federal monitoring process, and (3) "devolvement" (return to state control) of the responsibility for the educational services to handicapped via (a) changing the statutory language or (b) placing the bill in a separate or combined block grant. "Related services" may be modified so that the schools will no longer be required to pay for medical consultation services. Since new regulations will vary from state to state, physicians need to be cognizant of local guidelines.

Classroom Management

The wide range of special education services for learning disabled children, including full-time special education programs, self-contained classrooms, learning disability classrooms within a regular school, and "resource" (remedial or special class) placement, may no longer be as readily available in the years ahead. Despite their widespread use in recent years, there exists little documented evidence of their proven value. As McCarthy (1982) has emphasized, "research on the efficacy of remedial procedures is either conflicting, confusing, or absent. Good special education teachers will determine what works best for each individual child." It seems likely that in the near future, only more severely involved children will be able to receive special services in full-time or self-contained classes and that mainstreaming or resource room help will be the major programs in force. The pediatrician can assist in finding additional sources of special help for learning disabled students by arranging for tutoring after school, using "people resources" (such as a retired teacher, a teen-ager with interest in helping young people, or a parent of a handicapped child). Learning disabled children can improve in a variety of settings, if they are given the opportunity to achieve, receive praise, and avoid repeated failure.

Behavior Management

Medications such as methylphenidate, amphetamines, and pemoline may be useful adjuncts in the management of children with attention deficit disorders, but they should not be a primary therapy for children with specific learning disabilities. Behavior modification with small, structured, well-organized programs (particularly if carried over at home) may be extremely useful.

Controversial Therapies

Unproven means of therapy for learning disorders include optometric exercises, perceptual motor training, sensory integration therapy, various vitamin regimens, and special diets. There are no well-controlled scientific studies that have unequivocally shown the merit of any of these programs, and their use may mask the specific educational needs of the child. The pediatrician can assist families in his practice by becoming aware of the advantages and disadvantages of various forms of therapy and pointing out the available options.

CONCLUSION

The natural history of learning problems is variable. Most children improve, in spite of or because of special education programs. However, learning problems may well persist into adult life (Kahn, 1980). For example, dyslexic adults may have life-long difficulty reading driver's tests, telephone books, menus, dictionaries, instruction manuals, and street signs. Such individuals appropriately select vocational opportunities that require little in the way of reading skills. Only a few colleges have developed programs, which use a highly structured approach, to teach learning disabled students.

Pediatricians can assist their learning disabled patients and families at various stages throughout life, from early identification, careful diagnosis, long-term management, vocational guidance, and general moral support. A skilled teacher and a concerned, helpful pediatrician are two of the learning disabled child's best allies.

REFERENCES

Culbertson, J. L., and Ferry, P. C.: Learning disabilities. Pediatr. Clin. North Am., *29*:121–136, 1982.

Galaburda, A. M., and Kemper, T. L.: Cytoarchitectonic abnormalities in developmental dyslexia: A case study. Ann. Neurol., *6*:94–100, 1979.

Heilman, K. M., Tucker, D. M., and Valenstein, E.: A case of mixed transcortical aphasia with intact naming. Brain, *99*:415–426, 1976.

Kahn, M. S.: Learning problems of the secondary and junior college learning disabled student. J. Learn. Disabil., *13*:40–44, 1980.

Mattis, S., French, J. H., and Rapin, I.: Dyslexia in children and young adults: Three independent neuropsychological syndromes. Dev. Med. Child. Neurol., *17*:150–163, 1975.

Meadows, A. T., et al.: Decline in IQ scores and cognitive dysfunctions in children with acute lymphocytic leukemia with cranial irradiation. Lancet, *2*:1015, 1981.

McCarthy, J.: Cross currents and prevailing winds. Learning Disabil., *1*:3–10, 1982.

Scholom, A., and Schiff, G.: Relating infant temperament to learning disabilities. J. Abnorm. Child Psychol., *8*:127–132, 1980.

Appendix A

Developmental Assessment: Office Developmental Screening

Ernest E. Smith, M.D.

Developmental assessment is a major component of child health care. Cumulative information regarding the developmental, psychological, cognitive, and interactive areas of child and family life is acquired through the many health promotion and acute care visits of early childhood. By providing frequent contacts and continuity of care for children and their families, the pediatrician is in a strategic position for early identification and initial evaluation of developmental difficulties.

While pediatricians acknowledge the importance of developmental assessment, they seldom use standardized methods of evaluation and then only after evidence of developmental difficulty has been established by other criteria (Smith, 1978). Frequently, pediatricians evaluate children's development only by informal clinical assessment and parental recall of milestones, even though both methods have proven inadequate (Bierman et al., 1964; Korsch et al., 1961). Some pediatricians do not routinely perform developmental assessment because of the belief that early identification and evaluation are useless because intervention techniques are futile. However, many studies have suggested that intervention techniques at an early age can have short- and long-term benefits for the child and family (Frankenburg et al., 1981).

In a busy primary care office or clinic setting, formal and extensive developmental appraisal of all children is unrealistic; however, reliable and efficient office/clinic screening procedures can be established. Such a screening program should be effective in identifying developmental problems or alerting the physician to potential problems during the health promotion visit and useful in the initial evaluation of concerns raised by parents, preschool teachers, physicians, and other referral sources regarding a particular child's developmental status.

Developmental screening should cover the full spectum of developmental problems encountered in young children. Quantification of abilities in the motor, problem-solving, communication, and self-help areas is readily accomplished by standard screening instruments. Of equal importance but frequently overlooked are the qualitative aspects of the child's performance, including temperament, activity level and attention span, self-awareness and self-regulation, ability to play, response to success and frustration, and compliance with appropriate parental expectations. Success or failure on individual test items must be supplemented with observation and information regarding how the child uses his skills to learn, interact with others, satisfy needs, and develop independence.

Office developmental screening involves more than the administration of a screening instrument. Developmental assessment, whether it be a screening procedure or comprehensive evaluation, should be based on data gathered through interviewing, observation of the child, and appraisal of parent-child interaction. Information obtained from standardized instruments such as screening questionnaires and tests is imperative; however, it is crucial that such data are coordinated with other available knowledge about the child and family. Office personnel such as secretaries, nurses, and pediatric nurse practitioners can be trained to administer developmental screening questionnaires and tests. However, the pediatrician should be the individual who synthesizes information from all sources so that the child and family are understood as unique, and recommendations can be discussed in a clear manner with the parents.

The interview is a productive method of identifying problem areas, gathering developmental data, and gaining impressions of family-child interaction. During each health promotion visit, parents should be asked if they have any questions or worries about their child's development or behavior and if their child's abilities are comparable to those of other children his age. A helpful technique to elicit developmental information is to have the parent describe a typical day for the child. The parent is asked "How does Susie spend her day?" and encouraged to describe as precisely as possible the child's activities, mood, interaction with family members and peers, and responses to discipline. A description of the child's motor abilities, play, language, self-help skills, and home environment is effectively obtained in this manner. Table 1 includes several screening questionnaires that are available to assist in gather-

Table 1. SCREENING INSTRUMENTS

Title, Author, and Publisher	Age Range	Comments
	General—Interview	
Denver Prescreening Developmental Questionnaire (PDQ) (Frankenburg, Doorninck, Liddell, and Dick, 1977) Ladoca Project and Publishing Foundation	3 months to 6 years	Provides information about personal/social, fine motor-adaptive, language, and gross motor skills. Useful as first stage screening to identify children who should be more thoroughly screened by the Denver Developmental Screening Test. Should be used only with parents who have at least completed high school. Approximately 30% of children screened will need to take the Denver Developmental Screening Test. Takes parents 5–15 minutes to complete.
Developmental Profile II (Alpern and Boll, 1980) Psychological Development Publications	Birth to 9 years	Parental interview inventory which depicts child's functional developmental age level in five areas: physical scale, self-help age, social age, academic age, and communication age. Takes 20–40 minutes to administer.
Preschool Attainment Record (Doll, 1976) American Guidance Service	Birth to 7½ years	Behavior rating scale that measures physical, social, and intellectual competencies. Takes 10–20 minutes to administer.
Revised Developmental Screening Interview (Knobloch, Stevens and Malone, 1980) Department of Pediatrics, Albany Medical College	1 to 26 months	Items are based on the Revised Gesell and Amatruda Developmental Scales with assessment in areas of gross motor, fine motor, adaptive, language, and personal/social skills. Takes 15–30 minutes to administer.
Vineland Social Maturity Scale (Doll, 1982) American Guidance Service	Birth to 30 years	By parental interview, areas of assessment include self-help, self-direction, occupation, communication, locomotion, and socialization. Takes 20–30 minutes to administer.
	General—Test	
Denver Developmental Screening Test (DDST) (Frankenburg, Dodds, Fradal, Kazuk, and Cohrs, 1975) Ladoca Project and Publishing Foundation	Birth to 6 years	Provides information in the personal/social, fine motor-adaptive, language, and gross motor areas. Information obtained by performance of tasks and by parental report. Takes approximately 20–30 minutes to administer.
Denver Developmental Screening Test—Short Form (Frankenburg and Dodds, 1978) Ladoca Project and Publishing Foundation	6 months to 6 years	Consists of the same developmental items as the Denver Developmental Screening Test with only selective items being administered. Serves as a first stage screening process to identify children who will need to be screened more thoroughly by the Denver Developmental Screening Test. Takes 5–7 minutes to administer.
Goodenough-Harris Drawing Test (Draw-A-Man) (Harris, 1963) Psychological Corporation	3 to 16 years	Figure drawings are an important part of any screening battery. They are usually non threatening to the child and help establish rapport. Drawings can lead to verbal expressions of feelings and also can reveal a great deal regarding self image, level of cognitive and emotional development, adjustment to family and environment. Takes 5–10 minutes to administer.
Slosson Intelligence Test (Slosson, 1963) Slosson Educational Publications	2 weeks to adult	Test is poorly standardized and does not use a satisfactory method of computing IQ's; however, it serves as an adequate screening device. Has age scale format for assessment of language, fine motor, gross motor, and reasoning skills. Takes 10–20 minutes to administer.

Table 1. SCREENING INSTRUMENTS *(Continued)*

Title, Author, and Publisher	Age Range	Comments
	Behavior	
Kohn Problem Checklist (Kohn, Parnes, and Rosman, 1976) The William Alanson White Institute, New York, New York	3 to 6 years	Screening scale for evaluating behavior problems of preschool children. Behavior checklist with 49 items and 2 dimensions: Apathy-Withdrawal and Anger-Defiance. Takes 10–15 minutes to administer.
Kohn Social Competence Scale (Kohn, Parnes, and Rosman, 1976) The William Alanson White Institute, New York, New York	3 to 6 years	Screening scale for evaluating the social competence of preschool children. Behavior checklist with 64 or 73 items and 2 dimensions: Interest-Participation versus Apathy-Withdrawal and Cooperation-Compliance versus Anger-Defiance. Takes 10–15 minutes to administer.
Preschool Behavior Questionnaire (Behar and Stringfield, 1974) The Learning Institute of North Carolina, Durham, North Carolina	3 to 6 years	Useful screening device for evaluating behavior problems of preschool children. Behavior checklist involves 30 items and 3 scales: Hostile-Aggressive, Anxious-Fearful and Hyperactive-Distractible. Takes 5–10 minutes to administer.
	Temperament	
Behavioral Style Questionnaire (McDevitt and Carey, 1975) Psychology Department, Terry Children's Psychiatric Center, New Castle, Delaware	3 to 7 years	Dimensions and characteristics similar to Infant Temperament Questionnaire.
Infant Temperament Questionnaire (Carey and McDevitt, 1977) Dr. Carey, Media, Pennsylvania	4 to 8 months	Parents rate infant's behavior on checklist of statements. Dimensions include activity, rhythmicity, approach, adaptability, intensity, mood, persistence, distractibility, and threshold. Results used to identify clinically relevant traits of difficult, easy, slow-to-warm-up, and intermediate child. Takes approximately 30 minutes to administer.
Perception of Baby Temperament (Pedersen et al., 1979) Child and Family Research Branch, National Institutes of Health, Bethesda, Maryland	2 to 12 months	Card sort procedure which assesses how parents perceive infant on five temperament scales: positive mood, rhythmicity, activity, approach, and adaptability. Takes approximately 15 minutes to administer.
Toddler Temperament Scale (Fullard, McDevitt and Carey, 1978) Department of Educational Psychology, Temple University, Philadelphia, Pennsylvania	1 to 3 years	Dimensions and characteristics similar to Infant Temperament Questionnaire.
	Home Environment	
Nursing Child Assessment Training Questionnaire, University of Washington, School of Nursing	Infant to 9 years	Parental checklist covering child's experiences in the home, i.e., use of toys, interactions with parents, discipline. Takes 10–15 minutes to administer.
	Perceptual Motor/Drawing	
Bender Visual Motor Gestalt Test (Bender, 1938) American Orthopsychiatric Association, Inc.	5 to 12 years	Useful in evaluating visual motor abilities. Consists of 9 cards with geometric designs that child copies. Takes approximately 5 minutes to administer.
Developmental Test of Visual Motor Integration (VMI) (Beery, 1967) Follett Publishing Company	2 to 15 years	Useful for evaluating children's visual-motor abilities. Consists of 24 geometric designs that child copies. Takes approximately 10 minutes to administer.

Table 1. SCREENING INSTRUMENTS *(Continued)*

Title, Author, and Publisher	Age Range	Comments
	Parent-Child Interaction	
The Massie-Campbell Scale of Mother-Infant Attachment Indicators During Stress (AIDS) (Massie and Campbell, 1977) Children's Hospital and Medical Center of San Francisco	Birth to 18 months	Designed for use during infant's pediatric examination. Scale includes six basic attachment modalities: gazing, vocalization, touching, holding, affect, and proximity.
	School Readiness	
ABC Inventory to Determine Kindergarten and School Readiness (Adair and Blesch, 1965) Research Concepts, Muskegon, Michigan	4 to 6 years	Test items include language, reasoning, and motor abilities. Tasks involve drawing, copying, folding, counting, recalling of general information, recognizing colors, discriminating sizes, and understanding time concepts. Takes approximately 8–9 minutes to complete.
Boehm Test of Basic Concepts (Boehm, 1971) Psychological Corporation	5 to 7 years	A pictorial multiple choice test that measures various concepts (direction, amount, and time) considered to be necessary for school achievement. Useful in suggesting indicators of possible learning dysfunction. Takes approximately 30 minutes to administer.
Developmental Key for Assessing Children's Growth, Frank Porter Graham Child Developmental Center, University of North Carolina, 1974	Preschool to 1st grade	Information gained from long-term observation and performance of specific tasks. Areas assessed include social skills, attending skills, language development, emotional development, physical skills, and conceptual skills. Takes 10–15 minutes to administer.
McCarthy Screening Test (McCarthy) The Psychological Corporation	4 to 6½ years	Helpful in identifying children who are likely to encounter difficulties in school. Assesses language, concepts, visual perception, auditory memory, fine and gross motor coordination, and orientation in space. Takes approximately 20 minutes to administer.
Peabody Picture Vocabulary Test—Revised (PPVT-R) (Dunn and Dunn, 1981) American Guidance Service	2½ years to adult	A nonverbal receptive vocabulary test. Useful as a screening device for measuring extensiveness of vocabulary, particularly for children with speech and motor impairment. Takes 5–10 minutes to administer.
Preschool Screening System (Hainsworth and Hainsworth, 1974) Pawtucket, Rhode Island	3 to 6 years	Questionnaire which surveys learning skills involving physical, motor, perceptual, cognitive, speech, and language abilities. Takes 15–20 minutes to administer.
San Diego Quick Assessment (LaPray and Ross, 1969) Reproduced in Journal of Reading, *12*:305, 1969	Preprimer to 11th grade	Consists of graded word lists. Takes approximately 5 minutes to administer. A screening measurement of reading skill.
Wide Range Achievement Test (WRAT) (Jastak and Jastak, 1978) Guidance Associates of Delaware, Inc.	5 years to adult	A brief, limited screening instrument of academic skills. Contains reading, spelling, and arithmetic subtests. Takes approximately 20–30 minutes to administer.

ing information about parental concerns, the child's skills and behavior, parent-child interaction, and the home environment.

A number of developmental screening tests can be utilized to facilitate the pediatrician's observation of the child. Table 1 reviews some of these. It matters little which test is used as long as the examiner is trained to administer and score the items reliably. The pediatrician who interprets the results must be aware of the scope and limitations of the screening instrument.

Parent-child interactions can be systematically observed in the office or clinic. Rating scales of parent-child interaction are available (see Table 1); however, the examination room encounter also provides an excellent opportunity to evaluate the quality of these interactions. For example, the pediatrician can note whether the parent talked to the child during the examination, responded to the child's vocalizations, comforted the child, smiled at or praised the child, hugged or kissed the child, expressed anger or hit the child.

While developmental assessment is an integral part of all health promotion visits, screening questionnaires and tests need not be administered at each visit. The scheduling of such tests will depend on individual practice factors such as available testing personnel and the risk of developmental problems in the patient population. However, it is suggested that all children receive a standardized screening test during the following age periods: 1-3 months, 3-6 months, 9-12 months, 18-24 months, and during the third, fourth, and fifth years.

Screening methods should not be used to diagnose, label, or establish developmental levels. They alert one to potential problems that need more extensive evaluation of the child's development and life situation. When a screening method indicates possible developmental difficulties, the pediatrician must decide what to do next. The options include rescreening at

Table 2. PEDIATRIC OFFICE DEVELOPMENTAL SCREENING

I. Purpose and Scope
    A. Early identification and intervention
    B. Evaluation of specific concerns
    C. Assessment of developmental skills (quantity and quality) including behavior, temperament, and social interactions
II. Means of Obtaining Data
    A. Interview
        1. Inquire routinely about developmental concerns
        2. Interview for a day
        3. Parental questionnaires and checklists
    B. Observation of child
        1. Clinical
        2. Questionnaires and checklists
        3. Developmental screening tests
    C. Observation of parent-child interaction
        1. Clinical
        2. Checklists
III. Schedule
    A. Cumulative data obtained through health promotion and acute care visits
    B. Administer screening questionnaire or test at least once during following age periods: 1–3 months, 3–6 months, 9–12 months, 18–24 months, 2–3 years, 3–4 years, and 4–5 years
IV. Synthesis of Data
    A. Past history
    B. Physical and neurological exam including assessment of hearing and vision
    C. Developmental information from IIA, B, and C
    D. Individuality of child and family
    E. Do not label or diagnose from screening data
IV. Management
    A. Inform parents of results and use data for anticipatory guidance
    B. Rescreen in 1–2 months if difficulties are mild and involve single area of concern
    C. Refer to developmental specialist if mild difficulties persist on rescreen or if initial screen demonstrates moderate-severe and/or multiple problems

a later date to see if difficulties persist, performing a more in-depth developmental evaluation, or referring the child to a developmental specialist for further evaluation. The decision will depend on the following factors: the seriousness of the difficulty; historical predisposing factors that place the child and family at risk such as difficult neonatal course, poor home environment, and excessive parental concern; results of other observations regarding physical and neurological status; vision acuity and hearing ability; and the expertise and interest of the pediatrician. If a child is demonstrating questionable or borderline delays and the history and physical exam reveal no other concerns, a rescreen might be scheduled in one to two months. If a child is demonstrating significant difficulties or questionable delays with a poor quality environment or if parental concern is excessive, referral is probably indicated. Table 2 reviews the important aspects of a pediatric developmental screening progam.

The direct effect of routine developmental screening is early identification of and intervention in developmental difficulties so that the child's abilities are enhanced and the family is supported in developing an understanding of the child's skills and limitations. In addition, parents are interested in their children's abilities and enjoy the opportunity to see if they are progressing normally. Screening provides parents anticipatory guidance regarding developmental steps and skills they can encourage and indicates to parents that the pediatrician is interested and knowledgeable regarding the developmental and behavioral aspects of child health care.

REFERENCES

Bierman, J. M., Connor, A., Vaage, M., and Honzik, M. P.: Pediatricians' assessments of the intelligence of two-year olds and their mental test scores. Pediatrics, *34*:680, 1964.

Frankenburg, W. K., Thornton, S. M., and Cohrs, M. E. (Eds.): Pediatric Developmental Diagnosis. New York, Thieme-Stratton, Inc., 1981.

Identification and Referral of Young Handicapped Children: The Physician's Role. The University of the State of New York, The State Education Department, Albany, New York, 1982.

Korsch, B., Cobb, K., and Ashe, B.: Pediatricians' appraisals of patients' intelligence. Pediatrics, *27*:990, 1961.

Provence, S.: Developmental Assessment. *In* Green, M., and Haggerty, R. J. (Eds.): Ambulatory Pediatrics II. Philadelphia, W. B. Saunders Co., 1977.

Sattler, J. M.: Assessment of Children's Intelligence and Special Abilities. Boston, Allyn and Bacon, Inc., 1982.

Smith, R. D.: The use of developmental screening tests by primary-care pediatricians. J. Pediatr., *93*:524, 1978.

Appendix B

The Well-Equipped Office

Lawrence F. Nazarian, M.D.

A pediatrician starting a practice is confronted with an overwhelming list of practical decisions to be made, many of which are not discussed during training. Equipping an office can be one major area of challenge.

Visiting well-established offices should be an initial step in planning one's own equipment list. Pick places with practice styles similar to the format which will be followed in the new office. Survey several practices, since different people may solve the same problems in varied ways, and one solution may appear more comfortable than another. This advice also applies to the established practitioner, who might profit from fresh ideas.

Another good source of information is the physician's supply house. Finding a reliable dealer who is interested in providing personal service for many years as well as making sales should be done early in practice. This consultant can keep the physician abreast of new products while tailoring purchases to specific requirements.

As far as possible, names of specific brands or manufacturers have been omitted from this chapter to avoid making endorsements or recommending outdated products. In a few instances, names are given to allow the reader to find unusual products.

THE OFFICE LABORATORY

A large percentage of the testing needed in daily practice can be done well in a modestly equipped office laboratory. For those tests that cannot be done on site, a procedure for getting work done elsewhere must be worked out. In some cases, the patient can be sent directly to a hospital or private facility. Specimens can also be obtained in the office and taken by the physician to the hospital when he makes rounds. Some laboratories will make a pick-up at the end of the day. Be aware of which specimens can be tested a day or two later and which need processing within hours.

Testing can be done by the physician, a laboratory technician, a medical assistant, or a nurse. Office personnel are often eager to learn new procedures that will make their jobs more interesting. Sometimes an assistant can do most of a test, with the physician finishing up. For example, the doctor can quickly add his experience to a urinalysis by reviewing the microscope slide and combining his observations with those of the assistant.

Whatever other equipment is added, the office laboratory must have a suitable workbench, adequate shelves and cabinets, proper plumbing, and a refrigerator. A Bunsen burner will receive constant use, especially for flaming platinum loops. If it is impractical to install a gas line, one may substitute an alcohol lamp. There is an electrical device which is handy for sterilizing loops (Bacti-Cinerator, Sherwood Medical Industries, St. Louis). The loop is placed into a heated cavity within an insulated cylinder. At the heart of the laboratory is a good binocular microscope. Proper investment in and care of this instrument will pay dividends in ease of operation and accuracy of observation for years to come.

Urinalysis

Dipsticks for chemical testing have made urinalysis quick and efficient. For everyday use, the most practical stick is one that tests for protein, sugar, ketones, blood, and pH. Strips for occasional need, such as bilirubin testing, can be bought separately.

The protein portion of the sticks is very sensitive and can give false positive readings. Confirmation with 20 per cent sulfosalicylic acid is helpful. A small amount of urine is put into a test tube and several drops of the acid are added. The amount of turbidity resulting correlates with the concentration of protein in the urine, with a negative specimen remaining clear. If urine sugars other than glucose are suspected, a tablet giving a Benedict reaction should be used.

A glass hygrometer is inexpensive and accurate in determining specific gravity and can add valuable information to the work-up of a child who may be dehydrated or have diabetes insipidus or renal disease.

Centrifugation of urinary sediment adds enough to the urinalysis for selected patients to

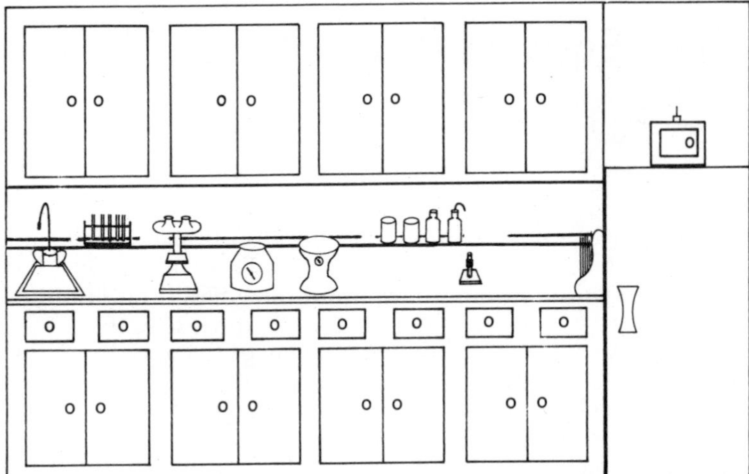

Figure 1. This office laboratory is 13 feet long by 6 feet wide. Cabinets and drawers allow for ample storage and a long shelf keeps reagents and smaller pieces of apparatus handy. The counter is 3 feet high and provides working space while accommodating a sink, microscope, urine centrifuge, hematocrit centrifuge, Bunsen burner and rack for papers. A small incubator fits on top of the refrigerator.

make the purchase of a urine centrifuge worthwhile. Some models can be adapted to spin both urine and blood for hematocrits, although a physician with a busy office may prefer separate units. Careful use of a balancing tube will prolong the life of the centrifuge, and a drop of bright dye in the water of the "dummy" will avoid confusion.

A common problem with refrigerated urine is cloudiness caused by the precipitation of crystals, usually urates. These crystals will interfere with a proper microscopic examination but can be eliminated by holding the centrifuge tube under a stream of hot water until the turbidity clears. This procedure should be done before spinning.

Stool Analysis

The most frequent stool test, other than culture, is the examination for blood. Many substances in a child's stool can look like fresh or degraded blood, and stools with occult blood can look normal. Tablets, slides, and solutions that employ the guaiac reaction are readily available and easy to use. Special care should be used in the interpretation of these tests, as timing and spread of color are important. Freshness of reagents is particularly relevant to these tests. If there is doubt about the sensitivity of the reagents, a small amount of blood from a discarded hematocrit tube can be mixed with some stool to create a positive control.

Fat stains can be used in the office to look for excessive globules of fat. Microscopic examination for parasites can also be done. Pinworm preps are easily made using special plastic strips or ordinary cellophane tape. A drop of immersion oil on the slide and another rubbed into the nonsticky side of the tape will enhance the clarity of the preparation.

In most cases of disaccharide malabsorption, intestinal bacteria break the double sugars down to create acid stools with a higher concentration of glucose. The pH can be tested by touching the watery periphery of a stool on a diaper with pH testing paper. The appropriate pad on a urinary dipstick can also be used. A pH below 5.0 is excessively acidic. Glucose testing paper or the glucose testing pad on the urine stick can be used in a similar manner. Anything more than a trace of glucose suggests malabsorption.

Hematology

Many hematological values can be obtained by the practitioner in the office laboratory.

A centrifuge for doing hematocrits will be used often. Duplicate tubes of blood should be collected and careful attention paid to sealing the ends. A chart for reading the hematocrit can be taped to the wall or cabinet directly above the machine. Sometimes other tests, such as the mononucleosis spot test, require plasma as provided by this centrifuge. There are instruments that will measure hemoglobin also, although the hematocrit is usually adequate for daily practice.

Free erythrocyte porphyrin is assuming greater importance in the diagnosis of iron deficiency and lead poisoning and a new machine, called the hematofluorometer, is available to measure this substance. The cost is high, but this tool may be appropriate for some practices.

Medical students of recent years are sometimes surprised to find that a white blood cell count can be done by hand. Quick and accurate counts are easily done with white cell pipettes, diluting fluid, a hemocytometer, and a hand counter. A rough assessment of the ratio of mononuclear to segmented cells can be made with high-dry search of the specimen in the counting chamber.

An accurate differential count and evaluation of cell morphology, including erythrocytes and platelets, require a Wright-stained slide. Regular stain can be used, but some newer rapid stains for blood smears are available (Hemal Stain, Hemal Stain Company, 397 Main St., Danbury, CT 06810; La Mar Dip Stain, La Mar Laboratories, Inc., 3240 Lawson Blvd., Oceanside, NY 11572).

Sickle cell preps can also be done in the office. One method involves a solubility technique in which blood is mixed with a reducing substance such as sodium hydrosulfite. If a turbidity results which makes it impossible to see newsprint clearly through the solution, sickle hemoglobin is present. A variation of the same technique uses reducing agents and dye to produce different colors, depending on the patient's hemoglobin complement.

Many practitioners do erythrocyte sedimentation rates in the office. Standard tubes, a rack for holding the tubes vertically, and a timer to signal the end of an hour will enable one to do the test using an aliquot of blood drawn by venipuncture. There is a micro sedimentation technique that requires only a finger prick. Special equipment is needed, but the technique is not complicated (available through the Clay-Adams Division of the Becton-Dickinson Company, Parsippany, NJ). The values obtained through this technique are not exactly the same as with conventional methods, but a meaningful correlation can be made with a little experience.

Nasal smears for eosinophils can be useful in the diagnosis of allergy and are done with either the Hansel stain or the Gugol blue stain.

Blood Chemistry

There are limits to how much blood chemistry can be done in the average office, and the practitioner should make sure he can get specimens to an outside laboratory efficiently. A variety of collecting tubes should be available and special directions should be followed. Sometimes it is best to have the blood drawn at the outside laboratory, although one should know in advance that the technicians are used to working with children.

One chemical value that can be obtained in the office is a blood glucose level. Reagent sticks that will provide an approximation of blood glucose are very easy to use, although timing is important and the sticks should not be stale. A more objective method involves the use of a machine that reads the strip and translates the intensity of color into a numerical value. These instruments are of moderate cost and are currently being used by many diabetic patients at home.

There is a machine available for office use which measures serum bilirubin in newborns (Unistat bilirubinometer, American Optical Company, Buffalo, NY 14215). The technique is simple, requiring four capillary tubes of blood. A physician who has many babies returning to hospital laboratories after discharge for follow-up bilirubin determinations might appreciate the convenience of this device. A standard is supplied to allow calibration of the machine and to ensure a satisfactory level of accuracy. Cost is approximately 2000 dollars.

Bacterial Studies

Investment in a small incubator, platinum loops, and culture media will allow the practitioner to do most of his cultures right in the office.

Throat culture is the most frequent bacteriological procedure done by pediatricians. Agar plates containing 5 per cent sheep blood can be inoculated directly with a long swab and then streaked with a platinum loop. Two cultures can be put on a plate with plenty of room for streaking. Beta hemolysis will become readily noticeable overnight, although some physicians will re-read the plates after an additional 24 hours at room temperature. One should become familiar with the gray, often translucent colonial morphology of the streptococcus, as opposed to the opaque, enameled colonies of the beta-hemolytic staphylococcus and the colonies of hemolytic gram-negative bacteria.

Since most beta-hemolytic streptococci grown from throat cultures are group A, many physicians will not take the extra step of using a Bacitracin disc to establish the grouping, although some will use the disc on follow-up cultures that appear positive. The correct procedure involves subculturing some of the beta-hemolytic colonies from the original plate, using a second plate; the Bactracin disc is then added. If the original culture is streaked widely, the Bactracin disc may be put on it directly. Assuming that the beta-hemolytic colony is predominant, without much overgrowth of other bacteria, successful grouping may be possible on that original plate, saving an additional step and a day of waiting. It would be worthwhile for an individual physician to group his beta streptococci for a while just to see how many are indeed group A in his locale. Variations of the basic agar plate technique are available, with special media such as coated slides.

In infants, a thick purulent nasal discharge can be caused by beta Streptococcus, and nasal cultures can be performed the same way throat cultures are done. The addition of an optochin (ethyl hydrocuprein) disc to the nose culture will identify those alpha-hemolytic bacteria which are pneumococci. Many clinicians believe that this organism can cause significant nasal infection in the very young.

Haemophilus influenzae is a major pathogen in children, and some office laboratories culture for this organism. Getting this bacterium to grow on artificial media and identifying it are not as easy as with other pathogens, and consultation with a bacteriologist is advised before deciding to include this organism on one's office list.

Wounds, boils, paronychiae, and similar lesions can be cultured and a penicillin disc can be applied at the initial plating. Since most of these conditions are caused by staphylococci or streptococci, identification is easily made the next day.

Culturing of urine has a few special requirements but is within the capability of the office laboratory. Specimen collection must be done properly to minimize contamination, and parents need guidance. It is handy to have a supply of instruction sheets which specify that (1) a first morning specimen is desirable, (2) the collecting jar should be run through the dishwasher or cleaned with soap and water and boiled, (3) the child's genital area should be thoroughly washed, (4) a midstream specimen is best, and (5) the specimen should be brought in immediately or put in the refrigerator until brought in. Leave room on the slip for the child's name and doctor's name, specify whether a urinalysis as well as culture is desired, and have the parent bring the slip in with the specimen. Mystery specimens have a way of being dropped off by parents in transit.

Younger children will require collection bags, and most offices will supply these to parents. Give out two at a time, since the first is often contaminated with stool or falls off. After many years, certain anatomical differences have been recognized and bags are now designed specifically for boys or girls.

Since the quantitative aspects of urine cultures are important, a calibrated loop is needed to inoculate the plate. A loop that holds exactly 0.01 ml of urine is practical, and the final colony count is obtained by counting colonies and multiplying by 100. Often, a positive culture will have colonies too numerous to count covering the plate.

The same blood agar plates used for throat cultures will serve well for urine cultures, although more selective media, some with chemical indicators, can be used. There are dipslides coated with media, special containers of media on which urine-soaked filter paper is applied, and other variations.

Cultures with mixtures of bacteria are probably contaminated. Those with intermediate numbers of bacteria usually bear repeating. Plates with large numbers of a single colony type probably represent significant infection. When good collection technique is used, most plates are clearly positive or negative.

Identification of the specific organism is beyond most office laboratories but is usually not necessary. If such information is needed in a patient with recurrent infections, the plate can be sent to an outside laboratory. Sensitivity testing can be done with selected discs, although most uncomplicated infections can be treated successfully with the usual antimicrobial agents of choice. It is good practice to get another culture after a few days of therapy to document efficacy of the treatment. If that culture is positive, sensitivities should be done. Cultures after therapy and in succeeding months are also important.

Stool cultures require special techniques and will need transport media and delivery to an outside laboratory. Some laboratories will supply mailers that parents can send directly from home.

Cultures for gonorrhea also need the facilities of a larger laboratory, although the specimens are collected in the office. Proper transport media incorporating chocolate agar and a CO_2-generating tablet should be on hand, and directions should be followed carefully to keep the organism viable. Gram stains of exudate can add information in the work-up of venereal disease, and the solutions for Gram staining should be part of the office laboratory.

Blood cultures are assuming greater importance in ambulatory pediatrics in light of recent studies on occult bacteremia in small children.

Proper blood culturing requires sophisticated techniques beyond most office laboratories; however, collecting bottles can be kept in the office, inoculated there, put into the incubator, and taken the next day to the larger laboratory.

Viral Studies

Culturing of viruses can be done only in highly specialized laboratories, but if such a facility is nearby, specimens can be collected in the office and transported on appropriate carrying media. Likewise, serological studies such as rubella titers, acute and convalescent viral titers, and hepatitis antibody studies must go to outside laboratories, but the blood can be drawn in the office. Some of these specimens can be mailed.

The infectious mononucleosis spot test has established itself in offices as a quick and accurate way to diagnose this common illness. More than one test is available, with some evidence that the most sensitive test is one employing horse erythrocytes.

Mycoplasma infection has been recognized as a common cause of respiratory illness in children, and a rapid cold agglutinin test can be performed in the office. Two hematocrit tubes of blood are emptied into a small test tube along with two tubes of 3.8 per cent sodium citrate as an anticoagulant. The tube is stirred in a beaker of ice cubes and water and the tube is held up to a light and slowly rotated. Definite agglutination of the cells correlates with a significant cold agglutinin titer. The specimen can be warmed and reexamined, then chilled again to confirm the agglutination. It may take five days or more for a titer to develop, and there are both false negatives and false positives. Nonetheless, the test can be very helpful, especially in establishing an infection pattern in the community.

Fungal Studies

A 10 per cent potassium hydroxide solution is used to prepare slides of skin scrapings and hair which might contain fungal elements. Media for culturing fungi are available and can be used to establish the presence of Candida or dermatophytes. Three common fungal culture media are Sabouraud's agar, Mycosel agar, and dermatophyte test medium. A Wood's lamp will cause fluorescence of the skin lesions of tinea versicolor and scalp infections caused by Microsporum. This same instrument can be used in the examination of the cornea with fluorescein.

Pregnancy Testing

Pregnancy testing on urine has become much more accurate in recent years, and a number of tests are available. The pediatrician should become familiar with one test and might well discuss the nuances of technique with an obstetrical colleague.

Charging for Laboratory Tests

Several factors go into the determination of an appropriate charge for a laboratory procedure. The amount of time involved, both by staff and physician, should be examined, as well as the cost of supplies. Check the fees set by local hospital and private laboratories as well as what other physicians are charging. In general, office laboratory fees are lower than those set by others, while still being fair to the physician. Some offices will set a lower fee if the test is part of an office call. It is worth the time to find out which insurance carriers will cover office laboratory work; often the patient will not know.

TESTING OF SPECIAL SENSES

Vision Testing

Much valuable information on vision can be obtained with simple equipment. Eye charts come with letters, illiterate E's, and pictures. Letter charts should be used when possible, since picture charts do not give as accurate an assessment. In the preschool child, however, picture charts may be the only practical means of evaluating acuity subjectively, and they do fulfill the critical function of detecting major differences in acuity between the two eyes. Eye charts require an unobstructed 20-foot hallway, although a 10-foot distance can be used and the denominator doubled. Children enjoy wearing a black "pirate" eye patch, which facilitates testing of individual eyes. More than half of the three-year-olds and almost all four-year-olds will be able to cooperate on an eye chart exam.

The eye chart tests only distance vision. Because of their great accommodative powers, children rarely have problems with near vision. One may, however, obtain inexpensive cards for near vision testing.

Muscle balance can be tested by way of the corneal light reflex and the cover test. Color vision testing requires only a book of testing plates.

An alternative way of testing vision is to use a multipurpose machine which can evaluate near and distance vision, muscle balance, and color vision in one compact location. Physicians who have used these machines find that most five-year-olds have sufficient concentration for accurate testing, although younger children may not. Saving space is the major advantage of an eye testing machine. The cost of one popular model at this writing is approximately 1000 dollars.

Hearing Testing

Since an audiometer will receive continual use in a pediatric office, it makes sense to invest in a good machine and have it recalibrated periodically. Special earphones that shut out background noise are an option worth considering unless a soundproof room is available. Make sure the standard cushions are included inside the special earphones. Most five-year-olds and many younger children will cooperate in pure tone audiometry. Crude testing in the office can be done with simple noisemakers, such as a small bell, and one may obtain a commercial kit of calibrated noisemakers for use with younger children.

Measurement of eardrum compliance with a tympanometer adds a valuable dimension to the evaluation of middle ear function. This instrument does not require active patient participation and is not affected by cerumen. The tester must be trained in proper technique, however, and appropriate interpretation of the test patterns takes some study. Although the tympanometer is expensive, many offices consider it essential.

For years, audiology laboratories have accurately measured hearing in babies and developmentally impaired children with a technique that measures brainstem evoked potential. This method requires very expensive and intricate equipment. A small unit designed for office testing which employs the same principle is now commerically available for approximately 5000 dollars, a fraction of the cost of the laboratory model. The physician contemplating such a purchase should seek the advice of an audiologist as to whether or not this new machine would be likely to measure hearing accurately under the specific conditions in which he would be using it.

In fact, all the equipment used for hearing evaluation is expensive, complex, and subject to constant technical change. Consultation with an audiologist is strongly recommended as part of the shopping process.

Removal of cerumen is often necessary and can be accomplished with a metal irrigating syringe and a kidney basin. If several drops of wax softener are instilled and allowed to work for a few minutes, removal is usually easy.

THE EXAMINING ROOM

The equipping of an examining room will reflect the individual style of each physician. Some general suggestions, however, will apply to most situtations.

Examining tables which are designed for adults are too low for the comfortable examination of a child and will cause the rapid onset of back pain in the physician. Besides being high enough, the table should be well padded, covered with a durable fabric, and incorporate a large amount of storage space.

Tables that incorporate scales and length-measuring devices may be worth their cost to some individuals. A separate infant scale can be put on a shelf in the room, perhaps in a corner, without taking up much space. Add a tape measure and infants and small children can have their lengths, weights, and head circumferences taken quickly. There are more sophisticated devices for measuring length, such as commercial or homemade boxes with sliding foot plates.

A larger scale will be needed for older children who can stand and may have to be put in a hall or separate room. Height measurements can be done efficiently and accurately with a wooden yardstick that has been fixed vertically to the wall, with its lower end exactly two feet from the floor.

Anticipate which pieces of small equipemt are used often and provide them for each room. The steps saved will make the expense worthwhile. For example, an otoscope and an ophthalmoscope in a wall unit which keeps the batteries charged will be used constantly. Tongue blades, culture swabs, reflex hammers, and similar tools should have their own niches within easy reach. It is helpful to have an adult stethoscope for obese children or teenagers with thick chest walls.

Provide a wall rack for papers such as educational handouts and blank instruction pads. Prescription pads can also be kept discreetly in such a rack, although some physicians prefer to carry their pads with them.

Another step-saver is an intercom for communicating with the front desk. Ground rules must be established to avoid an inappropriate rate of interruptions, but the entire office staff will function more efficiently when information can be exchanged this way.

Pediatricians are safety conscious and this orientation should be applied to the examining room. As much as possible, equipment should be kept out of the reach of the children. Search for sharp edges and protrusions that a toddler will inevitably find. Removable plastic plug covers for electric outlets will not only protect the children but will have a teaching impact on parents as well.

THE WAITING ROOM

Much variation exists among waiting rooms of different physicians, since needs are so diverse. The following suggestions have been found helpful in practical experience.

Some source of diversion for the waiting child is necessary. Creation of an actual play area is possible, with such items as climbing toys and a small table with chairs. Space limitations may make such an area impossible, or high patient flow may create unhealthy competition. Some parents feel uncomfortable about the sharing of toys among youngsters who may be harboring mysterious ailments of high contagiousness. In the right circumstances, however, a play area can be a genuine asset.

Books and magazines are an excellent source of amusement and avoid the problems associated with toys. For relatively little money the pediatrician can subscribe to a dozen magazines that cover the entire range from toddler to adult. A list of children's magazines is found at the end of this chapter. Books can be bought, obtained through children's book clubs, or brought from home when they are outgrown. Books can be carried into the examining room, since it is not unusual for a child to express disappointment when the doctor arrives because his mother has not finished reading to him.

Children love to watch fish in an aquarium. Not only do the fish amuse and occupy waiting children, but they can also be used in the clinical assessment of a febrile or lethargic child. The toddler who is carried over to the aquarium and reaches out toward the fish or babbles excitedly despite his illness is providing valuable information about himself. It is critical to structure the aquarium in such a way that it cannot be pulled over, since children will inevitably climb and grab.

Provision of background music need not cost a great deal. A good FM radio tuned to an easy listening station can provide a soothing influence so often welcomed in the chaos of a crowded waiting room.

Many pediatricians have a second waiting room for adolescents or for patients who are detained for a while. All physicians should provide a quiet place to allow patients who are unusually upset or have other special needs to wait. A conference room which is usually used for consultations can double as an auxiliary waiting room for these families.

As mentioned above, teaching aids can be put in the waiting room. A bulletin board allows the physician to display timely announcements that come along and may allow parents to share such information as babysitting services offered or desired.

THE TELEPHONE

Few physicians use the telephone as extensively as pediatricians do, and there are as many telephone systems as there are variations in practice style. A system structured to the needs of an individual office can lead to a smooth operation that is satisfying to patients and staff. Local telephone companies and private firms will provide communication consultants who can present the many options available and recommend an appropriate system.

Size of practice and frequency of incoming calls will determine how many lines are needed to avoid inordinate numbers of busy signals. Of course, adequate people trained to answer the phone must be there to staff those lines and avoid the complaint that no one answers the calls. The cyclical nature of pediatric practice will complicate these decisions, as telephone traffic will vary with the incidence of infectious disease in the community. But a system designed to handle a "busy average" day will usually work without being wasteful, and staffing patterns can be adjusted seasonally.

An additional incoming line with a number known only to selected individuals is a must.

One use of this line is to serve as an emergency channel if a patient has a real crisis during heavy telephone traffic on the regular lines and just cannot get through. Patients should be taught to call the answering service in such an eventuality, and the answering service can then use the unlisted line to get the office. Although this mechanism will not be used often, it is of great comfort to parents to know that it exists.

Hospital staff and other physicians can be given the unlisted number as well so that they can get through quickly when critical information needs to be transmitted. Spouses should be discouraged from using that line for routine calls. A ring which is different from that of the regular lines can be installed on the "hot line."

Still another line for outgoing calls is worth considering. Simply marked "out" on its selection button, this line allows staff to make calls without tying up regular lines.

Some physicians have a calling hour which works well for them. Others have found this system impractical. For those calls which come in during the working day, it is handy to have a location where slips requesting telephone calls can be put on a spindle of some sort and where patient charts can be placed nearby. It is worth having pads of uniform pre-printed call slips to avoid the hodgepodge of pieces of paper of every size and shape filling up the spindle. The slip should have lines for the patient's name and phone number, date and time, and a phrase or two describing the problem. Some room should be left for the doctor to jot down his reply or prescription directions. There should be a box marked "chart"; the slip can be filed in the chart afterwards if this box is checked. Some physicians will jot down on the chart itself the essence of the call as they are talking. For all but the most transient problems, a notation in the record can be immensely valuable later on. If slips and pertinent charts are placed in a location near the examining rooms, calls can be made between patients or when there is a lag, avoiding a large backlog at the end of the session.

A tape device can be installed that will automatically come on when all lines are filled and instruct the patient to call back in a little while or to call the answering service if a genuine emergency exists. The same machine can give a similar message over the lunch hour if the office chooses to shut off all calls but emergencies. At night, the recording will tell the patient how to reach the physician on call.

Paging devices, some of which just beep and some of which are more elaborate, give the physician who is on call but away from the office an additional measure of freedom.

APPOINTMENTS, BILLING, AND REGISTRIES

Appointment and billing systems are subjects beyond the scope of this chapter. The practitioner is well advised to look at a number of existing situations for ideas and to consult freely with relevant advisors, such as an accountant. A few practical ideas may be of use to the reader.

Especially in a busy office, appointment books can quickly fill with routine examinations. Demand for this service is quite variable; when school nurses send home physical forms and when summer camp is looming, everyone wants a check-up. At other times, such as midwinter, far fewer requests come in. It is a good idea to encourage parents to make appointments for physicals in the month of their child's birthday. This arrangement will balance things considerably; forms can be filled out when necessary, using the data from the last check-up, assuming it was not too long ago.

If the appointment sheet is filled with well child visits, ill children must be sandwiched in and a very hectic situation may ensue. One can color-code appointments in advance and put in only the number of well child visits that will allow sufficient time for the acutely ill. For example, a green check mark can be put in front of four time slots on a given afternoon, designating those times for older children's physicals. Four more slots might be preceded by a blue check, which means well baby examinations belong there. The other spaces receive a red check and are used for sick and follow-up visits. When all the well child slots are filled on a given day, no more physicals are scheduled. By trial and error, one can soon judge how many red spaces are needed at various times of the year and how many blue spaces will be required to keep the babies coming in on time. The remaining time goes to the older children. This system has the disadvantage of putting check-ups on older children into the future a bit; but it has the decided advantage of allowing sufficient time for sudden illness or injury, a feature that makes good sense to parents.

It is also a good idea to put aside the same block of time each week for conferences or other long visits. This block ensures that the time will be available if needed. If not filled in advance, this time can be used for last minute illness appointments.

One feature of billing worth keeping in mind is the "super-bill." This form contains on it enough identifying, financial, and diagnostic data to allow it to be used as a charge slip, a submission form for insurance purposes, and a receipt for the patient, since a carbon copy is generated. Lines at the bottom can be filled in with the next appointment.

An age-sex registry will prove valuable in many ways. Every patient in the practice has name, address and birthdate recorded on a 3 x 5" index card—pink for girls and blue for boys. The cards are filed by sex and birthdate. When a new family joins the practice, new cards are made; when a family leaves, the cards are withdrawn. Naturally, it is easier to start such a registry with a new practice; but an established office can catch up by having clerical helpers, such as high school students, make cards for the patients already in the practice.

This registry allows the physician to keep a constant eye on the size of the practice. It can also be used as a research tool. One can quickly find the names of all children of a given age who might be the subjects needed for a study.

A variation on this theme is the morbidity or disease index. If the physician codes each visit, he can keep track of the kinds of problems he is treating and can also generate a list of all children with a given condition. Such a tool is invaluable if, for instance, one wants to do an intervention study on children who are at higher risk for otitis media. The index can be simplified by including only those patients who have chronic conditions. A fair amount of clerical work is involved in these systems, although a computer will make things much easier.

TEACHING AIDS

Teaching is an important part of all medical care and assumes special importance in pediatrics, with its emphasis on prevention of problems and anticipatory guidance. Of course, teaching should occur every time the physician discusses an element of normal nutrition, growth, or development or gives instructions on the care of a sick child. Certain aids can be used to reinforce or amplify oral instructions.

Written handouts can be found in infinite variety, but for routine well and illness care the physician should consider writing his own. A one-page sheet custom-written for each well baby visit will contain the specific salient points each physician feels are important for that particular age. This material will reinforce what is discussed at the visit and will also reflect the individual style of that physician. The sheet given at the four-month visit may have a large section on feeding, while the eighteen-month sheet may concentrate on discipline. Reinforcement of the need to pick up a bottle of syrup of Ipecac can be given. Some parents will refer to the handouts frequently and remark years later on how helpful they were. Others will drop them in the parking lot. The physician needs to know the characteristics of his own population, but many parents will profit from a later leisurely review of the doctor's instructions on, for instance, a relaxed approach to toilet training, especially if the original discussion was held in the context of struggling with a crying toddler. One may also choose to write sheets on certain aspects of illness, such as fever and diarrhea.

In the course of practice other kinds of written material will be called for frequently. The physician will save much time if he has readily available copies of such items as reducing diets, lactose-free diets, and instructions on choosing a good car seat. Pamphlets on subjects such as sex education, which require more extensive treatment than one sheet can give, should be available to parents who request them. Bibliographies of books on subjects such as divorce or helping a child deal with death are also very helpful.

These written materials are not a substitute for the physician's personal advice and guidance. They are, however, useful in an adjunct role.

Some physicians have found value in educational presentations such as self-contained slide shows or short videotaped programs. A machine can be put into the waiting room with either a fixed format or a choice of programs. Anticipatory guidance can be given, or a common illness such as otitis media can be explained. As with written material, the physician should consider putting together his own audiovisual presentation.

One should not overlook the value of a well-placed poster or two. A brief but important point brought to the attention of a parent at a receptive moment might make an impact.

THE OFFICE LIBRARY

Hardly a day will pass without the physician needing to look something up in a reference book. A relatively small library can provide the answers to most questions immediately, especially if it is kept current. Naturally, a reference library is not a substitute for ongoing self-education. It can, however, supply a critical piece of information in the midst of a busy day.

Prescribing information is required frequently and is in constant need of updating. A current textbook of pediatric therapeutics can describe the treatment of an unusual disorder or supplement the physician's approach to something common. *Physician's Desk Reference,* which is a compendium of information supplied by pharmaceutical manufacturers, readily answers questions about dosage, concentration, bottle size, adverse reactions and similar practical matters. To round out the references on prescribing, the physician is well advised to subscribe to one of the brief, practically oriented loose-leaf letter-journals that come frequently and often seem to have that elusive fact needed in a given situation. Some of these journals deal exclusively with drugs and therapeutics, while others are general in scope and can help in many clinical situations.

Infectious diseases commonly pose questions, and many pediatricians turn first to the American Academy of Pediatrics *Report of the Committee on Infectious Disease,* commonly called the *Red Book.* More extensive coverage of specific disorders is found in a textbook of infectious diseases, one of which is worth purchasing. County and state health departments mail infectious disease newsletters and a file containing these updates can be invaluable.

Skin conditions are encountered frequently in pediatrics. Although many are easily recognizable, some are quite challenging. A textbook of pediatric dermatology will be consulted often and gratefully. Pictures in a textbook can be used to teach parents, especially if different phases of a condition can be demonstrated.

Information on poisoning and on plant ingestion is often needed in a hurry, and books on these subjects should be available. Plant books with many pictures are especially helpful.

Unusual eye findings come along often enough to warrant the acquisition of a textbook of pediatric ophthalmology, especially one written for the pediatrician.

Indeed, a case could be made for specialized texts in many other areas, such as orthopaedics and endocrinology, and each physician should determine his own specific needs. Of course, one must not overlook the general pediatric references. No office library is complete without a current textbook of general pediatrics, which will be consulted repeatedly. The handy "peripheral brain" from training days will also see heavy use, although more current versions can be obtained from several sources, as well as books that catalog practical tables and charts of every description.

Finally, the pediatrician should have a file drawer in which he can store, in an organized fashion, the latest guidelines on child abuse reporting, the directory of area nursery schools, normal laboratory values from the local hospital, and the myriad other pieces of information that should be within reach when they are suddenly needed.

EMERGENCY EQUIPMENT

Some physicians will need emergency equipment more often than others, depending on the nature of their practices and the proximity of a hospital or other emergency facility. Certain basic items should be considered.

A bag and mask should be available to provide artificial respiration, with a small oxygen tank and proper connectors. Oropharyngeal airways are also necessary, and some physicians would add a laryngoscope with several sizes of blades and endotracheal tubes.

Intravenous solutions, tubing and needles, at least on a small scale, should be handy, as well as vials of intravenous glucose and bicarbonate solutions. In lieu of an intravenous pole, one may install an ordinary lamp hook in the ceiling of a treatment or examining room. The seriously dehydrated child or the diabetic patient with hypoglycemia may well require intravenous therapy urgently.

Several drugs should be kept with the emergency equipment, including diazepam and phenobarbital for seizures, epinephrine, and vials of antibiotics and parenteral corticosteroid. A table of dosages should be kept in the same place.

Other drugs, tracheotomy equipment, and additional pieces of apparatus can be considered by each physician. But whatever the make-up of the emergency cart, office staff must check it frequently and should participate in periodic drills to make sure things will run smoothly in an actual emergency.

Eye injuries present regularly and their care is facilitated by an eye tray, on which is kept irrigating solution, fluorescein strips, mydriatic drops, antibiotic preparations, and patches. Some physicians will include ear medications as well, but it is best to keep items for eye care separate to avoid inadvertent use of ear drops in the eye.

There are specialized surgical instruments that can be extremely helpful to the pediatrician. For example, a reverse forceps (Hegenbarth clip applying forceps) will facilitate the removal of foreign objects from the nose. When the sides are pressed together, the tips move further apart, allowing movement of the tips beyond the object. An instrument shaped like a clamp with finely pointed, angled tips will make the removal of splinters much easier (Peet splinter forceps). The physician's supply house representative can help in the selection of these and other useful surgical tools, including the proper instruments and accessories for simple suturing and a small autoclave.

THE OFFICE COMPUTER

Computer technology is moving into most aspects of life, and the medical office is no exception. Office applications are in their early stages at this time, but the field is advancing quickly. Because there are so many vendors, large and small, international and local, the physician must shop slowly and carefully, looking at many demonstrations, including those already set up at other offices.

Practice size will be an important determinant of which system is best. The other major factor will be the spectrum of services expected from the machine.

At present, the main applicability of computers is to financial matters. Patient accounts are easily entered into the computer, which can then supply data on any patient's status, including the period of time a balance has been due. Bills can be generated and insurance forms can be printed out automatically. Lists of accounts meeting certain criteria can be compiled quickly. Productivity of different providers in the same office can be calculated, and the number of times a given procedure has been done is easily obtained.

Clinical information can be entered and retrieved later for purposes of treatment or research. For instance, all children who should receive an influenza immunization can be identified prospectively and a list can be printed when needed. All children with seizure disorders can be identified instantly if they are coded as they present to the office.

Systems are available which can make appointments and print out the day's schedule and all the charge slips in a few minutes. At present there has been little use of computers for storing the medical record. A few experimental programs exist, but they are generally too complex and expensive for office practice.

The practitioner should educate himself in basic computer technology. For instance, he should know the differences in capability between a "mini" and a "micro" computer, as well as the advantages of a hard disc over a floppy disc. The machines themselves constitute the "hardware." Capacity and availability of servicing are critical in this area. "Software" refers to the specific program which is introduced into the machine and enables it to perform. Applicability to the office's needs is most crucial in choosing a software package. Some companies provide complete systems, including staff education, servicing, and changeover from the previous arrangement. Others sell components of the total system.

The physician who does some homework will ultimately be able to obtain a system that will meet his needs and his budget. There is no question that offices in the future will run more smoothly and efficiently because of this exciting tool.

MAGAZINES FOR CHILDREN

Turtle. Ages 2–6. 1100 Waterway Boulevard, Indianapolis, IN 46206.

Highlights for Children. Ages 2–12. 803 Church Street, Honesdale, PA 18431.

Humpty Dumpty's Magazine. Ages 3–8. 685 Third Avenue, New York, NY 10017.

Children's Playmate. Ages 5–8. 1100 Waterway Boulevard, Indianapolis, IN 46206.

Ranger Rick's Nature Magazine. Ages 5–12. 1412 16th Street, N.W., Washington, D.C. 20036.

Child Life. Ages 7–11. 1100 Waterway Boulevard, Indianapolis, IN 46206.

Jack and Jill. Ages 7–11. 1100 Waterway Boulevard, Indianapolis, IN 46206.

National Geographic World. Ages 8–12. 17th and M Street, N.W., Washington, D.C. 30036.

Boy's Life. 9 years to young adult. P.O. Box 61030, Dallas-Fort Worth Airport, Dallas, TX 75261.

Seventeen. Teen and young adult. 850 Third Avenue, New York, NY 10022.

REFERENCES

Bass, L. W., and Wolfson, J. H.: The Style and Management of a Pediatric Practice. Pittsburgh, University of Pittsburgh Press, 1977.

Convey, H. D., and McAlister, N.: Computers in the

Practice of Medicine, Volumes I and II. Reading, MA, Addison-Wesley Publishing Company, 1980.

Garb, S.: Laboratory Tests in Common Use, 6th Ed. New York, Springer Publishing Company, Inc., 1976.

McClelland, C. Q., Burns, A. E., and Staples, W. I.: The office laboratory in pediatric practice. Pediatr. Clin. North Am., *21*:195, 1974.

North, A. F., Jr.: The office laboratory in pediatric practice. Review and commentary. Pediatr. Clin. North Am., *21*:213, 1974.

Sparer, C. N.: Organizing the physician's office. Pediatr. Clin. North Am., *28*:537, 1981.

Widmann, F. K.: Clinical Interpretation of Laboratory Tests, 8th Ed. Philadelphia, F. A. Davis Company, 1979.

Appendix C

Ambulatory Pediatric Drugs

Barton D. Schmitt, M.D.

This chapter summarizes information on drugs commonly used in ambulatory pediatric care. Most drugs for emergencies and uncommon chronic diseases have been excluded. For convenience in calculation, dosages are given on a *per dose* rather than a *per day* basis (an exception being the anticonvulsants). The adult (or older adolescent) dose that is listed is the standard dose, not the maximum dose. To help the less experienced clinician, the drugs are listed by symptom or illness, rather than alphabetically. A physician should not prescribe a drug without being aware of the potential side effects. The physician is also responsible for keeping abreast of changes in indications or dosage. When effective nonprescription drugs are available, they are listed and marked with an asterisk (*). While these drugs are usually not less expensive than equivalent prescription drugs, they can save a phone call or visit to the physician.

One cannot survey the drugs prescribed in our country without realizing that we are a greatly overmedicated society. Many people believe that there is a drug for every symptom. Some physicians prescribe a drug during every office visit. Some 95 per cent of people with colds leave their physician's office with a prescription. Over 10 billion dollars per year is spent on over-the-counter drugs for fever, colds, and coughs—many of them unnecessary. Physicians write prescriptions to shorten the office visit or to avoid counseling, listening, or parental pressure. To counteract this prescription dependency in our country, we must educate our patients. Mild symptoms do not require any medication, and moderate symptoms often respond to home remedies. Drugs are not essential to recovery from most illnesses.

ANTIBIOTICS

1. **Amoxicillin** 15 mg/kg/dose t.i.d. (Adult 250-500 mg/dose)
   Products: 125 and 250/5 ml; 250, 500 cap.
2. **Ampicillin** 20 mg/kg/dose q.i.d. (Adult 500 mg/dose)
   Products: 125 and 250/5 ml; 250, 500 cap.
3. **Cephalosporins**
   Cefaclor (Ceclor), Cephalexin (Keflex) or Cephradine (Velosef) 10 mg/kg/dose q.i.d. (Adult 250 mg/dose)
   Products: 125 and 250/5 ml; 250, 500 cap.
4. **Dicloxacillin** 5-10 mg/kg/dose q.i.d. (Adult 250 mg/dose)
   Products: 62.5/5 ml; 125, 250 cap.
5. **Erythromycin** 10 mg/kg/dose q.i.d. (Adult 400 mg/dose)
   Products: 200 and 400/5 ml; 200, chewable, 250 and 400 tablcap.
6. **Nitrofurantoin** 1.5 mg/kg/dose b.i.d. prophylaxis for UTIs (Adult 100 mg/dose)
   Products: 25/5 ml; 50, 100 cap.
7. **Pediazole** 10 mg/kg/dose of erythromycin q.i.d. (Adult 400 mg/dose)
   Product contains: 200 mg erythromycin and 600 mg sulfisoxazole/5 ml
8. **Penicillin V** 10 mg/kg/dose q.i.d. (Adult 500 mg/dose)
   Products: 125 and 250/5 ml; 250, 500 tab.
   Bicillin L-A contains 1.2 million units of benzathine penicillin G in 2 ml
   Bicillin C-R contains 900,000 benzathine and 300,000 procaine penicillin in 2 ml

Strep Throat Rx	Wgt	Pen V p.o.	Benzathine Pen IM
	<30 lb.	125 q.i.d.	300,000
	30-60 lb.	250 q.i.d.	600,000
	60-90 lb.	500 q.i.d.	900,000
	>90 lb.	500 q.i.d.	1,200,000

9. **Sulfisoxazole** 30 mg/kg/dose q.i.d. (Adult 1 gm/dose)
   Products: 500/5 ml; 500 tab
   Prophylaxis for recurrent AOM 30 mg/kg/dose b.i.d. for 2-4 months
10. **Trimethoprim** 5 mg/kg/dose b.i.d. (Adult 160 mg TMP/dose)
   Products: 40/5 ml; 80, 160 tab. (e.g., Bactrim, Septra)
   (Products contain 1:5 ratio of trimethoprim: sulfamethoxazole)

ALLERGIES

1. *Antihistamines*
   Hydroxyzine (Atarax) 0.5 mg/kg/dose t.i.d. (Adult 25-50 mg/dose)
   Products: 10/5 ml; 10, 25, 50, 100 tab.
   Diphenhydramine (Benadryl) 1 mg/kg/dose t.i.d. (Adult 50 mg/dose)
   Products: 12.5 mg/5 ml; 25, 50 cap.
   Brompheniramine and **Chlorpheniramine** 0.1 mg/kg/dose t.i.d. (Adult 4 mg/dose)
   Products: 2 mg/5 ml, 4 mg tab., 8 and 12 mg extended-release tab.
   *Chlortrimeton, Dimetane, and Teldrin are nonprescription antihistamines not combined with decongestants.
2. *Theophylline*
   Initial loading dose: 6 mg/kg/dose P.O. or I.V. in 50 ml saline over 20 minutes (Adult 300 mg/dose)
   Maintenance dose: 1 year–8 years 5 mg/kg/dose q 6 hours
   8–16 years 4 mg/kg/dose q 6 hours
   >16 years 3 mg/kg/dose q 6 hours (Adult 200 mg/dose)

   Products: Elixicon 100/5 ml, Slophyllin 27/5 ml, Somophyllin 90/5 ml
   Slophyllin or Somophyllin tabs 100, 200, 250
   Sustained-released theophyllines at 1.5 × the above dosages q 8 hours or 2 × the above dosages q 12 hours.
   Slo-Phyllin Gyrocaps 60, 125, 250 mg bead-filled capsules q 8 hrs.
   Theo-Dur Sprinkles 50, 75, 125, 200 mg q 12 hrs.
3. *Adrenergic Agents*
   Metaproterenol 0.4 mg/kg/dose t.i.d. (Adult 20 mg/dose) 10 mg/5 ml, 10 or 20 mg tabs
   Terbutaline 0.05-0.1 mg/kg/dose t.i.d. (Adult 2.5 mg/dose)
   (Not FDA approved for use under 12 years of age)
   Products: 2.5 and 5 mg tabs
   1:1000 **aqueous epinephrine** 0.01 ml/kg/dose SQ (Adult 0.3 ml/dose)
   Susphrine 0.005 ml/kg/dose SQ (Adult 0.15 ml/dose)
4. *Steroids*
   Prednisone 1.0 mg/kg/dose b.i.d. (Adult 40 mg/dose) 2.5, 5, 10 mg tabs
   Beclomethasone nasal aerosol 1-2 inhalations per nostril b.i.d.

GENERAL DISORDERS

1. *Anemia* (Iron Deficiency)
   Prophylactic Elemental Iron 1.0 mg/kg/dose daily (Adult 40 mg Fe/dose) or Ferrous Sulfate drops (25 mg Fe/ml) 0.04 ml/kg/dose
   Therapeutic Elemental Iron 1.5 mg/kg/dose 3X/day (Adult 65 mg Fe/dose) or Ferrous Sulfate drops (25 mg Fe/ml) 0.06 ml/kg/dose 3 X/day (Adult 325 mg $FeSO_4$ tab/dose)
   Therapeutic Iron must be continued for 2 to 3 months.
2. *Fever*
   Home remedy for fever: Light clothing, reduced activity, cold fluid intake; sponging if T >104°F.
   Aspirin or Acetaminophen for T >102° F or discomfort (same dosage)
   <2 years 15 mg/kg/dose 4-6x/day
   >2 years 65 mg/year of age (Adult 10 grains or 650 mg/dose)

Brand	Concentration	2-4 mo	5-11 mo	12-23 mo	2-3 yr	4-5 yr	6-8 yr	9-11 yr	>12 yr
Tylenol drops	80 mg/0.8 ml	0.4 ml	0.8	1.2	1.6	2.4	—	—	—
Tempra drops	60 mg/0.6 ml	0.4 ml	0.8	1.2	1.6	2.4	—	—	—
Liquiprin drops	60 mg/1.25 ml	0.8 ml	1.6	2.4	3.2	4.8	—	—	—
Tylenol elixir	160 mg/5 ml (1 tsp)	—	½ tsp	¾	1	1½	2	2½	4
Tempra syrup	120 mg/5 ml (1 tsp)	—	½ tsp	1	1¼	1¾	2½	3	5
Chewable aspirin or Tylenol	80 mg tabs	—	—	1½	2	3	4	5-6	8
Adult aspirin or Tylenol	325 mg tabs	—	—	—	—	—	1	1-1½	2

Aspirin or acetaminophen suppositories: 325 and 650 mg for febrile children with vomiting or medication refusal.
Note: Aspirin is not to be used in children with chickenpox or influenza-like syndromes.

3. *Immune Serum Globulin (ISG)*
   Hepatitis exposure 0.02-0.03 ml/kg I.M. (Adult 2 ml)
   Rubeola exposure 0.25 ml/kg I.M.
4. *Motion sickness*
   Bonine 25 mg chewable tablets
   Dramamine 50 mg tablets and 12.5 mg/5 ml syrup
   Dosage: <6 years: 1 mg/kg/dose 1 hour before activity
   6-12 years: 25 mg
   >12 years: 50 mg
5. *PAIN, mild to moderate*
   Aspirin, Tylenol—see Fever for dosage.
   Codeine 0.5 mg/kg/dose q 4-6 hrs.
   PAIN, severe
   Meperidine 1.0 mg/kg/dose I.M. or I.V. (Adult 50 mg)
   Morphine 0.2 mg/kg/dose SQ or I.V. (Adult 10 mg)
6. *Restlessness* (Sedatives)
   Chloral hydrate 25 mg/kg/dose (Adult 1 gm/dose)
   500 mg/5 ml; 250, 500 mg capsules
   Benadryl 1 mg/kg/dose (Adult 50 mg/dose)
   12.5 mg/5 ml; 25, 50 mg capsules
   *Vodka 1 ml/kg/dose (Adult 45 ml/dose)
   Diazepam (Valium) 0.2 mg/kg/dose (Adults 5-10 mg/dose)
   Product: 2, 5 and 10 tabs.

SKIN DISORDERS

1. *Acne*
   Benzoyl peroxide 5% and 10% for pustules or papules*
   Retinoic acid 0.05% and 0.1% cream; 0.025% gel for comedones
   Tetracycline 500 mg. h.s. x1 month for severe papules
   Then reduce to 250 mg. h.s. *or* q. other night
   Product: 250 mg. tab.
2. *Bee sting*
   Papain (meat tenderizer) solution rubbed on for 15 minutes*
3. *Diaper rash*
   Home remedy: dryness, air exposure, cleanse skin with plain water, cleanse diaper with bleach (1 cup/cycle)
   Monilial superinfection: Nystatin cream t.i.d. (15 gm tube)
4. *Dry skin*
   Eucerin cream b.i.d.
   Special soap (Lubiderm, Alpha Keri, Neutrogena or Oilatum)*
5. *Impetigo*
   Topical Bacitracin ointment or Betadine ointment q.i.d.*
   Penicillin (oral or I.M.) or Dicloxacillin
   Note: Mercurial compounds are weak antiseptics.
   Many Staphylococcus and Streptococcus species are resistant to neomycin.
6. *Itchy rash* (e.g., poison ivy, insect bites, contact dermatitis)
   0.5% hydrocortisone cream (nonprescription) (15 gm tube)*
   or 1% hydrocortisone cream (prescription) (15 gm tube)
7. *Lice*
   Kwell: 1 oz/shampoo for 5 minutes
   RID (purified pyrethrins): 1-2 oz/shampoo for 10 minutes (also A-200 or R+C)
   Note: Repeat in 10 days; remove nits with fine-tooth comb
8. *Pustules*
   Antibacterial soaps—Dial, Lifebuoy, Safeguard
   Betadine skin cleanser (Bottle 4 oz.)*
   Chlorhexidine (Hibidens) 15% cleanser (Bottles: 4 and 8 oz.)*
9. *Ringworm* (or Athlete's foot)
   Tinactin cream or lotion b.i.d. (Bottle: 10 ml)*
   If not effective, clotrimazole or micronazole cream.
   For ringworm of the scalp, use griseofulvin
   Griseofulvin (microsize) 5 mg/kg/dose b.i.d. × 2-3 months (Adults 250 mg/dose)
   Products: 125/5 ml; 125 and 250 tabs

10. *Scabies*
    Kwell: Cover body surface; remove in 8 hrs (Repeat in 1 wk)
    Under age 1 year—remove in 4 hours (Repeat in 1 wk)
    Pregnant women: Eurax cream q 24 hrs × 2 (Repeat in 1 wk)
    Note: 2 oz. per adult usually permits 2 applications; one treatment adequate for asymptomatic contacts
11. *Sunburn* (Sunscreens)
    Key factor is Sun Protection Factor (SPF) (Range 2-15)
    Minutes of protection = SPF × 20 minutes.
    An SPF of 15 gives 5 hours of protection.
12. *Warts*
    Common warts: Duofilm in collodion 1x/day
    Home remedy: Adhesive tape—6½ days on, ½ day off
    Juvenile flat warts: 0.05% retinoic acid cream t.i.d.
    Plantar warts: 40% salicylic acid plaster (Mediplast) q.o. day*
    Venereal warts: 25% podophyllin in tincture of benzoin (wash off after 4 hours) q week by the physician
    Molluscum contagiosum: After puncturing the surface with a needle, Duofilm daily at home or 30% trichloroacetic acid in physician's office. (Wash off after 3 hours.)
    Note: Most warts resolve in 2-3 years without treatment.

EYE DISORDERS

1. *Corneal Abrasion*
   1% Cyclogyl—2 drops, antibiotic eye solution, and tight patching × 24 hours.
   Before treating, wash eyelids with soap and water.
2. *Eye Infections (Bacterial)*
   Products: 10% or 15% Sulfacetamide drops q.i.d. (15 ml bottle)
   10% Sulfacetamide ointment q.i.d. (3.5 gm tube)
   Erythromycin ophthalmic ointment q.i.d. (4 gm tube)
3. *Eye Irritation*
   Products: Visine, Murine 2, Clear Eyes, 20/20, Naphcon q 8-10 hours.
   Also: Wash eyelids and irrigate eyes.

NASAL DISORDERS

1. *Colds*—see Nasal Congestion, Sore throat, or Cough.
2. *Nasal congestion*
   Home remedies—warm water (or normal saline) nose drops followed by nasal suction or nose blowing.
   A. *Topical decongestants* (Caution: Don't use beyond 4 consecutive days)
      <2 years: Neosynephrine 1/8% nosedrops or spray q 3-4 hrs.
      2-6 years: Afrin pediatric nosedrops or spray 0.025% q 8-12 hrs.
      >6 years: Afrin adult nosedrops or spray 0.05% q 8-12 hrs.
   B. *Oral decongestants*—side effects of jitteriness, insomnia, and elevated blood pressure make topical delivery the preferred route.
   C. *Antihistamines*—for uncomfortable degree of profuse nasal discharge (Howard et al., 1979)
      (See Allergies for dosage)
3. *Sinus congestion*
   Vasoconstrictor nosedrops or spray (See Nasal congestion)
   Aspirin or acetaminophen
   Selected cases: Antihistamines or antibiotics

EAR DISORDERS

1. *Cerumen impaction removal*
   Home remedy: Colace, Debrox or mineral oil 3 drops b.i.d. × 3 days
   Then irrigate with bulb syringe, Water-Pik, etc.
   Avoid cotton-tipped applicators in the ear canal
2. *Earache*
   Home remedy: acetaminophen, aspirin, codeine, warm compress, eardrops while awaiting appointment for exam.

3. *Otitis Externa*
   Cortisporin or Colymycin otic suspension (not solution) 2 drops q.i.d. (10 ml bottle)
   Prevention: after swimming rinse ear canal with 70% isopropyl alcohol.

MOUTH DISORDERS

1. *Fever blister (cold sore)*
   Ice for 60 minutes initially
   Alcohol, 70% isopropyl b.i.d.
2. *Mouth Ulcers*
   Home remedy: 3% hydrogen peroxide in mouth for 3 minutes; acetaminophen tabs
   2% viscous xylocaine—mouth rinse × 5 minutes, then expectorate. Bottle: 100 ml
3. *Sore throat*
   Home remedy: hard candy or warm salt water gargle
   Unnecessary: throat lozenges or sprays
4. *Thrush*
   Nystatin suspension 1 ml q.i.d. in front of mouth
   Amount: 60 ml bottle

DENTAL DISORDERS

1. *Fluoride Prophylaxis (mg/day)*

	CONCENTRATION OF FLUORIDE IN WATER (ppm)		
Age	**<0.3**	**0.3-0.7**	**>0.7**
6 mo-2 yrs	0.25	0	0
2-3 yrs	0.50	0.25	0
3-16 yrs	1.0	0.50	0

Products: Fluoritab 0.25 mg/drop and 1 mg tab.; Pediaflor 0.5 mg/ml; Luride 0.125/drop nd 0.25, 0.5, 1.0 tab

2. *Toothache*
   Aspirin, acetaminophen, or codeine
   Oil of cloves (80% eugenol) 2-3 drops in cavity while awaiting dentist

RESPIRATORY DISORDERS

1. *Cough*
   Home remedy: corn syrup, honey, warm tea, cough drops, humidifier
   A. *Expectorants:* no proven benefit
   B. *Antitussives*
      Dextromethorphan 0.5 mg/kg/dose q.i.d. (Adult 30 mg/dose)
      Products: Robitussin—DM (15/5 ml), Romilar Children's (7.5/5 ml)
      Codeine 0.3 mg/kg/dose q.i.d. (Adult 20 mg/dose)
      Products: Robitussin A-C, Novahistine with codeine (10/5 ml)
2. *Croup*
   Home remedy: warm mist in shower or wet washcloth over nose/mouth
   Decadron (if severe) (Tunnessen, 1980)
   0.4 mg/kg/dose I.M. followed by same dose in 12 hrs and 24 hrs, I.M. or P.O. if needed.
   Products: 0.5 mg/5 ml elixir or 4 mg/ml injectable

CARDIAC DISORDERS

Prophylaxis for bacterial endocarditis with dental procedures
Penicillin V: loading dose P.O. 1 hour before procedure
Follow-up dosages P.O. q.i.d. × 2 days
Wgt <60 lbs Initial dose: 1 gm, follow-up dosages 250 mg
Wgt >60 lbs Initial dose: 2 gm, follow-up dosages 500 mg

GASTROINTESTINAL DISORDERS

1. *Constipation*
   Diet: bran, beans, fresh fruit, fresh vegetables, salads
   A. *Stool softeners*
      Mineral oil or milk of magnesia 1 ml/kg/dose b.i.d. (Adult 60 ml/dose)
      Maltsupex: infants—½ tbsp b.i.d.; 2-12 years—1 tbsp b.i.d.
      >12 years: 2 tbsp or 2 tabs b.i.d.
   B. *Laxatives* (rarely needed)
      Ex-Lax: 6-12 years: ½ square; >12 years: 1-2 squares
      Dulcolax 5 mg tablets: children 1 or 2 tablets; adults: 2 or 3 tablets (onset of action in 6-12 hrs)
      Dulcolax 10 mg suppositories: <2 years: ½ supp; >2 years: 1 supp. (onset of action: 15-30 min)
   C. *Enemas* (rarely needed)
      Mineral oil 4 oz.
      Hyperphosphate 1 oz/10 kg (Adult 4½ oz)
      Normal saline (2 tsp. salt/quart of water): 10 ml/kg (Adult 16 oz.)
2. *Diarrhea*
   Diet—high fluid intake (e.g., Gatorade or Infalyte) to prevent dehydration
   Apple, banana, carrot purees
   Note: Lomotil and anticholinergics are contraindicated due to side effects, especially sequestration of fluids (Portnoy et al., 1976).
   Traveler's diarrhea—Peptobismol 2 tabs (or 30 ml) q 30 mins × 8
   —Trimethoprim-sulfamethoxazole for bloody traveler's diarrhea—see *Antibiotics*
3. *Giardiasis*
   Furazolidone (Furoxone) 2 mg/kg/dose q.i.d. × 10 days
   Product: 50 mg/15 ml *Age:* under 6 years
   Quinacrine (Atabrine) 2 mg/kg/dose t.i.d. × 5 days (Adult 100 mg/dose)
   Product: 100 mg tab *Age:* any
   Metronidazole (Flagyl) 5 mg/kg/dose t.i.d. × 5 days (Adult 250 mg/dose)
   Product: 250 mg tab *Age:* over 12 years
4. *Pinworms*
   Antiminth 2 ml/10 kg × 1 dose (*Product:* 50 mg/ml suspension)
   Vermox 100 mg chewable tab × 1 dose (½ tab if <2 years)
   Povan 50 mg/10 kg × 1 dose (*Products:* 50 mg tab or 50 mg/5 ml suspension)
5. *Vomiting*
   Diet—small sips of clear fluids.
   Note: Antiemetic suppositories are not effective for vomiting associated with acute gastritis (Ginsburg and Clahsen, 1980).

UROGENITAL DISORDERS

1. Candidal vulvitis/vaginitis
   Nystatin vaginal suppositories or Lotromin 1% vaginal cream
   h.s. for 14 days. Also, 1% hydrocortisone cream for severe pruritus.
2. *Contraceptives.* Please refer to Chapter 8.
3. *Dysmenorrhea (Severe)*
   Ibuprofen (Motrin) 400 mg. q.i.d. × 1 or 2 days
   Other products: mefenamic acid or naproxen
4. *Dysuria*—due to vulvitis (without a urinary tract infection)
   Sitz baths for 15 mins. t.i.d. × 2 days
   Discontinue bubble baths
   Wash genitals with water (not soap).
5. *Menorrhagia.* See Table 8–3.
6. *Sexually transmitted diseases*
   Note: treat the sexual partner simultaneously.
   A. *Chlamydia* vaginitis or urethritis
      Tetracycline 500 mg q.i.d. × 7 days
   B. *Gonorrhea* vaginitis or urethritis
      Procaine penicillin 4.8 million units I.M. with Probenicid 1 gm orally before injection
      (**Note:** if diagnosis uncertain, use Chlamydia regimen)
   C. *Syphilis*—primary or secondary
      Benzathine penicillin 2.4 million units I.M.
   D. *Trichomonas* vaginitis or urethritis
      Metronidazole (Flagyl) 2 gm (8 tabs) as a single dose
      Product: 250 mg tab
7. *Urinary Tract Infection.* Please refer to Chapter 14.

SEIZURES

1. **Carbamazepine** (Tegretol) 15-25 mg/kg/*day* divided into 3 doses (Adult 200-300 mg/dose t.i.d.)
   200 mg tab.
2. **Diazepam** (Valium) 0.2 mg/kg/dose I.V. (over 1-2 min), or deep I.M. (Adult 10 mg/dose)
   Product Concentration: 10 mg/2 ml
3. **Dilantin**
   Loading dose: 15 mg/kg/dose I.V. (over 5-10 min) or P.O. (Adult 800 mg/dose)
   Maintenance dose: 5-8 mg/kg/day (1-2 × day) P.O. (Adult 300-400 mg/day)
   Products: 30 or 125 mg/5 ml; 30 and 100 mg cap, 50 mg/chewable tab
4. **Ethosuximide** (Zarontin) 20-30 mg/kg/*day* divided into 2 doses. (Adult 500-750 mg/dose b.i.d.)
   Products: 250 mg/5 ml; 250 mg cap.
5. **Phenobarbital**
   Loading dose: 5-10 mg/kg/dose I.M., I.V., or P.O. (Adult 200 mg/dose)
   Maintenance dose: 3-5 mg/kg/day (1-2 ×/day) P.O. (Adult 90-120 mg/day)
   Products: 20 mg/5 ml; 15, 30, 60, 100 mg tabs.
6. **Valproic acid** (Depakene) 15-45 mg/kg/*day* divided into 3 doses (Adult 250-750 mg/dose t.i.d.)
   Products: 250 mg/5 ml; 250 mg cap.

EMERGENCIES

1. *Analgesia for Procedures*
   Meperidine 1-2 mg/kg/dose I.M. (Max 50 mg)
   Promethazine 0.5-1 mg/kg/dose I.M. (Max 25 mg)
   Thorazine 0.5-1 mg/kg/dose I.M. (Max 25 mg)

All 3 agents can be mixed in 1 syringe. If patient has eaten in last 3 hours, defer until 3 hours have passed or empty the stomach. Observe closely for respiratory depression.

2. *Poisoning*
   Ipecac, syrup of: 15 ml, repeat in 20 minutes (Adult 30 ml/dose)
   Magnesium sulfate (50% solution) or Fleet's Phospho-soda.
   0.5 ml/kg/dose (Adult 30 ml/dose)
   Charcoal 30 gm mixed into a slurry.

REFERENCES

American Academy of Pediatrics, Committee on Drugs: Generic prescribing. Pediatrics, 57:275, 1976.

Asnes, R. S., and Grebin, B.: Pharmacotherapeutics—a rational approach. Pediatr. Clin. North Am., *21*:81, 1974.

Chilton, L.: Strategies for reducing prescription costs. Pediatrics, *68*:713, 1981.

Cohen, S. N., and Cohen, J. L.: Pharmacotherapeutics—a review and commentary. Pediatr. Clin. North Am., *21*:95, 1974.

Ginsburg, C. M., and Clahsen, J.: Evaluation of trimethobenzamide hydrochloride (Tigan) suppositories for treatment of nausea and vomiting in children. J. Pediatr., *96*:767, 1980.

Howard, J. C., Kantner, T. R., Lilienfield, L. S., et al.: Effectiveness of antihistamines in the symptomatic management of the common cold. J.A.M.A., *242*:2414, 1979.

Oral cold remedies. Med. Lett. Drugs Ther., *17*:89, 1975.

Portnoy, B. L., DuPont, H. L., Pruitt, D., et al.: Antidiarrheal agents in the treatment of acute diarrhea in children. J.A.M.A., *236*:844, 1976.

Stickler, G. B.: Polypharmacy and poisons in pediatrics—the epidemic of overprescribing and ways to control it. *In* Barness, L. A.: Advances in Pediatrics, 27. Chicago, Year Book Medical Publishers, 1980.

Tunnessen, W. W., and Feinstein, A. R.: The steroid-croup controversy: An analytic review of methodologic problems. J. Pediatr., *96*:751, 1980.

INDEX

Note: Page numbers in italics denote illustrations; t indicates tables.